The Biology of Cancer
a new approach

P. R. J. Burch

Professor, Department of Medical Physics,
University of Leeds

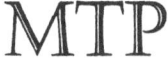

Published by

MTP PRESS LTD
St Leonard's House
St Leonardgate
Lancaster, Lancs
England

ISBN-13: 978-94-011-6605-8   e-ISBN-13: 978-94-011-6603-4
DOI: 10.1007/978-94-011-6603-4

Brandon Street, Edinburgh

The Biology of Cancer
a new approach

Contents

CHAPTER 1

Introduction

Of all the diseases that afflict mankind those described as 'cancer' evoke the strongest emotions. 'Cancer' connotes pain, protracted suffering, hideous growth and death. It is widely and justifiably feared. In medically advanced countries, *malignant neoplasms* (the official term for cancers) account for a substantial proportion of all deaths. Out of a total of 575194 deaths in England and Wales during the year 1970, some 117076—or 20·4 per cent—were attributed to neoplasms of one kind or another (Registrar General, 1972). Diseases of the circulatory system—mainly arteriosclerotic and degenerative heart disease—claimed many more victims, being responsible for some 50·6 per cent of all deaths, but our psyche evidently responds more to the manner of the disease than to the number of deaths it causes.

Many of us will have witnessed the deterioration of a close friend or relative suffering from an inoperable cancer: such an experience induces a sense of hopelessness and helplessness. The feelings of sorrow and distress can be a powerful stimulus to action and they often result in dedicated and tireless research efforts. At the same time, the very strength and depth of the commitment may sometimes be incompatible with the detachment that is needed for objective analysis and a wise strategy. Not too rigorously, we reason that if only we can discover the causes of cancer, then our problems will be solved and our agonies relieved. Remove the cause: prevent the cancer. The logic exerts an irresistible appeal.

It is widely assumed, particularly by experimental oncologists, that cancers are caused by environmental agents, such as ultraviolet and ionizing radiations, chemical carcinogens and oncogenic viruses. The concept of *spontaneous* malignancy—resulting from the intrinsic instability of complex biological structures such as genes—does not stir the emotions and it commands little support. Despite some loss of confidence, it seems that we still live in an age of 'environmental determinism'—to borrow Aldous Huxley's apt phrase. This pervasive philosophy may well conspire with our horror of cancer to convince us that, given sufficient effort, the causes of the disease are not only discoverable, but—and this is much more important—preventable.

In the West we seem to remain, against all the odds, essentially optimistic. We cannot permit the providence that rules over *us* to remain inscrutable: physical and chemical laws govern *our* universe and we have convinced ourselves that we possess a special knack in deciphering and exploiting these ordinances. Have we not unravelled the secrets of the atom and harnessed nuclear energy to our command? Have we not placed men on the moon? Surely, given a few more years, and some additional research funds, we shall also penetrate the mysteries of cancer? Can there be any serious doubts on this score?

These expectations are bolstered by so many recent successes within the field of biology (who has not heard of the double helix and the genetic code?), that we can scarcely doubt that a profound understanding of the nature and causes of cancer will emerge. Whether or not we shall welcome this knowledge remains to be seen.

In later chapters I shall argue, in opposition to the popular and prevailing view, that most of the deaths from cancer recorded in national mortality statistics cannot be attributed to external preventable factors, such as ionizing radiations, chemical carcinogens or infective oncogenic viruses. On the contrary, it appears to me that *internal*, and probably non-preventable *random events*, initiate changes that lead only too often, though perhaps not quite inevitably, to 'natural' cancer and death. That is to say, the 'cause' of most cancers in man is to be found, not so much in a hostile and inadequately controlled environment, but rather in the intrinsic properties of our biological constitution.

Should this general thesis prove to be correct, then the hope of eliminating cancer by attending carefully to the environment will have to be abandoned. I believe that, for excellent humanitarian reasons, and as a consequence of our success in combating infectious diseases, we have been trapped into a seductively simple, but largely unrewarding strategy. Of course, we cannot afford to relax our vigilance over the use and distribution of known and suspected carcinogens, but the time is ripe, I believe, for some radical and ruthless rethinking even if we have to sacrifice a few sacred cows in the process.

Problems of Definition

Many attempts have been made to define the terms 'tumour' and 'cancer' and the interested reader is referred to Willis's (1967) Chapter 1 for a fascinating and extensive discussion of the difficulties. Willis gives reasons for rejecting the views of his predecessors and essays the following definition himself: 'A tumour is an abnormal mass of tissue, the growth of which exceeds and is uncoordinated with that of normal tissues, and persists in the same excessive manner after cessation of the stimuli which evoked the change'.

I do not subscribe to the latter part of this definition, but rather than modify it at this stage I shall attempt in this book to describe those processes that are responsible for the initiation, development and maintenance of those disorders that clinicians and pathologists include under the term 'cancer'.

Definitions, I believe, should be pursued with the utmost diligence and scrupulousness when criteria and standards of diagnosis are being formulated, for it is most important that a pathologist in Melbourne, Australia, should concur with his colleagues in Edinburgh, Scotland, and in Houston, Texas. Eventually, precise and objective diagnosis might be facilitated by biochemical and immunological tests. Accurate diagnosis alone, however, will not elucidate the mechanisms of carcinogenesis.

The Idea of Crucial Evidence

A major embarrassment of cancer research is its sheer volume. No single person can hope to assimilate all that has been, and is being written, on this and neighbouring disciplines. (And what research in biology has *no* bearing on cancer?) Abstracting services have their value but they cannot record every detail. Reading and learning cannot be delegated: a new and creative idea, which is the product of a single mind, cannot spring from stores of unshared knowledge in other minds. Ideally, he who would integrate should be equipped, not only with a knowledge and understanding of what everyone else has accomplished in relevant fields, but also with an intimate personal contact with every practical aspect of the 'cancer problem' from the direct observation of patients, to the latest findings of molecular biology. Such a paragon never has existed and, we may hazard, never will. In any case, knowledge and practical experience alone are insufficient for synthesis which calls for the perception, description and explanation of previously unnoticed relations.

Because encyclopaedic knowledge and universal experience are unattainable, the identification of crucial evidence assumes special importance. We need to exploit particular observations that greatly limit the range of possible interpretations. Ideally, we would like to achieve a unique understanding of the fundamental nature of cancer. It goes without saying that this unique theory has to be internally consistent; in addition, it should explain all the reliable and relevant evidence as economically as possible. If it can make predictions that can be tested against further observations this will be a further advantage. In a rational world, a single unified theory will eventually oust a set of unconnected ones: above all, it should provide insight and understanding.

So far as I can see—and I shall argue the case in detail—two kinds of evidence, taken jointly, greatly restrict the range of tenable hypotheses of cancer. The first kind of evidence relates to the distribution, with respect to age, of the onset-rates and death-rates for cancers. The second relates to the distribution of the anatomical sites within a patient at which a neoplasm may be present. I have studied these kinds of evidence for over a decade, and I now believe that only one plausible interpretation survives out of the many that have been proposed. This surviving interpretation receives strong support from a wide range of independent observations, in many different fields of biology and medicine.

Cancer and Growth-Control

Despite the difficulties of definition, few will deny that a cancer is a growth that is inappropriate to the normal requirements of the organism. A theory of cancer will therefore be adjudged the more satisfactory if it can also account for *normal* growth and organization, as well as neoplastic development. That is to say, a general biological theory of the physiological and pathological aspects of growth is to be preferred to a set of unconnected hypotheses.

The theory described in this book is the outcome of collaboration with many colleagues, and it began, not with the problem of cancer, but as a theory of normal growth and *non*-neoplastic disease. Our first efforts were aimed at interpreting each so-called 'autoimmune' disease in terms of a specific breakdown in the *central system* that controls and coordinates the growth of the body. Gradually, we were able to extend this original theory to many diseases and conditions that do not usually attract the 'autoimmune' label. These included arteriosclerotic and degenerative heart disease; the menopause; meiotic non-disjunction of chromosomes resulting in conditions such as Down's and Klinefelter's syndromes; the psychoses, including schizophrenia and manic depressive psychosis; multiple sclerosis; psoriasis; ulcerative colitis; periodontal disease and clinical dental caries; Dupuytren's contracture; renal lithiasis; juvenile and late-onset diabetes mellitus; and also many conditions that usually appear under the umbrella term of 'ageing' such as the greying of hair, baldness, gingival recession, the loss of teeth, arcus senilis, spontaneous fractures and senile psychoses.

We first regarded carcinomas as belonging to a fundamentally different class of disease that is *initiated* by gene changes in the controlled, rather than the controlling cells (Burch and Burwell, 1965). However, when I was able to analyse the accumulating evidence for the age-distributions of those malignancies that have an appreciable incidence during childhood, it showed the same critical features as the corresponding evidence for non-malignant diseases. Finally, and only after various misgivings had been dispelled, I subsumed cancer under the same basic aetiological scheme (Burch, 1968(a), 1970(b)).

This new synthesis, which regards all diseases with reproducible age-distributions—including infectious diseases—as having the same fundamental mechanism of *initiation*, combines holistic with reductionist features. I seek to explain how normal growth and development are controlled and co-ordinated and I also attempt to define the basic genetics and the molecular components of control systems. Natural malignant neoplasms, and numerous other age-dependent diseases, result after *central* control cells have accumulated specific 'errors' through an intrinsic random process. These 'errors' destroy the normal *relations* between control and target tissues: the abnormal relations give rise to pathogenic interactions. In most neoplastic disorders, and notably carcinomas, cell division is stimulated in altered target cells.

CHAPTER 2

Some Earlier Theories of Neoplastic and Normal Growth

Many oncologists have been primarily concerned with the nature of carcinogens and with the changes that have to be produced in a cell to make it cancerous. Physical, chemical and biological carcinogens have been identified in bewildering profusion, but it has been suspected that they might all act via a final common pathway, to produce the same type of cellular disturbance (Horsfall, 1966). Proposed intracellular changes have included nuclear or cytoplasmic gene mutation, gene deletion, chromosomal mutation or deletion, changes in genetic regulatory mechanisms (epigenetic change), and viral infection and incorporation into the genome. The preoccupation with the 'cancer cell' has generally been accompanied by a neglect of biological phenomena such as: organization, induction, differentiation, growth-control, coordination, homoeostasis and self-recognition. Only a small minority of oncologists have considered that carcinogenesis might entail interactions between tissues.

Smithers (1962) labelled the philosophy prevailing among cancer workers as *cytologism*. In cytologism, a cancer is assumed to arise from a single cell that has undergone an all-or-none and essentially irreversible change. Smithers (1962) drew on pathological, clinical and epidemiological evidence in an attempt—not yet conspicuously rewarded—to exorcize cytologism. He contended that cancer represents a breakdown in organization; it is not a 'disease of cells' that can be encompassed by cytology alone.

Furth (1953, 1963) has also been a vigorous exponent of the notion that neoplasia represents a breakdown in intercellular communication, but his ideas, like those of Smithers, have had little impact on the direction of cancer research. Nevertheless, indications of a revival of interest in interactionist views can be seen in the recent appearance of a book *Tissue Interactions in Carcinogenesis*, edited by Tarin (1972(b)). The idea that carcinogenesis might be an indirect process, in which the 'target' tissue is transformed by another, is therefore neither new nor novel.

In this chapter I shall review only those theories that have a distinctive biological or immunological content.

Green's Immunological Theory of Cancer

One of the first theories to stress the importance of 'recognition' was introduced by the late H. N. Green in 1954. In his own words written in 1967: '. . . a theory must not treat the cancer cell as an entity on its own, but must account for its lack of "social" behaviour, and its relative lack of response to control mechanisms' (Green *et al.* 1967).

Burnet and Fenner (1949), in trying to explain why we do not normally form antibodies against our own tissues, had postulated that normal cells of the body carry *self-markers*. During embryonic life, self-markers are supposed to prevent the precursor cells of the immune system from synthesizing antibodies complementary to them: in other words, they somehow ensure immunological self-tolerance. Green (1954) adopted this idea and extended it to the cancer field, replacing the expression 'self-markers' by the equivalent, *identity proteins*.

Chemical carcinogens, he argued, produce a highly specific antigenic change in the identity-proteins carried by a cell and this acquired antigenicity elicits the formation of antibodies. Many cells succumb to the immune attack but some may adapt by deleting, in some degree, the synthesis of the modified identity proteins. Green (1954) went on to propose that this adaptational loss constitutes *in itself* the neoplastic change: gradations and progression correspond to the extent of the loss. (Deletion theories of carcinogenesis have enjoyed wide popularity: deleted genes, chromosomes, enzymes and antigens have each had their advocates.)

Identity proteins were regarded as complex molecules with tissue-specific, individual-specific, and species-specific components (Green, 1954). They are less specific than our 'tissue coding factors' (TCFs) which confer recognition properties on small groups of cells that often constitute minute elements of a conventional 'tissue'. In our theory, subtle morphological features, including distinctions between left and right, derive from the specificity of TCFs (Burch, 1968(a)). If we define a 'specific tissue' in terms of those cells in an individual that carry a distinctive TCF, then in the limiting case, a 'specific tissue' might consist of a single cell, such as a neurone.

Although Green formulated his hypothesis on the basis of experiments with chemical carcinogens and tumour-inhibiting compounds, he generalized it to cover the major types of neoplastic transformation (Green, 1954, 1958; Green *et al.*, 1967). In 1958, he stated that cells with incomplete identity proteins fail to be recognized by *growth-regulating* mechanisms. The idea of growth-regulating mechanisms external to a cell and much more specific than growth hormone—inasmuch as they recognize particular identity proteins—anticipates Burwell's (1963) theory which is described at the end of this chapter.

The Analogy of Graft-versus-Host

Tyler (1960) likened cancer to a graft-versus-host immunological reaction. He proposed that the malignant aspects of neoplastic disease depend on an immunological attack by some, or all, of the cancer cells, against normal self-tissues. In other words, the tumour cells are immunologically competent. The change in differentiation and the immune attack arise, according to Tyler, because the cancer cells lack one or more transplantation antigens. (This feature of Tyler's theory resembles the corresponding one of Green's. Identity proteins, which undergo loss, include transplantation as well as other antigens.) Tyler (1960) attributed the loss of transplantation antigens to the inactivation or loss of the corresponding gene(s).

Elaborating his theory, Tyler (1962) argued that an understanding of the phenomena of differentiation and normal growth must precede the under-standing of the biological nature of cancer. He assumed that a tumour can be initiated from a single cell if it suffers the loss, or inactivation, of *one* of its histocompatibility genes when the cell is heterozygous at the particular locus, or of *both* genes if the cell is homozygous. Burdened with these rigid assumptions, the theory cannot readily explain progression, regression, or the details of the age- and anatomical-distributions of cancers.

Kaplan and Smithers (1959) also used the analogy of the graft-versus-host reaction (*homologous disease*) to explain certain features of lymphoid tumours, including Hodgkin's disease in man. They attributed the wasting, anaemia, and lymphoid depletion observed in homologous disease in experimental animals, and lymphoid neoplasia in man, to an immune attack by lymphoid cells against haematopoietic cells. In homologous disease, the lymphoid cells of the *graft* attack the host: but in Hodgkin's disease, lymphocytic leukaemia, lymphosarcoma, reticulum-cell sarcomas and multiple myelomatosis, the patient's own aberrant lymphoid cells often attack self-tissues. Kaplan and Smithers (1959) suggested that tumour cells are more likely to become differentiated from normal lymphoid cells by the loss of 'antigens' than through the acquisition of new ones: they did not discuss the mechanisms of antigenic deletion.

Despite the attention paid to recognition relations, the three preceding theories shed no light on the multicentric origin of many tumours. The changes that initiate neoplastic growth—the loss of recognition factors of one kind or another—remain located in the cell that becomes neoplastic.

Furth's Theory

According to Furth (1953, 1963), neoplasia in general represents the break-down of a communication system that regulates the number of each type of cell. He found that the destruction of the thyroid in mice is followed by the formation of pituitary tumours. However, these tumours cannot be transplanted to normal mice and they are composed of cells that, both histologically and functionally, resemble normal cells (Furth and Clifton, 1966). Apparently, they constitute a hyperplastic response to an artificially modified hormonal milieu; nevertheless, after successive passages, they eventually acquire autonomy and become unresponsive to thyroid hormones. Although the development of these pituitary tumours may have little relevance to the pathogenesis of natural cancers in man, Furth's (1969) contention that neoplasia is *not* a mere multiplication of autonomous cells, but a disturbance of inter- and intracellular communications, seems to me to be an important concept. Despite this conceptual innovation, Furth (1969) still locates the *primary* carcinogenic change in the DNA of the 'target' cell and he regards hormones merely as powerful promoters or inhibitors of neoplasia. Hormones determine whether a cell, already transformed by a carcinogen (mutagen), will propagate a tumour.

Burnet's Theory: Immunological Surveillance

Burnet's (1970) theory of cancer is subsidiary to his concept of immuno-logical surveillance.

Following more-or-less traditional ideas, Burnet (1970) believes that malignant disease is *initiated* by one or more somatic–genetic changes, intrinsic to individual cells. These somatic–genetic changes, some of which might be point-mutations, are essentially random in character. The indi-vidual mutant cell, in its potentially cancerous state, begins to propagate a clone. According to Burnet, progress towards a detectable neoplasm depends on many local factors, one of the most important of which is immunological surveillance. Thymus-dependent lymphocytes (T-lymphocytes) are the main or exclusive agents of immunological surveillance and in Burnet's view they

their incidence with age. Nevertheless, the broad concept of 'immunological surveillance' could well prove to be substantially correct even if the details should require revision.

Theories of Growth-control

Concepts of growth-control, and of cancer, have tended to come together over the phenomenon of self-inhibition of growth. Several authors have believed that cells in a given tissue synthesize specific inhibitors, that, when present at a high enough local concentration, prevent the tissue from growing (Tyler, 1947; Weiss, 1950; Weiss and Kavanau, 1957; Rose, 1958; Druckrey, 1959; Bullough, 1962).

Tyler (1947) believed that complementary pairs of substances resembling antigen and antibody, are present in each cell: they constitute a system that forms the basis of cell structure. He regarded growth as consisting primarily in the formation of these complementary pairs of structural units: the process of growth was compared to that of antibody formation as conceived in the instruction theory of the immune response. In the instruction theory—which has now passed out of favour—the antigen acts as a template on which the configuration of the antibody is determined. Tyler (1947) also drew a parallel with the self-replication of genes. This had been described by Pauling and Delbrück (1940), in a remarkable anticipation of Watson and Crick, as the formation of substances that are both complementary and identical.

In Tyler's (1947) theory, differences in the rates of production of different 'antigens' are supposed to give rise to cytodifferentiation: all 'antigens' are present in all cells, but in widely differing amounts in different locations, and in the different tissues. We have already seen how this theory of normal growth was applied by Tyler (1960, 1962) to the problem of neoplasia. Although he was not explicit on the point, I presume that the loss of a transplantation antigen from a cell was supposed to leave the complementary antibody in that cell unpaired, and that this un-neutralized antibody accounts for the invasive properties of malignant cells. The ingenuity of this theory of growth, cytodifferentiation and cancer compels admiration; unfortunately, it founders on the multicentric origin of tumours.

Happily, its influence can be seen in Weiss's *template-antitemplate* theory of growth (Weiss, 1950; Weiss and Kavanau, 1957). Templates, specific to the cell type, are synthesized and normally confined within the cell, where they regulate growth-rate in proportion to their concentration. Each cell also produces antagonistic complementary molecules—the antitemplates—that can block templates. Antitemplates, unlike templates, diffuse freely out of cells into the extracellular space and circulation, and return back into cells. They are continually catabolized and excreted, but their loss is compensated by continuous production. When stationary equilibrium between the intra- and extracellular concentrations of antitemplates is reached, growth ceases.

This model has been subjected to extensive mathematical treatment and good agreement has been obtained between observed and theoretical curves of growth in relation to age (Weiss and Kavanau, 1957). But the model fails to account for many biological findings (see Chapter 3) that point to the existence of growth-controlling organs, including a 'comparator', *outside* the tissue that is under control (Burch, 1968(a)). Nevertheless, Weiss's theory invokes the concept of the negative feedback (homeostatic) control of normal growth.

Rose's (1958) theory is formally analogous to Weiss's. He again postulates that specific inhibition of normal growth results when a critical concentration of inhibitor(s), produced by viable cells, is reached and maintained: 'like inhibits like'. This theory suffers from the same limitations as Weiss's, for in both of them, growth is stimulated by a *deficiency* in the concentration of an inhibitor. Extensive evidence reviewed by Paschkis (1958) and Burch (1968(a))—see also Chapter 3—points to the existence of physiological agents that promote growth in a positive way: that is to say, an *increase* in their concentration *stimulates* growth.

The absence of mitotic promoters from the theories of Weiss and of Rose was remedied by Druckrey (1959) who introduced a two-stage system of feedback. The first stage is equivalent to Weiss's system of templates and antitemplates, but in the second stage, afferent signals flow from target cells to a 'higher' regulating centre. This centre exports mitotic stimulators when the concentration of afferent signals declines. In Druckrey's (1959) theory of carcinogenesis, cancer cells escape from the influence of either first-, or second-stage, mitotic regulators.

Bullough (1962) regarded none of the evidence for mitotic stimulators as critical and he argued that mitotic rate is controlled by a series of tissue-specific inhibitors. Although hormones may modulate mitotic rate, the ultimate control resides within the tissues themselves. Bullough (1965) and Bullough and Rytöma (1965) have isolated mitotic inhibitors which they call *chalones*. The epidermal, liver and kidney chalones have similar physical properties. Chalones are easily extracted, non–dialysable and water-soluble: they are destroyed by boiling and precipitated by alcohol. For maximum inhibitory action, the epidermal chalone requires the presence of adrenalin. It is tissue-specific, but neither species- nor class-specific (Bullough, 1965; Bullough et al., 1967).

At this juncture, it will be helpful to discuss Osgood's (1957, 1959, 1964) distinction between two main forms of mitosis: *symmetrical* and *asymmetrical*. Consider the healthy epidermis in a fully-grown person. In the steady state, the continuous loss of the horny layer of the skin is made good by cell division in the basal and Malpighian layers. On the average, a single division in the basal layer results in one cell that remains in the layer and another that migrates outwards towards the surface. This is *asymmetrical* mitosis. It maintains the *status quo* and the number of cells in the basal layer is conserved.

During normal growth, however, the area covered by the epidermis increases enormously and the number of cells in the basal layer must also increase because cell size does not change appreciably. From time to time a cell in the basal layer must give rise to two daughter cells, both of which remain in the basal layer until they, in turn, undergo mitosis. Divisions which in this way lead to a net increase in the number of cells in the basal layer are examples of *symmetrical* mitosis.

The same general principles apply to all those series of cells, including the erythrocytic, that exhibit a steady-state population while undergoing continual maturation, death and replacement. Further distinctions have been elaborated by Osgood (1957, 1959, 1964) but they do not concern us here.

The kind of mitosis that is inhibited by the chalones studied by Bullough and his collaborators probably belongs to the asymmetrical category. This form of mitosis is not characteristic of growth, if by 'growth' we mean a net, maintained increase in the number, or mass, of cells. Bullough and Rytöma (1965) suggest that in all examples of neoplasia, there is either a shortage of chalones, or a failure to react to whatever chalone is present. Both properties are local in origin, and, as such, they conflict with the age-incidence and the multicentric origin of natural cancers (see Chapter 7).

Burwell's thesis

In 1963, Burwell advanced a general theory of growth that led, via modifications, to the unified theory of growth and disease presented here and elsewhere (Burch and Burwell, 1965; Burch, 1968(a), 1970(a)).

According to Burwell (1963) 'The unity or the integrity of the body depends not only upon the interdependence of *different* tissues and organs but also, and perhaps equally importantly, upon the inter-relationship between the cells of any one differentiated tissue and cells of a *similar* differentiation, wherever they may lie in the body'. He maintained '. . . that in the mammal an essential function of lymphoid tissue is to establish and maintain *morphostasis* for many of its differentiated tissues'. (Morphostasis, following Weisz (1951), means '. . . the steady state condition that maintains a particular pattern'.)

Burwell's (1963) proposal clashed with the orthodox view that the function of the lymphoid system is *primarily* the recognition and elimination of *foreign* substances, although, as we have seen, the antigen–antibody analogy has often been invoked to explain the *specificity* of growth-control. Also, as far back as 1922, Carrel attributed growth-promoting properties to leucocytes of various kinds, both in tissue-culture preparations and in the process of wound-repair. From histological studies, Humble *et al.* (1956) concluded that the lymphocyte '. . . furthers the processes of growth and division of cells regardless of their nature'. Loutit (1962) has reviewed evidence that supports the commonly held opinion that the lymphocyte has a trophic or nourishing function. Metcalf (1964) demonstrated a striking parallel between the curves: (1) for the age-dependence of the rate of production of thymic lymphocytes in male C3H mice; and (2) for the age-dependence of the weekly increase in body weight. He proposed that lymphocytes or their breakdown products might be implicated in the control of mitosis.

Latterly, as described above, the function of *immunological surveillance* has been added to the repertoire of the lymphoid system (Burnet, 1970) and the idea has gained wide acceptance. The cells of the body are supposed to be scrutinized by agents of the lymphoid system: mutant cells that produce alien antigens are said to be identified and removed by an immunological mechanism (Burnet, 1959, 1970). But the notion that the lymphoid system— or at least one part of it—might be directly implicated in the more fundamental biological processes of growth-control has not been generally welcomed by immunologists.

The rather complicated details of Burwell's (1963) original scheme have since been replaced by a simpler notion involving a conventional negative-feedback system. We retain the key idea that one section of the lymphoid system regulates the growth of those tissues, notably endothelia, that are freely accessible to blood-borne cells (Burch and Burwell, 1965). In this revised control-system, the final effectors of symmetrical mitotis (mitotic control proteins or MCPs) are thymus-dependent small lymphocytes of the kind that feature in the rejection of allografts and in delayed hypersensitivity reactions (Burch, 1968(a); Burch and Burwell, 1965).

Advantages in Burwell's theory—Many advantages are explicit or potential in Burwell's (1963) theory:

(1) Immunology—especially transplantation immunology—becomes incorporated into the general biology of mammalian organisms. We see that allograft rejection is not an arbitrary device of the Almighty to frustrate the transplantation surgeon, but an inevitable consequence of the biological evolution of multitissue organisms (Burch, 1968(a)).

often succeed in aborting spontaneous cancers. Mutant cells in the developing clone carry not-self antigens that are recognized by thymus-dependent lymphocytes and the clone is eliminated by a mechanism that is entirely analogous to delayed hypersensitivity (Burnet, 1970). The efficiency of immunological surveillance is said to decline with increasing age because the thymus, which is supposed to be one of the main organs of surveillance, undergoes atrophy. This diminishing efficiency of surveillance with advancing age is said to be an important factor in the age-dependence of cancer incidence, and, indeed, for ageing processes generally (Burnet, 1970). As we shall see later, my own analysis of age-patterns does not support this contention.

A major omission from Burnet's (1970) theory is the failure to discuss how surveillance is exercised in those numerous tissues that lie behind blood-tissue barriers. If immunological surveillance is as important as Burnet (1970) believes it to be, it is difficult to imagine how tissues such as the central and peripheral nervous systems, articular cartilage and bone, can be left unsupervised.

Although my approach to cancer differs radically from Burnet's, I have also argued (Burch, 1970(a)) for a correction process that has certain affinities with the one proposed by Burnet. In my view, strand-switching gene mutations occur spontaneously in target cells, and these produce changes in the polypeptide components of the tissue coding factors (TCFs) of target cells. However, under normal physiological conditions, and provided the associated *mitotic control protein* (MCP) is non-mutant, these alterations in TCFs are reversed or eliminated by normal MCPs (Burch, 1970(a)). We can therefore regard normal MCPs—cellular or humoral—as exercising a monitoring-, or surveillance-function. When the normal MCP is cellular, it is carried by thymus-dependent lymphocytes, and hence in this instance, Burnet and I agree on the nature of the agent of surveillance. Burnet (1970), however, envisages that lymphocytes destroy mutant target cells through a delayed-hypersensitivity mechanism. In the absence of definitive evidence I remain non-committal on this point, and I would wish to leave open the possibility that TCFs might be restored to normal through an induction-type interaction—see Chapter 4.

My theory postulates that, when the mutant target cell lies behind a blood-tissue barrier, non-mutant humoral MCPs ($?\alpha_2$-globulins) function as the corrective agents.

In common with many others, Burnet's (1970) theory founders on the multicentric origin of cancers. Furthermore, the age-distribution of cancers reviewed in Chapter 7 gives no support to the idea that a progressive decrease of immunological surveillance is a major factor in the increase of

(2) The theory enables us to understand the significance of the elaborate anatomical pattern of lymphatics and the widespread distribution of lymphoid tissues throughout the body. These arrangements are eminently suited to the complex communication requirements of negative-feedback growth-control in mammals.

(3) A 'central' machinery is identified that can regulate and coordinate the overall growth of the organism.

(4) Specificity, which is the hallmark of developmental and morphological aspects of growth, is also *the* outstanding characteristic of the lymphoid system, which is able to distinguish 'self' from 'not-self' with remarkable facility.

(5) Growth regulation by a 'central' organ, using a negative-feedback loop, requires efferent and afferent pathways. These pathways are well-known features of lymph nodes.

(6) The extended theory provides a simple explanation of detailed evidence relating to various so-called autoimmune diseases, if we assume that each disorder arises from a specific breakdown in the central system of growth-control (Burch, 1968(a); Burch and Rowell, 1968, 1970).

(7) It explains the widely-recognized connections (Loutit, 1962) between lymphoid depletion on the one hand, and secondary disease, wasting and runting on the other. The failure of growth that follows: (a) the injection of cortisone in neonatal rats and (b) immunosuppressive prednisone therapy after kidney transplantation in children, is at once accounted for. Thus, rats stunted by cortisone show first a marked deterioration of thymic and splenic cells, followed by a slow rate of cell division in other organs (Winick and Coscia, 1968). In a series of children who received transplanted kidneys, the only patient who grew significantly during the first 9 months of follow-up was a boy who experienced no acute or chronic rejection episodes and needed only minimal immunosuppressive prednisone therapy (Fine *et al.*, 1970).

(8) As a corollary to (7), the theory explains the *increase* in general body size that follows the injection of syngeneic thymic tissue, at fortnightly intervals, into young mice (Flaks, 1967).

(9) The theory explains—indeed, it was partly based on—the complicated pattern of reactions within those regional lymph nodes that drain tissue allografts (Burwell, 1962).

(10) It enables us to understand the reason for the enormous variety of factors such as histocompatibility antigens, tissue-specific antigens and the many blood groups that characterize the outer (plasma) membranes of cells. The plasma membrane serves not only to regulate the entry and exit of metabolites to and from the cell: it also carries recognition factors that,

among other things, serve to identify mitotically competent cells to the specific effectors of cell-division.

This list is far from complete: other items are included in Burwell's (1963) original paper. One of the most attractive features of Burwell's proposal is its capacity to integrate what seemed previously to be a whole host of unrelated phenomena, into a unified and intellectually satisfying scheme. Nevertheless, we soon came to the conclusion that lymphocytes act as the effectors of symmetrical mitosis only for those tissues that are readily and normally accessible to blood-borne cells: another system is needed to control the growth of other tissues (Burch and Burwell, 1965).

What, then, controls cell division in those tissues—such as the central nervous system, articular cartilage and bone—to which lymphocytes are normally denied free access? A factor capable of penetrating the various types of barrier between such tissues and the blood must obviously be humoral. It seems extremely unlikely, however, that any of the major classes of immuno-globulins (IgG, IgM or IgA) can be held responsible. In Bruton's congenital agammaglobulinaemia, a syndrome in which these fractions are greatly depressed or absent, more-or-less normal growth occurs, apart from the absence of plasma cells. So far as we can judge, humoral effectors of mitosis in man seem generally to migrate on electrophoresis with the α_2-globulin serum protein fraction and in some instances, at least, to be α_2-macroglobulins (Burch and Burwell, 1965; Burch, 1968(a); Burch, de Dombal and Watkinson, 1969; Burch and Milunsky, 1969). The evidence for this conclusion, although bulky, is still largely circumstantial and more direct demonstrations will be needed for confirmation.

To a large extent, this book develops and extends Burwell's seminal idea to the biology of neoplastic growth.

CHAPTER 3

Is Normal Growth Regulated by a Central System?

Some of the most remarkable features of normal growth receive the least attention. No generally accepted answers have been given to basic questions such as: What mechanism ensures that we grow to a certain size and then stop? How is it that some parts of the body are related through left–right mirror symmetry whereas others are not? Individual organs follow characteristic growth curves that often differ widely from organ to organ (Brody, 1945): how then is a consistent balance maintained between them during normal growth? Claude Bernard (1865) used the expression *'ensemble harmonique'*. Widdowson (1970) refers to 'the harmony of growth'. The descriptions, though attractive, do not explain the underlying biological phenomena.

Certain organs and tissues—but not others—can regenerate in response to injury and partial removal. The phenomenon of *catch-up growth*—the ability of an organism to regain the normal growth curve after a period of starvation—indicates that something 'knows' what size the organism should be at a given age. Is each separate organ and tissue endowed with this 'knowledge' as postulated by Weiss in his template–antitemplate theory? Or do organs and tissues communicate with one another? Or is the growth of every 'target' organ and tissue regulated homeostatically by a system with a 'central' control?

The evidence to be reviewed in this chapter supports the last alternative. To account in such terms for the characteristic differences in the patterns of growth of individual organs and tissues, we have to postulate a separate control element for each distinctive 'target tissue'. In this context, 'tissue' connotes a much finer distinction than that used by histologists. Epidermis, for example, will comprise an immensely elaborate mosaic of distinctive elements. Elsewhere, I have estimated that the human body might consist of as many as 10^{10} 'distinctive tissues' (Burch, 1968(a)).

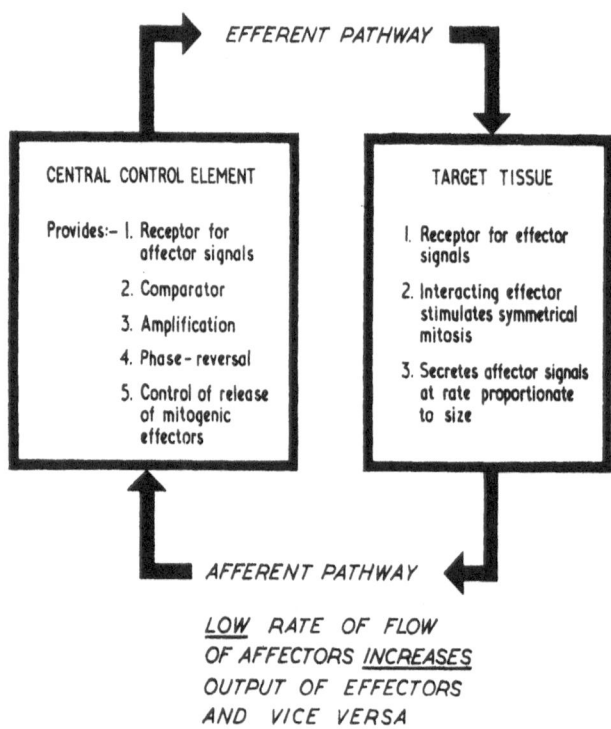

Figure 3.1 Basic requirements for the homeostatic or negative-feedback control of the growth of a target tissue by a central element

Figure 3.1 outlines the essential requirements of any homeostatic (negative-feedback) system of growth-control. In our theory, we call the effectors of symmetrical mitosis in target cells, mitotic control proteins or MCPs. (The distinction between symmetrical and asymmetrical mitosis was described in the last chapter.) MCPs may be cellular (carried on T-lymphocytes), or humoral, belonging perhaps, to the α_2-macroglobulin fraction. We call affectors from target cells and the labels that identify the cells to effector MCPs, tissue coding factors, or TCFs. The solution to problems of recognition—of target cells by effector MCPs and of central control elements by affector TCFs—is described in Chapter 4.

If symmetrical mitosis of cells in an organized tissue *in vivo* is stimulated by an effector signal from the central control, it follows that, in the absence of such signals, symmetrical mitosis must be inhibited. We have proposed that the inhibition of symmetrical mitosis in an organized tissue depends on the contact relations between contiguous cells (Burch 1968(a); Burch and Burwell 1965). Westermark (1971) has shown that such a mechanism—contact inhibition of mitosis, or, to use Dulbecco's expression, 'topo-inhibition'—functions even among cultures of normal, non-neoplastic, human glia-like cells. Castor's (1971) results for mouse embryo 3T3 cells are also consistent with the hypothesis that cell contact inhibits division in culture by limiting the free area and movements of the cell surface. However, high serum concentrations in the culture medium increase the cell density at which mitosis ceases. Virus-transformed 3T3 cells reach a higher population density than non-transformed cells before growth ceases (Castor 1971).

The elucidation of the mechanism of normal growth-control cannot but contribute to our understanding of neoplastic growth. If normal growth is indeed homeostatically regulated from the 'centre' it is almost tautologous to add that neoplastic growth arises from a defect or breakdown in the negative-feedback system. Our task is to define and locate the defect. Many, perhaps most, oncologists assume that the defect arises in a target cell. I shall argue, to the contrary, that natural cancers are always *initiated* by defects in central control cells.

Regenerative Growth of the Liver

In the rat, the species that has been most favoured for experiments on regeneration of the liver, the normal frequency of mitosis among hepatic cells in the mature animal is very low—about one cell in 10^4. However, surgical removal of two of the lobes of the liver triggers a wave of mitoses in the residual liver, followed by its rapid growth. Peak mitotic-rate occurs in parenchymal cells at about 24 hours after two-thirds partial hepatectomy and about a day later in littoral and ductal cells (Grisham, 1962). After the peak, mitotic-rate falls off at first rapidly and then asymptotically to normal levels as the regenerating liver approaches its original size at about 3 weeks. The literature of the subject has received several reviews: see Bucher (1963, 1967); Simpson (1963); Leduc (1964); and Gross (1965).

Two queries concerning regenerative growth have special importance in connection with my theory of growth-control: What stimulates liver cells to mitosis? What mechanism governs the extent of regeneration?

Reasoning from experiments with pairs of rats in parabiotic union, one of which was subjected to partial hepatectomy, Bucher (1963) tentatively suggested that a humoral factor regulates regenerative growth. Cells in the liver of the 'normal' partner undergo a marked increase in DNA synthesis in response to the ablation of the liver in its parabiotic partner (Bucher, 1963; Moolten and Bucher, 1967). Apparently, factors are released from the hepatectomized animal into the shared circulation, and these promote the growth of liver tissue in both animals.

Clearcut findings along these lines have been obtained by Sakai (1970), who used a different surgical procedure. He first established a simple parabiotic union between a pair of inbred Lewis rats. Two months later the abdominal cavities were opened and both aortae were freed. Silastic tubes were inserted into the aortae through the abdominal free canal, so that the lower part of each animal received blood from the upper section of its partner. Seven to eight days after this second operation, two-thirds partial hepatectomy, or sham-operation, was performed on one of the members of the parabiotic pair. A marked increase in DNA synthesis was seen in the liver of the non-operated animal at 24 hours after partial hepatectomy in its partner. Sakai (1970) concluded that his experiments convincingly demonstrated the existence of a humoral mechanism of regeneration that utilizes a shortlived factor. He was unable to determine whether the factor promoting regeneration is a diminution in concentration of an inhibitor, or the increase in concentration of a mitotic stimulator. Our negative-feedback theory of growth-control requires both factors—a decrease in the rate of flow of affector tissue coding factors (TCFs) from the diminished liver and an increase in the export of effector mitotic control proteins (MCPs) from the central part of the control system (Burch and Burwell, 1965).

The humoral theory of mitotic control receives further support from the observation that the initial wave of mitoses in parenchymal cells of the regenerating liver affects, predominantly, cells in the portal region (Bucher, 1963; Fabrikant, 1967; Melvin, 1968). In experiments with tritiated thymidine, it is not until 50 hours after partial hepatectomy that the percentage of labelled cells near to the central vein of a liver lobule rises to that of the (then falling) level of labelled cells in the portal region (Fabrikant, 1967). Moreover, when the direction of the blood-flow is reversed in a liver autograft of a partially hepatectomized dog, the uptake of tritiated thymidine occurs preferentially in cells at the centre of the lobule (Siegel et al., 1967). We can infer from these various experiments that the mitogenic factors in liver regeneration are blood-borne.

This conclusion is strongly reinforced by experiments in which heterotopic partial autografts of rat liver were studied before and after partial hepatectomy (Leong et al., 1964; Virolainen, 1964). Before partial hepatectomy, levels of DNA synthesis and of mitosis in well-established subcutaneous autografts of liver, resemble those in the primary organ. After partial hepatectomy, the increased DNA labelling and mitoses in the autografts follow the same time course as those in the residual liver, but at a lower level (Leong *et al.*, 1964). These studies show that portal blood *per se* is not essential to the regeneration of liver tissues: evidently the mitogenic factors become widely distributed through the systemic circulation. Neither is the increase in the rate of flow of blood through the residual liver of any appreciable importance to regeneration. This has been demonstrated by Thomson and Clark (1965) who altered the blood flow through the liver by surgical means. Regeneration was independent of changes in the rate of flow.

Fisher, Szuch and Fisher (1971) diverted the portal blood through a partial liver (syngeneic) transplant in a partially hepatectomized rat. The transplant receiving the portal blood responded in the same way as would the liver remnant in a non-transplanted host, whereas the response in the host liver remnant (in series with the liver transplant) was considerably diminished. Fisher *et al.* (1971(a)) concluded that in this series-arrangement of transplanted and host liver tissues, the transplant utilized most of the mitogenic humoral factor present in the portal blood, so that little was available to stimulate the host liver remnant. They found it impossible to reconcile these and related findings with the view that a reduction of inhibitor concentration—such as a chalone—in portal blood is responsible for the promotion of mitosis in the liver transplant. In my terms, the humoral MCP in the portal blood promotes mitosis by interacting with the parenchymal cells of the liver.

In cross-circulation experiments, Fisher *et al.* (1971(b)) showed that the humoral factor responsible for liver regeneration does not arise from the liver remnant. Cross-circulation between pairs of rats was established so that blood flowed from the left carotid artery of each member to the right jugular vein of its partner. The uptake of tritiated thymidine in the DNA of the unoperated liver of one rat, was studied in relation to the extent of removal of liver from its partner. Fisher *et al.* (1971(b)) found that the uptake in the unoperated liver increased in proportion to the amount of liver removed (including complete removal) from the cross-circulation partner.

Our theory predicts that regeneration of a specific tissue element will occur only if the rate of flow of residual affector TCFs exceeds a certain minimum value that is needed to maintain 'amplification' in the central control mechanism (Burch, 1968(a)). It is interesting to note, therefore, that 86 per cent partial hepatectomy in single rats produces a lower uptake of tritiated thymidine per mg DNA in residual liver, than in the liver of normal unoperated controls (Fisher *et al.*, 1968(b)).

From *in vitro* experiments, Paul *et al.* (1972) concluded that a 'positive control system' probably regulates DNA synthesis and cell division in foetal liver cells. They found that cultured liver cells from foetal rats responded to serum from partially hepatectomized rats by increased uptake of tritiated thymidine and tritiated leucine. Serum from a normal rat elicited no such response. Their findings were inconsistent with the idea that a 'negative control system', such as a chalone mechanism, would cause the increased uptake of DNA and protein precursors.

Some earlier and sadly neglected experiments carried out by Czeizel, Vaczo and Kertai (1962) are of great importance to the understanding of regenerative growth. These workers examined the effects of radiation and of bone marrow injections on liver regeneration in albino rats. In control animals, the extent of liver regeneration at one week after two-thirds partial hepatectomy was 90 per cent. A dose of 500 rads of x-rays delivered to the whole body, 24 hours after partial hepatectomy, reduced the equivalent regeneration to 60 per cent: when the residual liver was shielded from x-rays by lead, the comparable figure was 69 per cent. When, in addition, part of the bone marrow was also shielded from x-rays, the extent of regeneration at 1 week rose to 78 per cent. However, when syngeneic bone marrow (about 2×10^7 cells) was injected within two hours after irradiating the completely unshielded partially hepatectomized rat, regeneration reached 89 per cent at one week. This figure did not differ significantly from that (90 per cent) obtained with unirradiated control animals. If the bone marrow injected into irradiated animals was also irradiated (500R), then the extent of regeneration was only 57 per cent (Czeizel et al., 1962).

Injection of unirradiated bone marrow into unirradiated rats boosted 'regeneration' to give an overshoot—104 per cent at one week.

These ingenious experiments by Czeizel et al. yield some very important conclusions:

(1) The injection of unirradiated bone marrow into irradiated animals restores regenerative growth to normal.

(2) An excess of bone marrow given by injection produces excessive 'regeneration': bone marrow can therefore override the normal homeostatic control.

(3) Irradiation of the liver remnant itself (500 rads, x-rays) has little or no effect on its regeneration.

(4) Because 500 rads has little effect on protein synthesis in mammalian cells—but produces a marked impairment of their proliferative capacity—it appears that regeneration in irradiated animals requires proliferation of bone-marrow cells.

Davies et al. (1964) also performed experiments using radiation and bone marrow injections. They studied liver regeneration in the mouse, in relation to the chimaeric state of the animal. When an animal has received a dose of radiation that would ordinarily be lethal it can be rescued by an injection of bone marrow. Syngeneic bone marrow allows more-or-less complete recovery from the acute effects of such an irradiation, but injected allogeneic bone marrow often induces a wasting disease in the host animal, depending on the genetic relation between donor and host strains. Davies *et al.* (1964) found that the extent of liver regeneration relates not only to the chimaeric state, with syngeneic chimaeras generally showing better regeneration than allogeneic chimaeras, but also to the degree of lymphopenia. Severely lymphopenic animals, whether syngeneic or allogeneic chimaeras, showed poor liver regeneration after two-thirds partial hepatectomy.

These investigators pointed out that their findings were consistent with Burwell's (1963) theory that the lymphoid system maintains tissue size. In further tests of Burwell's theory, Davies *et al.* (1964) found that thymectomized, irradiated mice, when injected with syngeneic bone marrow, regenerated their liver more slowly than sham-thymectomized syngeneic chimaeras that had been treated similarly.

Eartl and Wieser (1971) studied changes in the thymus after partial hepatectomy in rats. A loss of thymus weight from about 450 mg at operation, to about 200 mg at 5 days post-operation was observed, followed by almost complete recovery at 10 days. Eartl and Wieser suggested that breakdown products of thymocytes might be utilized by the regenerating liver.

Experiments of special relevance to my main thesis have been carried out by Rabes, Hartenstein and Scholze (1970). They observed the mitotic rate in the liver of rats treated with diethylnitrosamine, a carcinogen that induces liver tumours. As long as the mitotic index in the parenchymal cells remained at the control level, the liver responded normally to partial hepatectomy, with about a tenfold increase in mitotic index 60 hours after the operation. However, when the mitotic index in the parenchymal cells of carcinogen-treated animals began to show an increase, marking the onset of neoplasia, the response to partial hepatectomy showed a corresponding decline. This suggests that the onset of carcinogen-induced neoplasia in these rats is accompanied by (perhaps caused by) a partial loss of normal growth-control.

Time-dependence of regenerative growth

Assume that the rate of secretion and flow of affector tissue coding factors (TCFs) is proportional to the mass, M_r, of the regenerating liver at time τ after partial hepatectomy. If the final mass of the fully regenerated liver is M_∞, then we shall assume that the regenerative stimulus at time τ is proportional to $(M_\infty - M_r)$. If we ignore the time-lags in the feedback-control, and if we assume the liver to be a homogeneous tissue from the point of view of the kinetics of regeneration, then

$$dM_\tau/d\tau = c(M_\infty - M_\tau) \qquad (3.2)$$

Which, integrated, gives

$$M_\tau = M_\infty \{1 - \exp(-c\tau)\} \qquad (3.3)$$

In view of the crudity of the assumptions, especially the one concerning the homogeneity of liver tissue, it is somewhat surprising to find (Spencer and Coulombe, 1966), that equation (3.3) describes the experimental results of Brues, Drury and Brues (1936) very accurately from $\tau = 1$ to $\tau = 12$ days after two-thirds partial hepatectomy. The value of the constant c in equation (3.3) was found to be 0·4 day^{-1} (Spencer and Coulombe, 1966).

Presumably, the agreement arises because the amount of non-parenchymal tissue (mainly littoral and ductal cells) is appreciably less than that of parenchymal cells, and because the remaining assumptions approximate fairly closely to reality.

It is even more surprising to find that the growth of the whole rat (white WAG/Rij), raised under specific pathogen-free conditions, gives a fairly good fit to equations of the form (3.2) and (3.3) over most of the lifespan (Grover, Block and Gross, 1970). Systematic departures of observations from equation (3.3) do occur, but they do not exceed 5 per cent.

Conclusions from studies of liver regeneration

The above findings and inferences from studies of liver regeneration support our theory of growth-control. Largely from studies of the age-dependence of diseases we deduced that a fixed number of stem cells, located mainly or wholly in the bone marrow, acts as the *comparator* in each growth-control element (Burch and Burwell, 1965; Burch, 1968(a)). This comparator determines the ultimate size of its target tissue. The dynamics of growth, from birth to maturity, depend also on the relation between the comparator stem cells, and the intermediate stations of the feedback control. Where the lymphoid control system is concerned it appears that at least two such stations are implicated: the thymus and regional lymph nodes (Burch, 1968(a))—see Figure 3.2. Whether the humoral control system utilizes similar intermediate stations is not yet clear although it seems likely.

In man, the number of comparator stem cells is probably fixed within about ±0·1 year of birth (Burch, 1968(a)). These stem cells are linked, via the intermediate stages of feedback, to the final executive (peripheral) control cells. Where target tissues such as the parenchymal cells of liver are concerned, the effectors of symmetrical mitosis (MCPs) are humoral, and

POSSIBLE STATIONS IN THE HOMOEOSTATIC CONTROL OF GROWTH

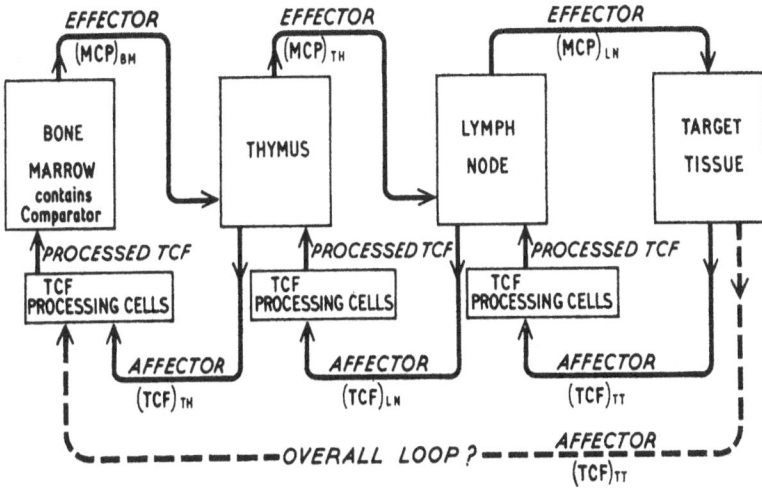

Figure 3.2 Outline of the possible series of feedback loops involved in the control of the growth of a target tissue by effector T-lymphocytes

the rate of their release from the final executive cells is governed by the homeostatic control. This control responds to the current size of the liver, and it 'measures' the differences between the 'correct' rate of flow of affector tissue coding factors (TCFs) and their actual rate of flow. At any stage during normal growth the liver remnant regenerates after partial hepatectomy to the size appropriate to the size of the animal. This implies that the number and effectiveness of the intermediate and executive growth-control cells also relate to the size of the animal. Under the experimental conditions imposed by Czeizel *et al.* (1962), the functioning of the executive cells depends on the integrity of the bone marrow.

If the sceptic feels that the experiments cited above on liver regeneration do not entirely rule out a contribution from neuronal stimulation, it should be mentioned that Mallet-Guy *et al.* (1956) and Clerici, Mozarelli and Privini (1964) have shown that sympathetic denervation of the liver has no effect on the response to partial hepatectomy.

Compensatory Growth of the Kidney

When one kidney is removed, an operation known as unilateral nephrectomy the other kidney usually undergoes a compensatory increase in size. Enlargement entails both an increase in the number of cells (*hyperplasia*), and an increase in their size (*hypertrophy*). Fox and Wahman (1968) have reviewed the early literature of this subject.

Similar compensatory changes are observed when one ureter is ligated: the contralateral kidney undergoes an increase in size—see, for example, Dicker and Shirley (1971). Two weeks after the ureter has been ligated the obstructed kidney shows signs of hydronephrosis (Dicker and Shirley, 1972).

Although compensatory growth of the kidney after unilateral nephrectomy has been less thoroughly investigated than regenerative growth of the liver, various experiments point to the existence of a central control mechanism located outside the kidney.

Wachtel and Cole (1965) studied the effects of radiation on the compensatory growth of the kidney in the growing rat. After uninephrectomy and x-irradiation to give an absorbed dose of 1000 rads in the exteriorized, contralateral kidney—with the remainder of the animal shielded—they observed no retardation of the growth of the whole body. A slight but significant decrement was seen in the compensatory growth of the kidney relative to that of unirradiated controls. However, when growing rats received a whole-body dose of 500 rads, with the exteriorized kidney shielded, Wachtel and Cole found that the growth of the whole body was retarded, the DNA content of the kidney was reduced, and compensatory growth of the kidney was markedly diminished. The latter effect was even more conspicuous when the kidney, as well as the body, was included in the radiation field. Wachtel and Cole (1965) concluded that the reduction in compensatory growth of the kidney after whole-body x-irradiation is due, in part, to an abscopal—that is, an indirect—mechanism. Irradiation of the remainder of the body produced a much greater deficit of growth than irradiation of the kidney itself.

Wachtel, Phillips and Cole (1966) studied the effects of both whole-body, and kidney-only irradiation, on the uptake of tritiated thymidine in the remaining kidney of nephrectomized rats. They again concluded that a 'systemic factor' is essential to compensatory hyperplasia. Wachtel, Cole and Rosen (1966) observed mitotic activity in the remaining kidney of rats after kidney-only, and whole-body irradiation. Following a dose of 500 rads to the whole body of uninephrectomized rats, they found no increase in mitotic activity in the remaining kidney, even when the kidney was shielded from x-rays. Direct irradiation of the kidney with a dose of 1000 rads, when the rest of the body was shielded, produced a slight but not significant reduction in mitotic activity. Only when the kidney received the very large doses of 2000 and 4000 rads was mitotic activity reduced to the level observed after a whole-body irradiation of 500 rads. These very high doses to the kidney also produced a significant decrease in whole-body weight 21 days after irradiation and unilateral nephrectomy. A dose of 1000 rads to the kidney alone did not suffice to reduce body weight. Apparently, very intensive damage inflicted by radiation on the remaining kidney has a general toxic effect; but doses of 1000 rads, or less, have little effect on compensatory hyperplasia. By contrast, the consequences of only 500 rads delivered to the whole body are severe.

Threlfall et al. (1966) studied the effects of unilateral nephrectomy in eight to ten-weeks-old, female C57 black mice. In unirradiated animals, the increases in weight and DNA content of the remaining kidney 21 days after operation, were about 56 per cent and 27 per cent respectively. After 600 to 700 rads of whole-body irradiation, these parameters were reduced to 30 per cent and 15 per cent respectively.

Fox and Wahman (1968) investigated the effects of radiation, and of injected spleen cells, on compensatory growth of the kidney in 10- to 12-weeks-old male and female mice of the strain CBA/J. Because they aimed to test our theory (Burwell, 1963; Burch and Burwell, 1965) their findings have a special relevance to this chapter.

They observed kidney weight, body weight, nucleated renal cell count, peripheral leucocyte count, and spleen weight at (generally) 2, 4, 7, 14, 25 and 45 days after left unilateral nephrectomy. Groups of animals were subjected to the following experimental procedures:

(1) left nephrectomy;

(2) whole-body irradiation (350 rads) followed by left nephrectomy half an hour to one hour after irradiation;

(3) whole-body irradiation (350 rads), then, in half an hour to one hour, intravenous injection of 10^8 syngeneic spleen cells, then, left nephrectomy within 1 hour;

(4) as in (3), except that the injected syngeneic spleen cells were taken from mice which, four days previously, had undergone unilateral nephrectomy;

(5) as in (3) except that the injected spleen cells were exposed to 1500 rads immediately after removal from donors;

(6) exposure and mobilization of the left kidney without surgical removal ('sham nephrectomy').

When the weight of the right kidney at 45 days after nephrectomy was compared with the weight of the removed kidney, the largest increase was seen in group (3)—mice that were irradiated and also received an intravenous injection of normal spleen cells. However, when the weight of the right kidney was compared with that expected for an animal of a given body weight, group (4) mice, receiving 350 rads and an intravenous injection of 'sensitized' spleen cells from nephrectomized mice, showed the largest increase. All irradiated groups showed a lower degree of compensatory growth than group (1), the unirradiated and uninjected group, from 0 to 14 days after nephrectomy.

Where body weight is concerned, the increases at 25 and 45 days were markedly higher in group (3)—which received 350 rads plus intravenous injection of normal 'unsensitized' spleen cells—than in all other groups. The nucleated cell counts at 25 and 45 days, the best criterion of hyperplasia (as distinct from hypertrophy), were much higher in group (1)—the unirradiated group—and group (4), which received 350 rads plus intravenous injection of 'sensitized' spleen cells from nephrectomized mice, than in all other groups.

Unirradiated animals showed a sharp increase in peripheral leucocyte count at two days, when it had risen from a starting level of 7000 to 14500 per mm^3, but at four days this had fallen to 10500 per mm^3. All irradiated animals suffered a sharp drop in leucocyte count, which reached a minimum at about four days, and then returned to normal levels at about 20 days. Spleen weight rose in unirradiated animals to a maximum at about seven days after uninephrectomy, whereas animals in all irradiated groups suffered first a sharp drop in spleen weight at two days, and then a gradual rise to the normal level.

Despite the difficulty of distinguishing clearly between hypertrophy, which is initiated rapidly, and hyperplasia, which should depend on the response of the central growth-control system, the findings of Fox and Wahman (1968) agree with our theory. Whole-body irradiation (350 rads) depresses leucocyte counts, spleen weight, and compensatory hyperplasia. The inhibiting effects of radiation on hyperplasia and the compensatory increase in kidney weight, can be offset by injecting spleen cells, and, more especially, by injecting unirradiated 'sensitized' spleen cells from nephrectomized mice. These latter 'sensitized' cells are evidently a direct or indirect source of mitogenic effectors and they are capable of inducing a larger increase in kidney weight at 40 days than is observed in unirradiated animals of group (1). It is also interesting and highly consistent with theory, that when *normal* spleen cells were injected into irradiated animals of group (3), the increase in whole-body weight at 45 days—some 36 per cent—was far higher than that found in the next highest group, the unirradiated animals of group (1), where the increase was about 22 per cent.

We are left in little doubt that syngeneic mouse spleen cells contribute in some way to compensatory hyperplasia of the kidney after unilateral nephrectomy, and also to the general increase in body weight of the growing animal. These experiments by Fox and Wahman on compensatory kidney growth in uninephrectomized mice usefully supplement those of

Czeizel *et al.* on liver regeneration in partially hepatectomized rats. Spleen cells in mice and bone marrow in rats promote these compensatory changes.

It is of incidental interest that electrolytic lesions in ventromedial hypothalamic nuclei of weanling male rats, which lower the levels of pituitary and plasma growth hormone, do not impair renal compensatory hypertrophy (Bernardis and Goldman, 1972).

Regeneration of Thymus

Chen (1971) investigated the relative efficiency of young and adult syngeneic spleen cells, and of bone-marrow cells, with respect to the induction of thymus regeneration. In one experiment, inbred mice (C57B1) received two exposures of 200 rads of x-rays, one week apart. At 20 days after the second irradiation, animals were killed and thymus weights were determined. The mean thymus weight of unirradiated control animals was 48 ± 8 mg; that of untreated irradiated animals was 19 ± 3 mg; that of irradiated animals injected with 15×10^6 adult spleen cells was 22 ± 7 mg; that of animals receiving 90×10^6 adult spleen cells was 23 ± 7 mg; that of animals injected with 15×10^6 newborn spleen cells was 42 ± 2 mg; and that of animals injected with adult bone-marrow cells was 68 ± 4 mg. These experiments of Chen (1971) show, therefore, that spleen cells from fully grown animals had little or no influence on thymus regeneration, whereas newborn spleen cells, from rapidly growing animals, had a marked effect and produced almost complete regeneration. Adult bone-marrow cells, in the dosage used, produced excessive regeneration and overgrowth of the thymus at 20 days.

Although not relevant to the immediate context, it is interesting to interpolate that adult spleen cells were about as effective as bone-marrow cells at reducing the incidence of lymphomas in irradiated animals (Chen, 1971).

Wound Healing

Research by van den Brenk *et al.* (1974) produced studies on the effects of radiation on the rate of contraction of a skin wound in the rat. Sublethal whole-body irradiation (570 rads) given just before wounding slowed down the onset of contraction by 2–3 days. No significant effects were seen when the same dose was given locally to the skin surrounding the wound. This abscopal effect parallels those seen in liver regeneration and compensatory kidney hyperplasia.

Affectors in Growth-control

If the growth of a tissue is controlled by a negative-feedback system, then affectors from the target tissue are necessary to signal its size. Consequently, if during regenerative or compensatory growth the level of affectors is raised artificially, it should inhibit the growth process. This feature of homeostatic control has been demonstrated experimentally by Saetren (1956, 1963). He found that kidney macerates spread in the peritoneal cavity, or in large subcutaneous pockets, inhibit mitosis in the half-kidney of a rat from which one-and-a-half kidneys had been removed. Such macerates did not affect mitosis in the regenerating liver. Similarly, liver macerates inhibited mitosis in the regenerating liver but not the kidney. In both instances, the inhibitor (affector) activity in the macerates rapidly decays. Macerates of spleen, testes and brain had no effect on regenerating liver or kidney. The inhibitor suffered little loss of activity if fresh whole kidneys were kept sterile at 1 °C for ten days. However, heating to 60 °C for ten minutes abolished the activity of the inhibitor. These findings of Saetren (1956, 1963) are in complete accord with the negative-feedback theory of growth-control. However, various subsequent experiments—see Spielhoff's (1971) review—have given apparently contradictory findings. Some organ homogenates have contained inhibitors, others stimulators. Spielhoff (1971) extracted inhibitors from liver and kidney homogenates but he was unable to demonstrate an organ-specific effect. The tissue-specific inhibitors demonstrated in macerates by Saetren (1956) were shown to be unstable and rapidly inactivated *in vivo*; it seems likely that they fail to survive various extraction procedures.

Dicker (1972) has studied the inhibition of compensatory renal growth in rats. He found that intraperitoneal injection of microsomes and/or supernatant fluid from a kidney homogenate (or the renal cortex) inhibited compensatory growth of the contralateral kidney. Dicker (1972) therefore confirmed the earlier experimental findings of Saetren (1956) and Roels (1969). An impressive volume of experimental evidence favours the idea that various forms of growth are regulated by a negative-feedback system.

The Connection between Regenerative and Normal Growth

Factors that affect regenerative and compensatory growth also affect the normal growth of the whole body, and to a similar degree. Radiotherapy during childhood, involving doses of several thousand rads to certain bones and bone marrow, produces growth impairment not only of the bone, but also of soft tissues such as muscle, breast and fat (Dawson, 1968). When the whole body receives sublethal doses of radiation in the region of 300 to 500 rads, depression of regenerative, compensatory and whole-body growth follows. A lower dose of whole-body irradiation (150 rads), is followed by an increase within 24 hours in the proportion of bone-marrow cells synthesizing DNA; Croizat, Frindal and Talians (1970) suggest that the bone marrow is stimulated by a compensatory mechanism. The stimulatory effect is also seen in marrow that is protected from radiation (Croizat et al., 1970). Factors that reverse the depressive action of large doses of whole-body irradiation, such as injections of unirradiated bone marrow or spleen cells, also restore regenerative, compensatory and whole-body growth.

Nevertheless, the compensatory response shows important limitations. For example, the amputation of a mammalian limb leads neither to its regrowth nor to a doubling in the size of the contralateral limb. Why is this? According to my theory, compensatory or regenerative growth of a specific tissue T, requires that an adequate amount of T should be left behind in the body to maintain the activation of its central growth-control element (Burch, 1968(a)). The liver and kidney each consist of a very large number of distinctive 'tissues' (recall the morphological complexity even of the liver) and we deduce that the cells of any one specific liver 'tissue' are, in general, distributed through the different lobes of the liver. Also, cells of some specific kidney tissues are represented, at least in man, in both the left and right organs. This conclusion follows from the occurrence of bilateral kidney stones in renal lithiasis (Burch and Dawson 1968(a)). In the development of autoaggressive disease, the simultaneous involvement of bilateral, or multiple sites, implies that the common target tissue, characterized by a specific TCF, is distributed at bilateral, or multiple anatomical sites. In baboons, however, in contrast to mice, rats, rabbits and dogs, no significant compensatory growth of the renoprival kidney was observed over periods ranging up to four months after unilateral nephrectomy (Dicker and Morris 1972).

The release of MCPs in effector form in the feedback system should normally be governed by the rate of flow of affector TCFs and their concentration at the receptors of the central control. A form of biological amplification is provided in the growth-control system by the clonal proliferation of cells from a progenitor stem cell; the synthesis and secretion of humoral MCPs provides another form of amplification. These processes of amplification are normally maintained by the affector TCFs (Burch, 1968(a)). The expected type of relation between the output of an effector MCP, either cellular or humoral, and the output of its related affector TCF, is illustrated in Figure 3.3. A minimum concentration (C) of TCFs is needed to maintain the clone of cells, whose peripheral members synthesize effector

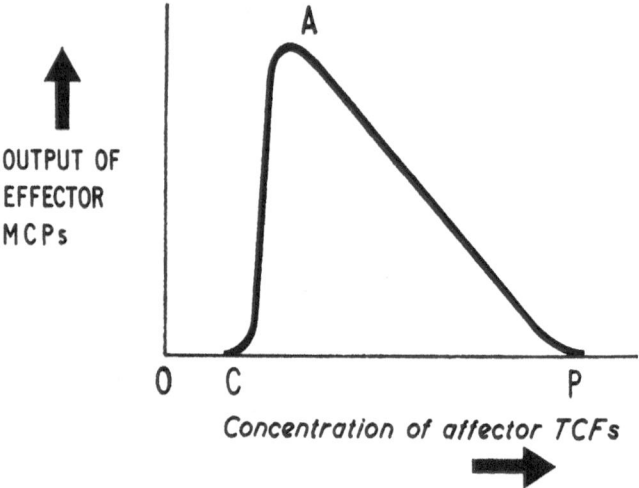

Figure 3.3 Expected relation in a negative-feedback system between the concentration of affector TCFs at the central receptors of the control system and the output of effector MCPs (Burch, 1968(a)); if the concentration of affector TCFs falls below the critical value C, the output of effector MCPs is not maintained and regenerative growth does not occur

MCPs. Below this concentration, the clone collapses and regeneration cannot occur. In most experiments on regenerative and compensatory growth, the working zone lies on the falling linear portion of the curve AP, where the output of each MCP is inversely related to that of its cognate TCF. At point P, the output of MCPs falls to zero and growth stops. It should be noted that the simple relations between time and regenerative growth given by equations (3.2) and (3.3)—see page 24—can be expected to apply only over the linear portion of the curve AP.

Although the amputation of a mammalian limb is not followed by its regeneration, compensatory changes have been observed to take place under certain experimental conditions within the tibia and the femur in rabbits (Hall-Craggs, 1968; Hall-Craggs and Lawrence, 1969). If the growth of the proximal epiphysis is arrested, either by destroying the epiphysial cartilage plate (experimental epiphysiodesis), or by the insertion of a staple to bridge the epiphysial cartilage, then the extent of growth of the distal epiphysis is increased. The increase, however, does not fully compensate for the decrease at the operated epiphysis. When the staple is removed, and the mechanical restraint on the growth of the proximal epiphysis is thereby relieved, nearly normal growth rates are restored at both proximal and distal epiphyses. Hall-Craggs and Lawrence (1969) concluded from their experiments that a direct relationship exists between the additional growth at the uninjured epiphysis and the deficiency of growth at the disabled epiphysis. Furthermore, the change in growth-rate appears to be limited to the experimental bone.

These observations suggest that some of the TCFs carried by cells at the growing proximal epiphysis of a femur of tibia of the rabbit, are also represented on cells at the distal epiphysis, of the same bone. It would be interesting to know whether the 'central' cells that control the growth of the femur and of the tibia are located solely in the bone whose growth they control, or whether they are dispersed through the body.

Dawson and Kember (1974) found that heavy x-irradiation (2400 rads) of the proximal cartilage plate of one tibia of a 4-weeks-old Wistar rat was followed by some degree of compensatory growth at the distal plate of the same bone. They thus confirmed the earlier work of Reidy et al. (1947) which demonstrated a similar effect in the tibia of a dog.

Murray and Huxley (1925) grafted a fragment of the left posterior limb bud of the 4-day-old chick to the chorioallantoic membrane of a chick of seven days' incubation. The graft was left for 5 days when it was recovered from the inverse side of the chorioallantoic membrane. It was then 0·75 cm long and had the clear general shape of a left femur, with a typical head and trochanter. At the distal end a small piece of free cartilage was found in the position of the patella (Murray and Huxley, 1925). This experiment suggests that the grafted fragment contained most, if not all, of the progenitor growth-control stem cells and femoral target cells needed for the development of a complete left femur.

Conard (1964) investigated the direct and indirect (abscopal) effects of x-irradiation on the growth of the tibia in the rat. Three groups of Sprague–Dawley male rats, 23 to 30 days of age, were studied: (1) the left leg was shielded from x-rays and the remainder of the body exposed; (2) the right leg only was exposed, and the remainder of the body shielded; and (3) unexposed animals were subjected to similar stresses. At 21 days post-exposure, and for doses from 200 to 600 rads, the decrement in tibial growth was about two to four times higher for indirect, than for direct irradiation. These results suggest that some of the growth-control cells whose proliferative integrity is essential to the normal growth of the tibia in the rat, lie outside the tibia. Part of the difference between direct and indirect irradiations was attributed by Conard (1964) to a decreased intake of food in the animals of group (1). It can be argued, of course, that the impairment of growth processes inflicted by the radiation was itself mainly responsible for the decreased food intake. But regardless of the interpretation of the significance of diet, Conard (1964) considered that direct irradiation has a pronounced effect on the growth of the tibia. This indicates that an appreciable proportion of the central growth-control cells responsible for directing the growth of the tibia are contained within the tibia itself.

This conclusion is consistent with those derived from the experiment ot Murray and Huxley (1925) with the chick femur; the stapling experiments of Hall-Craggs and Lawrence (1969); and the effects of x-irradiation (Reidy et al., 1947; Dawson and Kember, 1974). Of course, we cannot assume that the anatomical distribution of central growth-control stem cells follows the same plan in different species.

The Constant Number of Comparator Stem Cells

One of the outstanding enigmas of growth-control concerns the mechanism that preserves the constant number of comparator stem cells throughout postnatal life. The age-distributions of natural diseases give no indication that this number changes appreciably from around birth to the end of the lifespan (Burch, 1968a). Nash's (1970) experiments on the effects of radiation on the body weight of mice revealed only a small decrement, about 7 per cent at 63 days of age, after a dose of 400 rads delivered at 28 days of age. Cells in the bone marrow of mice that are capable of forming colonies of descendent cells are, however, very sensitive to radiation (Till and McCulloch, 1964). Only a few per cent of such cells can be expected to retain their proliferative capacity after a whole-body irradiation of 400 rads of x-rays. The relatively small effect of such an irradiation on body weight implies that all, or nearly all, the growth-control stem cells that are killed, are replaced by viable cells during the early phase of post-irradiation recovery.

Arguing in part from the observed dose-response relations for acute radiation death in mice (Upton et al., 1956), I have concluded that if every growth-control stem cell of a vital set is killed by radiation, recovery cannot normally occur and the animal dies because vital target cells cannot be regenerated (Burch, 1969(a)). (An injection of bone-marrow cells into a supralethally irradiated animal can, of course, often prevent acute radiation death.) The mathematical form of the dose-response curve for radiation-induced lethality suggests that the number of growth-control stem cells in a vital set might be of the order of 20 (Burch, 1969(a)). If fewer than 20 are killed, the animal survives and, if it is a young one, it will eventually attain a size not conspicuously less than that of an unirradiated animal. This raises the question as to how surviving growth-control stem cells 'know' which cells have been killed and where replacement is needed.

We might hypothesize that the 20 identical cells occupy a single region in which contiguous relations exist between each cell and its neighbours, at least one of which has an identical MCP. The loss of cells creates 'gaps' that are occupied by new cells arising from the division of one or more viable stem cells, with the same MCP. Opposed to this model is the evidence from experiments on partial body irradiation which indicate that growth-control stem cells are dispersed. We could explain these findings by proposing that a vital set of 20 growth-control stem cells is divided, say, into five dispersed subsets, each containing four cells. Alternatively, we can imagine that each growth-control stem cell normally resides in contact with a membrane, or some other acellular structure in the bone marrow that bears the characteristic MCP as a kind of 'imprint'. Destruction of the cell, and vacation of the site, would need to be followed by its reoccupation by a viable cell.

Support for the idea that the stem cells comprising each growth-control element are dispersed comes from some experiments of Mosier and Jansons (1970). The whole, or selected parts, of the head of the 1- or 2-day-old rat were irradiated by 220 kVp x-rays at dose-levels of 600 rads and 1000 rads. Irradiation of the whole head, with the remainder of the body shielded, leads to a pronounced retardation of the growth of the whole body including that of the tail. Mosier and Jansons (1970) found that bilateral, but not unilateral, irradiation of a short, narrow sagittal band was almost as effective as whole-head irradiation at producing retardation of the growth of body weight (both sexes) and of tail length (males only). The region vulnerable to radiation includes the hypothalamus, third ventricle, parts of the thalamus, limbic system and cerebrum—but not the hypophysis. If the effect of radiation is a direct one on the bone marrow in this region, then the ineffectiveness of unilateral irradiation suggests that growth-control stem cells in all or most elements are distributed on both sides of the midline. Indirect effects cannot be ruled out, although no evidence of nutritional disturbances, reduced food intake, or hypopituitarism had been obtained (Mosier and Jansons, 1970). The hypothesis of a direct effect on bone marrow has the advantage of explaining the dramatic difference between unilateral and bilateral irradiation. If growth-control stem cells of a given specificity on one side remain viable, they can populate the vacancies produced by irradiation on the contralateral side.

Patt and Maloney (1972) have demonstrated an intimate association of developing marrow tissue and newly formed bone, in heterotopic autologous marrow implants. Bone also plays a necessary role in the genesis of organized marrow structures within an evacuated medullary cavity (Patt and Maloney, 1972).

Experiments have been reported—see below—which suggest that certain extracellular tissues (or possibly, cell debris) might exert a specific inductive effect. Such findings also raise the question as to whether the incoming cell that occupies a vacant site in the bone marrow has always to carry exactly the same MCP as that of the imprint. We have to face the possibility that, in some instances at least, the imprinted MCP might be able to induce the synthesis of itself in a cell that previously had a different MCP.

Wolf and Trentin (1968) studied the distribution of erythrocytic and granulocytic *colony forming units* (CFUs) in heavily irradiated animals that had received injections of syngeneic bone marrow. They found that bone marrow stroma—either heavily irradiated or unirradiated—favoured the growth of granulocytic colonies even when the stroma was transplanted into the spleen, an organ that normally favours the growth of erythrocytic colonies. From these and other observations, they concluded that the stroma exerts a specific inductive influence on pluripotent colony forming units (Wolf and Trentin, 1968). These experiments show that mitotically competent cells in the stroma are not essential to its inductive action. They do not rule out the possibility of such an action by non-dividing cells, or by cellular debris.

Huggins *et al.* (1970) transplanted powdered, dehydrated, demineralized matrix of xenogeneic bone and tooth into guinea-pigs, mice and rats. Fibroblasts of the host animal were transformed into cartilage and bone, rat fibroblasts being the most susceptible. A specimen of decalcified human bone induced some cartilage formation in the subcutaneous tissue of a rat.

Slavkin *et al.* (1969) investigated the morphogenetic properties of the extracellular matrix material from rabbits' teeth. They cultured epithelial and mesenchymal cells within the matrix as explants on the chick chorioallantoic membrane. In addition to experiments with suspensions of rabbit incisor epithelial and mesenchymal cells taken from a 24-day embryo, they also observed the behaviour of epidermal and dermal cell suspensions from dorsal skin. During a ten-day period, cervical loop epithelial and mesenchymal cells, and dermal fibroblasts, migrated in contact with the extracellular matric of the tooth, became aligned and then differentiated as columnar cells of a protein-secretory type. Epidermal cells from dorsal skin did not differentiate under the influence of tooth matrix. Slavkin *et al.* (1969) claimed that their experiments were the first to show, *in vitro*, the differentiation of epithelial and mesenchymal cells in contact with an extracellular matrix, and in the absence of other types of cells. They assumed that the physicochemical properties of the exterior or interior surface of the matrix are responsible for the specific inductive action. Cells were not observed within the microdissected cervical matrix of incisor teeth, but membrane-bound cell extensions could be detected. Slavkin *et al.* (1969) were unable to decide whether these cell extensions, which include basal lamina (basement membrane), were responsible for the inductive effects observed in their *in vitro* experiments.

If 'imprints' in acellular structures in contact with bone marrow are essential to the proper organization of growth-control and erythrocytic elements, then we can readily understand why, as Crosby (1970) points out, normal haemopoiesis never becomes established at sites outside the marrow.

How the number of growth-control stem cells becomes fixed in the first instance is as intriguing as the maintenance of their number. This problem is but one among the many unsolved enigmas of embryogenesis and cyto-differentiation. We have proposed that some form of sequential change in gene-repression/gene-derepression occurs during embryogenesis to select, by stages, sets of genes that will synthesize specific MCPs (Burch and Burwell, 1965). In addition to the mechanism of sequential gene-selection, a 'counting system' has to ensure that, at each stage of embryogenesis, the correct *numbers*, as well as the correct types of cells are present. During the early cleavage divisions, contact relations between cells might furnish the signals or stimuli for the activation/inactivation of genes. An alternative, which is not mutually exclusive, is that DNA synthesis itself provides the stimulus to gene activation/inactivation; that is to say, the phenotypic state of a cell during early embryogenesis might be determined by mechanisms that have both intra and extracellular origins.

The experiments of Gurdon and Laskey (1970) show that the activity of nuclear genes depends on the state of the cytoplasm. However, if the 'state of the cytoplasm' is characterized by the presence of molecules with repressor- and derepressor-type function, it is difficult to avoid the suspicion that at least some of these are coded by nuclear genes. Hence, the overall state of the nucleated cell might depend on a two-way interaction between nuclear genes and the cytoplasm: the state of the cytoplasm can be influenced by other cells or molecules in contact with the plasma membrane.

From Grobstein's (1967) work it appears that, beyond the earliest stage of embryogenesis, progress from one stage to the next often depends upon two-way (reciprocal) interactions between, for example, 'embryonic MCPs' produced by mesenchymal growth-control cells and acting on target cells; and 'embryonic TCFs' synthesized by target, for example, epithelial cells, to act on mesenchymal control cells. The leading role in embryonic induction may often be played by mesenchymal elements (presumably 'embryonic MCPs') which can, for example, induce the appropriate differentiation (determined by the synthesis of an 'embryonic TCF') in adjacent epithelial cells. Such cells are thus enabled to step on to the next stage of differentiation. In this model, 'embryonic MCPs' act as primary inducers while 'embryonic TCFs' play a regulatory, or secondary inducer role. (I shall return to certain aspects of developmental problems in the next chapter.)

A vivid example of the directing role of mesoderm has been provided by Mayer and Fishbane (1972). In transplantation experiments using foetal mice, these authors showed that the pigmentary pattern of hairs formed in re-combination skin grafts was specific for the genotype of the mesodermal component of the hair follicle. The genotype of the epidermal, or ectodermal, component of the skin graft had no influence on the pigmentary pattern of the hair.

Whether the primary inducer in embryogenesis is humoral, as suggested by Holtfreter (1955), or whether it forms a part of the cell surface that interacts with the surface of the target cell, as suggested by Weiss (1958), or whether sometimes one and sometimes the other mechanism operates, remains unclear.

Some recent experiments on the induction of kidney tubules in mouse kidney mesenchyme by embryonic spinal cord, using interposed millipore filters are difficult to interpret in terms of a humoral inducer (Nordling et al., 1971). The lengthy transmission time observed for the inductive effect could be explained if cytoplasmic processes grow into the filter from both sides and make contact there (Nordling et al., 1971). On the other hand, extracts from mesenchymal tissues (MF) can replace intact tissue in the normal development of rat pancreatic epithelia in vitro (Levine, Pictet and Rutter, 1973). When MF is covalently linked to Sepharose beads, it promotes epithelial cytodifferention and cell proliferation; Levine et al. concluded that MF interacts with the epithelial plasma membrane.

Problems of Tissue Recognition

Fortunately, the details of embryogenesis and foetal development, which remain obscure, are inessential to the main thesis developed in this book. The means whereby normal growth is controlled during postnatal life are, however, fundamental to my argument.

In this chapter, I have reviewed evidence that bears on the nature and location of the growth-control system. I conclude that, in general, the growth of a target tissue is controlled homeostatically by a 'central' mesenchymal system that lies either partly, or wholly, outside that tissue. Factors that control symmetrical mitosis in target tissues are often systemic in character and originate outside the target organ. This raises the problem as to how the effectors of mitosis recognize their cognate target tissue. But the recognition problem arises in exactly the same manner along the afferent pathway: the affectors from the target tissue that signal its size have to locate their proper control element in the central system.

When we consider the formidable complexity of an organism such as man, with his countless target tissues, these two-way recognition problems assume immense significance. How can these subtle distinctions be made, with almost unfailing reliability, throughout the whole period of growth? Our solution to this problem has been described previously (Burch and Burwell, 1965; Burch, 1968(a)), but because it is so important to my general theory of growth and disease, including neoplasia, I shall discuss it again in the next chapter.

CHAPTER 4

Tissue Recognition in Growth and Disease

As yet, problems of tissue recognition, like those of the control of growth itself, have no generally accepted solution. In Weiss's theory of growth, templates combine stoichiometrically with antitemplates but the molecular basis of mutual recognition was not defined (Weiss and Kavanau, 1957). Tyler's (1947) 'pairs of structural units' resemble antigen and antibody. Stereochemical complementarity is implied, but Tyler did not elaborate on the details of growth-control. Druckrey (1959) postulated a 'higher' regulating centre in his theory of growth-control, but he did not discuss the mechanism whereby the mitotic stimulators released from that centre recognize their target tissue.

Burwell (1963) suggested that growth-control lymphocytes produce globulins that are complementary to tissue-specific factors released from differentiated tissue. The difficulty of this scheme is that complementarity between autoantibody and self-antigen is believed to be the basis of pathogenic autoimmune attacks. Some other molecular basis for recognition interactions in growth-control was called for. As an alternative, I suggested initially that circulating small lymphocytes recognize their target tissue through a 'weak immune-type' interaction with specific antigenic determinants borne by the constituent cells of the tissue: I regarded 'autoimmune' disease as a pathological deviation from the normal process of growth-control, and involving strong complementary and pathogenic interactions (Burch, 1963(a), (b)). I proposed that somatic gene mutation in lymphoid stem cells converts the normal 'weak' interaction between the lymphocyte and its target cell into the 'strong' interaction based on complementarity. These strong interactions were regarded as being analogous to those responsible for the rejection of allografts. In 1963, I was unable to propose a molecular basis for a 'weak', but necessarily highly specific, immune-type interaction. Nevertheless, I had an intuitive feeling that the evidence provided by autoimmune diseases, or, as I now prefer to call them, *autoaggressive* diseases, contained the solution to the genetic and molecular bases of mutual recognition in the control of normal growth.

Although several authors have considered the problem of tissue recognition in normal growth-control, analogous but even more neglected problems arise in the context of disease, particularly with regard to the anatomical distribution of lesions. Why are some cases of retinoblastoma bilateral at presentation, although the majority are initially unilateral and remain unilateral? (See Chapter 7.) Wood (1971) asks why only some of the 286 joints in the body are affected in an arthritic person? So far as I am aware, our theory is the only one that offers a general solution to the problem of the anatomical specificity of the lesions of natural disease.

Implications of the Age-Distributions of Disease for Recognition in Growth-Control

Burwell's (1963) theory of growth-control by the lymphoid system was strengthened by some unexpected properties of the age-patterns of disease.

Burnet's 'forbidden clone' theory

The motive for analysing the age-patterns of supposed autoimmune diseases arose out of the need to test certain features of Burnet's (1959(a)) 'forbidden clone' theory of autoimmunity.

Burnet (1959(a)) argued that, during embryogenesis, frequent gene mutations occur in precursor antibody-forming cells to generate a wide variety of antibody patterns. Should any of these antibodies combine specifically with the normal constituents of 'self', then a surveillance mechanism is supposed to intervene and to delete cells caught in the act of synthesizing such *auto*antibodies. Burnet (1959(a)) proposed that gene mutations will continue to occur randomly in stem cells of the antibody-forming series during the postnatal period, and that autoantibodies should arise from time to time. Occasionally, a mutant stem cell that produces autoantibodies will evade the scrutiny of the surveillance mechanism and propagate a clone of mutant descendant cells. Burnet (1959(a)) describes such clones, which should have been suppressed at their inception, as 'forbidden clones'. The cells in a forbidden clone, or their secreted humoral products, react strongly with normal target cells in the body to produce pathological consequences. In other words, a forbidden clone is the source of cellular or humoral autoantibodies; their strong interaction with target cells that bear complementary antigens gives rise to the symptoms and signs of autoimmune disease.

Burnet's (1959(a)) theory has one supremely important feature that cannot be overstressed. It enables us to understand how one, or a small number of random events, such as somatic gene mutations, can initiate a sequence of changes that subsequently involve many target cells at one, or multiple, anatomical sites. Although this capacity to account for widespread and multicentric lesions is more obviously relevant to non-malignant degenerative diseases such as osteoporosis, polyarthritis, the greying and loss of hair, and cardiovascular diseases, it is equally important to the understanding of the pathogenesis of multifocal tumours (see Chapter 7).

If Burnet's (1959(a), 1972) contention about the *random* nature of the somatic gene mutations that initiate autoimmunity is correct, then the age-distributions of such diseases should provide confirmation. That is to say, the age-specific prevalence, or onset-rates, of 'autoimmune' (autoaggressive) diseases ought to conform to stochastic laws. In testing this prediction we have to recognize that an interval must inevitably elapse between the time of occurrence of the last initiating somatic mutation, and the first appearance of symptoms or signs of the associated disease. The formation of a mutant stem cell has first to be followed by the growth of the forbidden clone, and then by the development of lesions in target cells of a severity that is sufficient to reveal the presence of disease. This interval between the completion of initiation and the first onset of disease is often called the *latent period*.

It soon transpired that the age-distributions of many non-malignant diseases confirmed Burnet's (1959(a)) proposals. Some of these diseases were (and are) widely regarded as 'autoimmune' while others had not attracted that label. Details of these findings are given in my book *An Inquiry Concerning Growth, Disease and Ageing* (Burch, 1968(a)) and in various papers by me and my collaborators. The age-distributions of malignant diseases are illustrated and discussed in Chapters 7, 9 and 10 of the present book. They exhibit the same remarkable statistical features as those of non-malignant diseases.

I found that the sex-specific and age-specific distributions of many diseases conform remarkably well to Yule statistics, or Weibull statistics, or a combination of the two (see Chapter 6 for details). In every instance where numbers of cases and the reliability of diagnosis were adequate, I found that the reproducible age-distributions of well-defined diseases could be explained if they are initiated by rather few random events. (The number of random events ranges from one, up to as many as 14 in rare instances—see Chapter 7.) The rates of certain of these events correlate in a very simple way with the ploidy of a particular chromosome (X or autosome 21)—see below. We can conclude, with some confidence, that forbidden clones are initiated by one or more random somatic gene mutations.

Unexpected findings

These aspects of my findings verified Burnet's (1959(a)) predictions. However, I had expected to find evidence for increasing rates during the growth phase; this expectation was not fulfilled.

Suppose a person has a set of lymphoid stem cells numbering L, and suppose that the mutation of a single specific gene, in any one of these L stem cells, will initiate the growth of a forbidden clone. Assume that the average rate of gene mutation is m, per gene at risk, per cell at risk, per year. If m is small, L is large, and the rate of back mutation is low, the average number of mutant cells formed over a period of t years will be Lmt. Provided L and m both remain constant with age, then Lmt will increase linearly with t.

I had expected that, during adult life, L would remain more-or-less constant and that Lmt would indeed increase linearly with t. However, I assumed initially that L would increase between birth and maturity, roughly in parallel with the general growth of the body, and that Lmt would therefore increase supralinearly with age during the growth phase. An elaborate model was worked out on this basis (Burch, 1965).

Many disorders (especially carcinomas) have a very low incidence during childhood, but where the incidence is high enough, and numbers are adequate, they refuse to conform to the complicated model. Instead, and against expectation, they agree remarkably well with the simplest possible model in which *both L and m remain constant, from around birth, throughout postnatal growth and to the end of life* (Burch, 1966, 1968(a)).

This finding was welcome on account of its simplicity, but nevertheless, perplexing. Although the full complement of neurones, and also of oocytes in females, are known to be present at birth, the great majority of cell types increase in number very substantially between birth and maturity. The stem cells at risk of mutation with respect to the initiation of disease would seem, therefore, to belong to a special class for which constancy of number during growth is mandatory.

Another unanticipated finding concerned the rates of somatic mutation in males in comparison with those in females. Because men, on the average, are larger than women, I had expected that the number of stem cells in males would exceed the corresponding number in females. On this assumption, the average overall rates of somatic mutation in men would be greater than the corresponding rates in women. (This held the attractive possibility of accounting for the greater average longevity of women.) Unfortunately, I was unable to find any evidence to support this expectation. In those (many) instances where men and women suffer from the same form of a given age-dependent disease, I found that the average rate (Lm) of a specific initiating somatic mutation is either the same in both sexes, or it is twice as *high* in women as in men (Burch, 1963(a), (b); 1968(a); Burch and Rowell, 1965, 1968, 1970).

In the latter instance, a simple biological interpretation suggests itself in terms of the X-chromosome. I know of no other way in which cytogenetic-ally normal (XX) women differ consistently from normal (XY) men, in the quantitative ratio of two to one. If an initiating mutation involves a gene on the X-chromosome, and if *both* homologous genes in women are at mutational risk, then we can readily understand how the overall rate of somatic mutation in women can be twice that in men (Burch, 1963(a)).

Further cytogenetic support for a somatic mutation interpretation of random initiating events came from studies of the onset of childhood acute lymphocytic leukaemia and juvenile-onset diabetes mellitus in patients with trisomy 21, that is, Down's syndrome (Burch, 1968(a); Burch and Milunsky, 1969). These diseases are not only more common in Down's syndrome, their average age of onset is also earlier. The form of the age-dependence of early-onset acute lymphocytic leukaemia and of juvenile-onset diabetes mellitus indicates (see Chapter 6) that in both disorders, two mutations, in a single stem cell, constitute the initiating events. However, their average rate in Down's syndrome exceeds that in the general population.

Suppose these two events involve homologous genes on chromosome 21. The average rate of the first event will be 3/2 times higher in trisomy 21 than in members of the general population with two chromosomes 21. When the first event has occurred, two genes remain at mutational risk in trisomy 21 and one only in the general population. Hence, the average rate of the second event will be twice as high in trisomy 21 as in members of the general population. For this model, the overall rate of initiation, k (see Chapter 6) in trisomy 21 will be $3/2 \times 2$—that is, 3 times—higher than in the general population.

The age-patterns of early-onset acute lymphocytic leukaemia (Burch, 1968(a)) and of juvenile-onset diabetes mellitus (Burch and Milunsky, 1969), are remarkably consistent with this quantitative relation. This evidence and the commonly found sex-difference offer powerful support for the idea that the random initiating events are some form of somatic gene mutation. Obviously, the age of onset of diseases in populations of individuals with the rarer trisomies needs to be investigated.

Conflict with Lyon's hypothesis and agreement with cytogenetic evidence

My interpretation of the two-to-one sex difference conflicts with Lyon's (1961) hypothesis which asserts that one of the X-chromosomes in the cells of XX females is inactivated during an early stage of embryogenesis and condenses to form the Barr body. The choice between the paternally derived and the maternally derived X-chromosome is said by Lyon to be made randomly, and, once established, the pattern of inactivation is then transmitted without change to descendent cells. If Lyon's hypothesis applies to all cells in the female body, and if inactivation of one X-chromosome is always complete, then the above interpretation of the two-to-one sex difference would be untenable. However, we have good reason to believe that Lyon's hypothesis does not apply to stem cells in the bone marrow because Barr bodies cannot be detected in that location (Hamerton, 1964).

The direct cytogenetic evidence therefore harmonizes very satisfactorily with the proposal that the somatic mutation of an X-linked gene accounts for the relation $m_F = 2m_M$. Other, but not insuperable difficulties remain with this interpretation and they will be discussed in the next chapter.

The nature of the comparator

For the purpose of the immediate argument, the unexpected constancy of the number of stem cells at somatic mutational risk—from around birth to old age—constitutes the most significant feature.

Suppose that Burwell (1963) is correct, and that one of the functions of the lymphoid system is the control of the growth of certain tissues and the maintenance of their size during adult life. Such a scheme requires a negative-feedback arrangement in which effector mitogenic signals are sent out from the central control to promote the mitosis of cells in the target tissue. Also, affector signals must be secreted from the cells of the target tissue so that their rate of flow is proportional to the size of the target tissue. To assess the size of a target tissue, the central control utilizes a fixed 'yardstick', or standard reference, known as a *comparator*, which remains invariant with respect to growth and size of the target tissue. The function of the comparator is to provide a fixed standard whereby the rate of flow of affector signals can be measured. If the rate is too low, because the target tissue is too small, the output of mitogenic effectors must be increased to correct the deficiency.

These essential properties of a homeostatic or negative-feedback system can no more be dispensed with in a biological organism such as man, than in an electronic apparatus, say, that provides a regulated voltage output. A fixed reference of some kind must be contained in the central system that controls the growth of a man. Because we are based on cells, it would not be altogether surprising if a constant number of cells provides the growth-control comparator. Indeed, it is not easy to devise a more plausible alternative.

Such considerations led us to propose that the fixed number (L) of stem cells at somatic mutational risk in the initiation of autoaggressive disease, furnishes the comparator yardstick in the central control of growth (Burch and Burwell, 1965).

This proposal had the additional advantage of uniting several different phenomena within a single conceptual scheme. Connections between delayed hypersensitivity, certain forms of 'autoimmunity' (such as chronic discoid and systemic lupus erythematosus), immunological surveillance, allograft rejection and graft-versus-host reactions had long been recognized. In these several situations the common factor appears to be the thymus-dependent small lymphocyte, or T-lymphocyte, as it is generally called. But the idea that the same lymphoid system might also be involved in the central control of growth—an even more fundamental biological function—was revolutionary when it was first put forward by Burwell (1963). Nevertheless, proposals tending in this direction had been made earlier by Grabar (1957, 1959), who regarded autoantibodies as a pathological variant of agents that normally perform a physiological function; and by Cajano (1960, 1963) and Cajano and Faiella (1960), who similarly proposed that an equilibrium normally exists between lymphoid cells and parenchymal cells and that this equilibrium is disturbed in 'autoimmunity'.

My inferences from the age-patterns of disease about the biological significance of the constancy of the number of stem cells at somatic mutational risk were therefore in full accord with the essence of Burwell's (1963) theory of growth-control. So far, so good. In mid-1963, however, I believed the main challenge to be that of tissue-recognition: how does a mitogenic effector recognize the correct target cell or tissue? Until this thorny problem was solved agnosticism seemed to be the best attitude. All the same, it was undeniable that the lymphoid system is ideally equipped for the task of controlling growth because everyone agrees that the recognition of subtle distinctions between 'self' and 'not-self' is its hallmark. It was not unreasonable to suppose that the lymphoid system might also be able to distinguish between the different parts of 'self'. Our problem was to find a solution that allowed two contrasting molecular foundations for highly specific recognition interactions: first, a weak and non-damaging one for use in growth-control; and second, a strong, damaging interaction of the kind involved in the rejection of allografts, graft-versus-host reactions, delayed hypersensitivity and the production of the lesions of autoaggressive disease.

The specificity of disease in relation to genotype

Other features of the age-distributions of disease, together with the associated genetic evidence, raised some perplexing problems whose solution was less obvious than the one connected with the constancy of somatic mutation-rates during growth. Analysis had shown that well-defined diseases are restricted either to one, or a small number, of specific subgroups within a general population, where each subgroup is homogeneous with respect to the number and type of initiating somatic mutations. Where adequate genetic evidence could be called on, it indicated that the specificity of each subgroup is determined by predisposing genetic factors. The difficulties arose over my failure to find the following expected connections between the genetic predisposition to a disease and the number of initiating somatic mutations.

Consider the particular example of diabetes mellitus. Predisposition to diabetes mellitus is genetically determined, although as yet there is no general agreement on the exact nature of the diathesis. We have put forward a tentative scheme that satisfies the available evidence, but more critical tests are needed for verification (Burch and Milunsky, 1969).

Two forms of diabetes mellitus can be distinguished: the early-onset (juvenile) form that usually predominates up to about 20 years of age; and the late-onset form that predominates above 30 years of age (Burch, 1968(a); Burch and Milunsky, 1969). We also found that the juvenile form of the disease occurs earlier, on the average, and at higher incidence in the Down's syndrome population than in the general population (Burch and Milunsky, 1969). From the quantitative relation between the age-patterns in these two populations, we concluded (see above) that two somatic mutations at a locus on chromosome 21, in a single cell, initiate the juvenile form of diabetes mellitus (Burch and Milunsky, 1969). Five somatic mutations at (unknown) autosomal loci, in a single cell, initiate the late-onset form of the disease (Burch, 1968(a)).

The puzzle is: Why do we find no indication of genotypes requiring one, three or four somatic mutations to initiate diabetes mellitus? A simple example (Figure 4.1) illustrates the generality of the problem.

Consider a hypothetical situation in which disease arises from a cell that acquires three mutant genes, a_m, b_m and c_m. This is the sole requirement. In (i) of Figure 4.1, a person inherits each of the genes, a, b and c in their non-mutant form, but during life, gene a mutates spontaneously to a_m in a somatic cell, b to b_m and c to c_m. (Other sequences are equally effective.) This amounts to a three-step random process. But if a gene can mutate in a somatic cell, then the same type of change would also be expected to occur

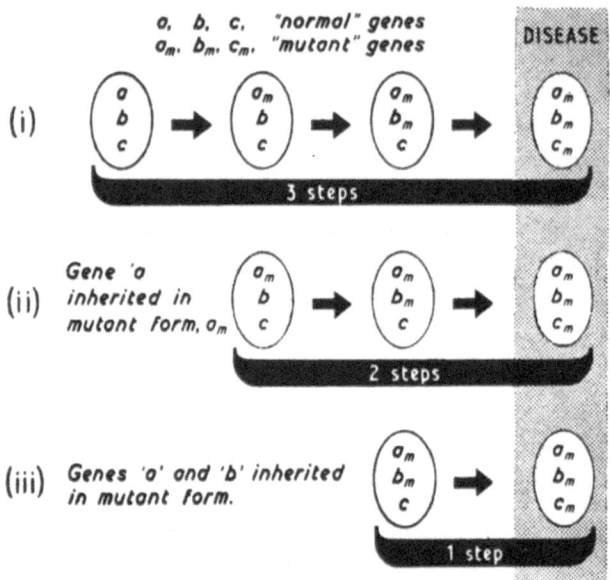

Figure 4.1 A possible scheme for the initiation of disease through the process of somatic gene mutation (see page 47)

in a germ cell. Suppose, as in (ii) of Figure 4.1, that a had already mutated to a_m in a germ cell so that the gene is inherited in its mutant form a_m. If b mutates in a somatic cell to b_m, and c to c_m, the disease-producing cell (a_m, b_m, c_m) will then be acquired through a two-step random process.

Similarly, if genes a and b are inherited in their mutant forms a_m and b_m respectively—as in (iii) of Figure 4.1—then the disease-producing cell should arise through a one-step random process of somatic mutation.

Generalizing the argument, if we find that a particular disease is produced in one group of people through the occurrence of r random somatic gene mutations, then we would expect to find $(r-1)$ other groups in which the same disease is produced by $1, 2, 3 \ldots (r-1)$ somatic mutations, respectively.

The example of diabetes mellitus described above, and many others described elsewhere and in Chapter 7, conflict with this expectation. How then can we resolve the problem of the 'missing genotypes'?

An answer came from a related question: What is the role of the genes that predispose to autoaggressive diseases such as diabetes mellitus? The argument led to the conclusion that predisposing genes perform a *dual* function; they specify products in two sets of cells: the '*central*' cells in which the initiating somatic mutations occur; and the '*target*' cells that are attacked as a consequence of the somatic mutations in the control set (Burch and Burwell, 1965; Burch, 1968(a)).

SCHEME WITH BIFUNCTIONAL GENES AND INTERACTION BETWEEN CENTRAL AND TARGET MACROMOLECULES

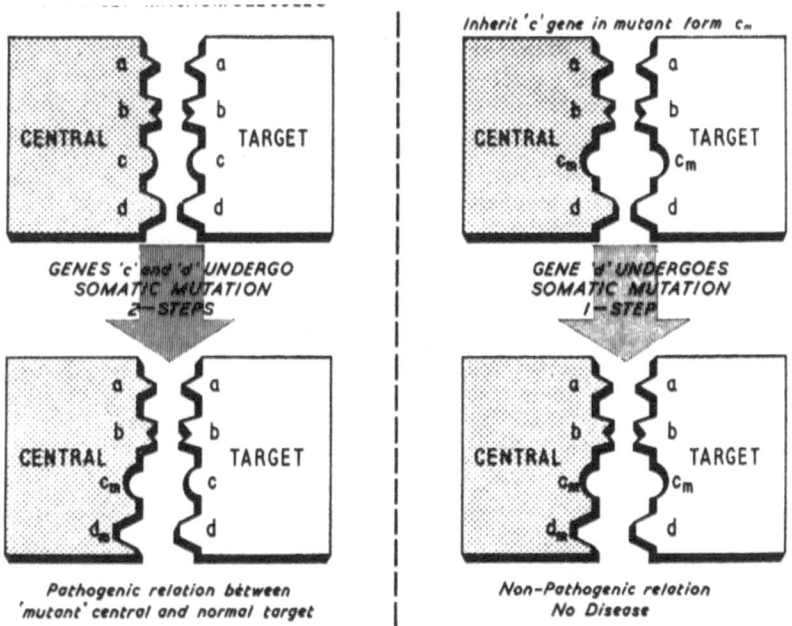

Figure 4.2 A scheme for the initiation of disease by somatic gene mutation; this avoids the difficulties of the scheme illustrated in Figure 4.1 (see page 48)

Figure 4.2 illustrates the thesis. Genes a, b, c and d specify components a, b, c and d of recognition proteins, both in central and in target cells. This relation of identity between recognition molecules in central and target cells is represented in the upper left part of Figure 4.2. Suppose genes c and d mutate in a central cell to c_m and d_m, which then specify mutant components c_m and d_m of the recognition molecule illustrated in the lower left part of Figure 4.2. Components c_m and d_m now complement c and d and the overall configuration a b c_m d_m bears a pathogenic relation to a b c d. This relation arises through a two-step random process of somatic mutation.

Now suppose gene c is inherited in its mutant form c_m—see Figure 4.2, upper right. This mutant gene specifies c_m in *both* central and target molecules. If gene d now undergoes somatic mutation in a central cell to d_m—a one-step random process—the configuration a b c_m d_m results in the central cell. However, it confronts the configuration a b c_m d in target cells and this relation is no longer pathogenic. Of course, the gene c_m in a target cell might back-mutate to c but such a mutation, in, say, one or a few target cells such as beta islet cells in the pancreas will have a negligible effect on the overall functioning of the pancreas.

In autoaggressive disease, initiating somatic mutations change the recognition relations between central and target factors with the result that the altered agents from the central system interact pathogenically with target cells. Predisposing genes help to determine these recognition relations by coding for, or indirectly determining, those factors (polypeptides, lipids, carbohydrates) between which recognition occurs. Various lines of argument show that these recognition factors include major and minor histocompatibility antigens, conventional tissue-specific antigens and more subtle determinants that distinguish one element of a tissue mosaic from another, and left from right (Burch and Burwell, 1965; Burch, 1968(a)). Our prediction (Burch and Burwell, 1965) that the major histocompatibility genes may associate with autoaggressive disease has since been abundantly verified.

However, in the present context, the most important prediction concerns the identity of recognition factors (especially polypeptides) in central and target cells. What, we must ask, is the *biological* purpose of this identity relation that applies to an astronomical number of tissue elements? We argued that the identity relation between macromolecules forms the basis of mutual recognition in growth-control (Burch and Burwell, 1965). A mitotic control protein (MCP) from the central control recognizes its cognate target cell, which carries tissue coding factor (TCF) molecules on its outer membrane. Similarly, affector TCFs secreted from target cells home onto MCP-bearing receptors in the central control system.

Mutual recognition in growth-control must be based, therefore, on 'self-association' interactions, that depend, in part at least, on London–van der Waal's *self-recognition* forces (Burch and Burwell, 1965). These forces are weak but highly specific: they are therefore admirably suited to mutual recognition in growth-control. (For discussions of the role of London–van der Waal's charge-fluctuation forces in biology see: Haurowitz, 1950, 1963; Jehle, 1963, 1969(a), (b); Jehle, Yos and Bade, 1958; Muller, 1951; Yos, Bade and Jehle, 1957. As early as 1922, Muller drew attention to the importance of 'auto-attractive' forces in biology, especially in connection with the pairing (synapsis) of homologous chromosomes (Muller, 1922).)

When we reflect that specific recognition interactions have to occur both at the central and the target regions of the negative-feedback system, we can appreciate the elegance and economy of nature's arrangement. An effector MCP locates its cognate TCF on the membrane of the target cell because certain polypeptide chains are common to both types of recognition molecule. In the same way, the TCF secreted from target cells finds the receptor

MCP in the central control through exactly the same type of self-recognition interaction. To use the same genes for mutual recognition purposes in a central element and its cognate target tissue is the most economical arrangement that could have evolved. The awe-inspiring morphological complexity of an organism such as man becomes less fearsome when we appreciate the extreme simplicity of the basic plan for the control of growth.

A wide range of molecules—from various dipeptides to insulin and haemoglobin—exhibit the phenomenon of self-association (Ruttenberg, King and Craig, 1966; Burachik, Craig and Chang, 1970; Deonier and Williams, 1970; Laiken, Printz and Craig, 1971). Although it is difficult to envisage how the self-association of complicated proteins occurs, the exquisite specificity of the mechanism has been demonstrated *in vitro* using 'light' chains of human immunoglobulins (Stevenson and Straus, 1968). If a mixture of heterogeneous light chains is allowed to associate in solution, specific dimerization occurs between monomers that have exactly the same electrophoretic mobilities. Mixtures of different Bence–Jones proteins in a suitable buffer solution give rise specifically to dimers made up of two identical monomers, with the same amino acid sequences (Stevenson and Straus, 1968).

It does not follow that the mutual recognition between MCPs and TCFs must depend on the direct association between the identical polypeptide components of each species, but neither can this be excluded. We have to bear in mind that non-protein components (for example, calcium and other ions, lipids and carbohydrates) might play an intermediate role in mutual-recognition interactions.

Recognition genes in central and target cells: the simple argument

Our conclusion (Burch and Burwell, 1965) that the genes that code for some or all of the polypeptide chains in a specific MCP also code for the corresponding chains in the cognate TCF, was derived, in the first instance, from the internal logic of the evidence for the age-distributions of disease as explained above. Having reached this conclusion by the hard route I then arrived at a simpler and more direct corroborating argument (Burch, 1968(a)), as follows.

Any alternative basis for mutual recognition between an MCP and its cognate TCF, would, by definition, require one set of genes to code for MCP molecules and a different set to code for TCF molecules. The total amount of DNA in the nucleus of a mammalian cell (about 6×10^{-12}g) would specify a haploid set of about 6×10^6 genes, assuming that each gene codes for a polypeptide chain with a molecular weight of 20000 daltons (Burch and Burwell, 1965; Comings, 1967). In view of the enormous demands on genetic information made by morphogenesis and the differentiation of numerous types of cell, it seems likely that a substantial proportion of the total gene set is devoted to these purposes.

For simplicity, let us assume that 10^6 genes, in appropriate combinations, code for a very much larger number of distinctive MCPs (see Figure 4.3).

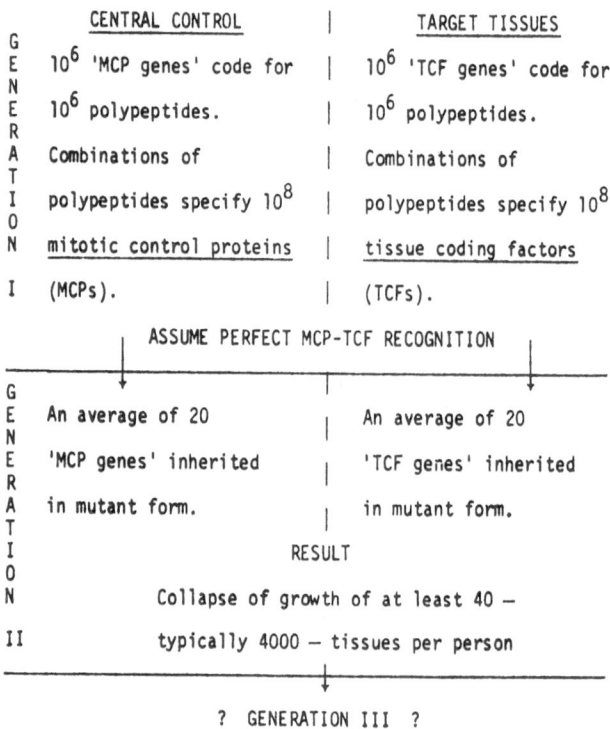

Figure 4.3 Consequences of a system that uses one set of recognition genes in central control cells and a different set in the cells of target tissues (see page 51)

This number might be as high as 10^{10} in man (Burch, 1968(a)). I have estimated that, for at least some MCPs and TCFs, and possibly all, the minimum number of genes involved in synthesizing the polypeptide components of a single recognition macromolecule is seven (Burch, 1968(a)). It follows, and the genetic evidence for pleiotropic genes gives ample confirmation, that certain genes are used to code for common components of many different MCPs and TCFs. We know, for example, that the major histocompatibility antigens are found on cell membranes in most tissues.

Suppose that an entirely different 10^6 genes, in appropriate combinations, code for TCFs. We shall assume, optimistically, that in generation 1 every

MCP is perfectly 'matched' to its cognate, but structurally dissimilar TCF. An outstanding property of genes, however, is their mutability. The point mutation of an MCP or TCF gene in a germ cell would often lead to an amino acid substitution in a polypeptide chain and the consequent distortion of at least one, and sometimes many distinctive types of recognition macro-molecules in an individual inheriting such a mutant gene. Changes of this kind would often destroy the stereochemical basis of mutual recognition between MCPs and TCFs.

In man, typical mutation-rates in germ cells for readily detectable disorders are of the order of 10^{-5} per gene, per gamete, per generation. Hence, if our system of MCPs and TCFs were perfectly matched for mutual recognition in generation 1, we would expect at least 40 mutant MCP–TCF genes per individual in the next generation. If any one or more of the mutant genes code for polypeptides in more than one MCP–TCF element, the number of specific tissues with impaired or disrupted growth-control could be very much larger than 40. In the succeeding generation, still more mutant genes would have accumulated.

With the disruption of so many growth-control elements, in so short a period, it is impossible to imagine how the species could survive. Occasionally, the disruption of the growth of even a single tissue, such as the erythrocytic could prove fatal.

I conclude that any species of complex organisms that relied on one set of genes for MCP coding, and a different set for TCF coding, could not survive. Any reasonable alterations in the quantitative values assumed for gene number or mutation-rate will not affect this conclusion.

To summarize: If the growth of the body is regulated by a central system, there can be only one workable genetic and molecular basis for tissue-recognition. The set of genes that code for recognition proteins (MCPs) in the central control system, also codes for corresponding recognition proteins (TCFs) in cells of the target, or controlled tissues.

An indispensable merit of this scheme is that it allows mutant genes to enter the gene pool without destroying the identity basis of growth-control. A mutant gene will code for the same polypeptide chain, with the same amino acid sequence, in an MCP and the cognate TCF: the relation of identity between the recognition portions of these molecules persists. Of course, if the other functions of the mutant polypeptide chain are not properly discharged, the mutant gene could prove lethal: however, the all-important identity relation between MCPs and cognate TCFs is *guaranteed*.

This identity principle makes very precise and brittle predictions. Thus, when we can isolate and purify the protein components of MCPs and TCFs, we should be able to establish the identity of corresponding amino acid sequences in the two species of macromolecules with complete, or almost complete, certainty.

At the time of writing, we have only slender empirical support for the identity principle; it is known that T-lymphocytes, which we believe to be the carriers of cellular MCPs, exhibit the same major histocompatibility antigens as many target tissues. It has yet to be shown, however, that these lymphocytes also carry the same tissue-specific antigens as their target cells.

Most important of all, the identity principle in growth-control should provide a secure foundation on which a more elaborate theoretical super-structure can be built: it constitutes a premise for many deductive arguments. In biology it is notoriously difficult to draw reliable conclusions from experimental evidence. Systems are often so complicated that alternative interpretations of experimental results abound. The genetic basis for mutual recognition in growth-control appears to me to be one of those rare bio-logical problems to which the possible solutions can, with some confidence, be narrowed to one.

In the remainder of this chapter I review the experimental evidence that bears on our theory of the control of normal growth.

Non-identity between humoral MCPs and TCFs

In a negative-feedback system of growth-control, the effector signals need to be distinguished from the affector signals. When the effector of sym-metrical mitosis is a thymus-dependent small lymphocyte and the affector is a humoral TCF, no difficulty of principle arises because the two types of signal are, morphologically at least, markedly dissimilar. However, when the target tissue lies behind a blood-tissue barrier, the effector of symmetrical mitosis (either final or intermediate) must be a humoral MCP, and the TCF affector secreted by the target cells is also humoral. We have concluded that some or all of the polypeptide components of related MCPs and TCFs must be identical. To satisfy the requirement for *dissimilarity* between effectors and affectors in the negative-feedback system, we have to postulate differences in any one or more of the following: (i) additional protein components *not* involved in mutual recognition between MCPs and TCFs; (ii) in the form of assembly of the molecules—for example, monomers, dimers, etc.; and (iii) in non-protein components such as lipids and/or carbohydrates (Burch and Burwell, 1965).

At least some humoral MCPs might prove to be α_2-macroglobulins: these proteins are complexed with carbohydrates. Their properties are discussed in greater detail later in this chapter. They may or may not include the major histocompatibility antigens. Because most cells in the body carry the major histocompatibility antigens these structures will convey no information as to tissue-specificity.

However, Van Rood et al. (1970) have found that the antibody activity of antisera HL-A2 and HL-A7b can be neutralized by whole serum from people carrying these histocompatibility antigens. Miyakawa et al. (1973) investigated soluble HL-A active substances in plasma using radio-immunoassay. Gel filtration of plasma yielded three fractions carrying HL-A alloantigenic, or HL-A common activities, or both. The high molecular weight fraction (2 to 8×10^5 daltons) migrated on electrophoresis in the α-globulin region. The electrophoretic mobility of the 48000 dalton fraction containing HL-A alloantigenic and common activities was found to be identical with that of papain-solubilized HL-A fragments prepared from the membranes of cultured lymphoid cells. Molecules in the 10000 daltons fraction carried only the HL-A common activities and not the alloantigenic activities. Astor et al. (1973) investigated the histocompatibility antigens HL-A2 and HL-A7 in lipoprotein fractions isolated from normal plasma. Both antigens were restricted to fractions containing lipoproteins of the HDL-3 subclass, having α electrophoretic mobility. Whether these fractions are merely shed from cell membranes, or whether they are actively secreted, has yet to be determined.

Stages of growth-control

Anatomical, serological and pathological evidence indicates that intermediate control stations exist between the central comparator and the final effectors of cell division (Burch, 1968(a)). In the control system that uses T-lymphocytes as effectors, the comparator stem cells probably reside in the bone marrow: the thymus constitutes the next link in the control system and exports lymphocytes to the spleen and regional lymph nodes: these organs in turn control the release of effector T-lymphocytes. Feedback loops exist between each stage (Burch, 1968(a)), but because an animal thymectomized at birth and kept under germ-free conditions can grow more-or-less normally, it seems likely that an overall feedback loop connects either the target tissue, or regional lymph nodes, to the 'central' comparator in the bone marrow (see Figure 3.2 page 25).

Such a scheme requires that the growth-control lymphocytes exported from the bone marrow to the thymus shall be distinguished (a) from lymphocytes exported from the thymus to the spleen and regional lymph nodes and (b) from effector cells migrating out of the regional lymph nodes to promote cell division in target cells. Consequently, distinguishing factors (protein or non-protein) must supplement the mutual recognition components that are common to MCPs and TCFs. At each stage of growth-control, cells require an identifying characteristic. These theoretical requirements harmonize well with the following experimental observations but they point the need for further investigations.

In mice of several strains, thymocytes carry an antigen (TL) that is not expressed on other types of normal lymphocyte (Boyse, Old and Stockert, 1966; Boyse, Stockert and Old, 1968). Leckband and Boyse (1971) have identified a small minority of thymocytes (in TL+ mice) that do not carry the TL antigen. They propose that these cells represent a stage in the differentiation of TL+ thymocytes into 'immunocompetent lymphocytes'. (Boyse *et al.* (1968) find, interestingly enough, that TL antigens are also carried by certain types of leukaemic cells, in many strains of mice, including those that are TL-negative for normal thymocytes.) The lability of the TL antigen is shown in the phenomenon of *antigenic modulation:* antibody to TL, in the absence of lytic complement, can convert a cell of the phenotype TL+ to TL− (Boyse, Old and Luell, 1963; Boyse, Stockert and Old, 1967; Old, Stockert, Boyse and Kim, 1968). How the synthesis of the TL antigen is switched on and off *in vivo* has not yet been determined, although Schlesinger and Hurvitz (1968) have shown that this occurs in the thymus, because, in suitable strain combinations, TL-negative cells become TL-positive after entering a thymus graft.

Potworowski and Nairn (1968) have demonstrated a lymphoid-specific antigen by immunofluorescence in all rat lymphocytes except those of the bone marrow. Order and Waksman (1969) irradiated Lewis rats (900 rads) and injected them with syngeneic, or (Lewis × BN)F_1 bone marrow. Cells of bone-marrow origin first appeared in the thymus 4 days after injection. When at 6 days cells from the repopulated thymus were injected into other partially irradiated animals, most of them homed to the irradiated marrow. However, after 6 days the capacity to home to the bone marrow rapidly declined: this decline coincided with a shift in size from large to small lymphocytes and the appearance of thymus-specific antigen (Order and Waksman, 1969).

Also consistent with the prediction of distinguishable MCPs at each stage of feedback control is the finding that heterologous antilymphocyte serum (ALS) prepared against circulating lymphocytes, is relatively ineffective against lymphocytes in the thymus and bone marrow (Jeejeebhoy, 1970). Colley, Wu and Waksman (1970) found that lymphocytes in the rat acquire peripheral properties sequentially, either during an intrathymic cycle of differentiation, or shortly after cells leave the thymus. The thymus-specific antigen (RTA) is not present on peripheral lymphoid cells.

We have to remember that at least two main populations of peripheral lymphocytes (T and B) can be distinguished, T-lymphocytes being thymus-dependent, and in our view the carriers of mitotic control proteins (MCP), while B-lymphocytes are concerned with the synthesis and secretion of humoral immunoglobulins. Raff (1970) has assessed the relative proportions of these two populations of cells in the thymus, lymph nodes, spleen and thoracic duct cells of mice. No B-lymphocytes were found in the thymus and they contributed only 5 per cent to thoracic duct cells: the percentage of T cells (carrying the θ antigen) in the spleen ranged from 35 to 50, and in lymph nodes from 65 to 85 (Raff, 1970).

The intermediate stages in the section of the growth-control system that uses humoral effectors have not been delineated. In some instances, circumstantial evidence suggests that mast cells either constitute, or are closely associated with, the cells that release the final humoral MCPs (Burch, 1968(a), (b)). Circulating basophilic granulocytes might represent an intermediate stage between stem cells in the bone marrow and tissue mast cells (Burch, 1968(a)).

However, another type of lymphocyte—distinct from B- and T-lymphocytes—might feature in the growth-control system that uses humoral effectors. McCormick et al. (1973) have reported the presence of α_2-macroglobulin (α_2M) molecules on the surface of human and mouse lymphocytes. Their studies suggested that α_2M might be associated with a special subpopulation of B, or non-thymus-dependent lymphocytes. McCormick et al. had not determined whether α_2M is merely passively adsorbed onto the surface of lymphocytes, or whether it is synthesized by them.

Tunstall and James (1974) cultured human peripheral blood lymphocytes in serum-free medium containing [^{14}C]glutamine and found that an appreciable amount of the [^{14}C]glutamine was recovered in α_2M, suggesting that the protein was synthesized by lymphocytes.

Trephocytes and Growth-control

Our proposals (Burch and Burwell, 1965; Burch, 1968(a)) that T-lymphocytes and mast cells act as the 'peripheral cells' of the two sections of the 'central' system of growth-control, were based mainly on transplantation and histopathological evidence. It is interesting that lymphocytes and mast cells had previously been credited with trephocytic (nutritive) and growth-promoting functions (Carrel, 1922; Liebman, 1947; Humble, Jayne and Pulvertaft, 1956; Loutit, 1962; Asboe-Hanson, 1964). Carrel was the first to break away from the influence of Metchnikoff and the preoccupation with the phagocytic and defensive roles of leucocytes. He directed attention to the growth-promoting properties of leucocytes in tissue culture and wound repair (Carrel, 1922).

Invertebrate trephocytes closely resemble the mast cells of vertebrates (Liebman, 1947). The main evidence for their trephocytic function comes from observations of their activity and aggregation at sites and periods of increased growth such as wound-healing, regeneration, metamorphosis, and sexual and asexual reproduction. Liebman (1947) stressed that invertebrate trephocytes '. . . are not merely nursing cells in the usual sense but that they appear to enter some close physicochemical relation with their surroundings or the object they nurture'. He had little doubt that the mast cells of verte-brates are trephocytes. This view is shared by Asboe-Hanson (1964),who contends that mast cells supply the fundamental material essential to any growth of the skin. Ehrlich, who first described the mast cells, also believed that they have a nutritive function.

In relation to the central thesis of this book it is noteworthy that mast cells have repeatedly been observed to congregate in the vicinity of spon-taneous and experimentally induced cancers—see Liebman's (1947) review. Although Liebman (1947) assumed that their role in this situation is defensive, I favour the opposite view: in appropriately mutant form, they *promote* the growth of carcinomas.

Although we have regarded T-lymphocytes and mast cells as being primarily sources of cellular and humoral MCPs respectively, this does not exclude the idea that these cells might also supply nutritive materials to target cells. Indeed, the two hypotheses complement one another. The penetration of mast-cell trephocytes into the eggs of certain invertebrates (Liebman, 1947) and the entry of lymphocytes into mammalian cells in tissue culture—the phenomenon of *emperiopolesis* discovered by Humble *et al.* (1956)—both support the trephocyte hypothesis. The fate of the T-lymphocyte, once it has stimulated symmetrical mitosis *in vivo*, is un-known. In theory, the cell must be either modified, or destroyed, to prevent it from stimulating further mitosis that would violate the homeostatic regulation of growth.

Metcalf (1964) has described a remarkable parallel between two curves: (a) for the age-dependence of the rate of production of thymic lymphocytes in male C3H mice; and (b) for the age-dependence of the weekly increase in body weight. He suggested that lymphocytes, or their breakdown products, might be connected with the regulation of certain forms of mitosis in tissue cells.

Specific Cellular Adhesiveness

Our theory of mutual recognition between MCPs and TCFs implies also mutual recognition among the target cells in an organized tissue. If cells of a similar differentiation, carrying similar TCFs, are artificially separated and then mixed with other cells in a suitable culture medium, reassociation should occur, like with like.

Sponges, and embryos from a wide range of species, can be dissociated into their component cells. If the intermixed cells are then allowed to commingle under suitable culture conditions, they eventually form aggregates in which tissues reconstitute in spatial relations resembling those of the intact sponge or embryo (Wilson, 1908; Holtfreter, 1948; Moscona and Moscona, 1952; Weiss and James, 1955; Towns and Holtfreter, 1955; Steinberg, 1962). A similar effect manifests during wound-healing. During the healing process, cells group themselves so that one tissue bears the proper spatial relation to its neighbours (Weiss, 1947). Organization can be restored therefore, at least to some extent, after an artificial disturbance. A vivid illustration of this phenomenon is provided by the re-establishment of the correct functional nerve connections following the experimental cutting of the optic nerve tract in fish—see reviews by Sperry (1963) and Gaze (1967).

Experiments along the above lines show, as theory predicts, that a cell of a particular differentiation can often recognize and adhere to a similar cell of a similar differentiation: this phenomenon is known as *specific cellular adhesiveness* or *selective cellular aggregation*. Furthermore, when cells of a similar differentiation adhere together to form an organized tissue, this tissue can recognize and establish the correct spatial relations with one or more neighbouring tissues. In addition to specific cellular adhesiveness, we have to account for the phenomenon of *specific inter-tissue adhesiveness*.

If mutual recognition between MCPs and TCFs depends on the identity of some or all of their protein constituents and the resulting London–van der Waal's self-recognition interactions, then mutual recognition between cells of the same differentiation, carrying identical TCFs, should also depend on a similar type of physicochemical interaction. The commonly observed genetic associations between autoaggressive diseases of dissimilar tissues, show that one or more polypeptide components of the TCF of one tissue can be shared with those of another tissue, of dissimilar differentiation (Burch, 1968(a)). If certain components of TCFs are identical in dissimilar but adjacent tissues, self-recognition interactions between the common components could readily account for specific inter-tissue adhesiveness.

From experiments on tissue reconstruction from dissociated cells, Steinberg (1962) concluded that the mutual anatomical relationships of tissues in an organ must be determined, in large part, by quantitative differences in mutual adhesiveness. Lilien (1969) found that when trypsin is used to dissociate embryonic tissue into single cells, reaggregation occurs in two phases. The initial one is non-specific and insensitive to inhibitors of macro-molecular synthesis. The second, specific, phase in the reaggregation of vertebrate embryonic cells, is sensitive to inhibitors of macromolecular synthesis such as lowered temperature, inhibitors of protein synthesis (for example, puromycin), and periodate, which reacts with *cis* hydroxyl groups and may destroy carbohydrate residues (Lilien, 1969). However, Lilien's (1969) conclusion that specific cellular aggregation depends on macro-molecular *complementarity* between macromolecular constituents at the cell surface is not supported by our analysis, which points to *self-recognition* interactions between *identical* components of macromolecular TCFs. Nevertheless, Lilien's (1969) conclusion that specific cellular adhesiveness results from interactions between surface macromolecules agrees entirely with our deductions, and also with Moscona's (1963) findings and con-clusions from experiments on the aggregation of sponge cells. Experiments of Ling, Horkawa and Fox (1970), and of Antley and Fox (1970) show that 'aggregation proteins' have a fairly rapid turnover and that the maintenance of aggregation of *Drosophila* embryonic cells depends on continuing protein synthesis.

Contact Inhibition

Our negative-feedback theory of growth-control requires that cells in an organized tissue will undergo symmetrical mitosis only when 'instructed' to do so by effector MCPs. Free cells, in a culture medium, often undergo apparently symmetrical mitosis in the absence of effector MCPs. What, then, is the basis of the non-mitotic state in the organized tissue?

When wandering non-malignant cells in a culture medium make contact with one another, then if the cells are of a similar differentiation, undulations of the cell membrane, and locomotory movements cease: this is known as *contact inhibition*. A related phenomenon is the *contact inhibition of cell division*. Certain kinds of cell such as mouse fibroblasts, under the appropriate conditions of culture, cease to divide when all of their edges make contact with their neighbours.

Various aspects of these phenomena have been described and reviewed by Abercrombie and Ambrose (1962), Todaro, Lazar and Green (1965), Castor (1968), Holley and Kiernan (1968), Pollack, Green and Todaro (1968), Schutz and Mora (1968), Fujii and Mizuno (1969) and Baker and Humphreys (1971).

Intimate cell-to-cell contact appears to have profound repercussions on cellular behaviour and metabolism. Arrested movement and inhibition of mitosis suggest that the whole economy of the cell can be drastically altered when its plasma membrane makes suitable contact with membranes of other similar cells. The mechanism of change has not been elucidated. Any one, or any combination of changes at the plasma membrane, such as transport properties, cooperative action and allosteric effects might be implicated. Contact relations affecting the outer surface of the plasma membrane could well modify the state of the inner surface, and in turn, this could influence the general metabolic state of the cytoplasm. Such sequences may require some time to take effect; Martz and Steinberg (1972) have found that high local cell density maintained throughout the G1 phase of the cell cycle often failed to produce immediate inhibition of cell division. If the resting, interphase cell represents one state, and the mitotic cycle leading to symmetrical mitosis constitutes another, then in principle, a switch-over between metabolic pathways could be achieved through a large enough change in the concentration of a single key metabolite. That a concentration change in one, or a few, key 'switching' metabolites might normally be controlled by the contact relations between the cell membrane and external MCPs and TCFs seems eminently plausible.

Predictions

Many predictions are implicit or explicit in our theory of recognition relations in growth-control. The obvious ones concerning the identity of some, and the non-identity of other components of MCPs and cognate TCFs, have been described above.

Transplantation antigens and disease

It will be recalled that the cellular MCPs and TCFs include transplantation antigens of various kinds, and that genes predisposing to autoaggressive disease encode for polypeptide chains in MCPs and TCFs. In the past, there has been a tendency to identify genetically based diseases with 'inborn errors of metabolism', to link this with the formula 'one gene, one enzyme', and to assume that defective or deficient enzymes must always be implicated in such diseases. Our theory predicts positive and negative associations between major and minor histocompatibility antigens, and tissue-specific antigens on the one hand (proteins that may have no enzymic properties), and age-dependent autoaggressive disease on the other (Burch and Burwell, 1965). Many associations with the major histocompatibility antigens have recently been reported—see Walford's (1970) review and numerous subsequent papers, especially in the *Lancet*.

Verified associations of HL-A antigens with the following diseases have been found: ankylosing spondilitis, acute anterior uveitis, coeliac disease, dermatitis herpetiformis, Hodgkin's disease, Reiter's syndrome, multiple sclerosis, myasthenia gravis, psoriasis and rheumatoid arthritis. Not all investigators have taken age-distributions into account. These sometimes imply genetic heterogenity: a given 'disease' may comprise two or more distinctive components (Burch, 1970(c)). Adult-onset Hodgkin's disease shows a bimodal age-distribution (MacMahon, 1966; Burch, 1968(a)). Very significantly, Forbes and Morris (1970) found that patients aged 15 to 34 years had a 45 per cent incidence of the W5 histocompatibility antigen, in contrast to 30 per cent for the older patients, and 16 per cent in 173 controls.

Even if proper corrections could be made for heterogeneity, it seems likely from the evidence available to date that we would seldom find a one-to-one relationship between (a) a major histocompatibility antigen and (b) a disease judged to be homogeneous with respect to initiating kinetics. This raises the possibility that the major histocompatibility alleles seldom predispose directly to an autoaggressive disease, but that they are closely linked to the actual predisposing genes, with which they are in linkage disequilibrium. That is to say, positive or negative associations frequently exist between the major histocompatibility and the predisposing alleles.

Somatic mutation and forbidden clones

Theory predicts that the cells in a forbidden clone will carry one or more antigens that are either absent from the MCPs and TCFs of the normal phenotype of the individual, or are present at a different 'dose'. Investigations of the phenotypic specificity of MCPs carried by lymphocytes and (?) basophilic granulocytes before, and after, the development of an auto-aggressive disease, could provide one of the most direct demonstrations possible of the reality of the somatic mutation of MCP genes, and the existence of forbidden clones.

Humoral MCPs, and violations of allelic exclusion

Mitotic control proteins (MCPs) incorporate the polypeptide chains coded by MCP genes, and very often, the gene at a given autosomal locus will be present in heterozygous arrangement. If the active form of a humoral mitotic control protein (MCP) is generally a *single* macromolecule, then in heterozygotes such a molecule needs to carry the allotypes specified by both homologous genes at such a locus. Thus, if the gene at an autosomal locus *a* has two alleles, *a1* and *a2* which code for the polypeptide chains (allotypes) a1 and a2 respectively, then a person heterozygous at this locus will need to incorporate both these chains in each relevant MCP macro-molecule. Where many serum proteins are concerned, the phenomenon of *allelic exclusion* operates, and any particular protein molecule incorporates a1 *or* a2, but not both types of polypeptide chain—see, for example, Albers and Dray (1969). Immunoglobulin-G molecules comprise two 'light' (L) and two 'heavy' (H) chains: identical L and identical H chains have always been found in the same molecule (Pernis *et al.*, 1965; Cebra, Colberg and Dray, 1966). For this and other reasons, I have concluded that immunoglobulins cannot, at least in isolation, act as humoral MCPs (Burch, 1968(a)).

From various indirect but consistent lines of evidence, we suggested that certain humoral MCPs might be found among the α_2-macroglobulin serum fraction (Burch and Burwell, 1965; Burch, 1968(a), (b)). It is intriguing, therefore, that the principle of allelic exclusion does not apply to the products from (at least) two autosomal loci that code for allotypes of rabbit serum α_2-macroglobulin; the Mtz1/Mtz2 and Mtz3/Mtz4 systems are both exempt from allelic exclusion (Knight and Dray, 1968(a), (b); Berne *et al.*, 1970; and Berne, Dray and Knight, 1972). In rabbits that are heterozygous at either or both of these loci, single α_2-macroglobulin molecules carry the allotypic specificities of all the inherited alleles. However, it is not yet known whether these allotypes are associated with the protein or the carbohydrate portions of the macromolecules. If the protein component proves to be implicated, further support will be given to the hypothesis that α_2-macroglobulins can act as humoral MCPs.

Genetic evidence, and the fairly commonly observed 2:1 (F/M) sex-ratio in somatic mutation-rates, shows that X-linked genes often code for MCP–TCF polypeptide chains (Burch, 1963(a), 1968(a); Burch and Rowell, 1965, 1968, 1970). It is not without interest, therefore, that Berg and Bearn (1966) identified an X-linked serum protein in man in which the associated antigen (Xm) appears in the α_2-macroglobulin fraction. They also found one family in which the daughter was Xm(a−), although both parents were Xm(a+). This anomaly can be explained—see Chapter 5—by our theory of *genetic dichotomy*, and the 'directed mutation' or 'allelic switching' of X-linked MCP genes during embryogenesis.

Lymphocytes of heterozygous individuals have been found to carry all the HL-A antigens represented by the diploid set of chromosomes (Tiilikainen, Kaakinen and Amos, 1970). Hence cellular MCPs, in accordance with theory, carry on their outer membrane the polypeptide chains associated with both alleles at an autosomal locus.

Humoral affector TCFs—Humoral TCFs, if secreted in the form of *single* macromolecules, will also need to violate the principle of *allelic exclusion*. Immunoglobulins (IgG, IgM and IgA), low density lipoprotein, haptoglobins, and α_1-aryl-esterase all show allelic exclusion (Alpers and Dray, 1969; Berne et al., 1970), and hence none of these serum proteins should comprise a complete humoral TCF.

We suggested that humoral TCFs are likely to be found in the α-lipoprotein fraction of the serum proteins (Burch and Burwell, 1965). Gilman-Sacks and Knight (1972) have recently found that high-density lipoprotein (HDL) molecules from a heterozygous (j^1 j^2) rabbit carry both j^1 and j^2 allotypic specificities on the same molecule. They believe that the allotypic specificities are due to differences in amino acid sequences, because lipid material is usually only weakly antigenic. Complete humoral TCFs might, therefore, be found in the HDL fraction of serum proteins. This possibility is further supported by the observations of Aster, Miskovich and Rody (1973) described above, who found that the (human) histocompatibility antigens HL-A2 and HL-A7 were recovered from plasma fractions solely of HDL-3 sublass of lipoproteins, with α-electrophoretic mobility. Although affector TCFs do not necessarily comprise all recognition components, the demonstration by Aster et al. of HL-A2 and HL-A7 antigens in HDL-3 lipoproteins agrees with the hypothesis that this subclass contains affector TCFs.

MCPs, TCFs and cellular differentiation

Because several fundamental properties of the normal target cells of higher organisms, such as the antigenic specificity of the plasma membrane, morphology, and physiological and biochemical function, all appear to be more-or-less inseparable; and because it is difficult to envisage a more basic and prior causal mechanism than the induction of TCF genes, I have proposed that TCFs, directly or indirectly, determine cellular differentiation (Burch, 1968(a)). The differentiation of a cell in a given situation is essentially a matter of the differential expression of its genome. Hence, TCF proteins, or subunits thereof, are likely to be responsible for selective gene derepression.

These arguments receive strong support from experiments designed to test the persistence of tissue-specific antigens in vitro. Dawkins, Aw and Simons (1972) found that cultures of chick and murine muscle cells retained muscle-specific antigen for prolonged periods. After repeated subculture, tissue-specific antigen persists, but only in cells with the morphological characteristics of muscle cells. Thus the presence of a tissue-specific antigen, which forms a part of the complete TCF, correlates with morphological differentiation.

Because an MCP and its cognate TCF have recognition polypeptide components in common, the many differences in the morphological and biochemical differentiation of mesenchymal growth-control cells on the one hand, and their target cell counterparts on the other, must derive from those genes that contribute to the unshared protein and/or non-protein components of MCP–TCF macromolecules.

Complexity of MCPs and TCFs

From the statistics for the age-distributions of disease I have suggested that, in some instances at least, the number of genes implicated in the synthesis of the common protein component of a single MCP and its related TCF, might be at least seven (Burch, 1968(a)). It does not follow that the number of separable polypeptide chains in a given MCP or TCF will be as high as this. We were the first to propose that an immunoglobulin 'light' (L) chain is encoded by two genes, one being responsible for the invariant or 'common' (C) section and the other for variable (V) section (Burch and Burwell, 1965). This proposal violated the generalization 'one gene, one polypeptide chain'. In our view, each distinctive V section of an L or H chain is the product of a distinctive gene. An H chain might well be the product of more than two genes. The idea that a single polypeptide chain can be encoded by more than one gene might well extend to the structure of MCPs and TCFs.

Rose and Bonstein (1970) have demonstrated three antigens specific for human tracheal mucosa, and another common to tracheal and oesophageal mucosae. This latter shared antigen migrated on immunoelectrophoresis as an α-globulin. Rose and Bonstein (1970) found that three carcinomas of bronchial origin reacted with one of the trachea-specific antisera.

α_2-Macroglobulins have a molecular weight of about 850000 daltons and an attractive morphological complexity 'resembling a graceful monogram of the two letters H and I' (Bloth, Chesebro and Svehag, 1968). Such complexity would seem to be well suited to the exacting demands of specificity in growth-control.

In view of the widespread distribution of the major histocompatibility antigens among the nucleated cells of the body, and the narrow distribution of classical tissue-specific antigens, the structure and the organization of MCP–TCF molecules are evidently planned on a hierarchial principle. It would not be surprising if in this respect, as in others, ontogeny recapitulates phylogeny.

From the viewpoint of our general theory of growth, invertebrates are fairly 'complex organisms' (but less complex than mammals) and hence they should possess relatively primitive forms of MCPs and TCFs with, perhaps, fewer polypeptide components than those of mammals. It follows that invertebrates should manifest a relatively primitive form of allograft rejection. Various recent observations show that this is indeed the case. Tissue incompatibility has been demonstrated in celenterates (Toth, 1967; Theodor, 1970). Rejection of first-set allografts, and an anamnestic response to second-set grafts, has been found in earthworms (Duprat, 1964; Cooper, 1969; Cooper and Rubilotta, 1969).

During ontogeny in mammals, the least specialized components of MCPs and TCFs, such as the major histocompatibility antigens that are represented in most tissues in the developed animal, would be expected to appear at an early stage. Edidin (1964) was able to demonstrate H-2 antigens in the nine-day mouse embryo, and Pellegrino, Pellegrino and Kahan (1970) extracted HL-A antigens from the spleen, lung, liver and kidney of human foetuses of three, four and five and a half months.

Relatively few genes are needed to characterize the main tissue types recognized in conventional histology. The X and Y chromosomes probably make an important contribution to this relatively crude level of cell differentiation (Burch, 1968(a)). In our theory, all the main morphological differences between men and women must stem, directly or indirectly, from the contribution of X and/or Y-linked genes to the relevant MCPs and TCFs. Several features point to the special status of the X-chromosome:

(1) For the proper functioning of a 'target' cell in mammals, X chromosome material, constituting approximately 5 per cent of the total genome, is required in the form of euchromatin to carry and transmit X-linked genes (Ohno, 1967; Hamerton, 1968): this requirement is maintained in the presence of sex chromosome abnormalities.

(2) Ohno (1967) has proposed that the X-chromosomes of all mammals are homologous in the sense that an X-linked gene that performs a specific function in one species, performs a similar function (and is also X-linked) in all other mammalian species (this proposal is highly consonant with our theory).

(3) In the *target* cells of normal (XX) women, one X-chromosome forms the Barr body; in karyotypes with two or more X-chromosomes, all X-chromosomes in excess of one form Barr bodies in target cells.

(4) We deduce that homologous X-linked MCP genes in *growth-control* cells are not subject to inactivation, but, in heterozygous females, one gene undergoes directed DNA strand-switching during embryogenesis (see Chapter 5).

(5) The X-chromosome is especially prone to non-disjunction during meiosis.

(6) X-linked genes commonly predispose to autoaggressive disease.

(7) X-linked genes undergo somatic mutation in males and females to

initiate, or to help initiate, various autoaggressive diseases; when this happens, only one X-linked gene undergoes somatic mutation in one stem cell.

This last property suggests that no MCP or TCF contains more than one X-linked polypeptide chain: by contrast, I deduce from the rates of somatic mutation in the Down's syndrome subpopulation that genes on chromosome 21 can contribute as many as three distinctive chains to an MCP and its related TCF (Burch, 1968(a)).

All the above properties of the X-chromosome are consistent with the view that X-linked genes commonly determine tissue type at the level of differentiation that can be recognized histologically (Burch, 1968(a)).

Morphological fine-structure

The morphological fine-structure within a tissue requires an enormous number of genes, many of which are autosomal. It is axiomatic that the size and shape of an organ is determined by the number, type and shape, of its constituent cells and extracellular tissue; and by the contact relations and orientation of one cell or tissue with respect to its neighbours.

My colleague Professor Jackson and I have studied in some detail the anatomical distribution of clinical dental caries in maxillary and mandibular incisor teeth (Burch, 1968(a); Jackson, 1968; Jackson and Burch, 1969, 1970). Our studies in this almost neglected field, and those of our colleague Fairpo (1968), show that, in a given environment, the anatomical siting of dental caries is genetically determined. We infer that odontoblasts probably constitute the target cells of the autoaggressive attack. Many genes are implicated in distinguishing the TCF of one type of odontoblast from that of another. The same principle will undoubtedly extend to other types of cells that help to determine the intricate architecture of organs such as bone, liver, kidney, brain, among others.

Because one set of odontoblasts will differ only slightly from another distinctive set, those components of TCFs that are responsible for morphological fine-structure are likely to be rather similar, one to another, in terms of molecular weight and amino acid sequence. The subtle differences could well be analogous to those seen between the variable (V) section of one immunoglobulin L chain and that of another. Fairly extensive regions of homology are interspersed with short variable sequences.

In the cells of higher organisms, repeating sequences of DNA have been discovered in which a high degree of homology exists between one sequence and the next. These quasi-repetitions occur within groups of related sequences that range from 50 up to 2 million repeats (Britten and Kohn, 1968; Walker, 1968). The range of the frequency of 'repetition' is therefore very wide, and the degree of homology in quasi-repeating sequences also differs considerably from one group to another (Britten and Kohn, 1968). I suggest (following Hood *et al.*, 1970), that genes in some of the longer 'repeating' sequences are likely to code for the variable sections of immunoglobulin L and H chains. Many other quasi-repeating sequences will need to be devoted to the synthesis of those polypeptide components of MCPs and TCFs that govern the fine-structural features of the morphology of tissues. We regard a classical 'tissue' as comprising a complex assembly of mosaic elements.

Studies of allophenic mice (Mintz, 1971) have led to conclusions strikingly similar to ours. (Allophenic mice are obtained by the experimental aggregation of cells from the early blastomeres of two different genotypes to form a single embryo in the uterus of a pseudo-pregnant mother.) Mintz (1971) concludes that any specific 'tissue' (such as all melanocytes) is clonally derived from a specific number (34 in the case of melanocytes) of primordial cells that are differentiated during embryogenesis. Hair follicles comprise some 150 to 200 clones. Thus each 'tissue'—as understood by ordinary histological criteria—consists of a specific number of *phenoclones* (Mintz, 1971). Whether studies of intratissue differences in allophenic mice detect the same degree of fine-structure as that which can be inferred from, say, the anatomical site-distribution of dental caries, remains to be seen. Nevertheless, it is interesting that these two markedly different and independent approaches should lead to virtually identical conclusions regarding the genetically determined phenotypic complexity (mosaicism) of conventional 'tissues'. Studies of neoplasia in allophenic mice (Mintz and Slemmer, 1969; Condamine, Custer and Mintz, 1971) also corroborate our conclusions regarding the cellular origin of malignant tumours in man—see Chapter 7.

Recapitulation

In case the central message of this chapter should have become submerged under the detail some reiteration of the main points may be helpful.

The chapter calls for nothing less than a radical reorientation of thinking about the fundamental nature of the processes of growth and age-dependent disease.

Instead of thinking exclusively in simple *action* terms: 'growth hormone controls growth', 'viruses cause leukaemia', 'smoking causes lung cancer', etc., we have to rethink in *relational* terms.

I contend that growth, beyond a certain stage of embryogenesis, is regulated by a homeostatic or negative-feedback system. Each distinctive target tissue in the body has its growth and size regulated by a central element of the control system. In man, the number of 'distinctive tissues' might be as high as $\sim 10^{10}$. *Recognition* relations assume a dominating importance in this system: mitogenic effectors have to recognize their correct target cells, and affectors, signalling the size of the target tissue, have to home onto their correct central controlling element.

Two independent arguments imply that only one solution to the genetic and molecular basis of mutual recognition in growth-control is tenable. The genes that code for some or all of the protein component of a specific recognition macromolecule (MCP) in a central controlling element, also code for the protein component of the corresponding recognition macromolecule (TCF) in the cognate target cell. This solution is therefore the simplest and, in terms of genes, the most economical one possible. Mutual recognition between MCP and cognate TCF, at both ends of the feedback loop, depends on the phenomenon of *self-association* which is probably based, at least in part, on London–van der Waal's *self-recognition* forces. The distinction between humoral MCPs and humoral TCFs derives from additional protein and/or non-protein components.

In 'natural' autoaggressive disease, which includes all forms of spontaneous pre-malignant and malignant change, the identity connection between an MCP and its associated TCF is replaced during initiation by complementarity between a mutant MCP and the TCF.

In the next chapter I discuss the possible genetic and molecular basis of this complementary and pathogenic relationship.

CHAPTER 5

The Nature of Initiating Somatic Mutations— Concept of Genetic Dichotomy

The notion of somatic mutation has found little favour among experimental biologists or clinicians. Burnet (1959(b)) has attributed this lack of appeal to the prevailing ethos: 'It is almost an inescapable characteristic of those educated in Western and scientific habits of thought to believe that effects have a definable cause and that undesired phenomena can always be prevented or cured . . . It is *diminishing* (Burnet's italics) to consider our helplessness in the face of the major limitations of life, the inevitable accident that sooner or later introduces a flaw into the copying of a genetic pattern'.

Gross chromosomal aberrations apart, somatic mutations suffer the further disadvantage—for the empiricist—of being invisible under both the optical and electron microscopes. Perhaps the most convincing demonstration of their reality would be the isolation of the protein products of a gene before and after somatic mutation. Such a programme cannot easily be carried out in connection with disease in man. Cancer-associated antigens might be considered good evidence for somatic mutation but such findings are indirect and, as we shall see, they can be quite misleading.

Statistical Properties of Random Initiating Events

My main reasons for inferring that some form of somatic gene mutation initiates the complex sequence of changes that culminates in autoaggressive disease have come from studies of the age-dependence of more than 200 malignant and non-malignant disorders in man. These studies have led to certain conclusions that may well apply to all 'natural' diseases that show a reproducible age-dependence.

(1) One or more *random* events initiate the process that gives rise to a specific autoaggressive disease. With a few rather special exceptions (see Chapter 7), the number and statistical character of the initiating events are the same, in different countries and different continents, for a given narrowly defined disease. The mathematical equations (see Chapter 6) that describe the age-dependence of these numerous diseases all derive from simple stochastic laws.

(2) The average rate of occurrence of a specific random initiating event is: (i) largely or wholly independent of ordinary environments; (ii) effectively independent of age, from within about $\pm 0 \cdot 1$ year of birth to the onset of disease, even when that occurs at the end of the normal lifespan; (iii) constant in genetically similar populations; however, even small differences in the base sequence of a gene that undergoes somatic mutation can be expected (see later) to affect the average rate: interpopulation differences of rates, especially between Japan and Western countries (see Chapter 7), may well arise in this way; (iv) either the same in females and similarly predisposed males, or, in certain instances, is twice as high in XX females as in similarly predisposed XY males; and (v) sometimes higher in persons with Down's syndrome than in cytogenetically normal persons: rate-differences observed for two forms of acute leukaemia in childhood (Burch, 1968(a)), and for early-onset (juvenile) diabetes mellitus (Burch and Milunsky, 1969), can be explained quantitatively if the somatic mutation of genes on chromosome 21 is required to initiate these diseases.

I cannot conceive that extrinsic factors such as infections, exposure to noxious chemical or physical stimuli, or episodes of acute mental stress, could account for all—or even any—of the above properties. The persistent conformity of the initiating events to simple stochastic laws, and the correlation of the average rates of certain of these events with the ploidy of chromosomes such as X and *21*, powerfully support the idea that nuclear genes undergo some form of spontaneous change. For reasons argued in the previous chapters and elsewhere (Burch and Burwell, 1965; Burch, 1968(a)), we concluded that these spontaneous changes occur in stem cells of the central system of growth-control. However, the exact mechanism of gene change has yet to be established. The sections that follow survey the evidence that bears on this problem.

Point Mutation and Rate of Mutation

Molecular biologists have familiarized us with the idea of 'point' mutation of genes in bacteria and their phages. Usually, a single base is either altered (transition or transversion), or deleted, or inserted. A transition or trans-version of a base in a structural gene often leads to the substitution of one amino acid for another in the associated polypeptide chain. We believe, however, that this type of point mutation cannot account for the gene changes that initiate autoaggressive disease (Burch and Burwell, 1965; Burch, 1968(a)).

In some autoaggressive diseases a single gene change can alter the normal identity relation between an MCP and its TCF into a complementary and pathogenic relation between the mutant MCP and the original TCF (Burch, 1968(a)). That a change in a single amino acid could *commonly* result in so specific a transformation seems unlikely. Moreover, the typical rate of those somatic mutations that initiate disease—of the order of 10^{-3} per gene, per cell, per year (Burch, 1968(a))—cannot easily be reconciled with the much lower rate of point mutation. Orgel (1963) has estimated that the rate of point mutation is of the order of 10^{-8} per nucleotide, per cell generation. The cell cycle time of myeloblasts is about 17 hours (Boll and Fuchs, 1970), so if we assume that a growth-control stem cell undergoes 5×10^2 divisions per year, then the point mutation-rate according to Orgel's estimate should be $\sim 5 \times 10^{-6}$ per nucleotide per year. Only if a point mutation of *any one* out of ~ 200 bases in a gene produces a 'complementary' polypeptide chain could we explain the typical rate of initiating somatic mutations. Such an hypothesis strains credulity.

Novick and Szilard (1950) determined the rate of mutation to resistance to bacteriophage T5 in *E. coli* (strain B/1). They varied the generation time of bacteria in their chemostat over the range of two to 12 hours. If the mutation-rate per generation is defined as ρ, and the generation time as τ, they found ρ/τ to be constant and equal to $1 \cdot 1 \times 10^{-4}$ year^{-1} at 37 °C. (This rate is within an order of magnitude of the typical rate of initiating somatic mutations in man.) At 25 °C the rate of mutation, ρ/τ, was halved. Novick and Szilard pointed out that if mutants arise as the result of an error in replication, it would be difficult to understand how the probability of mutation per cell division could be inversely proportional to the rate of growth. However, if the mutational process involves a unimolecular reaction then, at a given temperature, the rate of mutation per unit time would be constant—in accordance with observation (Novick and Szilard, 1950).

If a somatic mutation that initiates disease entails a unimolecular reaction, such as the dissociation of a gene complex, say DNA-protein, the constancy of average rates with age, and from person to person, becomes compre-hensible.

Of special interest are findings in mice (see Chapter 6) that point to at least two classes of germ cell mutation: one with a rate $\sim 10^{-6}$ to 10^{-5} per locus per gamete per generation; and another, involving histocompatibility genes (they are MCP–TCF genes), with a rate $\sim 5 \times 10^{-4}$ per locus per gamete per generation. For a typical breeding age of 150 days, this latter rate becomes $\sim 10^{-3}$ per gamete per year which corresponds to the rates estimated for initiating somatic mutations in man.

Induction by Radiation of 'Visible Mutations' in Mice

In addition to the preceding considerations, we have to bear in mind experiments by Russell (1964, 1965) in which ionizing radiation induced mutations in the germ cells of male mice. The average 'target size' for genes at seven specific loci that yield 'visible mutations', turns out to be $\sim 3 \times 10^5$ daltons, a value that approximates to the total DNA content of a typical structural gene (Burch, 1967). This estimate contrasts with the effective target area for the induction of presumed point mutations in yeast, which is some $10 \, \text{Å} \times 10 \, \text{Å}$, and corresponds roughly to the cross-section presented by a single base-pair (Mortimer, Brustad and Cormack, 1965).

If mature post-meiotic germ cells in mice are irradiated, and if a point mutation is induced in only one of the two strands of DNA of a structural gene, then we would normally expect that one-half of the cells of the inheritor of such a gene would carry the mutant gene, while the other half would be wild-type. Hence a visible character such as fur-type, or colour, would usually exhibit a mosaic pattern rather than the whole-body effect that results from a 'complete mutation'. Russell (1964) obtained no evidence for the induction by radiation of 'mosaic mutations' in mature germ cells, although occasionally, mosaicism is seen in the offspring both of irradiated and unirradiated animals. Hence, if the primary mutagenic event entails a change in a base of only one strand of DNA, then a 'correction' or 'repair' mechanism must function with 100 per cent efficiency to change the mismatched base on the antiparallel strand of DNA to the form that complements the 'mutant' base.

In other organisms, such as yeast, in which point mutations can be induced by agents such as nitrous acid, mosaics appear in high yield, ranging from around 50 to over 90 per cent, depending on conditions (Abbondandolo and Bonatti, 1970; see also the review by Nasim and Auerbach (1967)). Evidently the effectiveness of 'repair' mechanisms in yeast is much less than 100 per cent. A similar conclusion can be drawn from experiments with *Paramecium aurelia*. Kimball and Perdue (1967) found that the efficiency with which pre-mutational damage induced by x-rays is repaired in this organism changes markedly with the cell cycle. Hence, although repair mechanisms might function infallibly in mice, precedents are lacking.

I conclude that the type of complete mutation that is consistently induced by ionizing radiation in mice probably differs qualitatively from those point mutations that result in either complete or mosaic effects in other organisms. Because the genes at the seven specific loci studied in mice determine visible characters, they may well be MCP–TCF genes. Hence, the type of mutation induced in these genes by ionizing radiation might be similar to that which, in somatic cells, initiates autoaggressive disease.

Directed Mutation (Allelic Switching) of X-linked Genes?

We infer that 'directed mutations'—involving gene changes of the kind that initiate autoaggressive disease—occur at X-linked genes during embryogenesis, as the result of some form of induction mechanism (Burch and Burwell, 1965; Burch, 1968(a)). This inference comes in part from the commonly observed 2:1 (F/M) sex-difference in somatic mutation-rates. In several instances, it seems likely that the X-linked genes that predispose to disease also undergo somatic mutation to initiate the growth of forbidden clones (Burch, 1968(a); Burch and Rowell, 1965, 1970). To take the example of systemic lupus erythematosus, the characteristically high F/M sex ratio of affected persons, and the evidence for familial transmission, can be explained if three X-linked alleles, each with (generally) dominant expression, contribute to the predisposing genotype (Burch and Rowell, 1965, 1970). Three somatic mutations, each occurring, on the average, at twice the rate in females as in males, initiate this disease. We have proposed that, in this disease and some others, the predisposing X-linked genes themselves undergo somatic mutation (Burch and Burwell, 1965).

This proposal is not without its difficulties. Suppose the dominant predisposing allele at the Xa locus is $Xa1$ and that it can mutate, both in germ and somatic cells, to the alternative allele $Xa2$. Predisposed females will be either homozygous $Xa1/Xa1$, or heterozygous $Xa1/Xa2$. Suppose a forbidden clone is initiated by the transition $Xa1 \rightarrow Xa2$ in a growth-control stem cell. Only in homozygous females would we expect the rate of somatic mutation to be double that in hemizygous $Xa1/Y$ males. The rate of the transition $Xa1 \rightarrow Xa2$ in heterozygous females ought to be the same as the corresponding rate in males. Hence, in the population at large, which contains heterozygous and homozygous females in a ratio determined by the frequency of the $Xa1$ allele, the average rate of the somatic mutation $Xa1 \rightarrow Xa2$ in predisposed females ought to lie between one and two times the rate in males. So far, I have found no example of clearly intermediate rates.

To escape this difficulty we proposed that, in heterozygous $Xa1/Xa2$ females, the gene transition $Xa2 \rightarrow Xa1$ occurs in presumptive growth-control stem cells during embryogenesis as the result of a directing mechanism (Burch and Burwell, 1965). Such a transition can be described as *directed mutation* or *allelic switching*.

Whether or not directed mutation occurs at autosomal MCP–TCF genes remains to be determined.

Anomalous inheritance at X-linked loci

A mechanism of directed gene change can also account for anomalies in X-linked inheritance of the kind observed by Berg and Bearn (1966) in connection with the Xm system, and described in the previous chapter. In the same way, it can explain how Xg(a –) mothers can occasionally have Xg(a+) sons. The Xg(a+) blood group antigen behaves as an X-linked dominant character and hence mothers who are Xg(a –) should be geno-typically recessive $Xga - /Xga -$ at this X-linked locus. Because sons inherit their X-chromosome from their mother, we expect all sons of Xg(a –) mothers to be Xg(a –). In two out of over 1000 normal families studied by Sanger *et al.* (1964), Xg(a –) mothers had Xg(a+) sons only; in one family, both sons were Xg(a+), and in the other all three sons were Xg(a+). According to my theory, this could come about in several ways. The mothers might have been genotypically heterozygous $(Xga+/Xga -)$, but phenotypically Xg(a –), as the result of the directed gene transition: $Xga+ \rightarrow Xga -$ in presumptive growth-control stem cells during embryogenesis. This change would need to have been accompanied either by the same transition (induced?) in target (erythrocytic) cells, or by the inactivation of the chromosome carrying $Xga+$ in target cells. Alternatively, the directed mutation or allelic switching of X-linked genes might, at least in some instances, extend to males. If it does, a genotypically $Xga -$ male could become phenotypically Xg(a+) as the result of a directed gene transition during early embryogenesis.

Protan deficiency, which normally occurs only in homozygotes, manifests from time to time in heterozygous women. This phenomenon has been described as *change into dominance* (Jaeger, 1951, 1952). Our theory of directed mutation or allelic switching at X-linked MCP–TCF loci in heterozygous females during embryogenesis readily accounts for such anomalies.

Similarly, certain changes with time, or geography, in the sex-ratio of persons predisposed to autoaggressive disease might be attributed to allelic switching in heterozygous females (Burch and Burwell, 1965; Burch, 1968(a); Burch, de Dombal and Watkinson, 1969; Burch and Rowell, 1970). To take the example of late-onset diabetes mellitus, Freedman *et al.*

(1965) found a much higher prevalence in men than in women in a Hiroshima (Japanese) population. In Western populations, women are usually more prone to late-onset diabetes than men. However, in the nineteenth century, diabetes was more common in men; the sex-ratio (M/F) for standardized death-rates in England and Wales changed from 2 in 1861, to 1·2 in 1911, and 0·8 in 1936 (Fitzgerald, 1967). Such changes in the sex-ratio could be explained if the expression of genes on the X-chromosome can be altered in the manner postulated by our theory of allelic switching. The direction of allelic switching—that is, the choice between $Xa1 \rightarrow Xa2$ and $Xa2 \rightarrow Xa1$—is likely to be determined by an inductor molecule that is the product of one or more other genes. Changes in the frequency of these other inductor genes with time, due to migration, selection pressures, among other things, could account for an inconstant sex-ratio of predisposed persons.

The conclusion we draw from the complex behaviour of X-linked genes is that their expression is probably altered by inductive mechanisms during embryogenesis. It is very doubtful whether point mutations could be induced in this way; directed DNA strand-switching is a more plausible mechanism.

Tissue Compatibility in Allophenic Mice

Blastomeres from two (or more) genetically dissimilar cleavage-stage embryos can be aggregated *in vitro* and cultured to form a single embryo. At the morula, or blastocyst, stage the embryo is transferred to the uterus of a foster mother and allowed to complete its prenatal life. The resulting animal, a mosaic of two or more genotypes, is described as *allophenic*. Mintz and Palm (1969) examined erythropoietic cells in allophenic mice constituted from the two unrelated strains, C3H and C57BL/6. They found that in some mice, red cells of two types were present, some carrying the H-2^k antigen of the C3H strain and others carrying the H-2^b antigen of the C57BL/6 strain. Such allophenic animals will also accept skin grafts from both 'parental' inbred strains.

We are forced to conclude that certain changes occur during the embryonic development of allophenic mice that make otherwise incompatible tissues, mutually compatible. In other words, any given MCP of the C3H strain has to be compatible not only with its cognate TCF of the first strain but also with the corresponding TCF of the second strain. Similar requirements apply to MCPs of the C57BL/6 strain. One mechanism whereby such compatibility could be attained would be through the appropriate selection and induction by DNA strand-switching of compatible X-linked alleles that contribute polypeptides to the corresponding TCFs of both strains. Conceivably the need for a similar flexibility arises during the development of ordinary non-allophenic animals. If this is the case, the necessity for directed DNA strand-switching during embryogenesis can be understood. Whether the phenomenon extends to any autosomal MCP–TCF genes remains to be determined.

DNA Strand-switching Mutation

So far, I have been able to devise only one hypothesis of gene change that is consistent with the evidence relating to the random events that initiate autoaggressive disease. I have proposed that, instead of a change in a base or base-pair, there is a switchover of transcription from the regular strand of DNA to the base-paired, antiparallel strand (Burch and Burwell, 1965; Burch, 1968(a)). We call this a *DNA strand-switching mutation*. This hypothesis makes precise predictions although some sophisticated biochemistry will be needed to verify them.

The complementarity between the two strands of the Watson–Crick double helix hints at the possibility of some form of steric complementarity between the protein products of the two strands of DNA. In the stages of protein synthesis, transcription gives steric complementarity between messenger RNA (mRNA) and its DNA template; and the anticodon of transfer RNA (tRNA) complements the associated codon of mRNA. However, the hypothesis of DNA strand-switching also calls for some form of complementarity between at least some codons (or anticodons) and the side chains of their related amino acids (see Figure 5.1). This is a *minimum* requirement; the evidence and arguments that bear on it are presented below.

If this relation exists, then some form of stereochemical complementarity

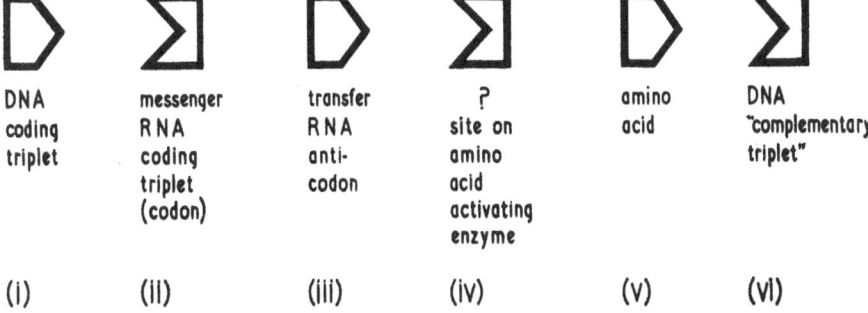

DNA coding triplet	messenger RNA coding triplet (codon)	transfer RNA anti-codon	? site on amino acid activating enzyme	amino acid	DNA "complementary triplet"
(i)	(ii)	(iii)	(iv)	(v)	(vi)

Figure 5.1 Type of steric relations required, for at least some codons and amino acids by the hypothesis of DNA strand-switching mutation

would necessarily exist between the side chain of one amino acid and the side chain of its 'complement'. We are ultimately concerned, however, with a specific relation between one protein and its 'complement' or, just conceivably, between their associated non-protein components, such as lipids and/or carbohydrates. The complicated folding of proteins adds a further dimension to this problem. But despite all the obscurities, the following facts are established—proteins can interact strongly with one another; protein antigens and complementary antibodies show strong affinity; and the recognition of an allograft by the host leads to graft rejection.

Informational Strand of DNA

In various bacteria and bacteriophages, certain parts of the genome are transcribed in one direction, along one strand of DNA, but other parts of the genome are transcribed in the opposite direction, along the antiparallel strand of DNA. Szybalski and co-workers have found that in bacteriophage λ, about 16 per cent of the genome can be transcribed in both directions. That is to say, both strands of DNA are transcribed, a phenomenon described as *overlapping convergent transcription* (Szybalski *et al.*, 1969; Szybalski, 1970; Nijkamp, Bøvre and Szybalski, 1971).

Lindstrom and Dulbecco (1972) studied the RNA transcribed from the SV40 virus in infected cells that allow the virus to replicate. They found that RNA sequences synthesized before the replication of viral DNA ('early' RNA), and sequences synthesized during the replication of DNA ('late' RNA), are transcribed from opposite strands of the SV40 DNA. The RNA synthesized *in vitro* has the same polarity as the 'early' *in vivo* RNA and it was shown to be complementary to the 'late' *in vivo* RNA.

Stampfer *et al.* (1972) described hybridization of labelled HeLa cell mRNA to HeLa cell nuclear RNA. Among the several (unresolved) possibilities considered by these authors is the idea that certain regions of DNA in HeLa cells might be transcribed in both directions. The discovery of 'palindromic' sequences of DNA (Wilson and Thomas, 1974)—see section on evolution of MCP–TCF genes, page 86—provides another possible interpretation of the results of Stampfer *et al.*

Genetic dichotomy and contrast with symmetric transcription

I call the non-simultaneous utilization of information from both strands of DNA at MCP–TCF loci, the principle of *genetic dichotomy*. This phenomenon should be contrasted with *symmetric transcription*, which appears to be the normal mode of transcription of mitochrondrial DNA in HeLa cells (Aloni and Attardi, 1971). In symmetric transcription, both strands of DNA are transcribed simultaneously. The phenomenon of genetic dichotomy, in common with the familiar process of asymmetric transcription, requires one or more signals to determine which strand of DNA is available for transcription, or, if both strands are transcribed, which product should be translated.

Associations between Amino Acids and Nucleotides and Synthetase Recognition Site on Transfer-RNA

On theoretical grounds, Woese (1962, 1967) predicted that the genetic code would display specific degeneracies, confined to particular positions in the codon. He conjectured that such an order, or logic, in the code might result from either of two mechanisms: (a) an interaction between an amino acid and a nucleotide grouping (simply related to the codon) either during one or more steps in translation, or at an early stage of evolution of the genetic code; or (b) interactions in the translation process that did not involve the amino acid—in other words an 'intercodon logic'.

Subsequent to the elucidation of the main features of the genetic code, which confirmed his basic ideas on specific degeneracies, Woese (1966) drew attention to simple correlations between (i) codon assignments and the chromatographic behaviour of associated amino acids; and also (ii) the codons that code for amino acids with related structures. Woese et al. (1966) demonstrated selective chemical interactions between amino acids and organic bases. They concluded that the codon assignments reflect an underlying pairing between each codon and its associated amino acid.

Nakashima and Fox (1972) found that microparticles composed of poly(G), poly(A), poly(U) or poly(C) respectively, combined with the same lysine-rich 'proteinoid', influence the condensation of the AMP-anhydrides of the four amino acids: glycine, lysine, phenylalanine and proline, respectively. Under appropriate experimental conditions, condensation favoured the amino acids whose codons are related to the homopolynucleotide in the microparticle. Thus, poly(G) favoured glycine; poly(A) lysine; poly(U) phenylalanine; and poly(C) proline. This represents, perhaps, the most direct experimental demonstration of a fairly specific association between amino acids and codons, or codon-like polynucleotides.

Arguing from the essential universality of the genetic code, Weinstein (1963) suggested ('at risk of committing heresy') that a stereochemical fit might exist between each amino acid and a group of nucleotides on its corresponding tRNA. The simplest version of my strand-switching theory predicts that the anticodon of at least some tRNAs should recognize the complex of amino-acid-plus-amino-acyl-tRNA-synthetase (Burch, 1968(a)). This prediction has been verified in the case of yeast $tRNA_1^{Val}$ (Mirzabekov *et al.*, 1971). By dissecting the tRNA molecule at specific regions, these workers were able to conclude that the dinucleotides AC in the anticodon loop, and the 5′-terminal G_1G in the CCA stem, constitute at least parts of two recognition sites of $tRNA_1^{Val}$.

It is suspected that the synthetase recognition sites of different tRNA molecules might reside at different positions, and it seems that the anticodon is not involved in every instance—see the review by Bhargava, Pallaiah and Premkumar (1970). Nevertheless, Squires and Carbon (1971) have shown in the case of three glycine tRNAs from *E. coli*, that base alterations at either of the first two positions of the anticodon—but not at the 'wobble' position— greatly reduce (10^{-4} times) the rate of the enzymic amino-acylation. Hence, in these three additional instances, the anticodon is evidently involved, directly or indirectly, in the recognition of the complex of amino acid with synthetase. Similarly, Saneyoshi and Nishimura (1971), by modifying with cyanogen bromide the base at the first position of the anticodon on the *E. coli* tRNA for glutamic acid, demonstrated that the anticodon region of $tRNA^{Glu}$ probably plays a part in synthetase recognition. Cyanogen bromide also caused the tRNAs for lysine and glutamine to lose acceptor activity. Again, this might have been due to modification of the base at the first position of the anticodon of $tRNA^{Lys}$ and $tRNA^{Gln}$ (Saneyoshi and Nishimura, 1971). Schimmel *et al.* (1972) measured the extent of binding of complementary oligonucleotides (triplets and tetramers) to free $tRNA^{Ile}$ from *E. coli*, and to $tRNA^{Ile}$ bound to its homologous isoleucyl–tRNA synthetase. They found that synthetase blocks the binding of complementary oligonucleotides both at the CCA sequence of the 3′ terminus of tRNA and at the anticodon section. This demonstration again accords with the idea that recognition of synthetase by tRNA involves the anticodon loop and bases at the 3′ or 5′ end of the tRNA molecule (Schimmel *et al.*, 1972). Soll (1974) and Yaniv *et al.* (1974) found that a single base substitution in the anticodon of a tryptophan-specific tRNA affected not only the coding specificity of the molecule, but also changed the amino acid acceptor specificity from tryptophan to glutamine.

Nirenberg *et al.* (1965) pointed out that amino acids that are structurally or metabolically related (such as being synthesized from a common precursor) often have similar codons. They argued that such relationships might reflect either the evolution of the code or, following Woese (1962, 1963) and Weinstein (1963), direct interactions between amino acids and bases in codons. Similar, but more elaborate arguments were advanced by Pelc (1965), who illustrated that simple differences in the structure of the side chain of an amino acid are accompanied by a difference of only one base in the codon. He favoured the hypothesis that a structural relationship exists between amino acids and codons and concluded that the probability that chance alone could account for the order in the genetic code would seem to be negligible.

Crick (1963, 1968) has opposed the preceding views and he considers it unlikely that every amino acid interacts stereochemically either with its codon or its anticodon. Nevertheless, his recent attitude towards stereochemical theories of the genetic code shows a softening in relation to his earlier condemnation of such ideas. In his 1968 paper, he states that it is essential to pursue the stereochemical theory, and that direct experimental proof of interactions between amino acids and codons is needed.

Woese (1969), replying to Crick (1968), argued that all-or-none specificities between oligonucleotides and amino acids would not have been needed for the evolution of the genetic code; a sufficient number of slight preferences would have sufficed. In this connection, Woese (1969) referred to the experiments of Leng and Felsenfeld (1966) which revealed a preference by AT-rich DNA for polylysine over polyarginine, and of GC-rich DNA for polyarginine over polylysine. (The codons for lysine are AA_G^A, and those for arginine are $CG_{A\ G}^{U\ C}$ and AG_G^A.) The case for a stereochemical basis underlying the genetic code is argued at length by Woese (1967).

Lacey and Pruitt (1969) carried out experiments and built molecular models to test the hypothesis that the genetic code evolved as the result of specific interactions between polypeptides and mononucleotides. They found that the addition of mononucleotides (except uridylic acid) to solutions of poly-L-lysine (of molecular weight about 100000) produced extreme turbidity. By analysing the effects of ionic strength, temperature, the molecular weight of the poly-L-lysine, and nucleosides in place of nucleotides, they concluded, however, that the specificity of turbidity formation depends on the nucleotide–nucleotide interactions, and not on interactions between amino acids and nucleotide bases. Although these experiments did not give the hoped-for result, they led Lacey and Pruitt (1969) to consider whether a structural arrangement could be devised that would give the genetic code stoichiometry of three bases to each amino acid residue in the polymer. Using space-filling models they found that, when the polyamino acid is in the form of an α-helix, it can be associated with a complementary strand of nucleotides, winding round the α-helix, in the required 3 : 1 stoichiometric relationship. Taking the example of poly-L-lysine, the lysine side chains intercalate between the first and second stacked nucleotides of a sequence of three AMP nucleotides, in their 'anti'-configuration. Generalizing, they proposed that in each codon, the side chain of the amino acid is inserted between the first and the second nucleotides of the codon.

Consequently, the third nucleotide does not come into direct 'contact' with the amino acid side chain and is therefore less important to the specificity of the codon. This feature of their model agrees with the present-day genetic code. Lacey and Pruitt (1969) were able to predict that the preferred codon for glycine (which has no side chain) would be the one with the greatest base stacking or self-associating tendency. This turns out to be guanylic acid, and hence their model correctly predicts the codon GGG for glycine.

Interaction between nucleic acids and proteins

A puzzle closely connected with the stereochemical relation between amino acids and codons is the nature of the interaction between nucleic acids and regulatory proteins. Although a λ-phage repressor is known to be a protein which binds tightly and specifically to λDNA (Ptashne, 1967), the molecular basis of its interaction with operator DNA has yet to be elucidated. It has since been shown, for two coliphage repressors, that when they bind to DNA they are in the form of oligomers, possibly tetramers (Pirrotta, Chadwick and Ptashne, 1970).

The exact role of histones and of non-histone DNA proteins in the regulation of gene activity in higher organisms also remains obscure. If the organization of MCP–TCF genes differs from that of genes synthesizing classical enzymes—as seems probable—the problems ahead assume an added complexity.

Stevens and Williamson (1973(a), (b)) have found that myeloma protein in mouse plasmacytoma cells represses the synthesis of the heavy (H) chain and thus provides for translational feedback control of immunoglobulin synthesis. This results from a specific interaction between the H_2L_2 myeloma protein and the mRNA that codes for the H-chain (Stevens and Williamson, 1973(b)).

DNA Strand-determination

What determines the transcriptional strand of DNA? If we knew the answer to this question, we would probably be able to cope with the further question: What brings about DNA strand-switching? Remembering that a very large number of genes are expected to code for MCPs and TCFs, the strand-determining factor needs to be as specific as the gene itself. This would seem to leave us with only three possibilities. Either the RNA, or the polypeptide chain product of the gene, or the RNA acting together with the polypeptide chain, would appear to have the requisite specificity.

We suggested that the polypeptide chain might complex with the non-. informational strand of DNA to block transcription from it (Burch and

Burwell, 1965). The association between polypeptide and DNA would presumably need to be analogous to that described by Lacey and Pruitt (1969) for polyamino acids and RNA, with three nucleotides per amino acid residue. Such a complex would leave the informational strand of DNA free for transcription. Dissociation of the complex between the non-informational strand of DNA and its associated polypeptide—an event which needs to obey unimolecular kinetics—would make it possible for the (previously) non-informational strand to be transcribed. If a polypeptide chain determines the transcriptional strand of DNA, completion of the 'mutation' would require translation of the resulting new mRNA and the association of the new polypeptide chain with the previous informational strand of DNA.

Unfortunately for this otherwise simple scheme, it is difficult to understand how associations between polypeptides and a single-strand DNA helix, of the kind described by Lacey and Pruitt (1969), could come about, and how they could survive the process of DNA replication. But we remain woefully ignorant of the organization of chromosomes in higher organisms, of the mechanisms that determine the repression and derepression of their genes, and how the informational strand of a derepressed gene is determined.

If persistent association of RNA with the non-informational strand of DNA should prove to be responsible for blocking transcription from it, we need to know what factors determine: (a) its non-release; and (b) the release of the RNA transcript from the informational strand. This scheme gives rise to no stoichiometric or stereochemical problems. Frenster (1965) has proposed a model in which a specific derepressor RNA hybridizes with the non-informational strand of DNA. Huang and Huang (1969) and Dahmus and Bonner (1970) have shown that in higher organisms, chromosomal RNA is required for the sequence-specific reconstitution of chromatin. Huang and Huang (1969) showed in their experiments with chick embryo cells that the chromosomal RNA is covalently linked to non-histone protein.

As a further alternative, effective DNA strand-determination might depend on the non-translation of the RNA from the non-informational strand. We would then need to postulate a mechanism for the recognition and immobilization, or neutralization, of the 'wrong' RNA.

In spite of our inability to construct a simple and fully convincing model the stubborn facts remain: DNA strand-selection occurs at transcription and it survives the process of DNA replication. For any scheme of DNA strand-determination a mechanism is needed to maintain the correct strand-determination at non-induced MCP–TCF genes in cells, such as germ and early embryonic cells, which need to transmit the correct information to daughter cells in which these genes will later become functional. It must be remembered, however, that the functioning MCP–TCF genes in any differentiated cell will constitute only a small fraction of the total number of functioning genes. Experiments relating to the *average* gene activity in whole cells may therefore have little or even no relevance to MCP–TCF genes. DNA strand-switching at genes that synthesize classical enzymes is unknown and not even suspected. Hence, the determination of the informational strand at such genes might involve a special mechanism that prohibits strand-switching and, therefore, differs from the one at MCP–TCF genes. Conceivably, the organization of the chromosome depends on the class of gene. Most genetic investigations on lower organisms such as bacteria and phages are likely to be more relevant to those genes in higher organisms that synthesize classical enzymes, than to MCP–TCF genes.

Genetic Dichotomy and Polymorphism

A most striking feature of human populations is the enormous range and subtlety of the morphological differences between individuals. The near-identity of monozygotic twins shows that most of these variations are genetically based. This seemingly unlimited variation (polymorphism) within populations constitutes a major embarrassment for orthodox genetics (Neel and Salzano, 1967). Genetic dichotomy, which provides at least two alleles at DNA strand-switching loci, offers a ready explanation of this extensive polymorphism.

Many genetically based diseases have a fairly stable frequency, despite the disadvantages they confer. With rather rare exceptions (for example, Huntington's chorea and familial intestinal polyposis) the frequency of genes that predispose to autoaggressive diseases is high, and usually lies within the range 0·2 to 0·8 (Burch, 1968(a)). That is to say, the frequency of predisposing MCP–TCF genes, as determined by the analysis of familial aggregations and the frequency of disease, tends to be near the value of 0·5, which yields the maximum frequency of heterozygotes (0·5).

Very often, predisposition to an autoaggressive disease entails the inheritance of autosomal genes in homozygous arrangement: the high gene frequencies are, of course, consistent with the hypothesis of heterozygous advantage. Probably, when a major allele (say *a1*) in homozygous arrangement predisposes to one disadvantageous autoaggressive disease, the homozygous arrangement of the alternative major allele (*a2*) predisposes to another disadvantageous disease. If the selection pressures against both diseases are similar, then the gene frequencies will be near to 0·5. From the Leigh and Wensleydale population survey for inflammatory polyarthritis (Lawrence, 1961), I concluded that approximately 50 per cent of those surveyed were at genetic risk. I proposed that the two homozygotes *a1/a1* and *a2/a2* predispose to the same disease (Burch, 1963(a)). Such a scheme readily accounts for the high and stable frequency of predisposed persons, because selection pressures would operate equally against both *a1* and *a2*. (It must be mentioned that the analysis of familial (including twins) evidence does not determine whether a predisposing gene, *a1* say, is homogeneous. Thus, *a1* might well comprise several alleles, differing only in one or a few nucleotides, but with an identical, or nearly identical, phenotypic expression in a given autoaggressive disease.)

The total number of MCP–TCF gene loci in the human genome could well be of the order of 10^6 (Burch and Burwell, 1965). If most of these have at least two alleles, and if they can undergo DNA strand-switching in germ cells, then the minimum number of possible distinctive genotypes would be $\sim 3^{10^6}$ If the polypeptide products of MCP–TCF genes combine, at least seven at a time, to produce in each person each of, say, $\sim 10^{10}$ MCPs and TCFs, we have no reason to be surprised at the unending variety of mankind.

Allogeneic and Xenogeneic Interactions

The principle of genetic dichotomy explains the molecular and biological mechanisms of host-versus-graft and graft-versus-host allogeneic inter-actions. In general, corresponding MCPs and TCFs of unrelated individuals will contain one or more component polypeptides that are the products of complementary, or near-complementary, strands of DNA. Consequently, the MCPs of certain mosaic elements of a given individual will generally bear a complementary and 'pathogenic' relation to the TCFs of the cor-responding mosaic elements of an unrelated individual. Hence, for appropri-ate combinations, allogeneic interactions provide a good analogy with autoaggressive (autoimmune) disease.

The principle of genetic dichotomy also explains a familiar paradox in immunology: The severity of the allogenic interaction between different inbred strains within the same species, exceeds that of the xenogeneic reaction between species, despite the greater antigenic disparity between, than within, species. Although corresponding MCPs and TCFs in one species (say, mice) will be expected to resemble fairly closely those of another related species (say, rats) the resemblance of corresponding amino acid sequences of MCP–TCF polypeptides will be less close than within a given species. It follows, therefore that the degree of complementarity between complementary polypeptide MCP–TCF chains will generally be greater within than between species. Hence, allogeneic interactions will be expected (as observed) to be more severe than xenogeneic interactions.

Evolution of MCP–TCF Genes

Our theory leads to an obvious prediction about the nature of the precursor MCP–TCF gene that was capable of undergoing effective DNA strand-switching (Burch, 1968(a)). *A priori*, we would not expect the polypeptide encoded by one strand of DNA to bear any special relation to the polypeptide encoded by the complementary strand. However, theory demands that the polypeptides derived from the complementary DNA strands of an MCP–TCF gene should perform closely similar biochemical, physiological and morphological functions.

These requirements suggested to me that the precursor MCP–TCF gene probably arose through gene duplication and inversion to give a 'double gene' as illustrated in Figure 5.2 (Burch, 1968(a)). With such a fusion, the messages from both (complementary) strands of DNA (ABB'A') would be identical. Such DNA, which reads the same in opposite directions, has been called 'palindromic' (Wilson and Thomas, 1974). However, the first point

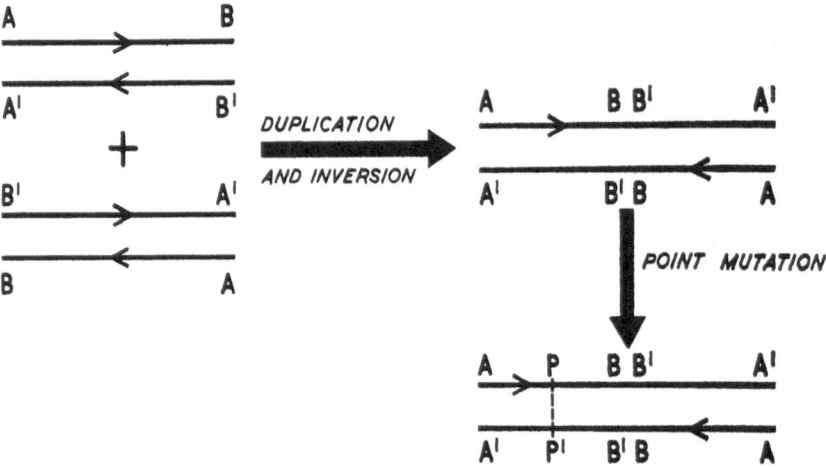

Figure 5.2 Proposed origin of precursor MCP–TCF genes (Burch, 1968(a)). AB and A'B' are complementary strands of DNA; duplication and inversion leads to the precursor gene ABB'A'; it reads the same for both directions of transcription: such DNA has therefore been called 'palindromic' (Wilson and Thomas, 1974)

mutation, P, that led to acceptable amino acid substitutions in both polypeptide chains would make them different. The sequences APBB'A' and ABB'P'A' are no longer exactly palindromic. Multiplication of 'acceptable genes'—and their further diversification through point mutation—had to occur to generate the complexity and diversity of MCP–TCF polypeptides in evolving organisms.

Large evolutionary progressions along the phylogenetic sequence probably required an increase in the number of polypeptide chains contributing to each MCP–TCF recognition macromolecule. Evolutionary change within a given class, could result from changes in those pleiotropic genes (such as histocompatibility genes) that code for polypeptide chains shared by many tissues. A single point mutation in such a pleiotropic gene might change the morphological character of many of the tissues in an organism.

According to my theory of the evolution of MCP–TCF genes, we would expect to find a large measure of reversed autocomplementarity between the two halves (AB and B′A′) of single-stranded DNA of existing MCP–TCF genes and their derived heterogeneous RNA (HnRNA) and mRNA transcripts. In view of the closely similar functions of 'complementary' MCP–TCF polypeptides, this reversed autocomplementarity of adjacent stetches of single-strand DNA would be expected to be detectable in contemporary DNA.

Flamm and his colleagues have reported a relationship of this kind in mouse satellite DNA (see Flamm's (1972) review). If this form of DNA is separated into two strands (L and H), reversed autocomplementary sequences are found within each single strand. These reversed sequences are less than 50 nucleotides in length and they occur, on the average, about every 1000 nucleotides within the satellite duplex (Flamm, 1972). However, these 'reversed sequences' are not found in guinea-pig α satellite (Flamm, 1972). It seems unlikely, therefore, that they have a direct connection with MCP–TCF genes.

A related phenomenon has been demonstrated in HnRNA from HeLa cells. Jelinek and Darnell (1972) found that 50s and 100s fractions of HnRNA each contain about 3 per cent double-stranded RNA: this probably exists as intramolecular loops ('hairpins') within large molecules. However, these long double-stranded regions were not found in mRNA (Jelinek and Darnell, 1972).

Palindromic DNA

Of special interest are the more recent findings of Wilson and Thomas (1974). They demonstrated that the rapidly self-associating fragments of single-strand DNA prepared from cells of higher eukaryotes form 'hairpin-like' structures. The 'turn-around' region of the hairpin is very small and/or is resistant to single-chain endonucleases. Lengths of the inverted repetitions AB, B′A′, that make up the hairpins range from about 300 to 6000 nucleotides, the most common being from 300 to 1200 nucleotides. Human (HeLa) cell chromosomes probably contain hundreds of thousands of palindromes, or near-palindromes, arranged in clusters of two or four, about 10 to 15 μm apart. The thermal stability of the hairpin structures from single-strand DNA suggests that the 'arms' of the hairpin AB and B'A' are near-perfect complementary sequences with, perhaps, less than one per cent base-pair mismatching (Wilson and Thomas, 1974).

At first sight, it is tempting to associate palindromes with functional MCP–TCF genes. Their number—of the order of hundreds of thousands in human DNA—corresponds with our guesstimate ($\sim 10^6$) of the number of MCP–TCF genes. Moreover, Ryskov et al. (1973) estimate that the number of families of palindromes in Ehrlich ascites (mouse) cell DNA is ~ 500, which fits in with the MCP–TCF attribution. Members of a given family of palindromes would be expected to contribute to the TCFs of the mosaic elements of a single 'tissue'. At this level of classification, the number of distinctive 'tissues' could well be about 500. Klein et al. (1974) find that only about six per cent of mRNA in HeLa cells is transcribed from repetitive DNA sequences. Only a small fraction of mRNA would be expected to be devoted to the synthesis of MCP–TCF proteins.

However, other evidence suggests that the Wilson–Thomas palindromes, of 300 or more nucleotides, are rather unlikely to be functioning MCP–TCF genes. Thus, failure of Jelinek and Darnell (1972) to find the longer double-strand hairpin RNA in the mRNA of the cytoplasm argues against the idea. Only short double-strand sequences of up to eight base pairs have been demonstrated so far in this cytoplasmic fraction (Ryskov et al., 1973). Moreover, the degree of perfection of the Wilson–Thomas palindromes, with perhaps less than 1 per cent base-pair mismatching, cannot easily be reconciled with functional MCP–TCF genes. Such perfection is attributed to the precursor MCP–TCF genes.

The isolation, purification and sequencing of MCP–TCF polypeptides will elucidate the types of DNA sequences that encode for them. When that formidable task has been accomplished the relation, if any, between Wilson–Thomas palindromes and MCP–TCF genes should be clarified.

Amino acid sequences (Cohen and Mistein, 1967) with the properties predicted by our DNA strand-switching theory have been demonstrated in the constant and variable regions of human κ immunoglobulin chains (Riley, 1973). Allowing a frame-shift of one base, and G:U base-pairing, Riley found two sequences of 11 amino acids (in the constant region) that imply short encoding palindromes of DNA in the κ light-chain genes. Many similar sequences of shorter length were found. Allowing no frame-shift, the two longest 'matching' sequences were each of seven amino acids, in the variable region (Riley, 1973). We argued that immunoglobulin chains are likely to be related to MCP–TCF polypeptides because, in our view, the primary function of immunoglobulins is endogenous defence against forbidden clones of mutant MCPs (Burch and Burwell, 1965).

Although diverse pieces of evidence favour our theory of the structure of MCP–TCF genes, definitive proof is lacking. Fortunately, the theory has the virtue of testability.

Conclusions

Autoaggressive disease is the price that multitissue organisms have to pay for extensive polymorphism. Polymorphism facilitates adaptation to different environments and it probably derives, to an important (but not exclusive) degree, from genetic dichotomy. Genetic dichotomy provides for the economic use of DNA inasmuch as it exploits the information from both strands of the double helix. For the individual, however, genetic dichotomy contains the seeds of destruction. When at certain genes, in certain cells, a spontaneous switch of transcription occurs to the 'wrong' strand of DNA, the resulting protein products lead to autoaggressive disease and ultimately to the demise of the individual. My theory implies that this demise is the outcome of a fundamental stereochemical relation between amino acids and codons. Others have argued that the genesis of self-replicating macro-molecules was contingent upon the existence of the same stereochemical relation, that enabled polynucleotides to marry polypeptides.

That the physicochemical basis of the origin of life should also ensure the death of the most highly evolved organisms has a certain ironical appeal. In the words of Albert Einstein (1949), 'A theory is the more impressive the greater the simplicity of its premises is, the more different kinds of things it relates, and the more extended is its area of applicability'.

Full corroboration of the theory of genetic dichotomy and DNA strand-switching will require the identification, isolation, purification and amino acid sequence analysis of 'complementary' MCP–TCF polypeptides. Mean-while, as shown throughout this chapter, a wide range of experimental evidence supports various predictions of the theory.

CHAPTER 6

The Age-dependence of Malignant Diseases: An Introduction

The age-dependence of malignant diseases in man has intrigued many investigators and inspired various theories of carcinogenesis (Muller, 1951; Fisher and Holloman, 1951; Nordling, 1952, 1953; Stocks, 1953; Armitage and Doll, 1954, 1957, 1961; Case, 1956(a), (b); Fisher, 1958; Burch, 1965, 1968(a), (b); Burnet, 1965; Curtis, 1967, 1969; Doll, 1968, 1971; Hems, 1968(a), (b); Mayneord, 1968; Ashley, 1969(a), (b), 1970(a), (b); Cook, Doll and Fellingham, 1969; Eyring, Stover and Brown, 1971; Knudson, 1971; and Hirsch, 1974). With few exceptions, investigators have concentrated their attention on adult-onset cancers, mainly carcinomas.

Curiously, the age-dependence of non-malignant diseases has been almost entirely neglected. This is the more intriguing because we find that the laws governing the age-dependence of malignant diseases are indistinguishable from those that govern non-malignant diseases (Burch, 1966, 1968(a), 1969(b), 1970(b); Burch et al., 1972, 1973). Moreover, these same laws apply with equal facility to the age-distribution of malignant and non-malignant diseases with onset in infancy, childhood and adolescence (Burch, 1968(a), 1969(b)). One set of simple premises covers all the diagnostically reliable examples of disorders with a reproducible age-pattern (over 200) that I have investigated so far. Following the dictum of the celebrated Occam I see no purpose in introducing more complicated alternatives.

The neglect of the age-dependence of non-malignant diseases is not wholly surprising. It follows, I suspect, from the ways in which the age-patterns of cancers have been generally interpreted: the same kinds of interpretation cannot plausibly be extended to non-malignant disorders.

The broad features of the age-dependence of many late-onset cancers point to a variety of possible stochastic interpretations. In each of these, two or more random events trigger a process that culminates in malignant change. Usually, the 'random events' have been identified with some form of somatic gene mutation. On the widespread assumption—stigmatized by Smithers (1962) as 'cytologism'—that a cancer grows from a *single* precursor cell, we can easily imagine that a few somatic mutations, affecting a single cell, could initiate a malignant transformation of that cell. Provided we adhere to the notion of a unicentric origin for a cancer, the age-distribution of many adult-onset carcinomas receive, therefore, a satisfactory interpretation.

When we turn to age-specific death-rates, for say, arteriosclerotic and degenerative heart disease, chronic rheumatic heart disease, and many other cardiovascular and cerebrovascular disorders, we discover, somewhat surprisingly, characteristics that closely resemble those for adult-onset carcinomas (Burch, 1963(b), 1974(a)). If we persist with the traditional approaches to the interpretation of cancer statistics, we find ourselves in an awkward dilemma. How can an anatomically extensive, non-neoplastic disorder, involving millions of target cells, arise from a few somatic mutations? This difficulty was recognized and described by Armitage and Doll (1954), who observed that the age-patterns of cerebral haemorrhage, coronary thrombosis and gastric ulcer resemble those of cancers. They found it difficult to believe that the pathogenesis of these non-malignant diseases could be similar to that of cancers, but they left the matter open and proffered no interpretation.

In 1963, I argued that the *stochastic* feature of the interpretation that had previously been given of the age-dependence of adult-onset cancers is valid, and that it is equally relevant to the age-dependence of various degenerative cardiovascular and cerebrovascular diseases (Burch, 1963(b), 1964). I proposed, however, that in these instances of degenerative disease, the random initiating events occur, not in cells of the target tissue—for example, of the heart or vasculature—*but in stem cells of the central system of growth-control.* Adapting Burnet's (1959) forbidden clone theory of autoimmunity (see p. 41), I argued that these various non-malignant degenerative diseases are also autoimmune, or, as I now prefer to call them, *autoaggressive* diseases. That is to say, the random initiating events should be identified with somatic gene mutations in growth-control stem cells: the resulting mutant stem cells propagate forbidden clones of cells. These latter cells, or their secreted humoral products, attack and damage the target tissue. In this way, we can readily understand how a few random events (or only one), occurring, say, in a single stem cell, can give rise to an elaborate sequence of changes and involve an astronomical number of target cells. The growth of the forbidden clone and its pathogenic products can therefore be looked upon as an (unfortunate) example of biological amplification.

Pursuing this new interpretation, and on studying the age-distributions of the hitherto neglected early-onset malignancies, I eventually reached the conclusion that 'natural' malignant diseases are *initiated* by exactly the same kind of mechanism as the non-malignant ones (Burch, 1968(a), 1969(b), 1970(a)). Such a mechanism offers, of course, a ready explanation of the multicentric origin of many cancers (see Chapter 7).

Thus, I have arrived at the somewhat ironical position where I contend that the original interpretations of the age-distributions of adult-onset natural cancers were mathematically correct—in so far as random initiating events were invoked—but were biologically false, because the events were allocated to the wrong class of cells, that is, to target cells, instead of central growth-control cells. Furthermore, I suspect that neglect of the problems posed by the age-distributions of non-malignant diseases was the direct outcome of the false biological assumptions concerning the nature of cancers. Turning concepts upside down can sometimes straighten them out. As a result of this turn-about, a genuinely unified theory of age-dependent disease can be formulated to explain in detail a vast accumulation of *quantitative* evidence—see Chapter 7.

Epidemiological Terms: Definitions

Unfortunately, the terms 'incidence' and 'prevalence' are sometimes used interchangeably and hence clarification is called for. I use *prevalence* to define the proportion of people in a population, at a given date, who are affected (and have been affected) by the disorder in question. (This proportion is sometimes called *point prevalence*.) Frequently, the chance that a person will have a given disease depends on age. *Age-specific prevalence*, or *age-prevalence*, refers to the proportion of people at a given date, in a specified age-group of the population, who are affected (and have been affected) by the disease in question. When sex-differences are found, we have to determine *sex-specific prevalence* and sex-specific and age-specific prevalence for males and females separately.

The terms 'incidence' and 'onset' are often used interchangeably. In view of the confusion between 'incidence' and 'prevalence' it is advantageous to use 'onset' rather than 'incidence' when referring to the first clinical diagnosis of the presence of disease. *Age-specific onset-rate* defines the proportion of people in a population, within a given age-group, who suffer the first onset of a given disease, per unit time (usually one year), over some given period of calendar time. Thus, if in the years 1958 and 1959, an average of 100000 men, aged 30 to 34 years, were alive in a defined population; and if 50 new male cases of disease A arose in that group during 1958 and 1959, then the average age-specific onset-rate of disease A in males aged 30 to 34 years was $50/(100000 \times 2)$, or 250 per million per year. This is a *sex-specific* and *age-specific onset-rate*: statistics for cancer are commonly expressed in terms of cases per 100000 per year.

Occasionally, I use 'incidence' in a non-technical sense—as for example, 'the incidence in relatives'—to mean the 'proportion of relatives affected'.

In some clinical series, the absolute size of the catchment population from which patients are drawn is not accurately defined—it might consist, for example, mainly of the City of Leeds together with some outlying districts of uncertain population size—and hence *absolute* age-specific onset-rates cannot then be obtained. However, in this example, the relative sex- and age-structures of the total population is likely to be very similar to that of the City of Leeds. Accordingly, relative sex-specific and age-specific onset-rates can then be calculated with sufficient accuracy using the known sex- and age-structures of the major part of the total catchment population.

Most diseases, and notably malignant ones, have been progressing some time before symptoms and signs become apparent. The age at which a disease can be said to have 'begun', or to have been 'initiated', depends on one's view of pathogenesis. I use the term *age-specific initiation-rate* in the same general way as age-specific onset-rate except that, in place of onset, I substitute the 'completion of initiation', which is the age at which the last initiating somatic mutation occurred in a growth-control stem cell. This is a theoretical concept and age-specific initiation-rates cannot be observed directly in ordinary, non-experimental, populations. The derivation of age-specific initiation-rate is described later in the chapter.

Earlier Hypotheses of the Age-distribution of Cancer

The early hypotheses attempted to explain the pathogenesis of adult-onset carcinomas. From Muller (1951) onwards, many investigators have observed that, over much of the adult age-range, sex-specific and age-specific onset- or death-rates (dP/dt) from various carcinomas are proportional to about the fifth or sixth power of age (t). (Chapter 7 illustrates the observed relations in detail. At this stage, I shall not distinguish between initiation-, onset- and death-rates, and dP/dt will be used to describe all three.) In mathematical terms we can write

$$dP/dt = a\ t^q, \tag{6.1}$$

where a is constant of proportionality that often differs from one population to another, and q has usually been regarded as being about 5 or 6.

Taking logarithms of both sides, we have

$$\log(dP/dt) = \log a + q \log t \qquad (6.2)$$

Hence, if we plot age-specific onset- or death-rates (dP/dt) on a logarithmic scale, against age at onset (t) on a logarithmic scale, and if the above relation holds, we shall obtain a straight line of slope q.

On the basis of certain plausible assumptions it can readily be shown that equations (6.1) and (6.2) would be obtained if the emergence of a cancer is the consequence of $(q+1)$ random events, each one of which occurs with equal but small probability per unit time, at any stage during life (Fisher and Holloman, 1951; Nordling, 1952, 1953; Stocks, 1953; Armitage and Doll, 1954; Burch, 1965, 1966).

At the outset, no consensus was reached about the biological nature of these random events. Muller (1951), Nordling (1952, 1953), Stocks (1953) and Armitage and Doll (1954) assumed that these random events occur in, or affect, a single cell (any one of many at risk) that becomes malignant when it has accumulated the full complement of random changes. Fisher and Holloman (1951) on the other hand, proposed that a critical colony, or compact group, of six or seven 'cancer cells' has to assemble before autonomous tumour growth becomes possible. Assuming that each 'cancer cell' incorporates a single somatic mutation, they derived equations (6.1) and (6.2), and hence they were able to account for the mathematical properties of the age-statistics of many cancers.

Following a suggestion of Platt (1955), Armitage and Doll (1957) introduced a new model to replace the earlier one (Armitage and Doll, 1954). Arguing that chemical carcinogenesis gives evidence for only two 'stages', *initiation* and *promotion*—rather than the six or seven they and others had postulated previously—they put forward a model that required only two random events for the appearance of a cancer. They proposed that the first random event in a cell is followed by the exponential growth of a clone of cells from that first mutant cell. The growth of a cancer then requires a further mutation in any one of these exponentially growing clonal cells. This two-stage model was able to give a fair fit to various cancer statistics although Ashley (1969(a)) has since shown that data for gastric cancer in women give a better fit to the earlier multistage 'power law' models.

J. C. Fisher (1958) criticized this two-stage model and argued that exponential growth is more characteristic of malignant growth itself than the hypothetical interstage hyperplasia. He considered that, in planar epithelial tissue, the number of mutant cells in a pre-malignant developing clone would be more likely to increase in proportion to the square of time. (The diameter of the disc of mutant cells would therefore increase uniformly with time.) For a model that involves two mutational steps, and an intermediate phase of clonal growth, age-specific initiation rates (dP/dt) would be proportional to t^3: for three mutational steps and two intermediate phases of clonal growth, dP/dt would be proportional to t^6. Proportionality of dP/dt to t^2, t^4, t^5, $t,^7$ t^8, t^{10} or t^{11} . . . could not be interpreted without modifying Fisher's model.

Rate of somatic mutation

A possible objection to the early multistage models of carcinogenesis is the high rates of somatic gene mutation they imply (Burch, 1965). I adapted J. C. Fisher's (1958) model in an attempt to avoid this difficulty and to account for the steep age-dependence of certain malignancies in terms of somatic gene mutation-rates that are similar to those observed in germ cells (Burch, 1965).

If we attempt to explain the steep age-dependence ($dP/dt \simeq t^5$) of chronic lymphatic leukaemia (or, indeed, coronary heart disease) in terms of a six-stage model, we become committed to somatic mutation-rates in excess of $2 \cdot 5 \times 10^{-4}$ per gene at risk per cell at risk per year (Burch, 1965, 1968(a)). Such rates are vastly higher than those that have been estimated for genes in human germ cells. In the units used for somatic mutation-rates, and assuming an average generation time of 30 years, observed germ cell mutation-rates lie between 5×10^{-8} and 4×10^{-6} per gene per gamete per year (Penrose, 1961; Fraser, 1962).

We are therefore confronted with two main alternatives: (a) we can reject the six-stage model and its associated high rates of somatic mutation: this was the course I first adopted (Burch, 1965); (b) we can accept the six-stage model and either ignore the contrast in mutation-rates between germ cells and somatic cells, or attempt to account for it. Latterly, I have accepted the multistage model and proposed a new theory of initiating somatic mutations (Burch, 1968(a), 1969(b)). Curtis (1969) proposed that some, but not all, of the steps in multistage models are mutational in character and Hirsch (1974) has generalized the model.

The discrepancy between the estimates of mutation-rates in germ and somatic cells might arise because, in most instances, the type of mutation scored in germ cells differs from that which occurs in growth-control cells to initiate disease. Estimates of mutation-rates in the germ cells of man have been based mainly on the sporadic emergence of individuals with relatively rare autosomal dominant disorders such as epiloia and Huntington's chorea; or with X-linked recessive disorders such as haemophilia and Duchenne muscular dystrophy (Penrose, 1961; Fraser, 1962). If the mutant genes that predispose to such disorders arise from point mutation—rather than from a DNA strand-switching mutation—the conflict over rates might be resolved.

Why then do we not detect high mutation-rates in germ cells attributable to DNA strand-switching mutations? One answer, I suggest, might lie in the technical difficulty of doing so and in the failure to appreciate the nature of the genetic predisposition to such relatively common autoaggressive diseases as, for example, inflammatory polyarthritis, diabetes mellitus, psoriasis, schizophrenia, Dupuytren's contracture and various carcinomas. Early- and late-onset forms of diabetes mellitus (Burch and Milunsky, 1969), both forms of psoriasis (Burch and Rowell, 1965), and schizophrenia (Burch, 1964(b)), almost certainly involve polygenic predisposition. Moreover, some predisposed persons do not manifest the disease until late in life and others not at all. In other words, the 'penetrance' of such conditions during the normal lifespan often remains incomplete. For these reasons, together with our current inability to identify the carriers of predisposing genes by objective tests, we cannot compare observed with expected segregation-ratios. Consequently, we are unable to calculate the rate at which genes in germ cells mutate to those alleles that predispose to the more common age-dependent disorders. At present, high rates of DNA strand-switching in germ cells would pass unnoticed.

Another answer is simpler. We cannot assume that the average rate of a given DNA strand-switching mutation will be the same in all types of cell. The rate of strand-switching at non-induced MCP–TCF genes in germ cells might well be much less than at induced MCP genes in growth-control cells. Alternatively, a correction mechanism might operate in germ cells.

With these several possibilities in mind, I no longer feel inhibited over accepting the very high rates of somatic mutation (up to $\sim 10^{-3}$ to 10^{-2} per gene per cell per year) demanded by multistage theories of the initiation of autoaggressive, including malignant diseases (Burch, 1968(a)).

As mentioned in the last chapter, observations of the rate of mutation at histocompatibility (MCP–TCF) loci in germ cells of mice point to high rates (Bailey and Kohn, 1965; Silver and Gasser, 1973). Bailey and Kohn found a frequency of mutation to histocompatibility of about 7×10^{-3} per gamete per generation. Uncertainty as to the number of loci at which mutation leads to graft rejection precludes reliable estimation of the average rate per locus. Egorov and Blandova (1972) estimated from their own and Bailey and Kohn's results that the rate at the H-2 locus is about 5×10^{-4}, but a contribution from induced mutations might be included in this value. They concluded that the mutation rate at the H-2 locus is, in any case, much higher than the average expected rate of spontaneous 'visible mutations', which range from about 10^{-6} to 10^{-5} per locus per gamete per generation, depending on the groups of loci tested.

With a typical breeding age of 150 days, the rate of mutation at the H-2 locus in the germ cells of mice ($\sim 10^{-8}$ per gamete per year) approaches the estimated upper limits of somatic mutation rates in man ($\sim 10^{-3}$ to 10^{-2} per gene per cell per year).

The Age-distributions of Malignant and Non-Malignant Autoaggressive Diseases: General Theory

The theory that follows was devised in the first place to explain the age-distributions of autoaggressive non-malignant, non-fatal diseases (Burch, 1966). When I subsequently found that the theory can also be applied to early- and late-onset malignant diseases my view of cancer was transformed (Burch, 1968(a), 1969(b), 1970). I shall here describe first the biological basis of the model, and then its mathematical consequences. In Chapter 7, I shall analyse age-statistics for malignant and pre-malignant diseases in terms of this model.

In general, the *shape* of the age-distribution of a well-defined auto-aggressive disease is found to be reproducibly similar in the populations of different countries and continents, and at different times (Burch, 1968(a), (b), 1969(b); Burch and Rowell, 1968, 1970; Burch, *et al.* 1969, 1973). This invariant property of shape contrasts markedly with the absolute levels of disease, which often differ widely from one population to another. To take the example of gastric cancer in men, the *shape* of the age-distribution is very similar in different countries. Over much of the age-range, age-specific initiation-rates are proportional to $t^6 \exp(-kt^7)$—see Chapter 7. However, in 1960 to 1963, the average age-specific death-rates at (for example) 50 to 54 years of age—in terms of deaths per 10^5 living persons per year—ranged from about 27 in England and Wales, 41 in United States (Caucasians), to 120 in Japan. Obviously, the *shape* of an age-distribution, and the *absolute rates* of onset for any given age-group, are properties that need to be clearly distinguished.

Biological basis

(1) A particular autoaggressive disease is confined to a genetically specific subpopulation that constitutes a fraction, S, of the general population. If the same disease occurs in males and females, the value of S may differ between the sexes. When a subpopulation with an abnormal complement of chromosomes such as Klinefelter's syndrome, or Down's syndrome, can be

delineated, the value of S for that subpopulation may well differ from that for the general population. For some diseases, 100 per cent of a particular population may be at genetic risk: in which case $S = 1$.

(2) A natural autoaggressive disease is initiated by the random occurrence of one or more (r) specific gene mutations in one or more (n) distinctive stem cells. Each distinctive stem cell belongs to a set of L similar growth-control stem cells (see Figure 6.1). The number (L) of stem cells in a set

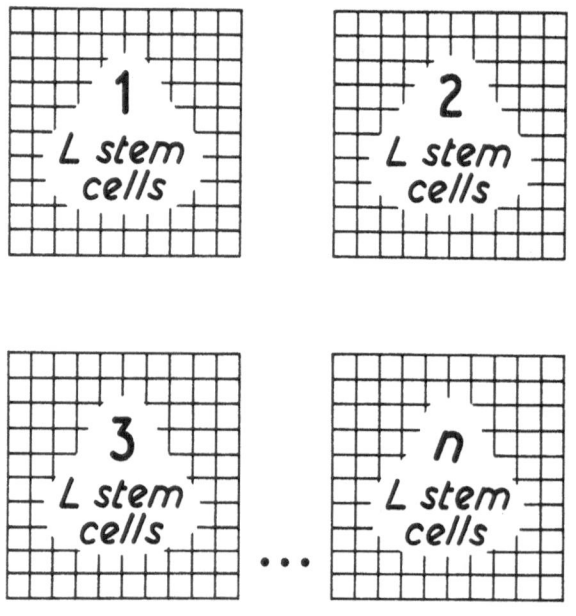

The L stem cells in compartment 1 synthesize
$(MCP)_1$ ... those in compartment n synthesize $(MCP)_n$

Figure 6.1 Outline of model of initiation for autoaggressive disease. In a genetically predisposed person, n distinctive sets of growth-control stem cells, each set containing L cells, are at somatic mutational risk; the process of initiation reaches completion when at least one cell in each of the n sets has acquired r specific somatic gene mutations

remains constant from around birth (generally within about $\pm 0 \cdot 1$ year of birth) to the onset of disease, even when this occurs at the end of the normal lifespan. The values of the integers r (mutations per cell) and n (number of sets of stem cells), are invariant for most specific and narrowly defined autoaggressive diseases in many, if not all, human populations. Where the same nominal disease (for example, acute lymphocytic leukaemia, diabetes mellitus, or psoriasis) occurs in more than one genetically specific sub-population, the values of n and/or r usually (though not always) differ from one subpopulation to the other. If the average rate of occurrence of a specific initiating somatic mutation is m per gene at risk per cell at risk per year, then in ordinary environments, m stays effectively constant from age $t=0$ (at around birth) to the onset of disease. Initiation is measured on a time scale that starts $(t=0)$ with the completion of the induction of the relevant MCP-TCF element. The age at which this occurs is probably not the same for all MCP-TCF elements, but appears usually to be within about ± 0.1 year of birth. Differences in the value of m between genetically dissimilar populations can be expected and are observed (see Chapter 7). (Different rates should be anticipated if a given MCP-TCF gene has slightly different base-sequences in different populations. (I define a kinetic constant $k=Lm^r$, where r has integral values 1, or 2, or 3, . . . etc., depending on the particular disease.

(3) When the full complement of r initiating somatic mutations has occurred in a growth-control stem cell, a forbidden clone of cells may proliferate from the mutant stem cell. In certain diseases, proliferation occurs only when a specific environmental factor—such as a micro-organism, or allergen bearing a particular antigen—is present in the host. The influence of micro-organisms in the classical acute infectious diseases has an all-or-none character; when they are absent, the potentially pathogenic forbidden clone, or clones, remain suppressed; when they are present in the non-immunized host a newly initiated forbidden clone can proliferate (see Chapter 8).

(4) In all diseases, an interval or *latent period* elapses between the occurrence of the last initiating mutation and the first appearance of symptoms or signs. The duration of this latent period can often be affected quantitatively by various environmental factors, notably infective agents, allergens and drugs, and also, perhaps, by severe mental stress. In the class of autoaggressive disease in which mutant T-lymphocytes constitute the primary pathogens, the average latent period in a given environment is twice as long in females as in similarly predisposed males. In the class of autoaggressive disease in which humoral factors ($?\alpha_2$-macroglobulins) act as the primary pathogens, the corresponding latent periods are of equal duration in the two sexes. The form of the distribution of the latent period in natural autoaggressive disease is unknown. In chemical and radiation carcinogenesis (see Chapter 9) the distribution of the age of onset of a tumour with respect to time (τ) after initiation can be described by the general equation 6.12 (page 103). The parameter t is replaced by τ, and an allowance needs to be made for an interval, assumed to be constant, during which the tumour grows from one or n mutant target cells to detectability.

Age-specific Prevalence of Chronic Non-fatal Conditions

If the average overall age-specific mortality-rates in the predisposed sub-population closely resemble those in the general population, both before and after the onset of the chronic condition, and if a single somatic mutation in any one stem cell out of a set of L stem cells initiates the disease, then Poisson statistics are relevant to the age-specific prevalence P_t of the initiated chronic condition at age t (Burch, 1966, 1968(a)). Hence

$$P_t = S\{1 - \exp(-kt)\} \qquad (6.3)$$

In this equation and equations (6.4) and (6.5) below, $r = 1$ and hence $k = Lm$.

If a single somatic mutation in each of n distinctive and independent stem cells is needed to initiate the disease, then, provided the conditions specified above hold, we have

$$P_t = S\{1 - \exp(-k_1 t)\}\{1 - \exp(-k_2 t)\} \ldots \{1 - \exp(-k_n t)\} \qquad (6.4)$$

If $k_1 = k_2 = \ldots k_n = k \ (= Lm)$, we have the Yule equation

$$P_t = S\{1 - \exp(-kt)\}^n \qquad (6.5)$$

Suppose r independent somatic mutations in a single stem cell are needed to initiate a single forbidden clone. Provided $mt \ll 1$ at all t of interest, the average number, $\bar{N}_t$, of cells per person with r specific mutations at age t, will be

$$\bar{N}_t = L \, (mt)^r \qquad (6.6)$$

The actual number, N_t, of cells per person with r specific mutations will have a random (Poisson) distribution and because $L \gg 1$, the average value of N_t at high t may readily exceed unity. Putting $k = Lm^r$, the probability that a predisposed person will have at least one such mutant cell at age t is given by: $1 - \exp(-kt^r)$.

Hence, if the disease is confined to a subpopulation S, the age-specific prevalence, P_t, of people in the general population who have at least one specifically mutant cell, and therefore at least one initiated forbidden clone, will be given by (Burch, 1965, 1966)

$$P_t = S\{1 - \exp(-kt^r)\} \qquad (6.7)$$

If r independent somatic mutations in each of n distinctive stem cells initiate the disease then, for the above provisos

$$P_t = S\{1 - \exp(-kt^r)\}^n \qquad (6.8)$$

Graphs of representative functions described by equations (6.3) to (6.8) are illustrated in Figures 6.2 to 6.4.

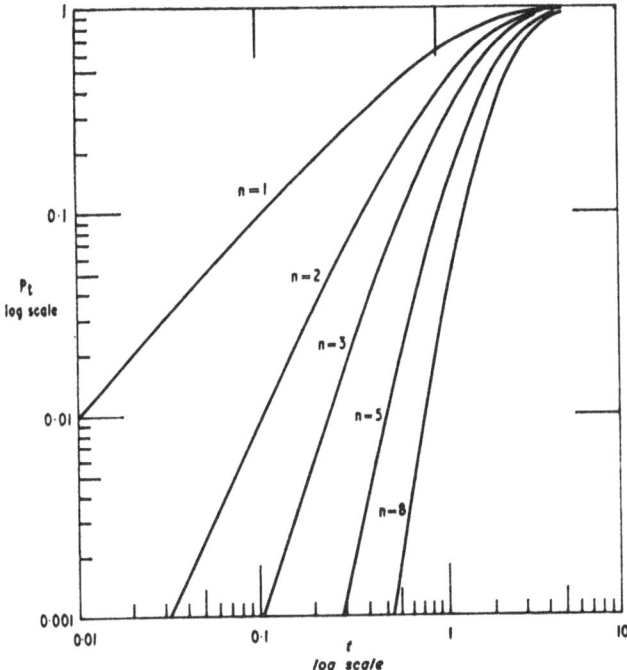

Figure 6.2 Curves of the function: $P_t = \{1 - \exp(-t)\}^n$. Log–log scales. Values for k and S in eqn. 6.5 are put equal to unity. Curves retain the same shape, regardless of the values of k and S. All curves approach $P_t = 1$ as t becomes large. The initial slope of each curve at low t is n

If we plot P_t on a log scale, against t on a log scale, then in Figure 6.2 we find that the slope of log P_t against log t is always n at low values of kt. As kt tends towards, and then exceeds unity, the slope of each curve decreases and eventually, when $kt \gg 1$, the slope tends to zero. In Figure 6.3 we see a somewhat similar behaviour, where an initial slope of r changes to a final slope of zero. However, the transition in slopes is much more abrupt than in Figure 6.2. Figure 6.4 shows a change from an initial slope of nr to a final slope of zero, where the abruptness of the transition (for a given total number of initiating events) is intermediate between that of the curves in Figures 6.2 and 6.3.

One great advantage of using log–log scales for prevalence curves and age-specific initiation curves—equations (6.9) to (6.12)—is that, if we use a consistent grid size, the curve of a given function *remains invariant in size and shape* regardless of the numerical values of k and S. Hence, if these curves are reproduced on tracing paper, then provided the horizontal-vertical alignment of the tracing is maintained, any given position of a

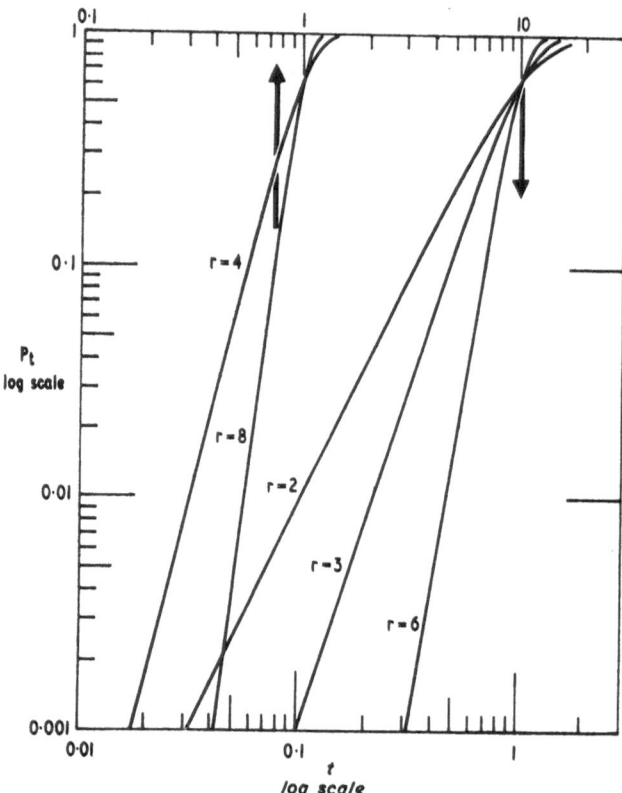

Figure 6.3 Curves of the function: $P_t = 1 - \exp(-kt^r)$. The initial slope of each curve at low t is r, but for $r \geqslant 2$, the transition to zero slope at high t is much more abrupt than for the corresponding curves in Figure 6.2

tracing on the graph paper will represent one version of the appropriate function, with a particular value of k, and a particular value of S. Moving the tracing paper up and down, parallel to the ordinate (P_t or dP/dt), corresponds to a change of S; moving it left and right, parallel to the abscissa, corresponds to a change of k—high values to the left and low to the right. These properties greatly facilitate curve-fitting when using graphical methods (see below).

Age-specific initiation-rates of chronic conditions

We obtain the age-specific initiation-rate, dP/dt, of a non-fatal auto-aggressive disease by differentiating the appropriate prevalence equation. When a single somatic mutation initiates disease we differentiate equation (6.3)

$$dP/dt = k \, S \, \exp(-kt) \tag{6.9}$$

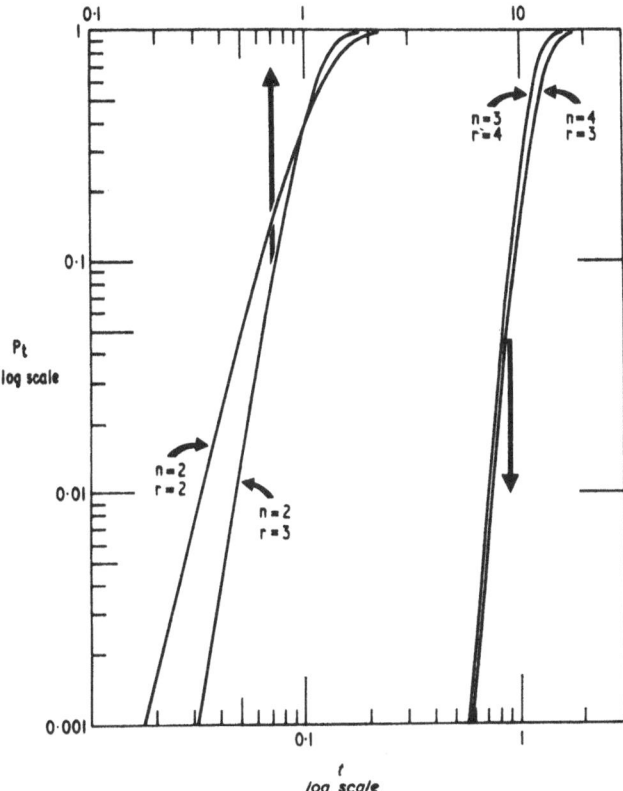

Figure 6.4 Curves of the function: $P_t = \{1 - \exp(-kt^r)\}^n$. The initial slope of each curve at low t is nr. The curve for $n=4$, $r=3$ (right) makes a more gradual transition to zero slope at high t than the curve for $n=3$, $r=4$

For initiation by a single somatic mutation, in each of n distinctive growth-control stem cells, we differentiate equation (6.4)

$$dP/dt = \{n\,k\,S\,\exp(-kt)\}\{1 - \exp(-kt)\}^{(n-1)} \qquad (6.10)$$

This is a Yule or 'homogeneous birth' equation.

For initiation by r independent somatic mutations, in a single growth-control stem cell

$$dP/dt = r\,k\,S\,t^{(r-1)}\exp(-kt^r) \qquad (6.11)$$

This is a Weibull equation; however, in this biological model, r is restricted to positive integers.

Finally, for initiation by r independent somatic mutations, in each of n distinctive growth-control stem cells

$$dP/dt = \{n\,r\,k\,S\,t^{(r-1)}\exp(-kt^r)\}\{1 - \exp(-kt^r)\}^{(n-1)} \qquad (6.12)$$

This general equation includes the special cases represented by equations (6.9) to (6.11).

Graphs of representative functions described by equations (6.10) to (6.12) are shown in Figures 6.5 to 6.7.

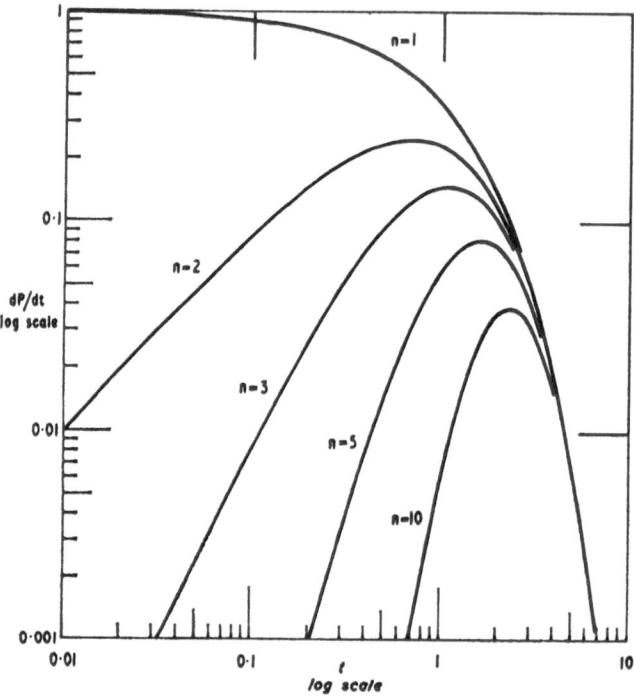

Figure 6.5 Curves of the function: $dP/dt = \{\exp(-t)\}\{1 - \exp(-t)\}^{(n-1)}$. When $n = 1$ we have $dP/dt = \exp(-t)$ which gives a straight line on a log–linear graph but a curve on this log–log graph. The initial slope of each curve at low t is $(n-1)$. At high t, all curves tend to the simple exponential, $dP/dt = \exp(-t)$

Equation (6.9) is a simple exponential function and in this special case, where only one somatic mutation is required to initiate the disease in a predisposed person, age-specific initiation-rates (dP/dt) are best plotted on a log scale, against age (t) on a linear scale. The result is a straight line of slope $-k$. In this instance we are unable to estimate the average latent period λ (except when $\lambda_F = 2\lambda_M$ and we know the relation between S_F and S_M), because the shape of the curve (a straight line) remains invariant with respect to λ. With the exception of this special case (in which $n = 1$, $r = 1$), and another to be considered later, all other curves of dP/dt versus t exhibit a mode. A mode is not always *observed*—at least for age-statistics

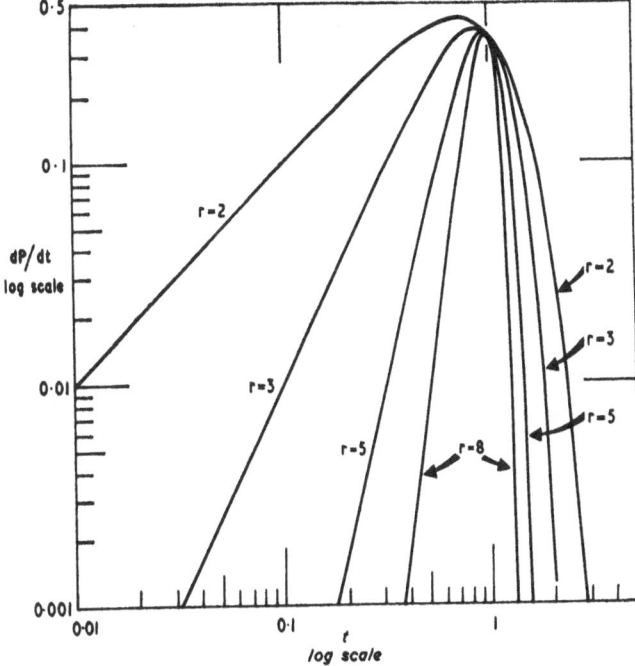

Figure 6.6 Curves of the function: $dP/dt = t^{(r-1)}\exp(-t^r)$. The initial slope of each curve at low t is $(r-1)$

that cut off at, say, 85 years of age—and in a few disorders, such as fractures of the proximal end of the femur in the cervical or trochanteric regions, a graph of log (dP/dt) versus log t shows no deviation from linearity up to 80 years of age (Burch, 1968(a)). When this occurs (because the value of k is relatively low) we are unable to assess values of k or S by curve-fitting.

It will be noticed that, for a given number of initiating somatic mutations, the sharpness of the mode is greatest for equation (6.11) and least for equation (6.10). Needless to say, the ability to interpret observations in terms of a particular theoretical curve, with explicit values of n and r, depends on the accuracy of the observations, the position of the mode, and the extent of the falling limb of the curve.

Age-specific initiation-rates of fatal conditions

Equations (6.9) to (6.12) relate strictly only to chronic, non-fatal diseases in subpopulations in which overall mortality-rates are the same as those in the general population. Mortality is assumed to affect members of the subpopulation and of the general population equally. In other words, the numerator (number of affected persons), and denominator (number of

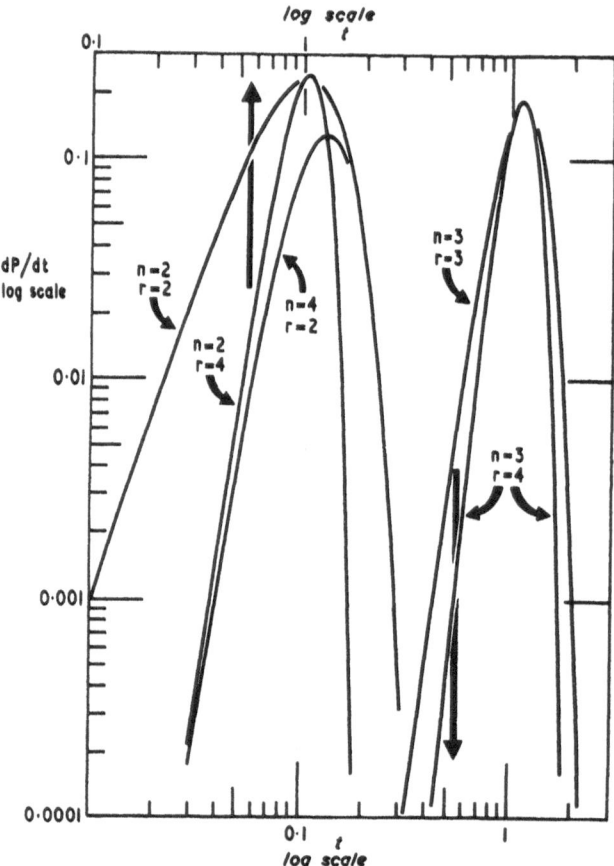

Figure 6.7 Curves of the function: $dP/dt = \{t^{(r-1)}\exp(-t^r)\}\{1-\exp(-t^r)\}^{(n-1)}$. The initial slope of each curve at low t is $(nr-1)$. The distribution for $n=2$, $r=4$ (left) is narrower than for $n=4$, $r=2$

people in population), in calculations of age-prevalence and age specific onset-rates, are assumed to be equally reduced by general mortality. In the case of fatal diseases, equations (6.9) to (6.12) should remain good approximations provided that: (i) the denominator (the size of the general population at age t) is not appreciably diminished by specific mortality in the subpopulation; and (ii) the numerator is not appreciably affected by selective mortality from other diseases that are positively or negatively associated with the subpopulation.

Generally, requirement (i) will be satisfied when $S \ll 1$, or when the penetrance of the fatal disorder at high t is low, regardless of the value of S. The following simple (extreme) example illustrates the distortion that can arise when neither of these latter provisos hold: Consider a disease that is instantly fatal (zero latent period), the kinetics of which conform to the Weibull model, described for non-fatal diseases by equations (6.7) and (6.11). Suppose every person in the population is at risk ($S = 1$) with respect to this fatal disease and that there are no other fatal diseases. Age-specific death-rates (which we shall now describe by dD/dt) give the number of deaths per unit time per surviving member of the population. At age t, the proportion of survivors is $(1 - P_t)$. Assuming a zero latent period

$$dD/dt = \{r \, k \, t^{(r-1)}\exp(-kt^r)\}/(1 - P_t) \qquad (6.13)$$

From equation (6.7)

$$dD/dt = r \, k \, t^{(r-1)} \qquad (6.14)$$

In this highly artificial model, age-specific death-rates remain proportional to $t^{(r-1)}$ and show no mode—statistical fluctuations apart—so long as some members remain alive.

Taking the more general case (with $n > 1$, $r > 1$, $S < 1$); assuming the average mortality from all diseases other than the one of interest is the same in the predisposed (S) and the general populations, we have, assuming a zero latent period

$$dD/dt = \{n \, r \, k \, S \, t^{(r-1)}\exp(-kt^r)\}\{1 - \exp(-kt^r)\}^{(n-1)}/(1 - P_t) \quad (6.15)$$

where $P_t = S\{1 - \exp(-kt^r)\}^n$.

Unfortunately, we are ignorant, as yet, about the details of positive and negative associations between different fatal diseases—except that such associations are common—and hence we cannot assume *a priori* that equation (6.15) will be relevant to a particular disease. To judge from observed mortality statistics for malignant diseases (see Chapter 7), it appears that inappreciable error arises if we treat the factor $(1 - P_t)$ as being effectively unity up to the highest age-groups. Hence, in most practical situations, we can regard the general equation (6.12) as giving a good approximation to age-specific initiation-rates for fatal malignant diseases.

To the non-mathematician, equation (6.12) may appear rather formidable. Our objective, however, is to formulate a theory with the simplest *biological* premises that are consistent with the evidence. The biological premises of equation (6.12) could scarcely be simpler: an autoaggressive disease is initiated in a genetically predisposed person, through r specific somatic gene mutations occurring randomly, in each of n independent growth-control stem cells. To date, this simple model appears to characterize adequately most, and perhaps all, well-defined diseases in man that have reproducible age-distributions.

Curve-fitting

If the initiation of a cancer could be observed directly, curve-fitting would be straightforward. We are presented, however, with sex-specific and age-specific onset-rates or death-rates from authorities such as cancer registries and the Registrar General for England and Wales. Accordingly, we have to correct for the latent period between initiation and onset, or initiation and death. Unfortunately, this cannot be done by rigorous mathematical methods because we are unable, as yet, to assess how latent periods are distributed in natural carcinogenesis. For the unavoidably non-rigorous curve-fitting I have found that graphical methods yield internally consistent results and provide a plausible interpretation of the initiation phase of carcinogenesis. A trial-and-error procedure can be applied to the majority of age-distributions to estimate an effective average latent period λ. This procedure depends on the fact that, on a logarithmic scale, an interval of ten years, say, occupies much more distance along the abscissa at low t than at high t.

Using graphical methods, if we overcorrect onset- or death-rates for latent periods, then the resulting points for age-specific initiation-rates will diverge progressively from the theoretical curve as we go from high t to low t: the overcorrected points will diverge above the theoretical curve and the discrepancy will be largest at lowest t. Conversely, if we undercorrect for latent periods, the subsequent points will lie beneath the theoretical curve, and the error will again be largest at lowest t. (Only one value of the latent period will yield a straight line at low t.) We aim to apply a correction that produces no systematic deviation of the points from the theoretical curve as we shift from high t to low t. This trial-and-error procedure works satisfactorily when we have an uncomplicated curve, with only one predisposed subpopulation, and adequate numbers at low t. Unfortunately, these conditions are not always satisfied, and when they are not, appreciable errors in estimates of latent periods may well arise. But fortunately, most reasonable values for the latent period correction have only a slight effect on the shape of the curve at high t. Except when the values of n, and/or r are high, and the accuracy of the statistics is low, graphical analysis often gives an unambiguous interpretation of the integers n and r.

In several non-malignant conditions and for polycythaemia vera (Figure 7.83), I have found that the only difference between the age-patterns in men and women is a 2 : 1 ratio in the average latent periods, with $\lambda_F = 2\lambda_M$. The magnitude of the latent periods and age-specific initiation-rates for both sexes are then easily assessed, because the curve of prevalence (or onset-rates or death-rates) for women lags behind the corresponding curve for men by an amount λ_M (Burch, 1964(b), 1968(a)). If after subtracting λ_M from the.

age at onset in men, and $\lambda_F(=2\lambda_M)$ from the age at onset in women, the resulting points fit one of the above stochastic equations, then interpretation is unambiguous. The existence of the relation $\lambda_F=2\lambda_M$ is of great theoretical importance, because when it applies, we find that λ_M and λ_F stay effectively constant from the age of 10 years, and perhaps earlier, to the end of the lifespan (Burch, 1968(a)). If intrinsic defence mechanisms contribute to the duration of λ_M and λ_F we can conclude that their efficiency changes little, or not at all, with age.

Some comment must be made about the values of S calculated from cancer statistics. If a cancer registry recorded the onset of a specific cancer in every affected individual within an accurately defined population; if initiation were invariably followed by onset; and if onset-rates were constant with time, then the resulting age-specific onset-rates could be analysed to give an accurate estimate of S for that population. Obviously, reliable diagnosis, completeness of registration, and precise definition of the sex- and age-structures of the population at risk are essential to accurate estimates of S. Similar considerations, together with some additional ones, apply when mortality statistics are analysed. Here, however, we are confronted with the further problem of survival between initiation and death. If the average interval (latent period) is long—as it is for several cancers—then some patients with an initiated cancer will die of another disease. Also, in the event of spontaneous regression, or cure, uncorrected mortality statistics will lead to an underestimate of S.

It follows from the preceding discussion that all estimates of S, based on either registry or death statistics, need to be treated with caution. Such estimates can only give the proportion of the population that, at birth, was at risk with respect to *recorded* onset or death from the disease in question.

Cancer Statistics: Cohort and Temporal Changes

Before cancer registries were established, evidence for the age-dependence of cancers came mainly from mortality statistics. Clinical and pathological series have provided useful information on a smaller scale. Even now, mortality statistics provide the largest numbers and the most comprehensive information about the geographical distribution of cancers. Nevertheless, mortality statistics have some obvious shortcomings where the theoretician is concerned. At the time of death, several diseases might be present, and it can be difficult to decide which was the actual cause of death. Also, a patient can develop a cancer but might be cured and die of another disease. In any event, the interval (latent period) between initiation and onset is shorter than that between initiation and death. Factors that reduce the size of the latent period corrections are welcome when we try to derive age-specific initiation-rates.

Errors of diagnosis and reporting, and different conventions of diagnosis, classification and reporting, will often be common both to onset- and death-rates. When death is followed by an adequate necropsy the most reliable diagnosis will be obtained. Errors in the size of the population at risk will affect both types of statistics. Random errors arising from small numbers will sometimes be larger in onset-, than in mortality-data, because certain cancer registries do not cover the whole population of a country. Incompleteness of registration is, perhaps, more likely to affect onset- than mortality-data.

Special problems arise when age-specific onset- or death-rates change with secular time. These become particularly complicated when, over one part of the age-range we find a decline with time, and over another part we find an increase (see Chapter 10).

Statistics are generally published in 'vertical' or 'cross-sectional' form: that is to say, age-specific onset- and death-rates at all ages generally refer to a particular calendar year. We can, however, fix our attention on the fate of people born, say, in a given year, or quinquennium, or decade, and determine age-specific onset- or death-rates throughout life for this particular cohort (Case, 1956(a). (b)). Longitudinal (cohort) analysis has been regarded by some as having greater validity than vertical studies. Of course, when age-specific rates are constant with time, both types of analysis yield the same result. Which method (if any) is preferable when rates change with time depends, however, on the cause(s) of the temporal trends and the objectives of the analysis.

Suppose the proportion (S) of the population predisposed to a given disease changes with time because gene frequencies drift. Then, if other time-dependent changes are absent, cohort or longitudinal studies would be needed to determine the value of S at a given date. (If S could be determined by, say, direct tests for specific MCPs and TCFs, corrections could be applied to vertical data.) In large populations, and in the absence of catastrophies and extensive immigration and/or emigration, abrupt changes of S with time are extremely unlikely, although slow drift is an inevitable concomitant of evolutionary change.

A much more common form of temporal change is that connected with diagnostic accuracy, due to the introduction of new techniques such as diagnostic x-rays, fibre optics, etc. Criteria and fashions of diagnosis also change and tend to affect all age-groups, although not necessarily to the same degree. They can occur relatively rapidly. In these circumstances, and with constant S, vertical studies will yield the correct *shape* of an age-distribution when underdiagnosis that is independent of age is involved, although the inferred value of S will be too small. When overdiagnosis is implicated, the resulting errors in the age-statistics will depend on the relative contributions of the different disease components.

The impact of an environmental carcinogen will depend on so many factors, such as the number of people exposed, sex, age, mode of action, and duration and intensity of exposure, that general comment serves little purpose. Problems of temporal (secular) change are described in Chapter 7, also in Chapter 10 where I consider at length the interpretation of statistics for lung cancer.

Conclusion

From the foregoing discussion I may have given the impression that the reliability of cancer statistics is so dubious, and the complications are so numerous, that no useful biological conclusions could possibly be drawn from them. When we actually examine the sex- and age-statistics for cancers in detail—as we shall in Chapter 7—we gain a somewhat different impression. For a given type of cancer, we find an astonishing degree of reproducibility in the fundamental parameters of the age-patterns, n and r, as we shift from country to country. Generally, the fit of age-statistics to the simple model described above, as judged by graphical analysis, is unexpectedly good. This form of analysis has about the right degree of accuracy and refinement for our present purposes and it is the one that has been widely adopted hitherto. Several minor approximations are involved, but a mathematically rigorous analysis is precluded because of the lack of precise information about the distribution of the latent period, and of associations between one fatal disease and another. Parameters n and r, because they are integers, can often be assessed exactly; values of k and S can usually only be estimated approximately and an objective measure of their errors is at present unattainable. Despite these limitations I believe that analyses of the age-distributions of malignant and pre-malignant conditions afford us a profound insight into the biology of cancer.

CHAPTER 7

Malignant Diseases: Sex- and Age-dependence, Genetics and Pathology

Percival Pott discovered the vulnerability of chimney sweeps to cancer of the scrotum in 1775. Since then, many have cherished the hope that the study of cancer incidence in relation to particular occupational, environmental, geographical and temporal factors might disclose the nature of carcinogenic agents. The connections found between ionizing radiations and disease in man, especially leukaemia; between aromatic amines and cancer of the bladder; and between asbestos fibres and lung cancer, represent outstanding successes for the epidemiological approach (Goldblatt, 1958). In Chapter 10, I discuss at length the association between cigarette smoking and cancer, especially lung cancer.

Using Cancer Statistics in Assessment of Cancer

The use of cancer statistics to aid the search for environmental carcinogens serves prophylactic objectives and therefore enjoys great prestige and popularity. It is a consequence of the widespread belief that exogenous agents cause the great majority of cancers. But as we saw in the last chapter, the relation of age-specific death-rates to age has inspired various theoretical approaches to the phenomenon of carcinogenesis. It is axiomatic that any hypothesis of carcinogenesis must be consistent with the age-distribution of cancer. Empirical regularities, such as the simple power-law relations referred to in the last chapter, invite interpretation. These relations, or the more precise alternatives considered in this chapter, have some kind of analogy with Kepler's empirical laws of planetary motion. Most theoreticians however, have not been content with a mere mathematical description of the regularities: they have also felt an urge to *explain* them in biological terms. To pursue the analogy with mechanics, a Newtonian synthesis ought to follow the Keplerian empiricism.

At the explanatory level we might maintain that, although the general features of age-distributions point to stochastic rate-determining mechanisms, they cannot help us to understand the biological and molecular aspects of carcinogenesis. In my view, an unimaginative attitude of this kind does scant justice to the remarkable and challenging features of the age-dependence, not only of malignant, but also of non-malignant diseases. Nevertheless, nagging questions persist: To what extent can we treat cancer statistics at their face value? Feinstein's (1968) discussion of the problems of diagnosis shows the need for caution (see also Chapter 10). Are the basic properties of age-dependence described in Chapters 5 and 6 genuine properties, or are they unreal idealizations? Are we being tricked by a gigantic series of highly repeatable artefacts? These questions can be answered in part by intensive and extensive studies of recorded age-dependence using diverse sources, but also, and perhaps more convincingly, by testing the predictions of theories that derive from the analysis of age-dependent disease. In this chapter, I show that theory is consistent not only with the observed age-dependence of many malignant diseases in man, but also with familial, genetic and pathological findings.

A major hazard of cancer statistics for the theorist—in addition to diagnostic error—is the heterogeneity within diagnostic categories, many examples of which will be encountered in this chapter. Ideally, whenever clear-cut clinical, pathological, histological, genetic, cytogenetic, immunological or biochemical distinctions can be drawn between groups within a given diagnostic category, the sex- and age-distributions for each group should be determined separately. When distributions exhibit effectively the same values of n, r and k, they can be combined; but when significant differences in any one or more of these parameters emerge, we can be confident we are dealing with biologically distinctive disorders. Different growth-control elements should be implicated, with distinguishable MCPs or TCFs. It does not follow, of course, that when the same values of n, r and k are obtained, we are necessarily dealing with biologically identical entities, but our conclusions about the values of these parameters will apply to each of the forms of the disease that can be distinguished on other grounds.

For the main types of malignancy, national mortality statistics are presented by age, crude site and sex, but they usually fail to discriminate between carcinomas and sarcomas, and between tumours at a given site that can sometimes be distinguished on clinical, pathological, histological, or other grounds. Some of these deficiencies are rectified in the statistics published by the Swedish Cancer Registry (1971) for the onset of tumours during the period 1959–1965. Where appropriate, I have availed myself of these more detailed statistics.

Fortunately, analysis of age-dependence is sensitive to certain kinds of heterogeneity. When the modal ages of age-specific onset-rates, or death-rates, for distinctive groups are well separated, a small contribution from an early-onset group can readily be detected in the presence of a large contribution from a late-onset group. However, when the age-dependence of distinctive groups is similar, but not quite identical, errors of interpretation will arise. Doubtless, errors of this kind are present in this chapter. The proffered interpretations should be regarded as hypotheses in need of further verification.

To avoid bias in the selection of data I have, where possible, relied primarily on mortality statistics for the four years 1960 to 1963 inclusive, from three populations: England and Wales, Japan and United States (Caucasian). These data are taken from the compilations of Segi and Kurihara (1964, 1966). The populations from which the data are drawn are large, and for most sites the reliability of diagnosis should be reasonably high. A wide range of environments is represented, especially within the United States, whereas Japan provides evidence for a distinctive genetic group.

For certain categories presented by Segi and Kurihara (1964, 1966): 'malignant neoplasms of the buccal cavity and pharnyx', 7th International Classification of Diseases (ICD) 140 to 148; 'malignant neoplasms of the breast', 7th ICD 170; and 'malignant neoplasms of the skin', 7th ICD 190 to 191; the heterogeneity of the types of cancer included within the single category has precluded age-analysis from mortality statistics. In several instances where numbers are adequate, and prognosis is good—giving a long interval, on average, between onset and death—I have been able to use data for onset from cancer registries. To illustrate or elucidate particular features, I have sometimes exploited special investigations.

In the interests of brevity, only important references to familial and genetic evidence will be quoted.

Analysis of Age-statistics for Malignant Neoplasms, by Sex and Site

National mortality statistics, as abstracted by Segi and Kurihara (1964, 1966), are presented in terms of 5-year age-groups, 0–4, 5–9, 10–14 years, etc., up to the highest age-group of 85 years and above. Strictly, these data should be plotted as histograms. To avoid this cumbersome form of presentation I have plotted the data as points, at a particular value of t, the estimated age at initiation. The point value of t is obtained from the midpoint of the age-group, minus a correction for latent period.

Consider the example of the age-group 40 to 44 years inclusive, of midpoint 42·5 years. If I apply a latent period correction of 3 years to allow for the interval between the end of initiation and death, the age-specific death-rate for this age-group is plotted as a point at $t = 39·5$ years. That is to say, an average age-specific death-rate for the age group 40 to 44 years, is treated in this example as an age-specific initiation-rate (dP/dt), at an initiation age t, of 39·5 years. Data for onset-rates are treated similarly: the latent period correction then refers to the interval between the end of initiation and onset.

Except when the slope of a curve of $\log (dP/dt)$ versus $\log (t)$ over an age-group is ± 1 or 0, some error is involved in approximating average rates to the midpoint. The error is generally small, especially at high t, and it will not seriously distort interpretation.

Data for men are symbolized by squares and those for women by circles; when the data for men and women are combined, triangles are used. A number next to a point represents the number of deaths (mortality statistics), or of cases (incidence or onset data). When error limits are shown, these are calculated from $N \pm \sqrt{N}$, where N is the number of deaths or cases.

In this chapter I attempt to characterize the major types of cancer in terms of the number of somatic gene mutations per forbidden clone, and the number of forbidden clones, that initiate the neoplastic process. Throughout, I interpret age-distributions in terms of my general theory of growth and disease. Thus, in every instance, I assume r initiating somatic mutations occur spontaneously in one or more (n) cells of the central system of growth-control of a predisposed person. As we shall see, almost all the epidemiological statistics and the pathological evidence are consistent with this simple assumption. A few apparent exceptions arise as the result, probably, of diagnostic error. Occasionally, ambiguities of interpretation are encountered because certain curves characterized by different values of n and r have similar shapes over a restricted range of t.

For each type of tumour I summarize, in tabular form, the parameters n, r, k and S used to fit the age-distributions shown in the accompanying figures. It will be recalled that k is a kinetic constant defined as Lm^r, where L is the number of growth-control stem cells at risk with respect to the formation of each of the n forbidden clones, and m is the average rate of occurrence, per stem cell, per year, of each of the r initiating somatic mutations; and S is the proportion of the population that appears to be at genetic risk with respect to recorded death (or onset) for the particular malignancy in question.

It will be appreciated that the values calculated for these several parameters depend on the accuracy of the input data; the reservations described in Chapter 6 need to be borne in mind.

Malignant Neoplasms of the Pancreas (7th ICD 157)

Cancer of the pancreas appears to be confined, in the main, to single groups of males and females that are homogeneous with respect to the kinetics of initiation (see Figures 7.1 to 7.4). Almost all the histologically verified cases in Sweden, 1959 to 1965, were described as 'adenocarcinoma'. Only 1·1 per cent came under the headings 'undifferentiated carcinoma', 'carcinoid' or 'sarcoma'. However, some 33 per cent of male cases and 30 per cent of female cases were not verified histologically.

In the data from England and Wales, and US Whites, the estimated modal age of initiation in men is about 85 years, and in women about 89 years. If these differences are genuine (which is doubtful—see below) they indicate that the average rate of initiation in women is lower than in men, or perhaps, that survival from carcinoma of the pancreas in old women is better than in old men. Survival statistics from California (1942 to 1956) for those aged 75 years and over show a slight advantage in favour of women, 7·3 per cent of whom survive one year, as opposed to only 2·9 per cent of men (Cancer Tumor Registry, 1963). This small advantage cannot account for the difference of about four years in the modal age of initiation but another factor might contribute: women who are genetically predisposed to cancer of the pancreas might be less susceptible to death from other diseases in old age, than corresponding men. When the mode occurs above the age of 80 years it is poorly defined. In Japan, however, the modal age of initiation occurs at 70 years in both sexes, and hence the rates of initiation are virtually identical in the two sexes. From the Swedish registry statistics, which are free from the complications of duration of survival, rates of initiation also appear very similar in both sexes, the modal age of initiation being at about 82 years for men and women.

From Table 7.1, we see that all the parameters for cancer of the pancreas in males and females in England and Wales are almost identical to the corresponding ones for US Whites. About 3 per cent of men, and 2–3 per cent of women, appear to be predisposed in these countries, whereas only about 0·6 per cent of men and 0·4 per cent of women are predisposed in Japan. These differences contrast with the findings for gastric cancer (see later) which is more common in Japan than in the Western countries. However, both for cancer of the pancreas and late-onset cancer of the stomach, the rates of initiation in Japan appear to be much higher than in

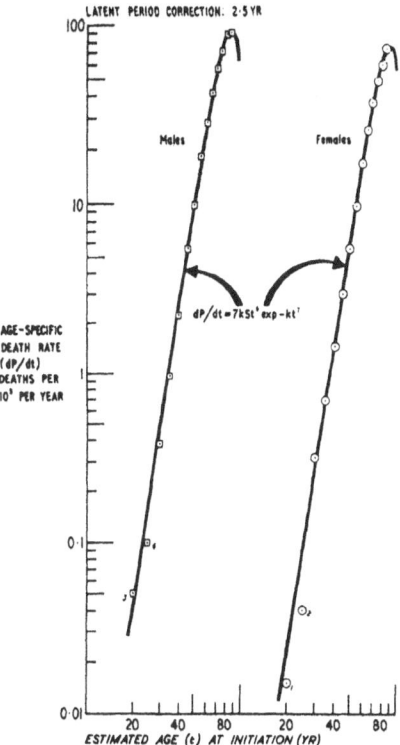

Figure 7.1 Sex-specific and age-specific death-rates from malignant neoplasms of the pancreas, England and Wales, 1960–63, in relation to estimated age at initiation (Segi and Kurihara, 1966)

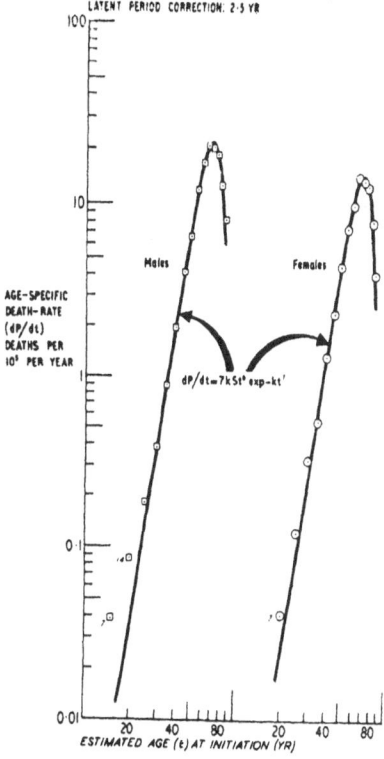

Figure 7.2 As for Figure 7.1. Data for Japan, 1960–63. For parameters describing the theoretical curves, see Table 7.1

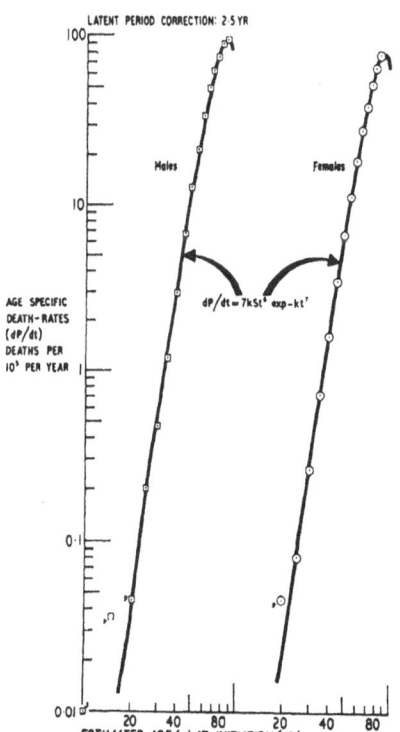

Figure 7.3 As for Figure 7.1. Data for US Whites, 1960–66

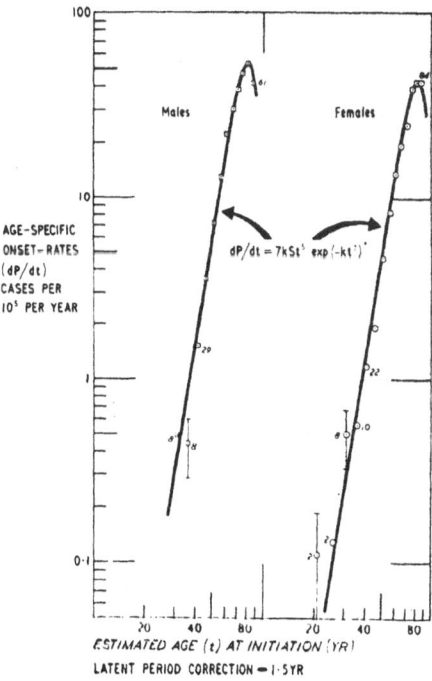

Figure 7.4 Sex-specific and age-specific onset-rates for adenocarcinoma of the pancreas, Sweden, 1959–65, in relation to estimated age at initiation (Swedish Cancer Registry, 1971). See also Table 7.1

Table 7.1 Malignant Neoplasms of the Pancreas

Population	Males ($n=1, r=7$)		Females ($n=1, r=7$)	
	k	S	k	S
Mortality statistics 1960–63				
England and Wales	$2\cdot7\times10^{-14}$ yr^{-7}	$3\cdot1\times10^{-2}$	$1\cdot9\times10^{-14}$ yr^{-7}	$2\cdot6\times10^{-2}$
Japan	$1\cdot0\times10^{-13}$ yr^{-7}	$6\cdot0\times10^{-3}$	$1\cdot0\times10^{-13}$ yr^{-7}	$3\cdot9\times10^{-3}$
US White	$2\cdot7\times10^{-14}$ yr^{-7}	$3\cdot1\times10^{-2}$	$1\cdot9\times10^{-14}$ yr^{-7}	$2\cdot7\times10^{-2}$
Onset statistics				
Verified adenocarcinoma Sweden 1959–65	$3\cdot4\times10^{-14}$ yr^{-7}	$1\cdot7\times10^{-2}$	$3\cdot4\times10^{-14}$ yr^{-1}	$1\cdot34\times10^{-2}$

Latent period corrections: 2·5 years (mortality statistics)
1·5 years (onset statistics)

England and Wales and US Whites. Values of S_M and S_F for Sweden refer only to verified cases of adenocarcinoma.

A steady increase in overall death-rates from cancer of the pancreas has been reported over the period 1950 to 1963, in each of the four populations considered here. These trends might be expected to distort the age-patterns as determined in vertical (cross-section) analysis; this depends, however, on the cause of the secular increase (see below and Chapter 10). In certain instances—see, for example, malignant neoplasms of the stomach (page 123) —opposite secular trends are observed in different populations. Nevertheless, vertical data for each population yield the same age-pattern. Thus, in these instances, at least, it appears that vertical analysis gives a biologically meaningful age-pattern despite the complication of secular trends.

Heredity

Although the age-distribution of cancer of the pancreas points clearly to a genetic predisposition, I have been unable to find reports of genetic or familial studies except for its occasional appearance in 'cancer families' (Lynch, 1967). However, carcinoma of the pancreas appears to associate with adenoma of the parathyroid. In a series of 241 patients with parathyroid adenoma, four had carcinoma of the pancreatic ducts and another four had carcinoma of the pancreatic islets (Kaplan *et al.*, 1971). In another series of 23 patients with parathyroid tumours, ten had neoplasms in other organs, including one patient with pancreatic islet cell carcinoma (Samaan *et al.*, 1974). This type of association is likely to have a genetic basis.

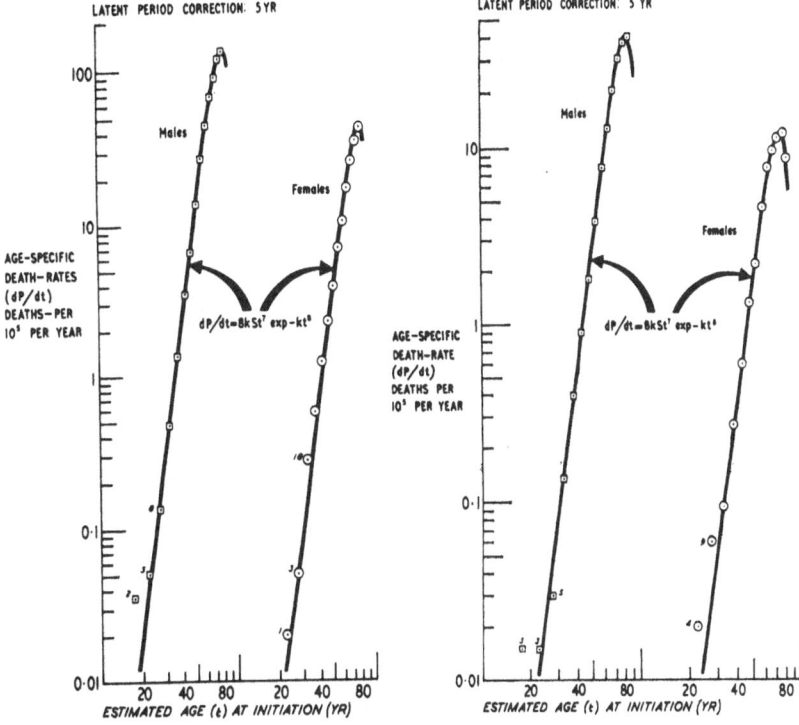

LATENT PERIOD CORRECTION: 5 YR

AGE-SPECIFIC
DEATH-RATES
(dP/dt)
DEATHS-PER
10⁵ PER YEAR

Males

Females

$dP/dt = 8kSt^7 exp-kt^8$

ESTIMATED AGE (t) AT INITIATION (YR)

Figure 7.5

LATENT PERIOD CORRECTION: 5 YR

AGE-SPECIFIC
DEATH-RATE
(dP/dt)
DEATHS PER
10⁵ PER YEAR

Males

Females

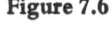
$dP/dt = 8kSt^7 exp-kt^8$

ESTIMATED AGE (t) AT INITIATION (YR)

Figure 7.6

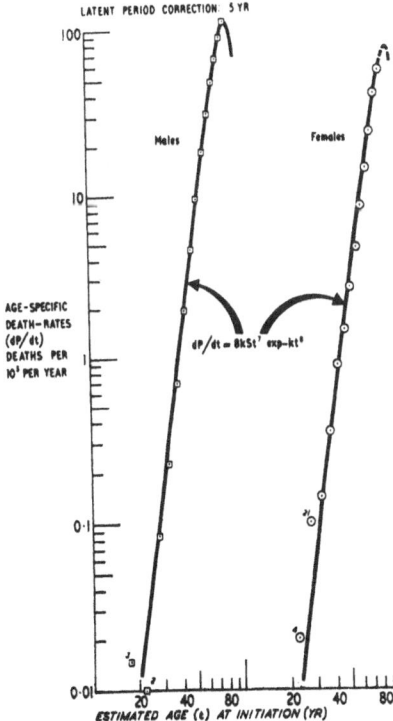

LATENT PERIOD CORRECTION: 5 YR

AGE-SPECIFIC
DEATH-RATES
(dP/dt)
DEATHS PER
10⁵ PER YEAR

Males

Females

$dP/dt = 8kSt^7 exp-kt^8$

ESTIMATED AGE (t) AT INITIATION (YR)

Figure 7.7

Figure 7.5 Sex-specific and age-specific death-rates from malignant neoplasms of the bladder and other urinary organs, England and Wales, 1960–63, in relation to estimated age at initiation (Segi and Kurihara, 1966). For parameters describing the theoretical curves see Table 7.2

Figure 7.6 As for Figure 7.5. Data for Japan, 1960–63

Figure 7.7 As for Figure 7.5. Data for US Whites, 1960–63

Malignant Neoplasms of the Bladder and Other Urinary Organs (7th ICD 181)

Fatal malignant neoplasms of the bladder and urinary organs appear to be confined to a group that is homogeneous with respect to the kinetics of initiation (see Figures 7.5 to 7.7). However, the mode occurs at high t and is poorly defined. As with cancer of the pancreas, cancer of the bladder is much more common in the two Western countries than in Japan.

In US Whites, the crude mortality-rates have been effectively constant over the period 1950 to 1963, at a level of just over six cases per 10^5 per year (males) and between 2·5 and 2·9 per 10^5 per year (females). A slight upward

Table 7.2 Malignant Neoplasms of the Bladder and Urinary Organs

Population	Males ($n=1, r=8$)		Females ($n=1, r=8$)	
	k	S	k	S
Mortality statistics 1960–63				
England and Wales	$4\cdot3\times10^{-16}$ yr^{-8}	$3\cdot7\times10^{-2}$	$4\cdot3\times10^{-16}$ yr^{-8}	$1\cdot2\times10^{-2}$
Japan	$4\cdot3\times10^{-16}$ yr^{-8}	$1\cdot1\times10^{-2}$	$9\cdot7\times10^{-16}$ yr^{-8}	$3\cdot1\times10^{-3}$
US White	$3\cdot5\times10^{-16}$ yr^{-8}	$3\cdot3\times10^{-2}$	?$1\cdot7\times10^{-16}$ yr^{-8}	?$2\cdot4\times10^{-2}$

Latent period correction = 5 years

trend can be seen in the crude rates in England and Wales (8·2 to 10·1 in males; 3·3 to 3·9 in females). A much more marked upward trend is seen in the Japanese statistics: 0·81 to 1·72 in males and 0·49 to 1·03 in females. (The units are per 10^5 per year.) Despite the substantial differences in these secular trends it will be seen from Figures 7.5 to 7.7 that all the data fit the same basic stochastic equation, with $n=1$ and $r=8$. It is exceedingly improbable, therefore, that the upward trends of death-rates in England and Wales, and Japan, can be attributed to a secular change in the true value of S, the fraction of the population that is genetically predisposed. Such changes would produce different degrees of distortion of the age-patterns in different countries.

In the Swedish Registry statistics for onset (1959–65), 96 per cent of tumours in the category ICD 181 were of the bladder. Some 22 per cent of tumours were described as 'papilloma of uro-epithelium', although it is stated that the borderline between papilloma and carcinoma is difficult to define (Swedish Cancer Registry, 1971). The age-dependence of these papillomas is less steep than that of the carcinomas; the age-patterns show irregularities that may well reflect, in part, the difficulty of differential diagnosis and they are not illustrated here.

Heredity

Morganti *et al.* (1965(b)) found four cases of carcinoma of the bladder in the relatives of 160 probands, and two in the relatives of age-matched controls. A much larger study is needed to test for significant familial aggregation. Fraumeni and Thomas (1967) described a family in which a father and three sons all had malignant tumours of the bladder: the mother died of metastatic adenocarcinoma of the colon. No common exposure to chemical carcinogens could be implicated.

Malignant Neoplasms of the Stomach (7th ICD 151)

At low *t* (below 25 years) we see from Figures 7.8 and 7.11 a clear indication of a contribution from an early-onset group of males in the Japanese and Swedish populations and in Figure 7.10 a suspicion of a very small, but corresponding contribution, in the data for US Whites.

The modal age of initiation for late-onset groups of males is about 80 years in England and Wales, 74 years in Japan, 90 years in US Whites and 82 years in Sweden. These differences cannot be explained by random errors and it is noteworthy that the data at high *t*—above 50 years of age, where departure from linearity becomes increasingly marked—fit the theoretical curves accurately, although the position of the mode differs from country to country. The close agreement with theory of all data from *t* = 50 years and upwards, suggests that systematic errors in the diagnosis and reporting of this cancer do not change markedly with age. Cook *et al.* (1969) concluded that the decrease in slope at high *t* is not in general an artefact due to under-diagnosis in the elderly. In this instance, 'clinical experience', which predicted a progressive underestimation of incidence with increasing age, seems to have been an unreliable guide (Cook *et al.*, 1969). Where lung cancer is concerned (see Chapter 10) marked overdiagnosis has occurred in the highest age groups in recent years, but this type of error is exceptional. Differences in the composition of populations at high *t*, arising in part from selective mortality from other diseases in the subpopulation predisposed to gastric cancer, could lead to differences in the position of the mode. If the theoretical requirements (see Chapter 6) for the validity of Equation 6.11 are not met, then the extent of the discrepancies might well differ from one population to another. The proportion of males at risk with respect to late-onset gastric cancer is so large (about 0·15 in Japan) that the approximate correction factor $(1 - P_t)^{-1}$ that allows for the distortion of the age-structure of the

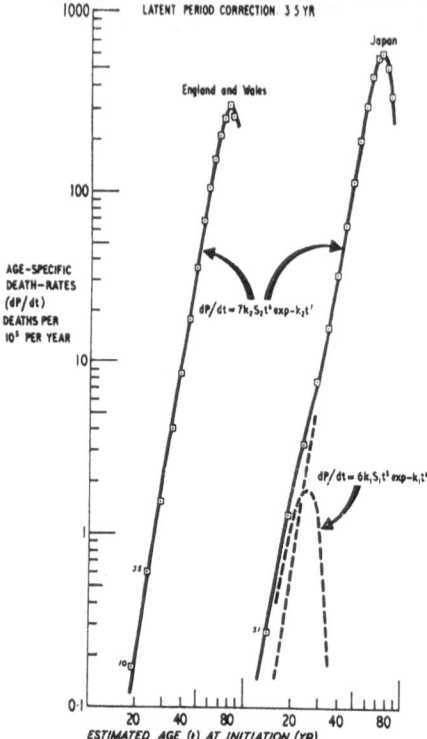

Figure 7.8 Age-specific death-rates (males) from malignant neoplasms of the stomach, England and Wales, 1960–63 (left panel) and Japan, 1960–63 (right panel), in relation to estimated age at initiation (Segi and Kurihara, 1966)

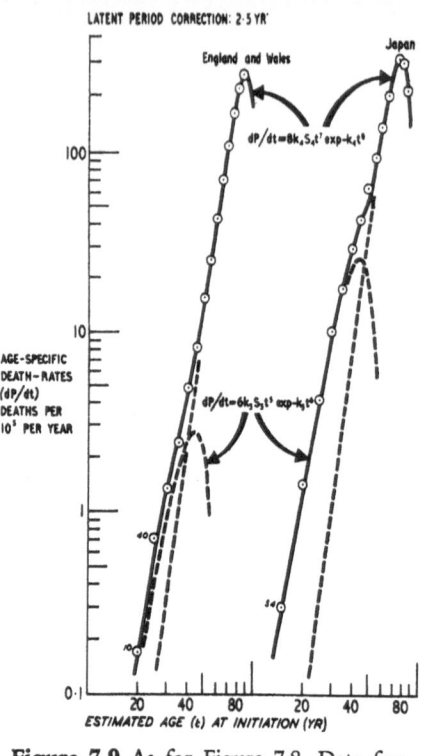

Figure 7.9 As for Figure 7.8. Data for women. See also Table 7.3

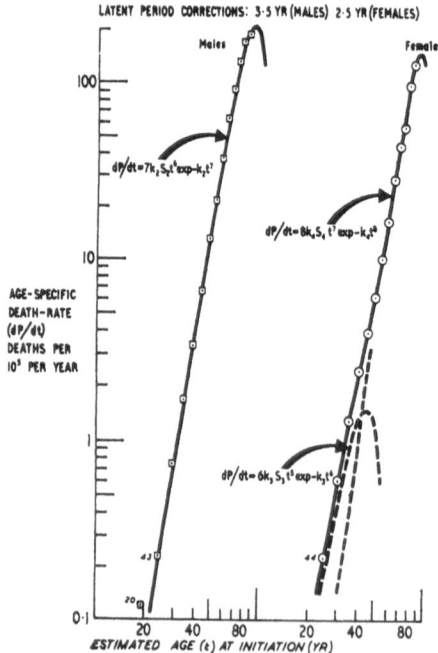

Figure 7.10 Sex-specific and age-specific death-rates from malignant neoplasms of the stomach, US Whites, 1960–63, in relation to estimated age at initiation (Segi and Kurihara, 1966). See also Table 7.3

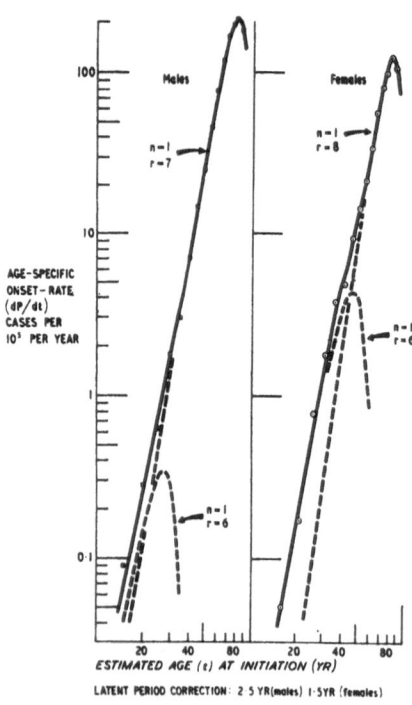

Figure 7.11 Sex-specific and age-specific onset-rates for adenocarcinoma of the stomach, Sweden, 1959–65, in relation to estimated age at initiation (Swedish Cancer Registry, 1971)

general population (see Equation 6.13) will be appreciable at high t. However, this source of distortion will tend to raise the modal age for the Japanese data relative to that for England and Wales, US and Swedish data. Selective mortality from other positively associated diseases in the subpopulation at risk would have the opposite effect. Because of these several uncertainties, the value of k cannot be derived reliably when the modal age occurs at high t.

Data for women, from all four countries, reveal two clearcut groups (Figures 7.9 to 7.11). Both groups differ kinetically and genetically from the male groups. The modal age of initiation for the early-onset group is very similar in all four populations: about 44 to 46 years. In the late-onset group, interpopulation differences appear in the modal age at initiation, roughly in line with those for men. These are about 87 years in England and Wales, 75 years in Japan, 91 years in US Whites and 83 years in Sweden.

It should be noted that the onset data for Sweden (Figure 7.11) relate only to adenocarcinoma verified cytologically and/or at necropsy with histological examination. Some 7414 males and 4355 females came into this category out of a total of 10 410 male and 6169 female cases of stomach cancer; 2906 male and 1741 female cases were not assigned to a histological type. The proportions of the Swedish population predisposed to cancer of the stomach (all kinds) will therefore be greater than those given in Table 7.3.

Secular trends

Of special interest are the secular changes of recorded death-rates from gastric cancer. In males of all ages in England and Wales, the crude rates fell steadily from 38·3 per 10^5 per year in 1950–51, to 34·0 per 10^5 per year in 1962–63; in the same units, the corresponding decrease for females was from 28·5 to 24·5 (Segi and Kurihara, 1966). A steady decline was also reported in US Whites, where the corresponding rates for males fell from 20·0 to 12·0, and for females, from 11·7 to 7·4. In Japan, however, the corresponding recorded rates climbed from 47·2 to 57·3 (males), and from 28·9 to 35·1 (females). In Sweden, crude rates for males fell from 43·2 per 10^5 per year in 1952–53 to 39·3 (same units) in 1962–63; for women the corresponding rates fell from 33·6 to 23·8 (same units).

Despite these contrasting secular trends, we see that the data for all four countries fit the same basic stochastic equations. The changes in reported mortality-rates cannot therefore be caused by secular changes in the true value of S, the proportion of the population that is genetically predisposed. A continuous fall in S with time in England and Wales, the United States and Sweden would distort the age-pattern in a direction opposite to that caused by a rise in S in Japan. Evidence for this distortion is absent. These secular

Table 7.3 Malignant Neoplasms of the Stomach

Population	Males				Females			
	Early-onset $(n=1, r=6)$		Late-onset $(n=1, r=7)$		Early-onset $(n=1, r=6)$		Late-onset $(n=1, r=8)$	
	k_1	S_1	k_2	S_2	k_1	S_1	k_2	S_2
Mortality statistics 1960–63								
England and Wales	?	?	4×10^{-14} yr^{-7}	$8 \cdot 2 \times 10^{-2}$	$1 \cdot 2 \times 10^{-10}$ yr^{-6}	$5 \cdot 5 \times 10^{-4}$	$2 \cdot 7 \times 10^{-16}$ yr^{-8}	$7 \cdot 8 \times 10^{-2}$
Japan	3×10^{-9} yr^{-6}	$2 \cdot 1 \times 10^{-4}$	7×10^{-14} yr^{-7}	$1 \cdot 5 \times 10^{-1}$	$1 \cdot 2 \times 10^{-10}$ yr^{-6}	$5 \cdot 3 \times 10^{-3}$	9×10^{-16} yr^{-8}	$8 \cdot 1 \times 10^{-2}$
US White	?	?	$1 \cdot 8 \times 10^{-14}$ yr^{-7}	$6 \cdot 4 \times 10^{-2}$	$1 \cdot 0 \times 10^{-10}$ yr^{-6}	$3 \cdot 1 \times 10^{-4}$	$1 \cdot 9 \times 10^{-16}$ yr^{-8}	$4 \cdot 6 \times 10^{-2}$
Onset statistics								
Verified adenocarcinoma Sweden, 1959–65	2×10^{-9} yr^{-6}	4×10^{-5}	4×10^{-14} yr^{-7}	$6 \cdot 5 \times 10^{-2}$	8×10^{-11} yr^{-6}	$9 \cdot 2 \times 10^{-4}$	$4 \cdot 4 \times 10^{-16}$ yr^{-8}	$3 \cdot 4 \times 10^{-2}$

Latent period corrections: 3·5 years, men, 2·5 years, women (mortality statistics)
2·5 years, men, 1·5 years, women (onset statistics)

changes show that the true value of S, the proportion of a population that is genetically predisposed to a specific form of gastric cancer, cannot be obtained accurately from analysis of these data.

It follows from these and many other statistics, that cohort (horizontal) analysis would give one form of age-distribution for one country, and a mathematically very dissimilar one for a country that showed an opposite secular trend in death-rates. I find, however, that vertical (cross-sectional) analysis gives a generally high degree of invariance of the shape of age-patterns for this and many other cancers. This striking consistency can hardly be accidental. It greatly limits the range of tenable hypotheses of secular change. One obvious hypothesis concerns the level of diagnosis. Whenever changes in recorded mortality-rates with time are due to changes in the accuracy of diagnosis, cohort analysis will always give a spurious indication of the kinetics of pathogenetic mechanisms in predisposed persons. When errors are due to underdiagnosis, then provided the degree of error is effectively independent of age, vertical analysis will reveal correctly the kinetics of pathogenetic mechanisms although the value of S will be underestimated. Other hypotheses of secular change will be discussed in Chapters 8 and 10.

Heredity

Many workers have concluded from studies of populations, families, twins and ABO blood-groups that genetic factors predispose to gastric cancer, although no accepted scheme of inheritance has emerged. In the light of the complexity revealed by the analysis of age-distributions this is scarcely surprising. Evidence for familial aggregations and genetic factors has been reviewed by Koller (1957), Graham and Lilienfeld (1959), McConnell (1966) and Lynch (1967); and described in original reports by Mosbech and Videbaek (1950), Videbaek and Mosbech (1954), Ashley and Davies (1966), Maddock (1966) Ashley (1969(b)), Lee (1971), Glober *et al.* (1971) and Creagan and Fraumeni (1973). This last report describes an inbred kindred in which twelve members of a family developed stomach cancer over four generations. Age at death ranged from 53 to 81 years. 'Recessive' (homozygous) inheritance at one or more autosomal loci might contribute to the genetic predisposition, but the differences in age-patterns between men and women imply that sex-linked factors are also involved.

In an ingenious study, Ashley and Davies (1966) and Ashley (1969(b)) showed that the high susceptibility to stomach cancer in Wales is associated with 'Welshness'—as indicated by surnames and the use of the Welsh language—rather than with residential area. They concluded that the enhanced susceptibility of Welsh people should be attributed to genetic factors.

A negative association between cancer of the stomach and colorectal cancer has been observed between many different communities (Haenzel and Dawson, 1965), and within a community by comparing the observed and expected frequency of individuals with primaries at both sites (Cook, 1966). Howell (1973) has shown that, depending on the choice of communities and countries, positive, negative and neutral relationships can be demonstrated between the death-rates for stomach and colonic cancers among the different communities. To account in genetic terms for the negative association *within a community*, we have to assume that one or more of the alleles predisposing to gastric cancer are negatively associated with one or more of those that predispose to colorectal cancer. To account for the 'inconsistency' in the intercommunity findings, we need to assume that the frequency of the other predisposing alleles, and/or their associations, differ from one population to another.

It should be mentioned that in Cook's (1966) study of multiple primaries he tested the following null hypothesis: when one cancer has occurred in a patient, the prevalence of a second cancer at another anatomical site is the same as the prevalence of that cancer when it occurs as a first cancer. A positive correlation was deemed significant if the observed number of second cancers exceeded the expected number at the level $P < 0.05$. A negative correlation was regarded as significant if the observed number of second cancers fell below the expected number at the level $P < 0.01$. However, some 561 site-to-site comparisons were made and hence many apparently 'significant' positive and negative associations would have arisen by chance alone. This type of study involves various other complications, but with appropriate precautions it has great potential for exploring the associations between different primaries.

Many investigators have found a raised frequency of blood group A in association with gastric carcinoma: the earlier literature has been reviewed by van Wayjen and Linschoten (1973). These latter authors studied in Holland 874 patients with gastric carcinoma and they found that the extent of the increase in frequency of blood group A differed with the site of the cancer. The increase above each of four control populations was highest for cancer of the antrum, intermediate for cancer of the corpus and least for cancer of the cardia and fundus.

The association of gastric carcinoma with blood group A is neither simple nor universal. Southwestern American Indians are predominantly (80 per cent) of blood group O. Nevertheless their incidence of gastric carcinoma is similar to that of non-Indians in the same region, and the frequency of blood group O in Indians with gastric carcinoma is also 80 per cent (Sievers, 1973). This suggests that in certain populations one or more of the MCP–

TCF genes that predispose to gastric cancer have a positive association with blood group A, but that in other populations the association is neutral.

Malignant Neoplasms of the Esophagus (7th ICD 150)

Certain of the data for cancer of the esophagus are highly anomalous. Thus, the data for US White males (Figure 7.14), cannot be fitted by a small number of basic equations, with plausible values of n and r. In the England and Wales female population (Figure 7.12), we see a marked excess of recorded death-rates above the theoretical curve at $t = 55$ years and below. A similar excess is seen in the data (Figure 7.13) for Japanese women. From $t = 30$ to $t = 80$ years for US White men, and below $t = 70$ years for US White women (Figure 7.14), we see a fluctuating excess of death-rates above the theoretical curve. However, in the Swedish Registry statistics (Figure 7.15) for verified cases of the similarly age-dependent adenocarcinoma (107 M, 63 F), squamous carcinoma (649 M, 370 F) and undifferentiated carcinoma (166 M, 88 F) combined, this type of discrepancy is absent. (Only two cases—1 M, 1 F—of sarcoma were reported but 114 male and 82 female cases were unspecified.) Apart from two wild points in the data for men at 60 to 64 years and 80 to 84 years, the fit to the theoretical curves is good.

The discrepancies in the mortality data almost certainly reflect diagnostic error. Willis (1960) reported a study of 1000 consecutive hospital necropsies at the Alfred Hospital, Melbourne, during the period July 1936 to December 1944. A clinical diagnosis of malignant disease had been made, or malignant disease had been discovered *post mortem*. The final diagnosis was established histologically by Willis or an associate. Where carcinoma of the esophagus was concerned, eight false–positive and 12 true diagnoses were found. Four of the eight false–positives were cases of carcinoma of the stomach.

If discrepancies arise mainly from confusion between cancer of the stomach and of the esophagus, then we might expect to see marked discrepancies in Figures 7.8 to 7.10 between recorded death-rates from cancer of the stomach and the theoretical curves. In fact, discrepancies appear to be small. However, cancer of the stomach is much more common than cancer of the esophagus and hence a small proportion of stomach cases transferred to the esophageal diagnosis introduces a relatively large error in the latter. To take the example of statistics for women in England and Wales 1960–63, the average recorded death-rate from cancer of the stomach in the age-group 40 to 44 years was 4·8 per 10^5 per year, whereas the corresponding rate for cancer of the esophagus was only 0·96 per 10^5 per year. The estimated error in the latter rate (from Figure 7.12) is about 0·46 per 10^5 per year; this represents less than 10 per cent of the rate for cancer of the stomach, but

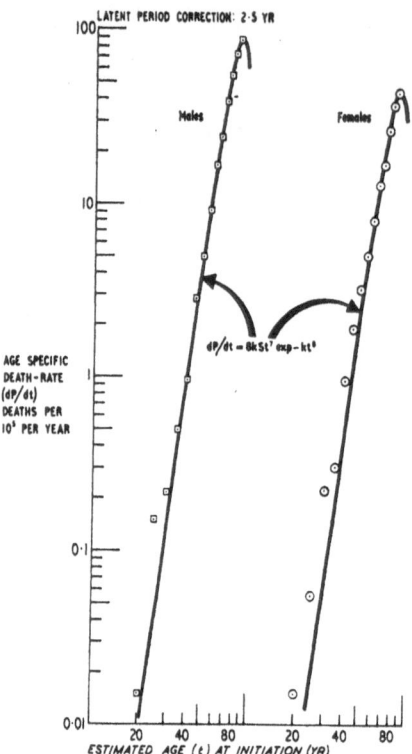

Figure 7.12 Sex-specific and age-specific death-rates from malignant neoplasms of the esophagus, England and Wales, 1960–63, in relation to estimated age at initiation (Segi and Kurihara, 1966)

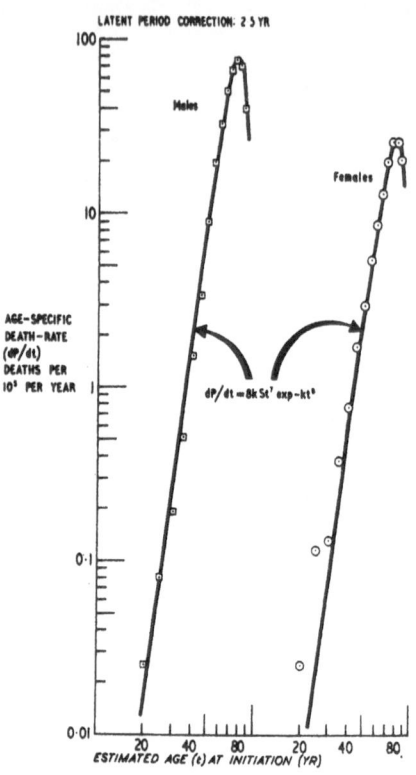

Figure 7.13 As for Figure 7.12. Data for Japan, 1960–63. See also Table 7.4

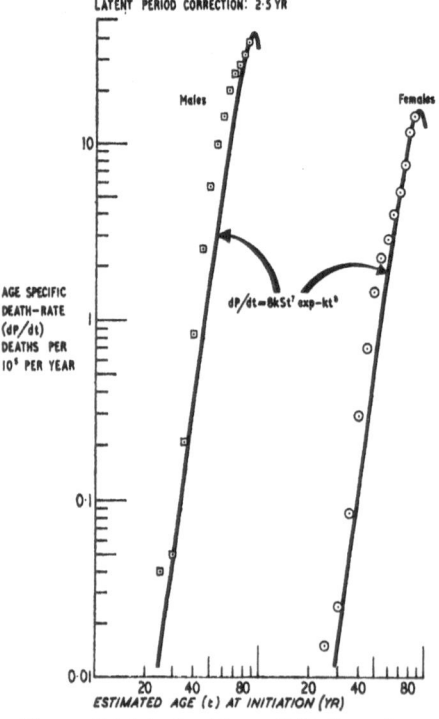

Figure 7.14 As for Figure 7.12. Data for US Whites, 1960–63

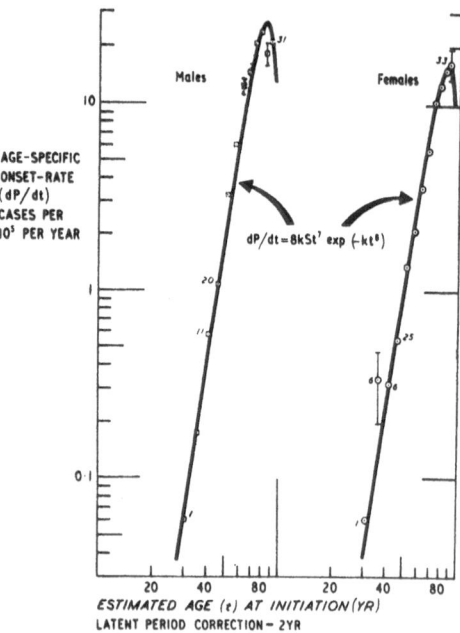

Figure 7.15 Sex-specific and age-specific onset rates for verified cases of adenocarcinoma, squamous carcinoma and undifferentiated carcinoma of the esophagus Sweden, 1959–65, in relation to estimated age at initiation (Swedish Cancer Registry, 1971)

92 per cent of the rate for cancer of the esophagus.

Although death-rates at high t show internal consistency, and appear to be fairly reliable in England and Wales, and Japan, the accuracy of k and S will, of course, depend rather critically on the extent of diagnostic error at high t.

If dietary carcinogens are of major importance we might expect to find a simple connection between death-rates from carcinoma of the esophagus and those for carcinoma of the stomach. From Tables 7.3 and 7.4 we see,

Table 7.4 Malignant Neoplasms of the Esophagus

Population	Males $(n=1, r=8)$		Females $(n=1, r=8)$	
	k	S	k	S
Mortality statistics 1960–63				
England and Wales	2.9×10^{-16} yr^{-8}	2.5×10^{-2}	2.9×10^{-16} yr^{-8}	1.3×10^{-2}
Japan	7.9×10^{-16} yr^{-8}	2.0×10^{-2}	6.4×10^{-16} yr^{-8}	7.2×10^{-3}
US Whites	2.0×10^{-16} yr^{-8}	1.3×10^{-2}	2.0×10^{-16} yr^{-8}	4.7×10^{-3}
Onset statistics				
Verified adenocarcinoma, squamous carcinoma and undifferentiated carcinoma, Sweden 1959–65	4.9×10^{-16} yr^{-8}	7.4×10^{-3}	4.9×10^{-16} yr^{-8}	4.3×10^{-3}

Latent period corrections: 2·5 years, mortality statistics
2·0 years, onset statistics

however, that the calculated values of S for gastric cancer are consistently higher in Japan than in England and Wales, whereas the reverse relation holds for cancer of the esophagus.

Heredity

Ashley (1969(a)) concluded that genetic factors are responsible for the raised susceptibility of Welsh people to esophageal carcinoma and that an X-linked gene or genes might be implicated. Pour and Ghadirian (1974) reported a remarkable familial aggregation: one Iranian pedigree, involving two first-cousin marriages, contained 13 members (over three generations) who died from cancer of the esophagus.

A rare autosomal dominant form of late-onset (~ 5 to 15 years of age) keratosis palmaris et plantaris (tylosis) is associated with carcinoma of the esophagus (Howel-Evans *et al.*, 1958; Shine and Allison, 1966). Howel-Evans *et al.* (1958) estimated that the risk of death from carcinoma of the esophagus in this syndrome is about 96 per cent by 65 years of age. If this estimated high degree of penetrance is correct, then the form of esophageal cancer associated with tylosis differs from that which makes the overwhelming contribution to national onset and mortality statistics.

Malignant Neoplasms of the Prostate (7th ICD 177)

Cancer of the prostate has the distinction of being the most steeply age-dependent of the common malignancies affecting men. The Swedish Registry statistics for 1959–65 show that almost all the verified cases (99·8 per cent) were adenocarcinoma: however, the histological type of some 29·1 per cent of cases was not specified.

Interpretation of the curve of $\log (dP/dt)$ versus $\log (t)$ in terms of n and r is difficult because it departs only slightly from linearity towards the end of the lifespan (Figure 7.16 to 7.19). Up to $t = 70$ years, dP/dt is approximately proportional to t^{11} (Figure 7.18b). Mortality statistics (Figures 7.16 and 7.17) hint at, but do not clearly define, a mode. Onset statistics, involving a smaller latent period correction (about 2·5 years as against 5 years) have a slight advantage over mortality statistics, inasmuch as some series show a mode. Data from cancer registries are graphed in Figures 7.18a, b and 7.19: some of those from the Birmingham registry (Figure 7.18b), covering an (unspecified) 6-year period, are included in the England and Wales data in Figure 7.18a. The Birmingham registry data generally, have the great advantage of extending the age-groups to 85 to 89 years, 90 to 94 years and 95+ years, but the numbers of cases of cancer of the prostate in the two highest groups are only 19 and 1 respectively (Waterhouse, 1974). In Figure 7.18b, the Birmingham data are fitted to the general equation 6.12 with $n = 3$, $r = 5$ in the left panel; and $n = 1$, $r = 12$ in the right panel. The rising limb (with large numbers) is better fitted by $n = 3$, $r = 5$; but the falling limb (with small numbers) is better fitted by $n = 1$, $r = 12$. The other registry and mortality data, which are almost or quite devoid of the falling limb, are fitted to the equation with $n = 3$, $r = 5$. At high t, one of the conditions for the strict applicability of the general equation 6.12, that is $(1 - P_t) \simeq 1$, is violated by some of the data. This violation is not apparent: the curves show the same shape regardless of the value of S, and hence other effects, such as selective mortality in the predisposed population, may cancel the expected distortion.

Recorded mortality-rates for Japanese men are about ten times lower than the corresponding rates for England and Wales and US Whites. The Japanese data are contrasted, in Figure 7.17, with those for Belgium, a country with very high rates. (The scale of dP/dt for the Belgian statistics is

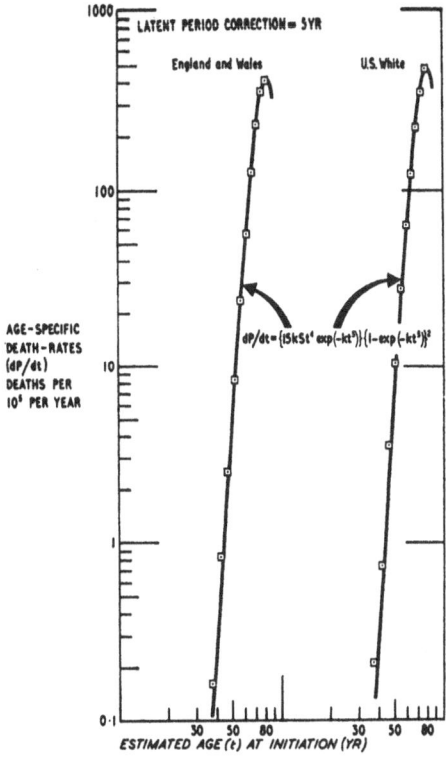

Figure 7.16 Age-specific death-rates from malignant neoplasms of the prostate, England and Wales (left panel) and US Whites (right panel), 1960–63, in relation to estimated age at initiation (Segi and Kurihara, 1966). See also Table 7.5

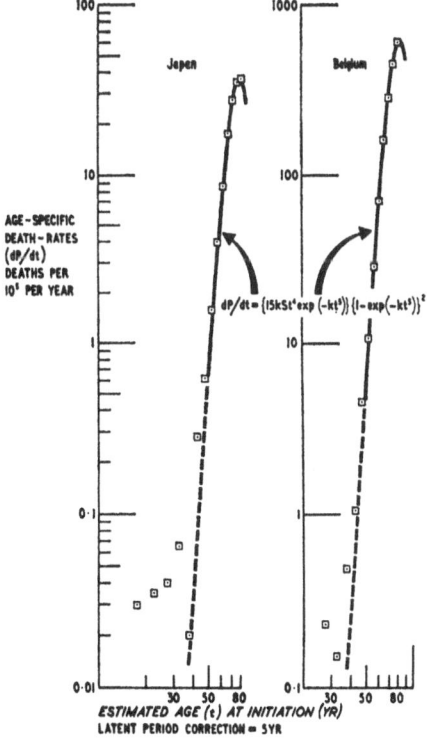

Figure 7.17 As for Figure 7.16. The ordinate for the Belgian statistics (right panel) is raised by one decade relative to that for the Japanese statistics (left panel)

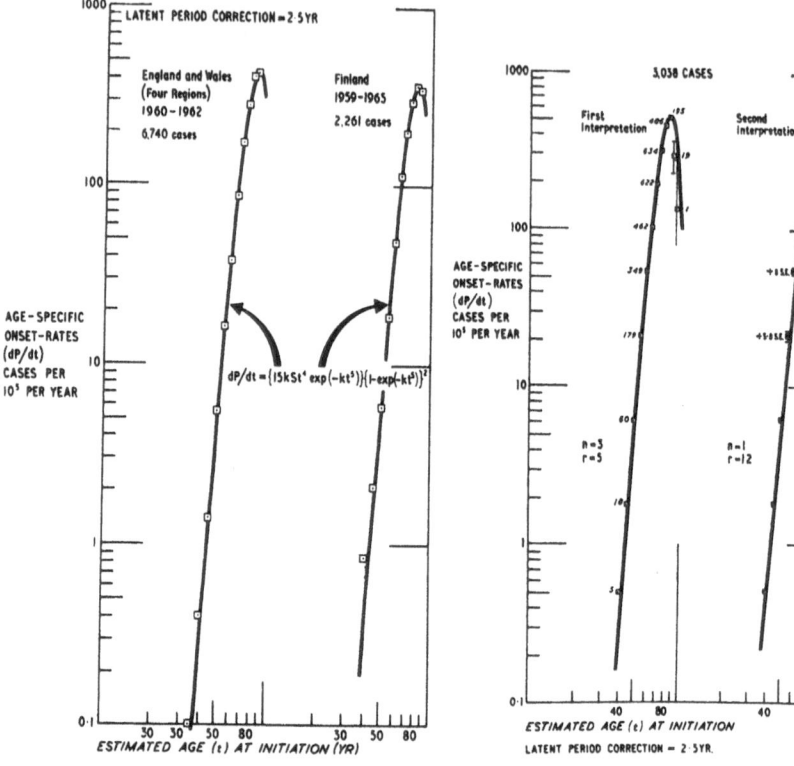

Figure 7.18a

Figure 7.18b

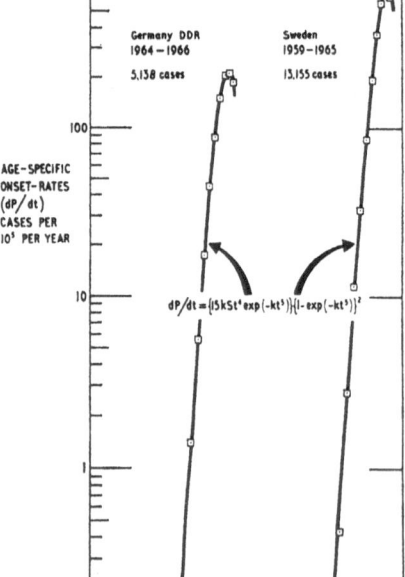

Figure 7.19

Figure 7.18a Registry statistics for age-specific onset-rates of malignant neoplasms of the prostate, England and Wales, 1960–62 (left panel) and Finland, 1959–65 (right panel), in relation to estimated age at initiation (Doll *et al.*, 1966, 1970)

Figure 7.18b Birmingham Regional Cancer Registry statistics (included in part in Figure 7.18a, left panel) fitted to the equation with $n = 3$, $r = 5$ (left panel) and to $n = 1$, $r = 12$ (right panel) (Waterhouse, 1974)

Figure 7.19 As for Fig. 7.18a. Data for German Democratic Republic, 1964–66 (left panel) and Sweden, 1959–65 (right panel) (Doll *et al.*, 1966, 1970)

displaced upwards by one decade relative to that for the Japanese statistics.) A large change in death-rates with time has been recorded in Japan. Crude rates (all ages) increased from 0·26 per 10^5 per year in 1950–51, to 1·25 per 10^5 per year in 1962–63. The corresponding changes for England and Wales are, in the same units, 14·5 to 16·7 and for US Whites, 15·3 to 15·8. Despite the large differences in the secular trends, the shapes of the age-patterns remain very similar. Most sets of mortality statistics show occasional deaths below 35 years of age and, as in Figure 7.17, the observed values of dP/dt in this age range are well above the theoretical curve. (Values for England and Wales and US Whites in this age-range are less than 0·1 per 10^5 per year.) If these occasional early-onset cases are genuine primary malignancies of the prostate they must differ genetically from the majority of late-onset cases.

The coincidence in the values of k and S derived from: (a) mortality statistics for England and Wales; and (b) registry statistics for four regions of England and Wales, demonstrates a satisfactory consistency between similar, though not quite identical, populations.

If three forbidden clones ($n = 3$, $r = 5$) are required to initiate clinical carcinoma of the prostate, then we would expect to find evidence of pre-malignant change. The phenomenon of 'latent carcinoma of the prostate' has been described by Franks (1954). He found this condition in 36 per cent of men aged 70 years and above, and in 70 per cent of those aged 80 years and above. In a study of autopsy records, Berg et al. (1971) found that 5·3 per cent of men aged 70 years and above had latent cancer of the prostate, although only a single section of each prostate was examined. On the basis of these observations, the connection between latent carcinoma of the prostate and overt carcinoma is not clear, because, even in the high-incidence countries Belgium and Sweden (see Table 7.5), less than 20 per cent of men appear to be at genetic risk with respect to the diagnosis of prostatic cancer. Either most cases of latent carcinoma of the prostate as recognized at autopsy are unconnected with clinically overt carcinoma, or latent carcinoma of the prostate arises from one and/or two forbidden clones, and more males are genetically predisposed to this condition than the fully malignant disease, which (probably) requires three forbidden clones. In principle, the choice between these alternatives could be resolved by determining the age-specific prevalence of latent carcinoma of the prostate.

Greenwald et al. (1974) studied cancer of the prostate among 838 patients with benign prostatic hyperplasia and 802 age-matched controls. Patients were followed for an average of 10·7 years; 24 developed prostatic cancer. Controls were followed for an average of 11·2 years; 26 developed prostatic cancer. This evidence suggests, therefore, that benign prostatic hyperplasia has little or no connection with carcinoma of the prostate.

Table 7.5 Malignant Neoplasms of the Prostate

Population	$(n=3, r=5)$	
	k $(10^{-10}\ \text{yr}^{-5})$	S
Mortality data 1960-63		
Belgium	3·7	$1·61 \times 10^{-1}$
England and Wales	3·9	$1·12 \times 10^{-1}$
Japan	4·8	$9·9 \times 10^{-8}$
US White	3·7	$1·33 \times 10^{-1}$
Cancer registries (Onset)		
England and Wales, four Regions 1960–62	3·9	$1·12 \times 10^{-1}$
Birmingham Region, six consecutive years	3·7	$1·45 \times 10^{-1}$
Finland 1959–65	4·5	$1·01 \times 10^{-1}$
German Democratic Republic 1964–66	5·2	$5·7 \times 10^{-2}$
Sweden 1959–65	4·5	$1·78 \times 10^{-1}$
(Alternative analysis— see Figure 7.18(b))	$(n=1, r=12)$	
	k Units: $10^{-24}\ \text{yr}^{-12}$	S
Birmingham Region, six consecutive years	8·1	$1·0 \times 10^{-1}$

Latent period corrections: 5 years, mortality statistics
2·5 years, onset statistics

Multiple foci

Byar and Mostofi (1972) examined by step-sections 208 total prostates removed surgically for 'early' carcinoma. In some 97 per cent, carcinoma was present either peripherally, or both peripherally and centrally; 80 per cent were clearly multifocal.

Heredity

Familial aggregations of carcinoma of the prostate have been reported by Morganti *et al.* (1956(a)), Woolf (1960), Lynch *et al.* (1966) and Lynch (1967). Thiessen (1974) found a significantly raised incidence of prostatic cancer in the fathers of women with breast cancer, in relation to the incidence in the fathers of controls.

Malignant Neoplasms of the Breast (7th ICD 170)

Several factors complicate interpretation of the age-dependence of breast cancer. Outstanding among these is the prolonged survival in at least one group of women—see Chapter 11. This particular complication can be circumvented by avoiding mortality statistics and relying instead on the fairly abundant data from cancer registries for age-specific onset-rates. However, difficulties that arise from the heterogeneity of the types of breast cancer are also present in the data published from registries.

On the basis of pathology, Haagensen (1971) distinguished the following forms of disease: (i) intraductal carcinoma; (ii) mucoid carcinoma; (iii) apocrine carcinoma; (iv) tubular carcinoma; (v) adenoid cystic carcinoma; (vi) carcinoma with squamous metaplasia, (vii) carcinoma with fibroblastic metaplasia; (viii) carcinoma with cartilaginous and osseous metaplasia; (ix) lipid-secreting carcinoma, and (x) carcinoma of no special type. This last category is by far the largest, constituting 70 per cent of Haagensen's (1971) series. It does not follow that each type of cancer that can be distinguished on pathological grounds will have a distinctive age-dependence, but because the mean ages of some of these groups differ, certain differences in the kinetics of initiation appear inevitable.

In Figures 7.20 to 7.23, registry data are (incompletely) analysed in terms of two main components: an early-onset group characterized by $n=1$, $r=8$ and a late-onset group, with $n=5$, $r=2$ (Table 7.6).

In most sets of data some degree of misfit is evident between $t=50$ and 60 years. We can conclude from the analysis of age-dependence—as well as from pathology—that more than two genetically distinctive groups of women are predisposed to breast cancers diagnosed under the broad category ICD 170.

The modal initiation age for at least one group occurs between $t=40$ and 50 years and this is responsible for 'Clemmesen's hook'. (Clemmesen (1948) was the first to draw attention to the peculiar shape of the curve of the age-specific onset-rates of breast cancer in relation to age.) To give some idea of the proportions of the female population that are predisposed to breast cancer, the numerical values of the parameters used to 'fit' the registry data in Figures 7.20 and 7.23 are listed in Table 7.6.

Whether the age-dependence for any group is actually represented by the equations with $n=1$, $r=8$ and $n=5$, $r=2$, will have to await studies in which attention is paid to age-at-onset in relation to the details of pathology. On the basis of an analysis of age-dependence, Hakama (1969) proposed that two groups contribute to breast cancer but this interpretation, in common with mine, represents an oversimplified view. Epidemiological

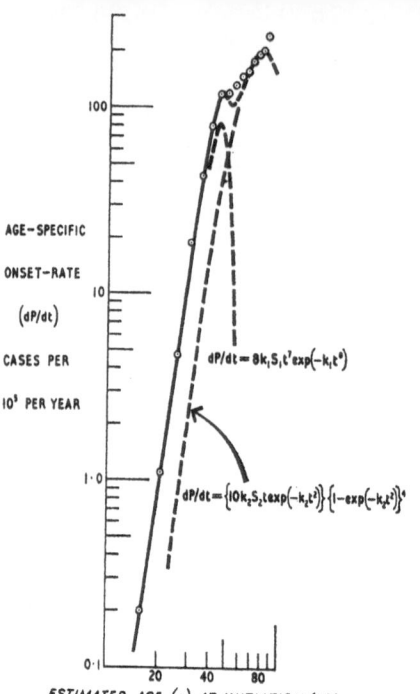

Figure 7.20 Age-specific onset-rates for malignant neoplasms of the female breast, England and Wales, 1960–62, in relation to age (Doll *et al.*, 1966). No particular attention should be paid to the theoretical curves, which give an oversimplified interpretation

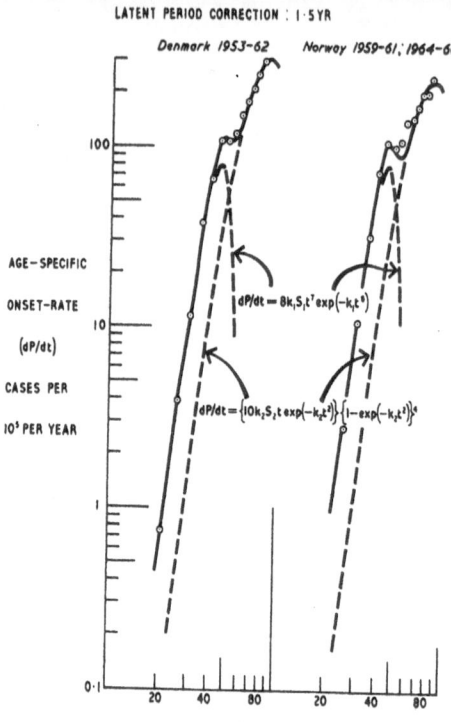

Figure 7.21 As for Figure 7.20. Data for Denmark, 1953–62, (left panel) aud Norway, 1959–61 and 1964–66 (right panel) (Doll *et al.*, 1966, 1970)

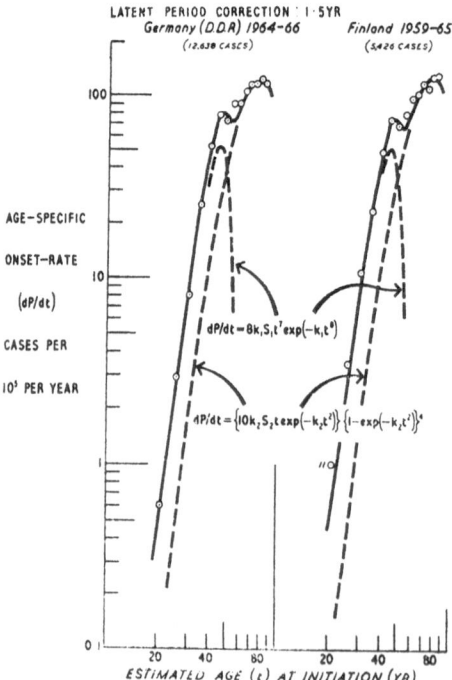

Figure 7.22 As for Figure 7.20. Data for German Democratic Republic, 1964–66 (left panel) and Finland, 1959–65 (right panel) (Doll *et al.*, 1966, 1970)

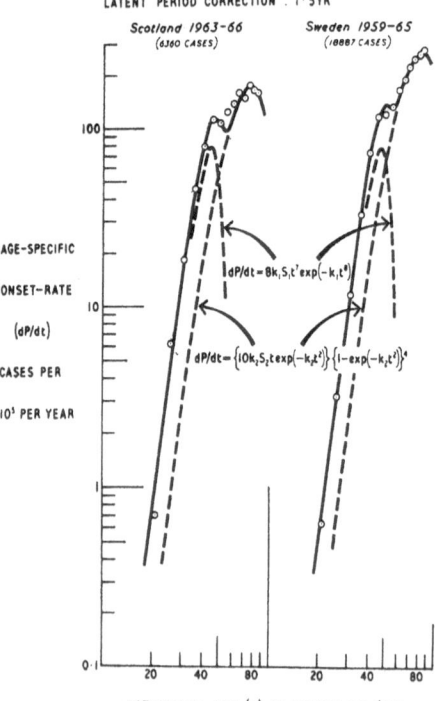

Figure 7.23 As for Figure 7.20. Date for Scotland, 1963–66 (left panel) and Sweden, 1959–65 (right panel) (Doll *et al.*, 1966, 1970)

Table 7.6 Malignant Neoplasms of the Breast (Female)

Cancer registry and period	Early-onset ($n = 1$, $r = 8$)		Late-onset ($n = 5$, $r = 2$)	
	k_1	S_1	k_2	S_2
Denmark 1953–62	$4 \cdot 2 \times 10^{-14}$ yr^{-8}	$1 \cdot 23 \times 10^{-2}$	$2 \cdot 3 \times 10^{-4}$ yr^{-2}	$1 \cdot 9 \times 10^{-1}$
England and Wales four regions 1960–62	$4 \cdot 2 \times 10^{-14}$ yr^{-8}	$1 \cdot 28 \times 10^{-2}$	$3 \cdot 0 \times 10^{-4}$ yr^{-2}	$1 \cdot 1 \times 10^{-1}$
Finland 1959–65	$4 \cdot 2 \times 10^{-14}$ yr^{-8}	$8 \cdot 1 \times 10^{-3}$	$3 \cdot 0 \times 10^{-4}$ yr^{-2}	$6 \cdot 6 \times 10^{-2}$
German Democratic Republic 1964–66	$4 \cdot 2 \times 10^{-14}$ yr^{-8}	$8 \cdot 3 \times 10^{-3}$	$3 \cdot 0 \times 10^{-4}$ yr^{-2}	$6 \cdot 6 \times 10^{-2}$
Norway 1959–61 1964–66	$4 \cdot 2 \times 10^{-14}$ yr^{-8}	$1 \cdot 23 \times 10^{-2}$	$2 \cdot 4 \times 10^{-4}$ yr^{-2}	$1 \cdot 4 \times 10^{-1}$
Scotland 1963–66	$5 \cdot 0 \times 10^{-14}$ yr^{-8}	$1 \cdot 20 \times 10^{-2}$	$3 \cdot 1 \times 10^{-4}$ yr^{-2}	$8 \cdot 6 \times 10^{-2}$
Sweden 1959–65	$4 \cdot 2 \times 10^{-14}$ yr^{-8}	$1 \cdot 24 \times 10^{-2}$	$2 \cdot 6 \times 10^{-4}$ yr^{-2}	$1 \cdot 5 \times 10^{1}$

Parameters of curves used to give an approximate fit to data from Cancer Registries. (Oversimplified interpretation—see text)
Latent period correction $= 1 \cdot 5$ years

studies by Mirra, Cole and MacMahon (1971) in Brazil also support the concept that at least two distinctive groups of women are predisposed to breast cancer. For women who were under 50 years of age at the time of interview—but not for older women—a first pregnancy prior to the age of 20 was associated with a reduced risk of breast cancer. For women who were over 50 at the time of interview—but not for younger women—the risk of breast cancer correlated with body weight and with the index, weight/height^2.

Viadana et al. (1973) found that cancer of the breast is more aggressive in its metastatic spread in women under 50, than in those over that age. Fechner (1971) examined the age-distribution of women with infiltrating ductal carcinomas (a) with lobular involvement and (b) without lobular involvement. Numbers of cases in category (a) peaked at 40 to 49 years, but those in category (b) peaked at 60 to 69 years. Hence, early-onset, and late-onset cases of infiltrating ductal carcinomas show, on the average, different pathological patterns. The overall evidence gives strong support to the hypothesis that early-onset and late-onset cancer of the breast are genuinely different. However, it is probable that neither form is homogeneous.

Paget's disease of the nipple

From Figure 7.24 we see that the age-dependence of Paget's disease of the nipple differs from that of other forms of breast cancer. Furthermore, heterogeneity exists even within this narrow category. Haagensen (1971) gives the distribution of onset of cases by age for: (a) breast involvement; and (b) nipple only. The average age at onset for the latter group is higher than for the former. Numbers are small, but for breast involvement, the age-dependence can be represented by the stochastic equation in which $n = 4$, $r = 2$; for those cases in which the nipple only is involved, $n = 7$, $r = 2$.

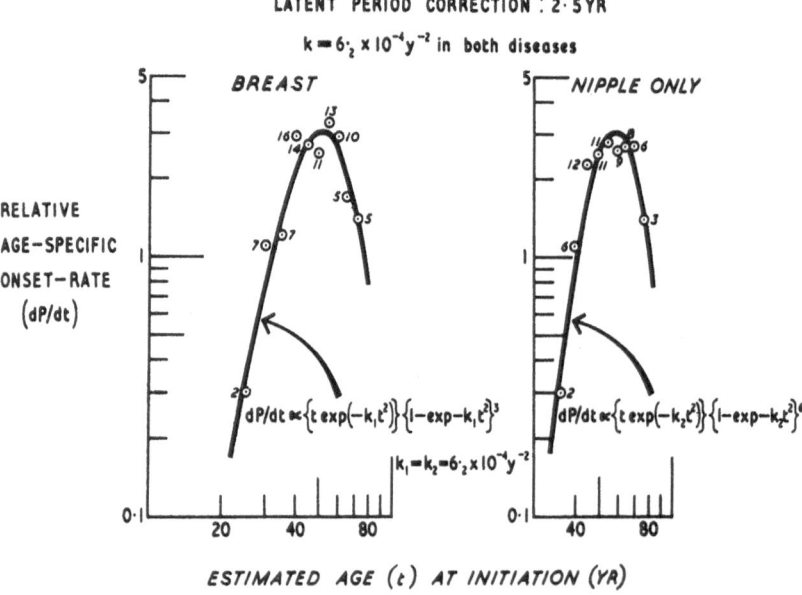

Figure 7.24 Relative age-specific onset-rates for Paget's carcinoma of the breast (left panel) and nipple only (right panel), in relation to estimated age at initiation (Haagensen, 1971)

Many pathologists have believed the disease of the nipple to be secondary to an already established intramammary tumour—see Willis's (1960) review. Willis himself regards Paget's disease as being primary to the nipple region and the frequently coexisting carcinoma of the breast to be an independent primary growth. My analysis of Haagensen's (1961) series implies two pathogenetically distinctive forms (at least) of Paget's carcinoma. The participation of multiple forbidden clones—and hence of multiple target tissues—in both forms of the disease helps to account for the many interesting features of the pathology reviewed by Willis (1960). He describes Paget's disease as a form of epidermal carcinoma *in situ* and argues that neoplastic change in the duct epithelium is concomitant. The latter feature, he points out, does not prove a ductal origin for Paget's disease. Indeed, certain cases—

those involving the nipple only—are not accompanied by neoplastic change of the ducts. The transitions observed between epidermal and 'Paget' cells probably represent the action of intermediate numbers of forbidden clones. Also noteworthy is the multifocal origin of the nipple changes, which are not continuous with carcinoma in a duct (Inglis, 1936).

Regardless of the pathology, we see that the modal initiation age for Paget's disease involving only the nipple is about 60 years. This peak will perturb the pattern described by the equations characterized in Table 7.6 and it helps to explain some of the discrepancies in Figures 7.20 to 7.23.

Heredity: multiple primaries: blood groups

Many population studies have revealed a higher incidence of cancer of the breast in the relatives of probands, as compared with controls—see the studies and reviews by Lilienfeld (1965), Post (1965), Lynch (1967), Papadrianos, Haagensen and Cooley (1967), Dmytryk (1971) and Vakil and Morgan (1973). In most surveys, the incidence of breast cancers in sisters of probands has been found to be about three times higher than in controls, or in the general population.

Anderson (1971) studied 500 breast cancer patients with positive family histories of the disease. The study group was on the average younger, and had a higher incidence of bilaterality, than patients with negative family histories. Among the familial group, those with an early diagnosis (under 45 years) had a higher incidence of bilateral disease than those with a later diagnosis. Also, patients with an early diagnosis had higher frequencies of blood group O, benign breast disease, and ovarian cysts and tumours; those with later diagnosis had higher frequencies of blood group A, diabetes, obesity, hypertension and uterine disorders. The risk of breast cancer in relatives of patients with bilateral disease was some three to four times higher than in the relatives of patients with unilateral breast cancer. Anderson (1971) suggests that there are at least two genetically distinctive types of breast cancer. In a continuation of his study, Anderson (1972) has found that for bilateral cases, the risk in first degree relatives is five times higher than in controls; when cases are both bilateral and premenopausal, the corresponding risk is nine times higher. These later findings further support the distinction between early-onset and late-onset breast cancers.

In a series from the Johns Hopkins Hospital, eight cases (1·7 per cent of the total) were found to have bilateral breast involvement at the first diagnosis; in another 34 cases (6·9 per cent of total) the second breast subsequently developed a primary malignancy (Lewison and Nato, 1971).

Doubt exists as to whether the incidence of cancer at other sites is raised in the relatives of women with breast cancer. Jacobsen (1946) obtained a positive finding, and Macklin (1959) a negative one. Moore *et al.* (1965) examined necropsy cases for synchronous multiple primaries and they found that tumours of the breast associated positively with those of genital organs. Schoenberg, Greenberg and Eisenberg (1969) give a critical review of the earlier extensive literature; in their own study of 19394 cases of breast cancer they found that second primaries of the large intestine, corpus uteri and ovary were significantly more frequent than expected on the null hypothesis, and that cancer of the pancreas was significantly less frequent than expected. Schottenfeld and Berg (1971) found cancer of the female breast to be significantly positively correlated with cancer of the opposite breast, ovary, larynx (three cases only), thyroid (seven cases), soft-tissue sarcomas (five cases) and bone sarcomas (three cases). However, in contrast to Schoenberg *et al.* (1969), they found a significant negative association with cancer of the corpus uteri (six cases).

Li and Fraumeni (1969) described four families in which soft-tissue sarcomas in children had occurred in association with breast cancer and other neoplasms in young adults. Of the ten cases of carcinoma of the breast, the age at diagnosis was known in six of them; 22, 24, 28, 32, 33 and 80 years. Among the remaining four cases the age at death was known in three: 32, 40, 41. Because the modal age at initiation for the early-onset group in Figures 7.20 to 7.23 occurs at about 46 years, it is possible that these four families, with a generally very early age of onset of breast cancer, have a rare gene or genes which predispose not only to a very early-onset form of breast cancer, but also to soft-tissue sarcomas, mainly rhabdomyosarcomas.

Berg, Hatter and Foote (1968) reported an increased risk of breast cancer in women who had developed a major salivary gland carcinoma; seven cases were observed against 0·9 expected. Moertel and Elveback (1969) failed to confirm this finding; four cases of breast cancer were observed by them where 4·7 were expected. From the California Tumour Registry, Dunn *et al* (1972) found eight cases of breast cancer among Caucasian women with carcinomas of major salivary glands where 4·2 were expected. If the three sets of data are pooled, the excess risk (19/9·8) is statistically significant ($P < 0·01$).

Complicated associations were found by Lynch *et al.* (1972) in a study of 34 families, in which two or more members had breast cancer. In 12 of these families, 11 women and 12 men out of a total population of 256 had adenocarcinoma of the colon. In another six families, five women and six men out of 80 persons had gastric carcinoma. Ovarian carcinoma occurred in five families of cases of endometrial carcinoma. In others, a high incidence was found of the combined category: brain tumours, leukaemia and sarcoma.

Hormones and breast cancer in males

Gutierrez and Williams (1968) have demonstrated distinctive patterns of ketosteroid excretion in women with breast cancer and they believe that proneness to the disease can probably be detected before its onset.

Lilienfeld (1965) suggested that the change in the slope of the age-pattern at $t = 45$ years arises because entry into the menopause decreases susceptibility to breast cancer. De Waard, De Laive and Baanders-Van Halewijn (1960) proposed that ovarian estrogenic activity has aetiological significance for breast cancer prior to the menopause, but that after the menopause, estrogenic activity of adrenal origin is responsible.

In view of these suggestions, the age-specific death-rates from breast cancer in men have a special interest. Segi and Kurihara (1964, 1966) do not give these statistics, but Schottenfeld, Lilienfeld and Diamond (1963) have extracted death-rates for US men, by race and by decennial age-groups, for the period 1949 to 1958.

To compare mortality statistics for men with those for women, data for the latter (England and Wales, US Whites) have been fitted in Figure 7.25 to the sum of two stochastic functions, using the same values of k_1 and k_2— see Table 7.7. Although these parameters are fictitious (for example, the true average latent period between initiation and death is much longer than 2·5 years), the similarity of the form of the age-patterns suggests that the kinetics of initiation of comparable forms of breast cancer in predisposed members of both sexes are similar or identical. The proportion of late-onset cases is higher among men than women.

The similarity of the kinetics supports the majority view (see Wynder *et al.*, 1960) that sex hormones play no part in the *initiation* of breast cancer,

Table 7.7 Comparison of Parameters describing Mortality Statistics for Malignant Neoplasms of the Breast in Men and Women

Population and sex	*Early-onset* $(n=3, r=3)$		*Late-onset* $(n=1, r=8)$	
	k_1	S_1	k_2	S_2
Women, England and Wales 1960–63	9.6×10^{-6} yr^{-3}	1.7×10^{-2}	2.2×10^{-16} yr^{-8}	7.3×10^{-2}
Women, US White 1960–63	9.6×10^{-6} yr^{-3}	1.5×10^{-2}	2.2×10^{-16} yr^{-8}	6.4×10^{-2}
Men, US White 1949–58	9.6×10^{-6} yr^{-3}	1.0×10^{-4}	2.2×10^{-16} yr^{-8}	1.2×10^{-3}

(Oversimplified interpretation—see text)
Latent period correction $= 2.5$ years

Figure 7.25 Age-specific death-rates, cancer of the breast, 1960–63, England and Wales (left panel) and US White (right panel) in relation to age (Segi and Kurihara, 1966). The theoretical curves are used as a guide to the age-specific death-rates from cancer of the breast in males (see Figure 7.26). The latent period correction is unrealistic

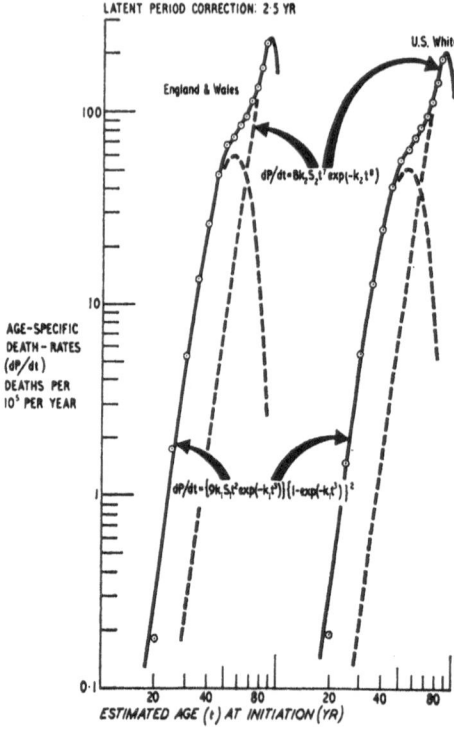

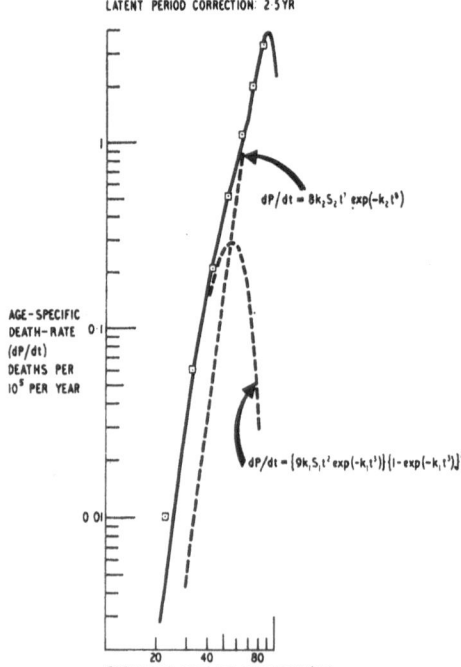

Figure 7.26 Age-specific death-rates, cancer of the breast in US White males, 1949–58, in relation to age (Schottenfeld et al., 1963). The data are fitted to theoretical curves, with the same values of n, r and k, as those used in Figure 7.25 to fit death-rates among women

although once the cancer is initiated, they can affect its course. Nevertheless, the approximate proportions of predisposed males (as fractions of the total male population) are very much less than the corresponding proportions of females—see Table 7.7.

On a genetic interpretation, the preponderance of predisposed females is intriguing, because it must derive ultimately from X- and/or Y-linked factors. Fortunately, we can narrow the choice. Jackson *et al.* (1965) were able to make a rough estimate of the incidence of breast cancer in patients with chromatin positive (*XXY*) Klinefelter's syndrome. They estimated, albeit from only three cases of breast cancer, that the incidence in Klinefelter's syndrome approximates to that in women. Harnden, Maclean and Langlands (1971) found that of 150 cases of breast carcinoma in males, five were chromatin-positive and of these, three were confirmed to have an *XXY* sex chromosome constitution. They estimated that breast cancer in chromatin-positive males is about 20 times more frequent than in *XY* males. Scheike, Visfield and Petersen (1973) found that nine out of 242 male cases of breast cancer were chromatin-positive. In this series, the incidence of breast cancer in chromatin-positive males was again about 20 times higher than in normal men and one-fifth of that in women.

These findings provide a vivid illustration of the importance of chromosomal- and hence of genetic-complement, to the predisposition to disease. However, detailed interpretation of the findings presents difficulties, because Klinefelter's syndrome associates positively with dizygotic twinning, diabetes mellitus and, perhaps, other disorders (Burch, 1968(a)). The presence of the *Y* chromosome appears to have rather little or no influence on the predisposition to breast cancer; the complement of two, as opposed to one *X*-chromosome, evidently plays the main predisposing role insofar as sex-differences are concerned. This still leaves us with a baffling problem in genetics, the resolution of which probably lies beyond the scope of traditional concepts.

Consider first the simple hypothesis that an *X*-linked allele *Xb1* predisposes to early-onset breast cancer. Assume that ~ 2 per cent of females are predisposed, and that the gene has a classical dominant effect. Then the frequency of the *Xb1* allele would be $\sim 10^{-2}$. (If autosomal factors also contribute to predisposition, then the frequency of *Xb1* would have to be higher.) On traditional grounds, the frequency of predisposed hemizygous males would be of the order of 10^{-2}—half that of women—in contrast to the observed frequency, which is of the order of 10^{-4}.

We can resolve this disagreement by resorting to the hypothesis of induced DNA strand-switching at *X*-linked genes during embryogenesis. Here we are embarassed by too many options. In theory, this discrepancy of a factor of ~ 100 can be resolved if induced DNA strand-switching in growth-control stem cells occurs during embryogenesis as follows: (a) through the double-transitions: $Xb2/Xb2 \rightarrow Xb1/Xb1$ in genotypically homozygous females and in XXY Klinefelter's syndrome; and/or (b) through the transition $Xb1 \rightarrow Xb2$ in XY males. In mechanism (b), we have to explain how the presence of a second X-chromosome generally prevents the transition: $Xb1 \rightarrow Xb2$. Various possibilities exist, the simplest, perhaps, being one in which a mutual interaction occurs between an inducer complex and both X-chromosomes in XX or XXY individuals. To test these hypotheses, we shall need to be able to identify 'available' Xb alleles in germ and somatic cells.

Anatomical factors

In view of the theoretical importance of the anatomical distribution of the lesions of disease, the distribution of cancer between the left and right breasts has particular interest. Wynder et al. (1960) found in their series of 632 US White women that the left breast was affected in 51 per cent, the right in 47 per cent, while 2 per cent had bilateral lesions. (Many unilateral cancers of the breast are, of course, multicentric in origin—see Warner, 1969; Gallagher and Martin, 1969; Kern and Brooks, 1969; Kern and Mikkelsen, 1961.) The slight bias to the left breast appears to be real. Garfinkel, Craig and Seidman (1959) reviewed the literature of the subject and examined additional series from cancer registries: the overall left/right ratio for 15931 American cases was 1·04. This bias differs significantly from unity, with $P = 0.02$. Among 18173 cases from seven countries the left/right ratio was 1·13 (Schottenfeld et al., 1963).

Interestingly, the ratio shows age-dependence. Above the age of 70 years, the ratio for Danish, and US White and Negro women is reversed, with 732 left and 783 right cases, giving a right/left ratio of 1·07. In an Australian series of 119 cases of breast carcinoma in women aged between 35 and 45 years the left breast was involved in 74 instances and the right in 45, giving a left/right ratio of 1·64: numbers are rather small, but the ratio differs significantly from unity $(P < 0.02)$ (Singer et al., 1972). The age-dependence of the laterality of lesions gives further support to the idea that at least two distinctive subpopulations of women are predisposed to breast cancer.

An overall predilection for the left breast of men is also observed. From a review of the literature Crichlow (1972) found a left/right ratio of 590/552, or 1·07.

Gynecomastia also tends to affect the left breast more frequently than the right. Among 127 cases, the left/right ratio was 1·2 and 26 cases (20 per cent) were bilateral (Schottenfeld et al., 1963). Scheike and Visfeldt (1973) give several reasons for suspecting that, in certain men, gynecomastia is a pre-malignant state.

According to our theory, the anatomical distribution of the lesions of natural autoaggressive disease is genetically determined (Burch, 1968(a); Jackson, 1968; Jackson and Burch, 1970). Studies of twins provide cor-roboration (Fairpo, 1968). Early-onset cases of breast cancer are associated with a bias to the left breast, while late-onset cases, with a different genetic predisposition, have a bias to the right breast. Differences between selected subpopulations in the frequencies of the alleles that determine (a) the form of breast cancer; and (b) the site-distribution, can also account for differences of laterality observed between: single and married women; women in the US and other countries; one region and another within the US; one ethnic group and another within the US; and between US males and females (Garfinkel et al., 1959).

Wynder et al. (1960) studied the distribution of lesions not only for laterality, but also with respect to the quadrant of each breast. An approxi-mately symmetrical distribution between left and right was found, with the highest prevalences (about 20 per cent) in both the right upper outer and the left upper outer quadrants; and the lowest prevalences (3 per cent) in the right lower inner and left lower inner quadrants. Singer et al. (1972) also described the distribution of carcinoma, by quadrant, in their series of 119 patients. The upper and outer quadrants were involved in 55 per cent; lower and outer in 18 per cent; upper and inner in 13 per cent; and lower and inner in 5 per cent.

Peniston and McBride (1970) studied the distribution of carcinomas in 148 patients with bilateral cancer of the breast. Of the known locations in the first breast to be affected, 35 per cent were in the upper outer quadrant; in the second breast 34 per cent of carcinomas presented in the upper quadrant. The lower quadrants, inner and outer, had the lowest prevalences, ranging from 1·1 to 4·1 per cent. Distributions were similar in first and second breasts. In theory, the location of the affected target tissue depends on the distribution of target TCFs and these in turn reflect the systematics of morphogenesis.

Segi et al. (1957) found that the laterality of hypolactation is associated with the laterality of breast cancer. This points to an association between those MCP–TCF alleles that determine: (a) the anatomical distribution of hypolactation; and (b) at least one form of breast cancer. Post (1965) has reviewed the extensive evidence for genetic factors in hypolactation, which appears to be yet another autoaggressive condition.

Chorlton, Hughes and Larkin (1969) reported that the distribution of the P blood groups in patients whose cancer occurred in the right breasts, differed significantly ($0·02 < P < 0·05$) from that in patients with cancers in the left breast; the distribution of the ABO blood groups in patients with affected upper distal quadrants differed significantly $(0 \cdot 02 < P < 0 \cdot 05)$ from that in patients with lesions in the other quadrants. A larger series is needed to confirm these intriguing associations between antigenic determinants on cell membranes and the anatomical distribution of breast cancer. They resemble those described above in connection with carcinoma of the different regions of the stomach.

Theories that locate initiating somatic mutations in target cells, rather than central growth-control stem cells, lead one to expect a simple association between the incidence of cancer and the size of the target tissue (Burch, 1965). In view of the overall bias of breast cancer to the left breast, we have to note that, in the American women studied, 13 per cent had a larger left breast and 8 per cent had a larger right breast (Wynder et al., 1960). At first sight this might appear to account for the bias in the distribution of cancer to the left breast. However, it fails to explain the bias to the right breast for those aged 70 years and above. In fact, the idea that the size of the breast ought to correlate with cancer incidence cannot be sustained, because women with infantile breasts have the same risk of developing cancer as those with large pendulous breasts (Wynder et al., 1960).

Pre-malignant hyperplasia

Willis (1960) emphasized the structural variability seen within a given mammary carcinoma. He also directed attention to Cheatle's important studies of pre-invasive carcinoma in which duct epithelium shows carcinomatous change *in situ*. Forms ranging from simple papilloma to areas of invasive carcinoma may coexist in a single breast. Humphrey and Serdlow (1962) found large duct epithelial hyperplasia in 69 per cent of breasts removed for carcinoma. A similar type of hyperplasia was also present in eight out of 14 benign breast lesions excised one to 13 years *before* the development of carcinoma. In a later study, duct hyperplasia was examined in fibrocystic disease (Humphrey and Swerdlow, 1968). In six out of 14 patients with severe large duct hyperplasia, carcinoma eventually developed. Kern and Brooks (1969) found fibrocystic disease in 71 per cent of breast cancer cases; it was nearly as common as in the benign breasts. Of 42 cases with atypical duct hyperplasia, 24 were found in patients in the cancer group (Kern and Brooks, 1969). In a retrospective case-control study, Black et al. (1972) found that women with some degree of atypical ductular changes in benign breast lesions had a five times greater risk of developing breast cancer than women with no evidence of atypical changes.

Wellings and Jensen (1973) studied 60 whole breasts by a quantitative three-dimensional method that enabled them to identify and count foci of hyperplasia, dysplasia and neoplasia. Five breasts were removed for cancer and six were contralateral to a mammary cancer; the remainder were from random autopsies of women, 25 to 96 years of age. In one breast containing a primary invasive carcinoma, 91 separate foci of ductal carcinoma *in situ* were identified; in another breast, contralateral to mammary carcinoma, ten such foci were counted. Less advanced, but still hyperplastic lesions, were often observed: in one breast not associated with mammary carcinoma, 156 such foci were counted. Wellings and Jensen (1973) found that all the small foci of ductal carcinoma *in situ* were confined to terminal ductal-lobular units.

A multicentric origin for breast cancer is also favoured by Kern and Mikkelsen (1971). In their view, transition from hyperplastic to neoplastic epithelium occurs and multiple foci coalesce to form larger tumours. Their studies of the pathology of small carcinomas of the breast did not support a broad field effect; they argued that, in their series of patients, the individual neoplastic masses must have started from small foci or fields because surrounding breast tissue showed no unusual degree of atypia (Kern and Mikkelsen, 1971). Izuo *et al.* (1971) examined the nuclear DNA content of epithelial cells in hyperplastic lesions of 15 patients with cystic disease of the breast. Among the eight patients who subsequently developed carcinoma, three had had an aneuploid distribution of DNA in five hyperplastic lesions.

These various findings for pre-malignant change indicate that one or more forms of breast carcinoma, in common with both types of Paget's disease of the nipple, require more than one forbidden clone for their initiation.

Malignant Neoplasms of the Thyroid (7th ICD 194)

Mortality rates for malignant neoplasms of the thyroid are low in all three populations (Figures 7.27 to 7.29 and Table 7.8). Onset-rates obtained from registry statistics are appreciably higher than death-rates especially below 55 years of age. Swedish Cancer Registry statistics (1959–65) show that the age-dependence of the onset of thyroid adenocarcinoma is much less steep than for fatal cases and it follows approximately the curve characterized by $n = 1$, $r = 3$; however, more than one group may be implicated. The age-dependence of the onset of 'undifferentiated carcinoma' is similar to that of fatal cases although numbers are too small (90 M, 150 F) to define the age-pattern reliably (Swedish Cancer Registry, 1971).

Most deaths above $t = 50$ years should probably be attributed to anaplastic carcinoma, which is rapidly lethal (Woolner *et al.*, 1961). The somewhat erratic departures in observed death-rates above the theoretical curves at $t < 40$ years might be due to occasional deaths from papillary carcinoma of

Figure 7.27

Figure 7.28

Figure 7.29

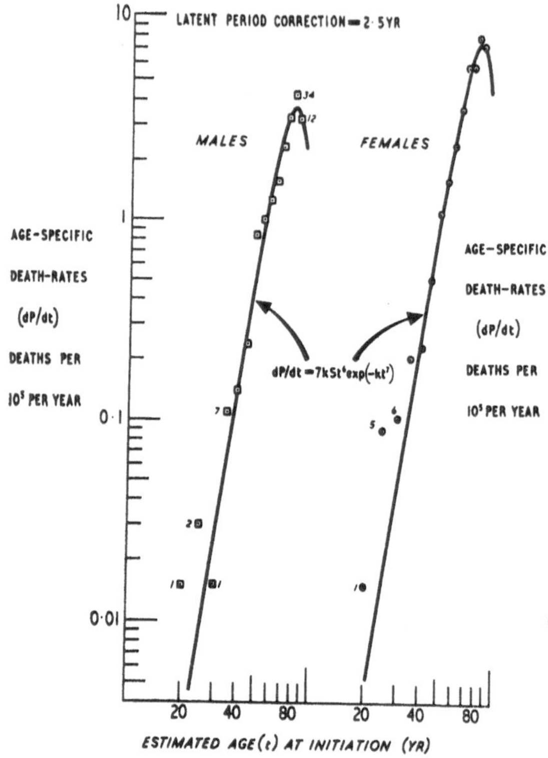

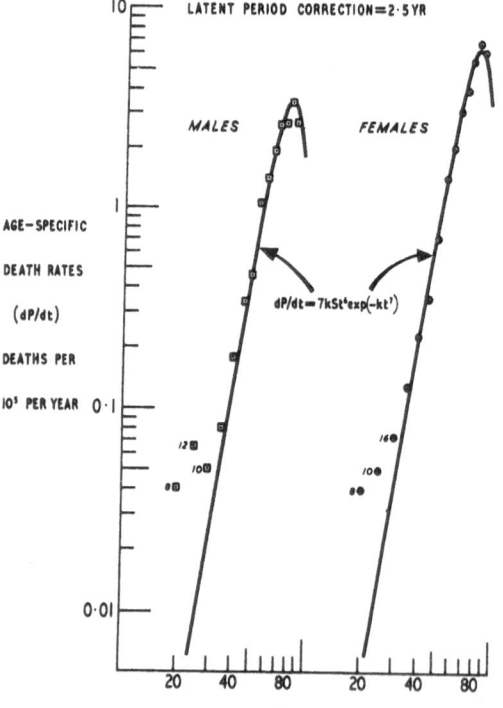

Figure 7.27 Sex-specific and age-specific death-rates, malignant neoplasms of the thyroid, England and Wales, 1960–63, in relation to estimated age at initiation (Segi and Kurihara 1966). See Table 7.8

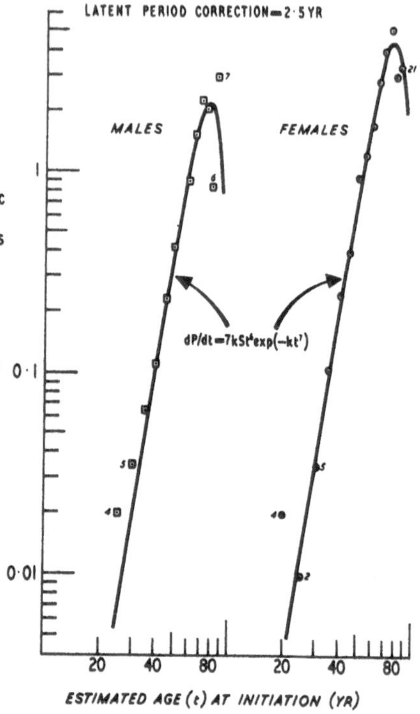

Figure 7.28 As for Figure 7.27. Data for Japan, 1960–63

Figure 7.29 As for Figure 7.27. Data for US Whites, 1960–63

the thyroid. This is a slow-growing cancer of the thyroid, with a good prognosis, that is seen predominantly in children and young adults (Woolner et al., 1961). In Finland, Franssila (1973) found relative survival rates at 5 years of 83 per cent for papillary and 54 per cent for follicular carcinoma.

Table 7.8 Malignant Neoplasms of the Thyroid

Population	Males ($n=1$, $r=7$)		Females ($n=1$, $r=7$)	
	k	S	k	S
Mortality statistics 1960–63				
England and Wales	3.8×10^{-14} yr^{-7}	1.2×10^{-3}	3.8×10^{-14} yr^{-7}	2.4×10^{-3}
Japan	5.3×10^{-14} yr^{-7}	6.6×10^{-4}	5.3×10^{-14} yr^{-7}	1.4×10^{-3}
US White	3.8×10^{-14} yr^{-7}	1.1×10^{-3}	3.8×10^{-14} yr^{-7}	2.0×10^{-3}

Latent period correction $= 2.5$ years

Both benign and malignant forms of thyroid tumours are more common in females than in males. For the fatal disease, we find in all three populations, $S_F/S_M \simeq 2$ (Table 7.8). Such a ratio suggests that one or more X-linked genes with dominant effect, together with autosomal genes, predispose to anaplastic carcinoma of the thyroid.

Heredity: multiple primaries

Genetic factors are suspected in connection with medullary carcinoma of the thyroid, which shows some striking familial aggregations and sometimes occurs in association with phaeochromocytoma—a combination known as Sipple's syndrome (Woolner et al., 1961; Williams, Brown and Doniach, 1966; Catalona et al., 1971; Melvin, Miller and Rashajian, 1971; Hill et al., 1973 and Pearson, Wells and Keiser, 1973). Familial medullary carcinoma of the thyroid is usually bilateral and a majority of phaeochromocytomas, when present, are also bilateral. A large kindred studied by Pearson et al. (1973) had 21 members (10 men, 11 women), all with bilateral medullary carcinoma of the thyroid. Ten of these patients also had phaeochromocytomas, six of which were bilateral. The parathyroid glands of 20 of the patients were examined and in 12 instances abnormalities (hyperplasia and/or adenoma) were found (Pearson et al., 1973).

In a large-scale study, Wyse et al. (1969) found that thyroid cancer patients have an increased risk of developing a second primary malignant neoplasm. Out of a total of 687 patients, 117 had one or more primaries at sites other than the thyroid. One patient had four primaries in all (thyroid, endometrium, breast, and basal cell carcinoma of the skin); eight patients each had three primaries (Wyse *et al.*, 1969). Berg *et al.* (1971) found that at autopsy, patients with thyroid cancer had a significantly higher prevalence of latent cancers (all sites) than in cancer patients generally; five latent cancers were observed, whereas 1·1 were expected.

Jensen, Norris and Fraumeni (1974) reported an association between familial arrhenoblastoma, a rare ovarian neoplasm, and thyroid adenoma. They concluded that the association is genetic in origin. A mother had an ovarian tumour (type not determined) and nodular goitre; both daughters had arrhenoblastoma of the ovary and one had a nodular goitre. Their maternal grandmother and great grandmother both had a nodular goitre; the goitre of the grandmother was found to be a follicular adenoma. The files of the US Armed Forces Institute of Pathology revealed 14 cases of arrhenoblastoma, four of whom had thyroid abnormalities (two of which were shown to be adenomas); the type of abnormality in the other two was not ascertained (Jensen *et al.*, 1974).

Anatomical aspects

Woolner *et al.* (1961) reported an interesting anatomical distribution for papillary carcinoma of the thyroid. Foci were found on the right side in 229 patients, on the left in 149, and in the isthmus or pyramidal lobe in 29. In 44 patients, the carcinoma was bilateral. Multiple, apparently separate, foci were found in the two lobes (Woolner *et al.*, 1961). I need hardly add that this evidence for multifocal and bilateral origins points once again to a 'central' location for the initiating somatic mutations. In a study of medullary carcinoma of the thyroid, Hill *et al.* (1973) found bilateral involvement in 30 patients, unilateral in 21 and undertermined laterality in another 21 patients.

Malignant Neoplasms of the Ovary, Fallopian Tube and Broad Ligament (7th ICD 175)

Earlier theories of the age-dependence of cancers were devised to interpret a simple power-law relation between age-specific death-rates and age (see Chapter 6). Ironically, a strict relation of this kind seems almost never to arise in practice, although if the age-range of observations is sufficiently truncated, it may appear to do so. Complicated distributions, such as those seen in Figures 7.30 to 7.32, impose severe tests on quantitative theories of carcinogenesis and they are, therefore, specially important. Most of the theories of age-dependence proposed so far fail to account for such distributions.

The malignancies included within the broad category 7th ICD 175,

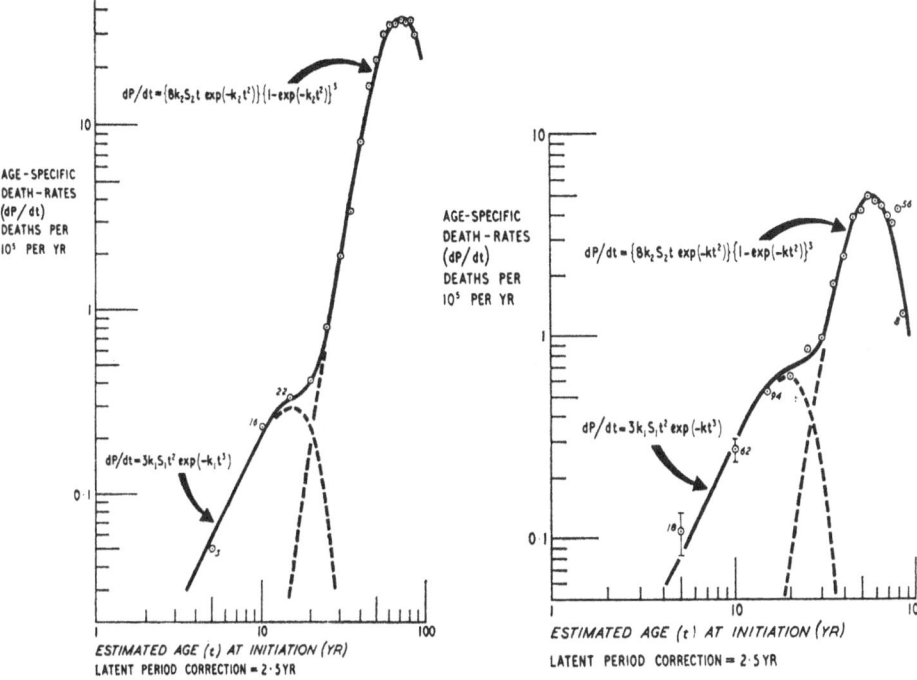

AGE-SPECIFIC DEATH-RATES (dP/dt) DEATHS PER 10^5 PER YR

$dP/dt = \{8k_2 S_2 t \exp(-k_2 t^2)\}\{1-\exp(-k_2 t^2)\}^3$

$dP/dt = 3k_1 S_1 t^2 \exp(-k_1 t^3)$

ESTIMATED AGE (t) AT INITIATION (YR)
LATENT PERIOD CORRECTION = 2·5 YR

Figure 7.30

AGE-SPECIFIC DEATH-RATES (dP/dt) DEATHS PER 10^5 PER YR

$dP/dt = \{8k_2 S_2 t \exp(-kt^2)\}\{1-\exp(-kt^2)\}^3$

$dP/dt = 3k_1 S_1 t^2 \exp(-kt^3)$

ESTIMATED AGE (t) AT INITIATION (YR)
LATENT PERIOD CORRECTION = 2·5 YR

Figure 7.31

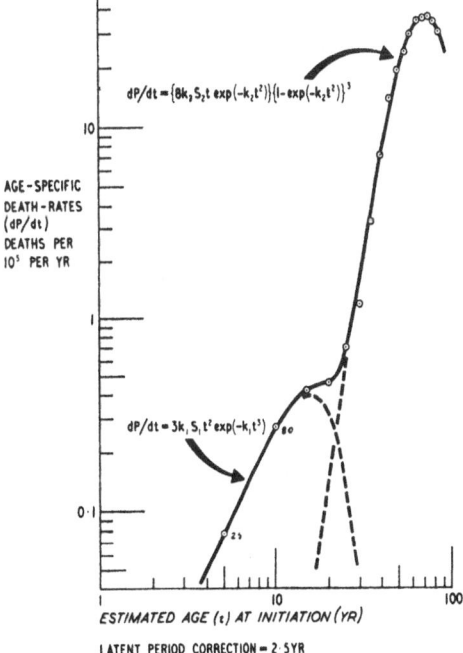

AGE-SPECIFIC DEATH-RATES (dP/dt) DEATHS PER 10^5 PER YR

$dP/dt = \{8k_2 S_2 t \exp(-k_2 t^2)\}\{1-\exp(-k_2 t^2)\}^3$

$dP/dt = 3k_1 S_1 t^2 \exp(-k_1 t^3)$

ESTIMATED AGE (t) AT INITIATION (YR)
LATENT PERIOD CORRECTION = 2·5 YR

Figure 7.32

Figure 7.30 Age-specific death-rates, malignant neoplasms of the ovary, Fallopian tube and broad ligament, England and Wales, 1960–63, in relation to estimated age at initiation (Segi and Kurihara, 1966). See Table 7.9

Figure 7.31 As for Figure 7.30. Data for Japan, 1960–63

Figure 7.32 As for Figure 7.30. Data for US Whites, 1960–63

appear to be confined, in the main, to two genetically distinctive groups of women. However, this represents an oversimplification. Primary carcinoma of the Fallopian tube contributes from about 0·2 to 0·5 per cent of all primary malignancies of the genital canal (Novak and Woodruff, 1967). In registry statistics from Sweden, 5293 cases were recorded with onset of malignant neoplasms of the ovary (7th ICD 175·0) during the years 1959–65, and only 69 cases with malignant neoplasms of the Fallopian tube (7th ICD 175·1); 4416 of all the cases were described as adenocarcinoma.

I have analysed the age-distribution of 232 cases of primary carcinoma of the Fallopian tube reported prior to 1955 and reviewed by Sedlis (1961), and of 75 cases published after 1955 and reviewed by Schiller and Silverberg (1971). Making a latent period correction of 5 years, the distribution of onset-rates by age can be fitted to the equation with $n = 5$, $r = 2$, with a mode at about $t = 50$ years, in contrast to about 70 years for carcinoma of the ovary in Western countries (Figures 7.30 and 7.32). In view of the inferred large number of initiating forbidden clones ($n = 5$), it is scarcely surprising that carcinoma in situ is commonly observed in the Fallopian tube (Ryan, 1962; Schiller and Silverberg, 1971). In 11 of the 76 cases reviewed by Schiller and Silverberg (1971), the tumour was limited to the tubal mucosa; one of these cases was bilateral.

Of particular interest are the contrasts and similarities between the statistics (7th ICD 175) for Japan on the one hand (Figure 7.31), and those for England and Wales and US Whites on the other (Figures 7.30 and 7.32). In the three populations, the values of n and r ($n = 1$, $r = 3$ for the main 'early' group; $n = 4$, $r = 2$ for the main 'late' group) are the same, and they give rise to the same general pattern of bimodality. However, the magnitude of k_1 in the Japanese population is appreciably less than in the other two; the early-onset cases appear, on the average, at a later age in the Japanese population. The estimated modal age of initiation for the early-onset group in Japan is about 19 years, in contrast to 15 to 16 years for England and Wales, and US Whites. When we turn to the late-onset group, we find the position reversed: the modal age of initiation in Japan is about 58 years, but 72 years in England and Wales and 73 years in US Whites. In other words, k_2 for Japan (4.9×10^{-4} year^{-2}) is markedly higher than for England and Wales (3.3×10^{-4} year^{-2}) and US Whites (3.2×10^{-4} year^{-2}).

This reversal in the ranking order between k_1 and k_2 is interesting because it is inconsistent with the idea that a general carcinogen in Japan, say, is responsible for the relatively high values of k_2 and other kinetic constants associated with various other malignancies. Generally, it appears that differences in the magnitude of kinetic constants, both between countries and racial groups, are more likely to be genetic than environmental in origin.

Table 7.9 Malignant Neoplasms of the Ovary, Fallopian Tube and Broad Ligament

Population	Early-onset ($n = 1, r = 3$)		Late-onset ($n = 4, r = 2$)	
	k_1	S_1	k_2	S_2
Mortality statistics 1960–63				
England and Wales	$1 \cdot 77 \times 10^{-4}$ yr^{-3}	$4 \cdot 4 \times 10^{-5}$	$3 \cdot 3 \times 10^{-4}$ yr^{-2}	$2 \cdot 1 \times 10^{-2}$
Japan	$9 \cdot 4 \times 10^{-5}$ yr^{-3}	$1 \cdot 16 \times 10^{-4}$	$4 \cdot 9 \times 10^{-4}$ yr^{-2}	$2 \cdot 2 \times 10^{-3}$
US White	$1 \cdot 71 \times 10^{-4}$ yr^{-3}	$6 \cdot 0 \times 10^{-5}$	$3 \cdot 2 \times 10^{-4}$ yr^{-2}	$2 \cdot 0 \times 10^{-2}$

Latent period correction $= 2 \cdot 5$ years

Point mutations in corresponding MCP–TCF genes, giving rise to occasional alterations of base sequence, could account for differences in the average rates of DNA strand-switching, as well as for characteristic morphological differences between, for example, Japanese and Caucasians. However, this evidence for the ranking of k_1 and k_2 in different populations is inconclusive because early-onset ovarian cancers are a very heterogeneous group (Li, Fraumeni and Dalager, 1973). The differences in k_1 might arise from differences in the relative proportions of the several types of early-onset tumour, in different populations. Details of the age at death, by type of ovarian cancer (Li *et al.*, 1973), give no support, however, for this alternative interpretation.

Recorded death-rates for the category ICD 175 in Japan have risen by more than a factor of two between 1950 and 1963. The crude rate of $0 \cdot 79$ per 10^5 per year in 1950–51 rose to $1 \cdot 69$ per 10^5 per year in 1962–63. In England and Wales, and US Whites, a small increase—about 10 per cent—was recorded over the same period. These secular changes, and especially those in Japan, complicate the interpretation of S, but it is noteworthy that the calculated value of S_1 for Japan is about double that for the other two populations, whereas the value of S_2 for Japan is almost ten times lower than the corresponding values for the other two populations. (Note that the values of S_1 and S_2 for England and Wales closely resemble those for US Whites.) Despite the large differences in absolute rates between Japan and the other countries, all the data give impressive fits to equations of the same basic form, with the same values of n and r.

Heredity: multiple primaries

I have found no reports of large-scale studies of familial aggregations of cancer of the ovary, although occasional families with conspicuous aggregations have been described (Graham, Graham and Schueller, 1964; Liber,

1950; Lewis and Davison, 1969; and Li *et al.*, 1970). Furthermore, this malignancy sometimes features in 'cancer families' (Savage, 1956; Lynch *et al.*, 1966; and Lynch, 1967). It is worth noting that the incidence of multiple primary malignancies is significantly higher in 'cancer families' than in the general population (Moertel, Dockerty and Baggenstoss, 1961; Lynch, 1967). In a family studied by Cannon and Leavell (1966), seven out of nine siblings developed at least one ovarian malignancy; and one sibling had carcinoma of both ovaries. From an epidemiological study, Joly *et al.* (1974) concluded that certain women are predisposed both to ovarian cancer and low fertility.

Schottenfeld and Berg (1971) assessed the risk of metachronous primary carcinoma of the breast in 921 women with carcinoma of the ovary: this was three to four times higher than in the general population based, however, on a total of only seven cases.

Pathology in relation to multiple initiating forbidden clones

In view of the conclusion that the late-onset form of ovarian cancer is initiated by four forbidden clones, we would expect to find clear evidence for pre-malignant, hyperplastic conditions, initiated by three, or even fewer, forbidden clones. Willis's (1967) comments on the pathology of ovarian tumours, are, therefore, very pertinent. He believes that the great majority of malignant tumours of the ovary arise from cystadenomas. All gradations of structure can be seen from active papilliferous cystadenomas, to invasive papillary, cystic, or solid carcinomas. Willis (1967) refers to the development of invasive growth in one part of an elsewhere benign serous or mucinous tumour. Evidently, one, two or three forbidden clones promote a benign growth, but only when the fourth clone is initiated and propagated does invasive carcinoma develop from specific foci.

A majority of ovarian carcinomas are either bilateral at origin or become bilateral (Novak and Woodruff, 1967; Willis, 1967; Dyson, Reilly and Steele, 1971). Some 20 to 30 per cent of cases of carcinoma of the Fallopian tube are also bilateral (Sedlis, 1961; Schiller and Silverberg, 1971). Such cases are generally attributed (Sedlis 1961) to the formation of separate primaries, rather than to metastasis, for the following reasons: (a) bilateral tumours often occur in the absence of metastasis at other sites; (b) the tumours on both sides often show symmetrical development and equal size; (c) various stages of development of carcinoma from normal epithelium can be seen on both sides; and (d) implants in the endometrium are not seen, although they would be expected if metastic spread occurred from one uterine horn to the opposite one. A further reason for believing that bilateral tumours of the Fallopian tube represent separate primaries is that out of the 11 cases of carcinoma *in situ* (limited to tubal mucosa) reviewed by Schiller and Silverberg (1971), one was bilateral.

Malignant Neoplasms of the Large Intestine and Rectum (7th ICD 153 and 154)

Analyses (not shown here) of the age-dependence of death-rates for the categories Seventh ICD 153 and 154 considered separately, can be made in terms of the same basic equations. That is to say, the types of forbidden clone (as characterized by the parameters n, r and k) needed to initiate a cancer in these two parts of the intestinal tract appear to be the same. The location and character of vulnerable target TCFs within the colon and rectum would appear to be determined by similar genetic factors. Accordingly, data for the two categories have been combined.

Most cases belong to a late-onset group characterized by $n=1$, $r=8$ (Figures 7.33 to 7.37, Tables 7.10 and 7.11).

Although the values of k_3 for males and females in this group appear to be identical in Japan, where the initiation mode at $t=78$ years is clearly defined, mortality data for England and Wales, and US Whites, suggest that $k_{3,M} > k_{3,F}$. However, in these latter populations, the positions of the modes (86 to 91 years) can be inferred only approximately from the change in slope of $\log dP/dt$ versus $\log t$ at high t: the mode itself is not revealed directly in the mortality statistics. The suspicion that the apparent positions of these modes might be misleading is supported by an analysis of cancer registry statistics for *onset* in four regions of England and Wales, 1960–62, and in Sweden, 1959–68—see Figures 7.36 and 7.37, and Table 7.11. These onset data suggest that for both populations $k_{3,M} = k_{3,F}$.

Survival data (California Tumor Registry, 1963), together with the onset statistics, reveal a source of bias in the position of the initiation mode inferred from mortality statistics. Relative survival-rates from cancers of the large intestine and rectum at 1 year after registration, are only a little over 50 per cent, but beyond 1 year the survival curve becomes much less steep (see Chapter 11). For the group aged 75 years and above, the relative survival of men 5 years after registration is 22·4 per cent, but for women the corresponding proportion is 29·1 per cent (Californian Tumor Registry, 1963). Hence, a larger proportion of women with late-onset colorectal cancer survive into the highest age-groups of 80 years and above. This differential survival will have the effect of raising the apparent modal age for women above that of men when mortality statistics are analysed.

From death-rates in England and Wales, and the US White population, $S_{3,F}$ appears to be higher than $S_{3,M}$, by about 19 per cent. The absolute

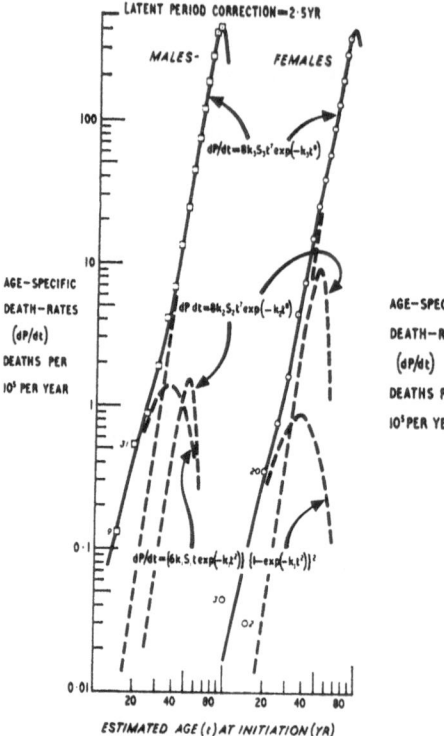

Figure 7.33

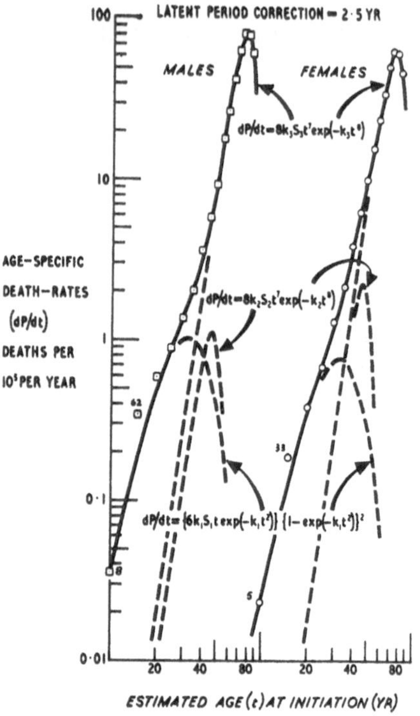

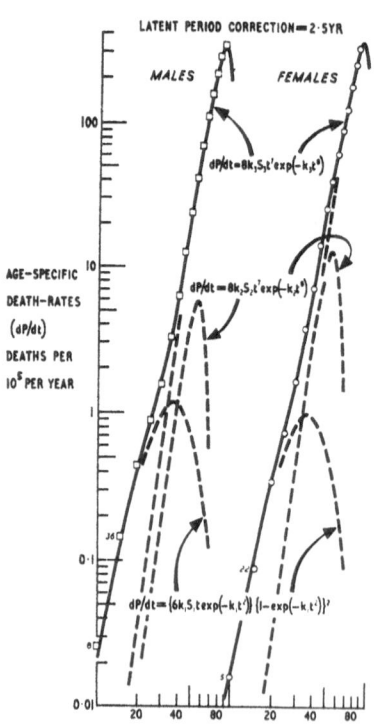

Figure 7.34

Figure 7.35

Figure 7.33 Sex-specific and age-specific death-rates, malignant neoplasms of the large intestine and rectum, England and Wales, 1960–63, in relation to estimated age at initiation (Segi and Kurihara, 1966). See Table 7.10

Figure 7.34 As for Figure 7.33. Data for Japan, 1960–63

Figure 7.35 As for Figure 7.33. Data for US Whites, 1960–65

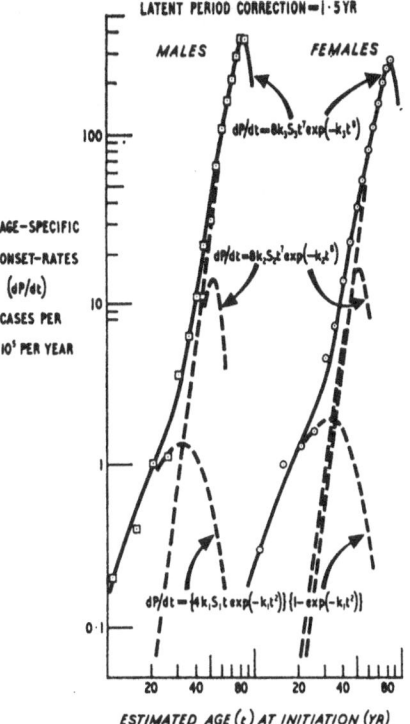

Figure 7.36 Sex-specific and age-specific onset-rates, malignant neoplasms of the large intestine and rectum, four regions of England and Wales, 1960–62, in relation to estimated age at initiation (Doll *et al.*, 1966). See Table 7.11

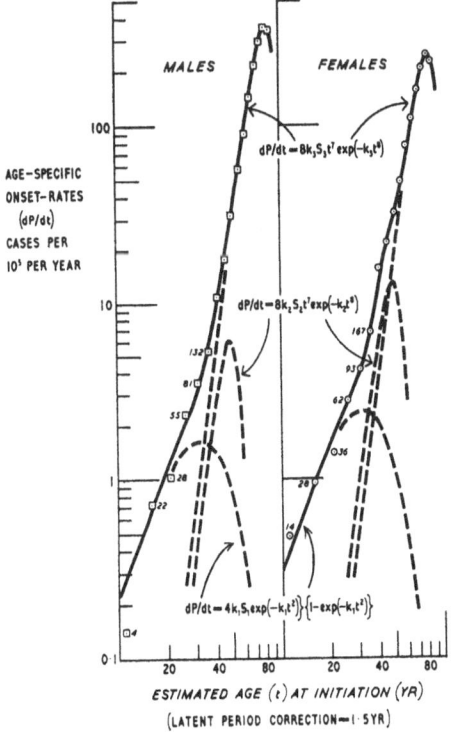

Figure 7.37 As for Figure 7.36. Data for Sweden, 1959–68 (Swedish Cancer Registry, 1971)

Table 7.10 Malignant Neoplasms of the Large Intestine and Rectum
(Analysis of Death-Rates)

Population and group	Males		Females	
Early-onset ($n=3$, $r=2$)	k_1	S_1	k_1	S_1
England and Wales	$1{\cdot}04 \times 10^{-3}$ yr^{-2}	$3{\cdot}5 \times 10^{-4}$	$1{\cdot}04 \times 10^{-3}$ yr^{-2}	$2{\cdot}7 \times 10^{-4}$
Japan	$1{\cdot}37 \times 10^{-3}$ yr^{-2}	$3{\cdot}1 \times 10^{-4}$	$1{\cdot}37 \times 10^{-3}$ yr^{-2}	$2{\cdot}4 \times 10^{-4}$
US White	$1{\cdot}04 \times 10^{-3}$ yr^{-2}	$3{\cdot}6 \times 10^{-4}$	$1{\cdot}04 \times 10^{-3}$ yr^{-2}	$3{\cdot}4 \times 10^{-4}$
Mid-onset ($n=1$, $r=8$)	k_2	S_2	k_2	S_2
England and Wales	$1{\cdot}4 \times 10^{-14}$ yr^{-8}	$2{\cdot}8 \times 10^{-4}$	$1{\cdot}4 \times 10^{-14}$ yr^{-8}	$1{\cdot}8 \times 10^{-3}$
Japan	$3{\cdot}7 \times 10^{-14}$ yr^{-8}	$1{\cdot}8 \times 10^{-4}$	$3{\cdot}7 \times 10^{-14}$ yr^{-8}	$3{\cdot}7 \times 10^{-4}$
US White	$9{\cdot}0 \times 10^{-15}$ yr^{-8}	$1{\cdot}1 \times 10^{-3}$	$9{\cdot}0 \times 10^{-15}$ yr^{-8}	$2{\cdot}5 \times 10^{-3}$
Late-onset ($n=1$, $r=8$)	k_3	S_3	k_3	S_3
England and Wales	$2{\cdot}9 \times 10^{-16}$ yr^{-8}	$1{\cdot}25 \times 10^{-1}$	$1{\cdot}9 \times 10^{-16}$ yr^{-8}	$1{\cdot}31 \times 10^{-1}$
Japan	$7{\cdot}1 \times 10^{-16}$ yr^{-8}	$2{\cdot}16 \times 10^{-2}$	$7{\cdot}1 \times 10^{-16}$ yr^{-8}	$1{\cdot}74 \times 10^{-2}$
US White	$2{\cdot}9 \times 10^{-16}$ yr^{-8}	$9{\cdot}4 \times 10^{-2}$	$2{\cdot}0 \times 10^{-16}$ yr^{-8}	$1{\cdot}08 \times 10^{-1}$

Latent period correction $=2{\cdot}5$ years

Table 7.11 Malignant Neoplasms of the Large Intestine and Rectum
(Analysis of Registry Data for Onset in Four Regions, England and Wales 1960–62; and Sweden 1959–68)

Group	Males		Females	
Early-onset				
($n=2$, $r=2$)	k_1	S_1	k_1	S_1
England and Wales	$1{\cdot}04 \times 10^{-3}$ yr^{-2}	$4{\cdot}3 \times 10^{-4}$	$1{\cdot}04 \times 10^{-3}$ yr^{-2}	$6{\cdot}4 \times 10^{-4}$
Sweden	$1{\cdot}04 \times 10^{-3}$ yr^{-2}	$5{\cdot}7 \times 10^{-4}$	$1{\cdot}04 \times 10^{-3}$ yr^{-2}	$8{\cdot}4 \times 10^{-4}$
Mid-onset				
($n=1$, $r=8$)	k_2	S_2	k_2	S_2
England and Wales	$1{\cdot}4 \times 10^{-14}$ yr^{-8}	$2{\cdot}5 \times 10^{-3}$	$1{\cdot}4 \times 10^{-14}$ yr^{-8}	$2{\cdot}9 \times 10^{-3}$
Sweden	$2{\cdot}6 \times 10^{-14}$ yr^{-8}	$1{\cdot}0 \times 10^{-3}$	$2{\cdot}6 \times 10^{-14}$ yr^{-8}	$2{\cdot}2 \times 10^{-3}$
Late-onset				
($n=1$, $r=8$)	k_3	S_3	k_3	S_3
England and Wales	$3{\cdot}5 \times 10^{-16}$ yr^{-8}	$1{\cdot}06 \times 10^{-1}$	$3{\cdot}5 \times 10^{-16}$ yr^{-8}	$7{\cdot}5 \times 10^{-2}$
Sweden	$4{\cdot}0 \times 10^{-16}$ yr^{-8}	$1{\cdot}02 \times 10^{-1}$	$4{\cdot}0 \times 10^{-16}$ yr^{-8}	$7{\cdot}1 \times 10^{-2}$

Latent period correction $=1{\cdot}5$ years

values of S_3 for England and Wales, which are only slightly higher than those in US Whites, are some six- to eight-fold higher than those in Japan. The faster kinetics of initiation in Japan are associated with much lower values of S_3 and hence of death-rates in the higher age-groups.

The onset data for four regions of England and Wales, 1960–62, show $S_{3,M} > S_{3,F}$, whereas mortality data, as we have seen, suggest the opposite. This discrepancy has several possible explanations: (a) women in the highest age-groups survive better than men; (b) the populations contributing to the two sets of statistics are not identical; (c) under-registration in the onset data which is suggested when we compare values of S_3 in Tables 7.10 and 7.11— this error might be more severe for women; and (d) mortality from colorectal cancer might be overdiagnosed in women.

Secular trends

Crude death-rates, to which the late-onset group makes the major contribution, have remained almost constant in US Whites over the period 1950 to 1963. In England and Wales, a steady decline has been recorded over this period; from 38·0 per 10^5 per year in males, 1950–51, to 29·4 in 1962–63; and from 36·2 to 33·3 (same units) in females. In Japan, marked increases have been recorded over this period: from 4·74 to 6·23 in males; and from 4·70 to 6·17 in females. Despite these contrasting secular changes in the three populations, we find, once again, that the same basic stochastic equations, with the same values of n and r describe the age-distributions of death-rates in 1960 to 1963. Cohort analysis would yield basically different age-distributions between the populations. Unless we are dealing with a coincidence of fantastically high order, we are justified in concluding that, from the biological viewpoint, vertical analysis again yields the 'correct' form of age-dependence, whereas cohort analysis would lead to spurious conclusions about the values of n and r. (I recognize, of course, that false conclusions can be drawn from a correctly defined age-dependence.)

Mid-onset group

The mid-onset group, with a mode in both sexes at about 53 years in England and Wales, 56 years in US Whites, 47 years in Japan and 49 years in Sweden, is sandwiched between the early- and late-onset groups, and is thus poorly defined. Consequently, the interpretation in terms of $n = 1$, $r = 8$ is vulnerable to small errors in the data. The parameters for this group must, therefore, be regarded as being probably incorrect—see the section below on association with ulcerative colitis, page 165—and little significance should be attached to the discrepancies in S_2 between Tables 7.10 and 7.11.

Early-onset group

The initiation of forbidden clones that lead to *death* in the early-onset group with a mode at $t = 30$ to 40 years (Figures 7.33 to 7.35), is described by the stochastic equation in which $n = 3$, $r = 2$. That is, two somatic gene mutations, in each of three independent growth-control stem cells, initiate this early-onset, fatal form of carcinoma. The average latent period between the initiation of the third clone, and death, is in the region of 2·5 years.

However, the initiation of forbidden clones that lead to the *onset* and registration of carcinoma of the large intestine or rectum (Figures 7.36 and 7.37) is described by the stochastic equation in which $n = 2$, $r = 2$. The latent period correction applied to the onset statistics is 1·5 years. Particular interest attaches to the age-dependence of onset and death in this early-onset group. The same value of k_1 is used to fit the mortality and the onset statistics. I conclude that two forbidden clones lead to an initially non-fatal form of cancer, but that a third forbidden clone, with kinetics of initiation similar to those of the other two, is needed to produce the condition that leads, after an average latent period of one to two years, to death.

These not uncommon situations, in which more than one forbidden clone is needed to promote a malignant transformation, have great biological interest. A 'target organ', such as the colorectal epithelium, will comprise a very large number of distinctive tissue elements, each with a distinctive TCF. In the colon/rectum, the cooperative action of two forbidden clones is needed to produce a diagnosable neoplastic condition in the early-onset group. In principle, a cooperative action between forbidden clones could occur at central, intermediate and/or peripheral locations. Also, cooperative effects might take place at the level of the transformed target tissue. Evidently, the distinction between a non-fatal and fatal early-onset malignant condition of the colon/rectum, derives from the differences between the action of two and three forbidden clones, all of which exert their effects at the periphery. But whether the qualitative distinction depends on the interclonal cooperative action, or on cooperation between transformed target tissues (or indeed, on both effects) remains unresolved.

Association with familial intestinal polyposis

A most interesting aspect of cancer of the large bowel and rectum is the association with familial intestinal polyposis. Before the advent of colectomy, familial intestinal polyposis generally terminated in fatal cancer. Reed and Neel (1955) gave the age-distribution of deaths from carcinoma in the patients from their series and from that of Dukes (1952). The absolute size and age-structure of the populations at risk are unknown, and to calculate relative age-specific death-rates, I have assumed that the age-structure of the populations at risk resembled that of England and Wales, 1946. Calculated relative age-specific death-rates, corrected for an average latent period of 2·5 years, are plotted against estimated age at initiation in Figure 7.38. (The

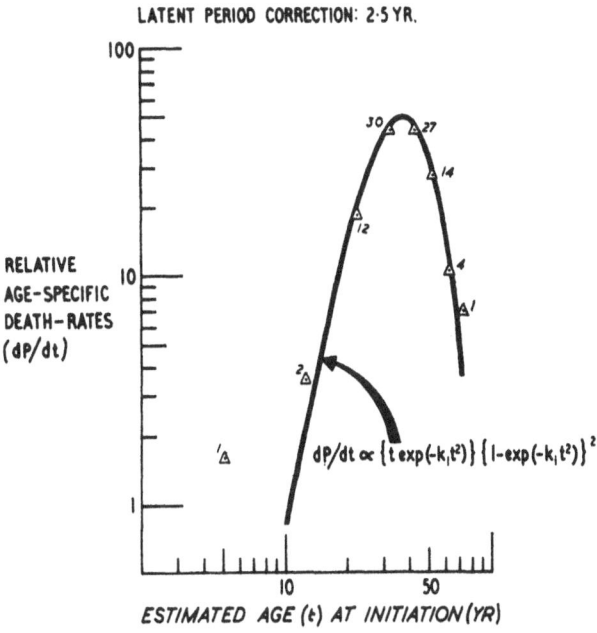

LATENT PERIOD CORRECTION: 2·5 YR.

$$dP/dt \propto \{t\exp(-k_1 t^2)\}\{1-\exp(-k_1 t^2)\}^2$$

RELATIVE AGE-SPECIFIC DEATH-RATES (dP/dt)

ESTIMATED AGE (t) AT INITIATION (YR)

Figure 7.38 Relative age-specific death-rates from colorectal carcinoma in two series of patients with familial intestinal polyposis, in relation to estimated age at initiation (Reed and Neel, 1955)

single case in the 5 to 9 years age-range of Reed and Neel's (1955) series, might belong to a very early-onset group, discernible in national statistics.)

From the concordance of the age-patterns we can conclude that the early-onset group of colorectal cancer defined in national mortality statistics by the parameters $n=3$, $r=2$, and in registry data by the parameters $n=2$, $r=2$, is either identical with, or it includes, those cases that arise in persons with familial intestinal polyposis.

We need to compare, therefore, the values of S_1 in Table 7.10—they represent the proportion of each population that is predisposed to, and dies from, early-onset colorectal carcinoma—with the frequency of familial polyposis. Reed and Neel (1955) attempted to deduce this latter frequency and they arrived at a figure of $1·2 \times 10^{-4}$ which, however, they believed to be an underestimate. This figure should be compared with the values derived from mortality statistics for US Whites: $2 \cdot 6 \times 10^{-4}$ for males and $3 \cdot 4 \times 10^{-4}$ for females (Table 7.10). These frequencies are probably consistent with Reed and Neel's (1955) estimate and hence it is likely that all persons in the early-onset group defined in Figures 7.33 to 7.37 had familial intestinal polyposis.

A word of caution is necessary. Since the early 1950s, many patients with familial intestinal polyposis have undergone colectomy and ileorectal anastomosis. This operation reduces the risk of subsequent cancer, although retention of the rectal stump is associated with a risk of rectal cancer (Lockhart-Mummery, 1967; Aylett, 1971). Mortality statistics can therefore be expected to show declining death-rates from colorectal cancer in patients with familial intestinal polyposis. Such complications are present in the statistics of Veale (1965) that describe the onset of cancer in patients with familial intestinal polyposis, some of whom underwent colonic resection. These statistics were analysed by Ashley (1969) who assumed that colonic resection completely eliminated the risk of neoplasia. This assumption is overoptimistic (Aylett 1971), and hence Ashley's (1969) estimate of the age-prevalence of cancer in familial polyposis is likely to be in error at high values of t. The initial slope of the derived prevalence curves—4·1 (males), 3·4 (females)—should not, however, be seriously overestimated. At low t, the expected age-prevalence (for conditions characterized by $n=2$, $r=2$ and $n=3$, $r=2$) should show a fourth to sixth power dependence on age, allowing for latent period. Ashley (1969) did not correct for latent period, which would slightly reduce the initial slope of his age-prevalence curve. Thus his findings at low t agree reasonably well with expectation.

McKusick (1962) distinguished at least six varieties of hereditary polyposis. A single autosomal gene (with dominant expression) is believed to be responsible for each form of polyposis. Familial polyposis of the colon is the form that is of chief concern to us here. That predisposition to fatal carcinoma of the colon in this group might be slightly more complicated than a single autosomal gene is suggested by the numerical value of the sex-ratio, $S_{1,M}/S_{1,F}$. This is about 1·3 (England and Wales), 1·3 (Japan) and $1 \cdot 0_6$ (US Whites) —see Table 7.11. In each population, therefore, $S_{1,M}/S_{1,F}$ exceeds unity, although only marginally in US Whites. Such a sex-ratio could be explained if, in addition to the major autosomal gene, an X-linked allele of high frequency, and recessive effect, is needed to predispose to carcinoma of the colon. If we assume a typical sex-ratio of $1 \cdot 2_5$, the average frequency of the predisposing X-linked allele (assuming conventional rules of inheritance) would be 0·8. The values of S_1 in Table 7.11 indicate that predisposition to the *onset* of carcinoma of the colon in four regions of England and Wales, and in Sweden, is more frequent in females. However, these conclusions rest on small numbers and they assume equal efficiency of registration for both sexes.

Dukes (1952) recorded two instances in which intestinal polyposis skipped a generation. Gates (1946) also believed that generation-skipping could occur. If an X-linked factor, in addition to the well-established autosomal genes, is needed to predispose to familial intestinal polyposis, then the phenomenon of generation-skipping can be readily explained.

It appears that the major gene that prediposes to polyposis in some families might also predispose to multiple osteomas and 'hard' and 'soft' surface tumours (Gardner, 1951; Gardner and Plenk, 1952; Gardner and Richards, 1953; Smith, 1958; Dukes, 1968; Hoffman and Brooke, 1970; Smith and Kern, 1973). The correlation between multiple polyposis and epidermal cysts in the same patient is virtually 100 per cent, except in very young patients in whom the penetrance of multiple polyposis is incomplete (Gardner and Richards, 1953; Smith, 1958). Two closely-linked genes with dominant effect would also account for this correlation (Gardner and Richards, 1953). Bone and subcutaneous abnormalities do not accompany familial polyposis in all families (Duke, 1958). Hence if we wish to retain the idea of a single predisposing gene, we have to postulate allelic differences between families.

Hoffman and Brooke (1970) described the first instance of an association between *malignant* osseous tumours and familial polyposis. Six of a family of 35 members were known to have developed polyposis coli. In addition, a mother and her son both developed sarcoma of the bone. Unfortunately, it was not possible to assess the condition of the mother's colon; the son died, at age 13, of pulmonary metastases without his colon being examined for polyps (Hoffman and Brooke, 1970). Prior to this report, Smith (1958) observed that the bony tumours associated with familial polyposis attain full size within a few years after detection and then remain dormant. Again, allelic differences between the predisposing genes are suggested, although the hypothesis of polygenes is not eliminated.

Age-distribution of onset of polyposis: importance to theory

Familial intestinal polyposis is not a congenital condition and hence the age-distribution of the emergence of polyps acquires special interest. Onset can be quite sudden. Lockhart-Mummery (1934) described a patient who had no polyps when first examined, but had extensive polyposis four years later. Dukes (1958) gave the age at onset in 38 cases: the average age at onset was 21 years, but these small numbers are inadequate for reliable age-analysis.

Fortunately, Asman and Pierce (1970) were able to determine the age at onset of polyposis in 73 members of a large Kentucky kindred consisting of

1422 members. In Figure 7.39, the relative age-specific onset-rates for polyposis in their series are fitted to the equation in which $n=1$, $r=2$ and $k_1 = 1·04 \times 10^{-3}$ year^{-2}. In view of the small numbers, the fit is most satisfactory: only one point lies more than one standard deviation from the theoretical curve.

We can conclude that polyposis in predisposed persons is initiated by a forbidden clone, propagated from a single growth-control stem cell that has acquired two somatic gene mutations. Moreover, the kinetics of initiation of this clone (as defined by k_1) are the same as those for the clones that initiate early-onset colorectal carcinoma.

These data for the onset of polyposis, and for onset and death from the associated colorectal cancer, have immense theoretical importance. The multifocal origin of the numerous polyps cannot be disputed. Figure 7.39

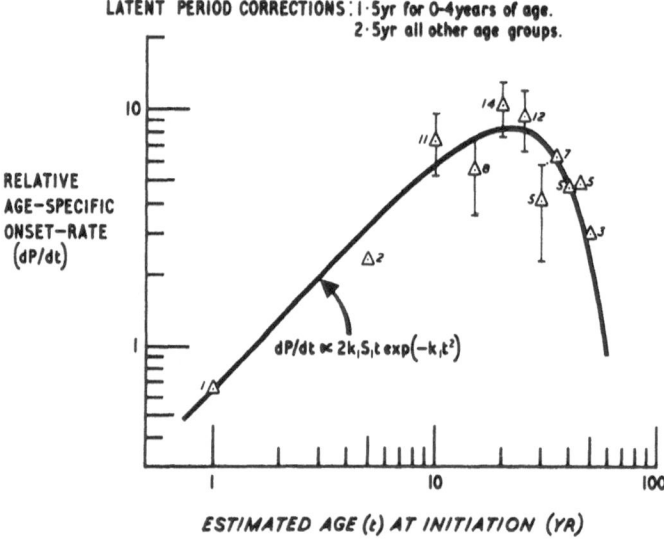

LATENT PERIOD CORRECTIONS: 1·5yr for 0-4 years of age.
2·5yr all other age groups.

RELATIVE AGE-SPECIFIC ONSET-RATE (dP/dt)

$dP/dt \propto 2k_1 S_1 t \exp(-k_1 t^2)$

ESTIMATED AGE (t) AT INITIATION (YR)

Figure 7.39 Relative age-specific onset-rate of intestinal polyposis in 73 members of a Kentucky kindred, in relation to estimated age at initiation (Asman and Pierce, 1970)

indicates that this widespread adenomatous, but pre-malignant condition, is initiated by two somatic gene mutations. These mutations occur at a constant average rate from birth, and when a growth-control stem cell in a specific cell population has acquired the two particular mutations, it propagates a forbidden clone of cells. Interactions between the products of this clone, and widely distributed colorectal epithelial cells that bear a complementary TCF, give rise to the formation of multiple polyps. Typically, some hundreds are observed (Smith and Kern, 1973).

Their carcinomatous transformation requires the formation of a second and independent forbidden clone ($n = 2$), but with the same kinetics—as defined by k_1—as the first clone. The products of this second clone must, therefore, interact with another distinctive set of colorectal epithelial cells, bearing a distinctive and complementary TCF. Conceivably, carcinomatous development in this situation requires an autoaggressive attack on *contiguous* elements of the epithelial mosaic. However, *death* from colorectal cancer does not occur until after a third, and independent forbidden clone has arisen, with the same kinetics ($k_1 \simeq 1.04 \times 10^{-3}$ year^{-2}) as the first two. Again, some form of synergism is probably implicated: contiguity between three distinctive elements of the attacked epithelium may well be necessary to produce the fatal form of the disease.

This is a vivid example of *progression* from adenoma, to malignancy and death. It is an equally convincing pointer to the *central* origin of the random events (somatic gene mutations) that initiate the sequence of changes that promote multifocal hyperplasia in the first place, and then lead to the induction of carcinoma. Collectively, these findings relating to familial intestinal polyposis and the progression to colorectal cancer strongly corroborate our theory of the age-distribution of disease (Burch *et al.*, 1973).

Papillary (villous) adenomas

In a clinicopathologic study of 219 papillary (villous) adenomas of the large intestine in 215 patients, Quan and Castro (1971) observed a high frequency (59 per cent) of carcinomatous change. Four patients had double lesions. The distribution of the age at onset of the adenomas, benign and with malignant change, is illustrated in Figure 7.40, where the data are fitted to the equation in which $n = 1$, $r = 7$. The connection between the benign and malignant tumours is obscure, although the average age of patients with benign adenomas, 57 years, was lower than that—65·1 years—of patients with malignant change (Quan and Castro, 1971). For analytical purposes, the age-dependence of the adenomas is needed by histological type, but these details were not given. Hence, the data in Figure 7.40 may result from more than one age-pattern. Some 35 of these patients (16 per cent) had additional cancers of the bowel and 105 (49 per cent) had associated adenomatous polyps. Quan and Castro (1971) suggested that these various neoplasms of the bowel might derive from a 'common genetic defect'.

Association of ulcerative colitis with cancer of the colon and rectum

The high risk of carcinoma of the colon and rectum in certain patients with ulcerative colitis is well established. MacDougall (1964) found that in distal colitis and proctitis the cancer risk was negligible, but that when

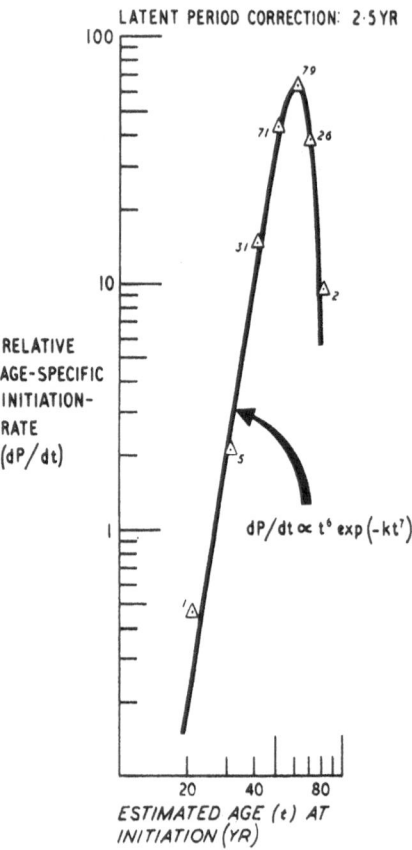

Figure 7.40 Relative age-specific onset-rate of papillary (villous) adenomas of the large intestine, in relation to estimated age at initiation (Quan and Castro, 1971)

the whole colon was involved, the risk of carcinoma was thirty times greater than in the general population. Similarly, de Dombal *et al.* (1966) estimated that the incidence of carcinoma of the colon was effectively zero in patients whose colitis was restricted to the rectum and left side of the colon, but in patients with total involvement of the colon, the estimated cumulative incidence of carcinoma was 56 per cent at 30 years after the onset of colitis, and appeared to be rising still. Furthermore, the average age of onset of cancer is much earlier in patients with ulcerative colitis than in the general population (Slaney and Brooke, 1959; MacDougall, 1964; Welch and Hedberg, 1965; Farmer, Hawk and Turnbull, 1971). From their own and other series, Slaney and Brooke (1959) calculated that the average age at onset of carcinoma in colitic patients was 42 years, in contrast to

63 years for previously healthy persons. The average age at onset of carcinoma in 37 colitic patients at the Cleveland Clinic was 40·1 years (Farmer et al., 1971).

The age-specific onset-rate of colorectal cancer in patients with ulcerative colitis raises interesting but difficult issues. One difficulty arises from a possibly high mortality (independent of colorectal cancer) associated with ulcerative colitis: selective mortality violates one of the requirements of our mathematical model (see Chapter 6). However, a recent study indicates that, in Denmark at least, mortality among ulcerative colitis patients is not as high as had been supposed (Bonnevie et al., 1974). In principle, any difficulties associated with selective mortality could be circumvented if the ulcerative colitis subpopulation could be defined, and if the age-specific onset-rate of colorectal cancer at age t could be assessed in relation to the surviving members of that subpopulation, rather than the general population.

From age-analysis, supported by independent clinical evidence, we can identify a further difficulty: *two* distinctive subpopulations (at least) are predisposed to ulcerative colitis as diagnosed in seven clinical series, from four different countries (Burch, de Dombal and Watkinson, 1969). The age-distribution of colitis in the early-onset group is described by the equation in which $n=1$, $r=2$, with a modal age of initiation at about 17 years, in each of the seven clinical series analysed. In the second subpopulation the age-distribution follows the equation with $n=1$, $r=6$ and a modal age of initiation at 50 years (Burch et al., 1969). At $t=40$ to 60 years, we found a large overlap between the two distributions. In the light of this further complication, an observation of Edwards and Truelove (1964) has special significance: '. . . none of the 56 patients age 60 or more at the start of colitis developed cancer'. MacDougall (1964) found no cases of carcinoma in those patients who first registered with ulcerative colitis at the age of 55 years and above. In the 112 cases reviewed by Slaney and Brooke (1959), only three of the colitic patients developed carcinoma above the age of 60 years.

This evidence prompts two suggestions: (a) the enhanced risk of carcinoma is largely or wholly confined to certain members of the early-onset subpopulation of ulcerative colitis patients; (b) the mid-onset group of carcinomas of the colon and rectum (Figures 7.33 to 7.37) is comprised of, or it includes, those cases that arise in the early-onset subpopulation of patients with ulcerative colitis.

To test (a) in detail, we would need to be able to allocate each colitis patient, to one of the two subpopulations. At present this cannot be done for patients aged, say, 30 to 70 years at the onset of colitis. To test (b), we would need to be able to define accurately the age-distribution of mid-onset colorectal cancer, both in the colitic and the general population.

If hypotheses (a) and (b) are both valid, then the initiation of colorectal cancer in the colitic group will probably *not* be represented by the equation with $n = 1$, $r = 8$ (as shown in Figures 7.33 to 7.37), because selective mortality in patients with ulcerative colitis should distort the age-pattern. Mortality and registry statistics are calculated on the basis of the age-structure of the *general* population, which has a lower age-specific mortality than that of the subpopulation of patients who develop ulcerative colitis. I find, however, that if statistics for cases of cancer of the colon in ulcerative colitis from various sources are combined (Slaney and Brooke, 1969; Edwards and Truelove, 1964; MacDougall, 1964; Welch and Hedberg, 1965); and if a 'pseudo-dP/dt' is calculated using the age-structure of the general population, a mode appears in the age-range 50 to 59 years. Mortality and registry statistics should define this sharp pseudo-mode fairly reliably and in Figures 7.33 to 7.37 they show a mode in the same age-range.

Tables 7.10 and 7.11 suggest that the frequency of persons in England and Wales predisposed to mid-onset cancer of the colon and rectum is about $(1 \text{ to } 3) \times 10^{-3}$. Previously, we estimated the frequency of people predisposed to colitis to be in the region of 10^{-3} (Burch *et al.*, 1969). Because a substantial proportion of the colitic subpopulation fails to develop cancer, it follows that other individuals might be predisposed to mid-onset cancer of the colon without being predisposed to ulcerative colitis. That is to say, not everyone predisposed to early-onset ulcerative colitis is predisposed to mid-onset colorectal cancer; and conversely, not everyone predisposed to mid-onset colorectal cancer is predisposed to ulcerative colitis. Predisposition to both conditions is polygenic and perhaps some, but not all, predisposing genes (alleles) are common to both conditions.

Multicentricity, multiple primaries, cancer families

Shands, Dockerty and Bargen (1952) refer to the striking multicentricity of adenocarcinomas in 40 surgically resected colons from patients who also had chronic ulcerative colitis. The distinction between hyperplastic and adenomatous polyps of the colon is described in detail by Lane, Kaplan and Pascal (1971); these authors favour the hypothesis that carcinoma of the colon arises from adenomatous, but not from hyperplastic polyps. Willis (1960) reviewed the extensive literature relating to multicentricity and he also described many of his own necropsies that, in his opinion, excluded the possibility of spread, or metastasis, from one part of the large intestine to another. Travieso, Knoepp and Hanley (1972) investigated the incidence of multiple adenocarcinomas of the colon and rectum in a large series from which they excluded patients with familial polyposis or ulcerative colitis. Thirty-four patients (1·6 per cent) had multiple synchronous adenocarcinomas and 13 (0·5 per cent) developed metachronous adenocarcinomas. Weir (1973) studied a series of 642 patients with cancer of the colon in which 26 (4 per cent) had synchronous colonic tumours and 22 (3·5 per cent) had antecedent or metachronous tumours; three patients developed a third tumour. In a series of 960 cases of colorectal cancer, from which patients with familial intestinal polyposis and ulcerative colitis were excluded, Ekelund and Pihl (1974) found that 6·5 per cent had multiple primary colorectal carcinomas: in 4·6 per cent the multiple primaries were synchronous.

Muir *et al.* (1967) reported a Maltese male who developed four synchronous primary carcinomas of the large bowel, two of the duodenum, carcinoma of the larynx, and multiple tumours of the face comprising keratoacanthomas and a sebaceous adenoma. No family history of malignancy was obtained. Schottenfeld *et al.* (1969) found that 4771 patients with index carcinomas arising in the colon or rectum subsequently developed primaries at other anatomical segments of the large intestine more frequently than expected (48 observed metachronous primaries; 15·3 expected). In the same series of 4771 patients, 142 developed primaries at sites outside the large intestine, as compared with 103·7 expected; second primaries of the skin, breast, and kidney and bladder, developed significantly more frequently than expected, by a factor of about two. Weir (1973) found in his series of 642 patients, 38 with 47 skin cancers (basal cell or squamous) and another 65 with 74 primaries mainly of the prostate, breast and genito-urinary system.

Cancer of the colon is diagnosed quite frequently in members of cancer families including Warthin's Family 'G'; some of these patients also develop a primary at another site, notably the endometrium (Lynch *et al.*, 1966; Lynch, 1967; Lynch and Krush, 1971). In a recent follow-up of Warthin's Family 'G', 53 of 114 malignancies in 96 persons were diagnosed as carcinoma of the colon (Lynch and Krush, 1971).

Cannon and Leavell (1966) described a family in which seven out of nine siblings had developed at least one malignancy; three had carcinoma of the descending colon, with age at diagnosis of 47, 50 and 58 respectively. Other families have been reported—see the literature review by Lynch (1967)— with a high incidence of carcinoma of the colon *not* associated with malignancies at other sites. A remarkable family, spanning four generations, was described by Dunstone and Knaggs (1972) in which 25 members (some still alive) had a certain diagnosis of colonic cancer; a further five may have had colonic cancer although there was some doubt over the diagnosis; 25 died with no suggestion of colonic cancer and 49 were alive with no evidence of the disease. No signs of polyposis were present and the mean age at death ranged from 42·6 years in generation IV (in which various members were still alive), to 61·7 years in generation II.

In a study from which persons with familial intestinal polyposis were excluded, Woolf (1958) found that, in the State of Utah, deaths from cancer of the colon among first-degree relatives (parents, siblings) of probands were three times more frequent than among matched controls. Macklin (1960) found that carcinoma of the colon in first- and second-degree relatives of probands was also three times higher than in controls. However, her series included one kindred with familial intestinal polyposis.

Hence the overall familial evidence is consistent with the hypothesis that genetic factors predispose to late-onset cases—which constitute the majority of colorectal cancers—as well as to the early- and mid-onset groups, associated with familial intestinal polyposis and ulcerative colitis, respectively.

Malignant Neoplasms of the Liver and Biliary Passages, Primary and Secondary (7th ICD 155 and 156)

The combined categories 7th ICD 155 and 156 extracted by Segi and Kurihara (1966) suggests a heterogenous group of diseases. This expectation is confirmed by statistics from the German Democratic Republic and Swedish cancer registries, in which ICD 155 is broken down into 155·0 'liver primary' and 155·1, 'gallbladder, extrahepatic bile ducts and ampulla of Vater'. Because these two categories exhibit different forms of age-dependence and because category ICD 156 gives a third form, mortality statistics as published by Segi and Kurihara (1966) for the combined classifications ICD 155 and 156 are not illustrated here.

In Figures 7.41 and 7.42, the German Democratic Republic and Swedish data for ICD 155·0 are fitted to the stochastic equation in which $n = 3$, $r = 3$.

A very small group, with onset predominantly at 0–4 years, is not illustrated in Figures 7.41 and 7.42. The rates in excess of the theoretical curve at low t, in all data except for males, German Democratic Republic, appear erratic and might therefore be due to diagnostic error. Both sets of data suggest that $k_M > k_F$ but the modes are not defined in the Swedish data and the suggestion is unreliable. However, S_M exceeds S_F in both countries. In the German Democratic Republic, $S_M/S_F \simeq 1·4$ and in Sweden, the corresponding ratio is about 1·7. An X-linked predisposing allele of frequency about 0·7 in the German Democratic Republic, and about 0·6 in Sweden, could account for these sex ratios. Because the absolute frequency of pre-disposed persons is in the region of 10^{-2}, predisposing autosomal as well as X-linked factors, need to be invoked. The higher values of S in Sweden could be attributed, at least in part, to the markedly lower values of k and

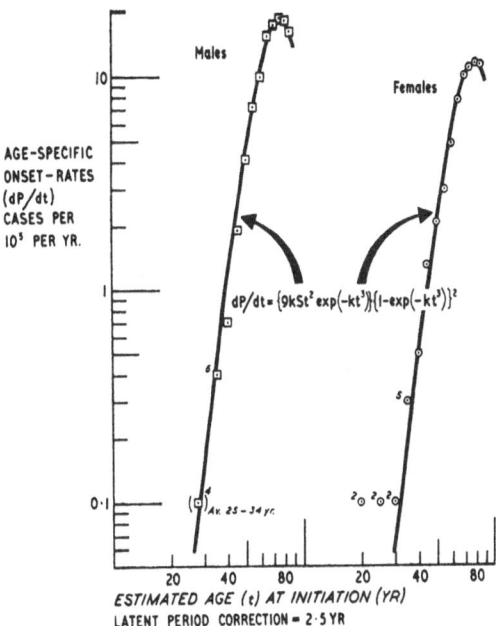

Figure 7.41 Sex-specific and age-specific onset-rates for primary malignant neoplasms of the liver, German Democratic Republic, 1964–66, in relation to estimated age at initiation (Doll *et al.*, 1970)

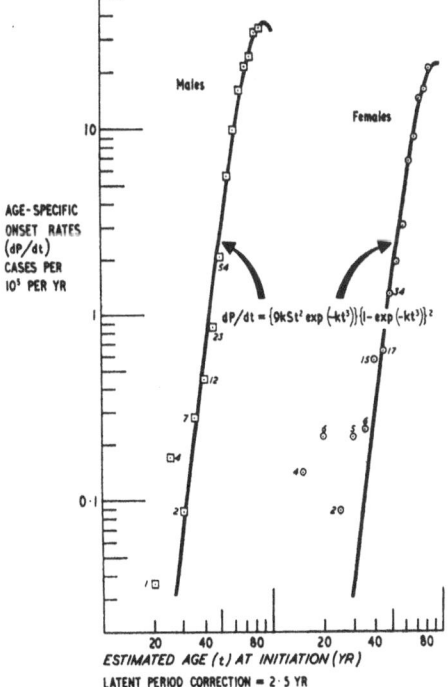

Figure 7.42 As for Figure 7.41. Data for Sweden, 1959–68 (Swedish Cancer Registry, 1971)

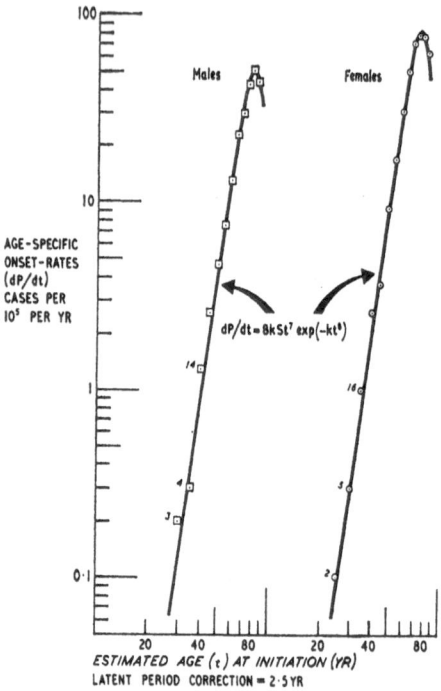

Figure 7.43 Sex-specific and age-specific onset-rates for malignant neoplasms of the gallbladder, extrahepatic bile ducts and ampulla of Vater, German Democratic Republic, 1964–66, in relation to estimated age at initiation (Doll *et al.*, 1970)

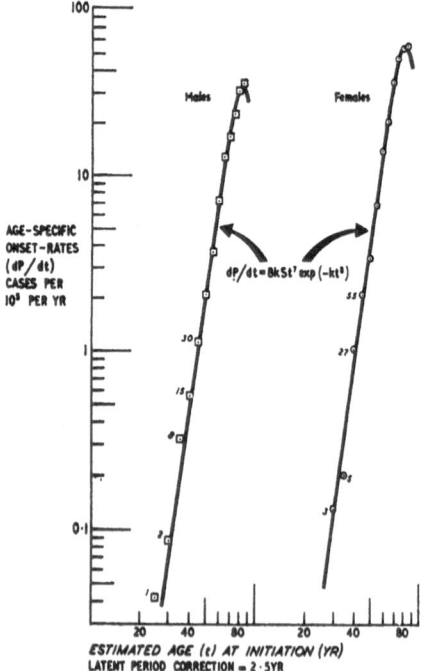

Figure 7.44 As for Figure 7.43. Data for Sweden, 1959–68 (Swedish Cancer Registry, 1971)

the consequent lower selection pressure against the predisposing genotype.

In Figures 7.43 and 7.44, the German Democratic Republic and Swedish registry data for ICD 155·1 are fitted to the equation in which $n = 1$, $r = 8$.

This is one of those rather rare cancers common to both sexes for which $S_F > S_M$. The small apparent sex-differences in k are unreliable, however, because the modal dP/dt is ill defined. From both the German and the Swedish statistics, $S_F/S_M \simeq 1·6$. On a genetic basis, this ratio could be attributed to a dominant-effect X-linked allele of frequency about 0·4. Again, it would be necessary to invoke one or more predisposing autosomal factors to account for the frequency of predisposed persons in the population. This frequency is higher in the German Democratic Republic than in Sweden, despite an apparently slightly higher value of k in the former country.

No clear indications of heterogeneity can be seen: the data fit the theoretical curves satisfactorily. However, small groups with modes at high t would be undetectable.

The incidence of primary carcinoma of the liver is high in the Bantu (Oettle, 1956), but the available data (Oettle and Higginson, 1956; Doll et al., 1966, 1970) for age-specific onset-rates are too scanty for reliable analysis of the age-patterns. However, below $t = 50$ years, the age-dependence is much less steep than in Figures 7.41 and 7.42.

Table 7.12 Malignant Neoplasms of Liver: Primary (7th ICD 155.0) (Analysis of Registry Statistics for Onset)

Population	Males		Females	
	k	S	k	S
German Democratic Republic 1964–66	$3·5 \times 10^{-6}$ yr^{-3}	$7·6 \times 10^{-3}$	$2·9 \times 10^{-6}$ yr^{-3}	$5·3 \times 10^{-3}$
Sweden 1959–68	$2·0 \times 10^{-6}$ yr^{-3}	$1·9 \times 10^{-3}$	$1·8 \times 10^{-6}$ yr^{-3}	$1·15 \times 10^{-2}$

Latent period correction $= 2·5$ years. Parameters $n = 3$, $r = 3$

Table 7.13 Malignant Neoplasms of the Gallbladder, Extrahepatic Bile Ducts and Ampulla of Vater (7th ICD 155.1) (Analysis of Registry Statistics for Onset)

Population	Males		Females	
	k	S	k	S
German Democratic Republic 1964–66	$4·9 \times 10^{-16}$ yr^{-8}	$1·4 \times 10^{-2}$	$7·3 \times 10^{-16}$ yr^{-8}	$2·2 \times 10^{-2}$
Sweden 1959–68	$3·7 \times 10^{-16}$ yr^{-8}	$9·2 \times 10^{-3}$	$4·0 \times 10^{-16}$ yr^{-8}	$1·6 \times 10^{-2}$

Latent period correction $= 2·5$ years. Parameters $n = 1$, $r = 8$

Table 7.14 Malignant Neoplasms of the Larynx (Tentative Analysis of Death-rates)

Population	Males				Females			
	Mid-onset $(n=3, r=4)$		Late-onset $(n=1, r=12)$		Mid-onset $(n=3, r=4)$		Late-onset $(n=1, r=12)$	
	k_2	S_2	k_3	S_3	k_2	S_2	k_3	S_3
England and Wales	7.7×10^{-8} yr^{-4}	3.4×10^{-3}	1.2×10^{-23} yr^{-12}	4.4×10^{-3}	1.5×10^{-7} yr^{-4}	3.7×10^{-4}	1.6×10^{-23} yr^{-12}	6.3×10^{-4}
Japan	7.7×10^{-8} yr^{-4}	2.7×10^{-3}	1.8×10^{-23} yr^{-12}	1.7×10^{-3}	1.5×10^{-7} yr^{-4}	2.2×10^{-4}	2.5×10^{-23} yr^{-12}	7.0×10^{-4}
US White	1.0×10^{-7} yr^{-4}	1.0×10^{-3}	1.0×10^{-23} yr^{-12}	2.6×10^{-3}	2.0×10^{-7} yr^{-4}	2.0×10^{-4}	1.0×10^{-23} yr^{-12}	4.0×10^{-4}

Latent period correction $= 5$ years.

Familial aggregations

Kaplan and Cole (1965) reviewed the earlier reports of familial aggregations of liver cancer and described a family in which three male siblings developed primary carcinoma of the liver. Other family studies have been described by Hagstrom and Baker (1968), Denison and Reynolds (1971) and Hagstrom and Ho (1972).

Malignant Neoplasms of the Larynx (7th ICD 161)

Several difficulties arise over the interpretation of the age-patterns of cancer of the larynx: (a) numbers of cases, especially of women, are small; (b) the age-dependence is complex, indicating two, and possibly three, distinctive groups with largely unresolved modes; (c) survival is relatively high; (d) because of (c), it would be advantageous to analyse registry statistics for onset, but because of (a), the data available from registries lack statistical accuracy. Accordingly, the interpretations shown in Figures 7.45 to 7.47 and Table 7.14 must be regarded as tentative.

No attempt has been made to characterize an early-onset group, which is relatively conspicuous in the data for males, England and Wales. For the mid-onset group, characterized by $n = 3$, $r = 4$, the value of k in females appears to be double that in males. Should this be confirmed, it would suggest that one of the four somatic mutations initiating the growth of each clone is of an X-linked gene (Table 7.14). Values of $S_{2,F}$ are rather similar in the three populations, but $S_{2,M}$ for England and Wales is more than treble that for US Whites. The characterization of the late-onset group ($n = 1$, $r = 12$) needs to be treated with great reserve and it is doubtful, for example, whether k_3 shows genuine sex-differences in England and Wales, and Japan. However, there is no doubting the large sex-differences in both S_2 and S_3 in all three populations. The highest ratio of S_M to S_F is seen in the mid-onset group of US Whites, where $S_{2,M}/S_{2,F} \simeq 19$. Male predominance can be explained if an X-linked recessive factor contributes to the polygenic predisposition for each group. According to the conventional rules, the frequency of an X-linked allele that would yield $S_M/S_F = 19$, is 0.05_3. The highest value of S_M is found for the late-onset group of males in England and Wales, with $S_{3,M} \simeq 4.4 \times 10^{-3} : S_{3,M}/S_{3,F} \simeq 7$. For $S_{3,M}/S_{3,F} \simeq 7$, the frequency of the predisposing X-linked allele (see above) is 0.14 and that of the predisposing autosomal contribution to this genotype would need to be about $4.4 \times 10^{-3}/1.4 \times 10^{-1}$, that is, 3×10^{-2}.

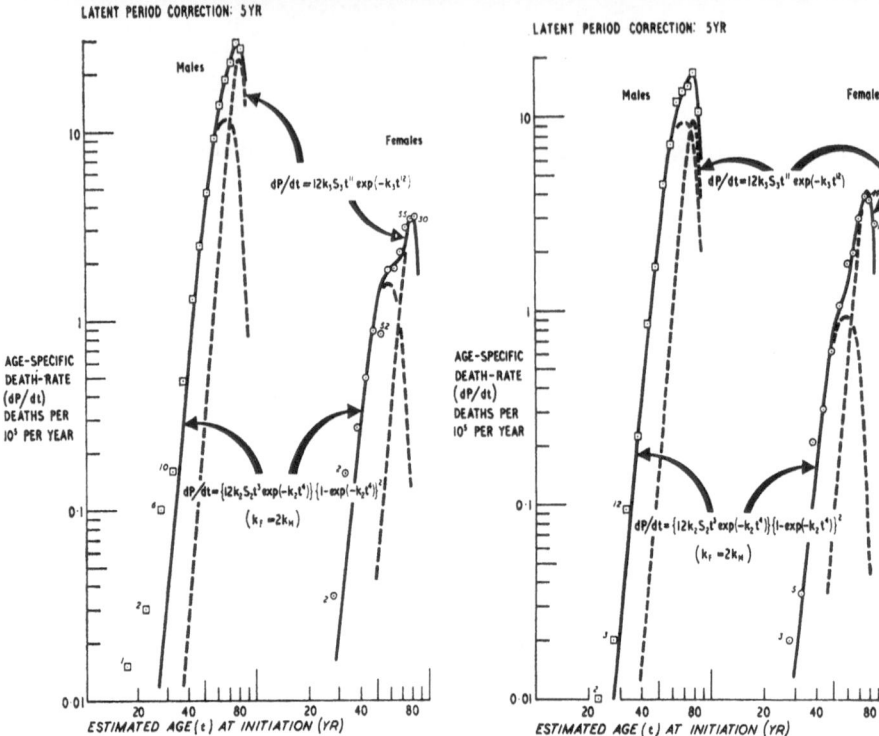

Figure 7.45 Sex-specific and age-specific death-rates from malignant neoplasms of the larynx, England and Wales, 1960–63, in relation to estimated age at initiation (Segi and Kurihara, 1966). See Table 7.14

Figure 7.46 As for Figure 7.45. Data for Japan, 1960–63

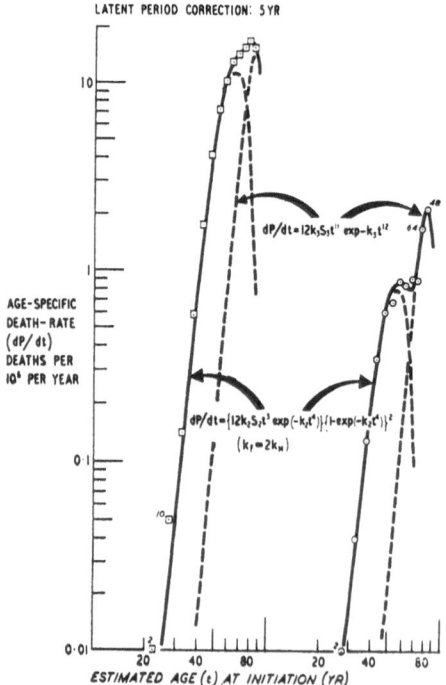

Figure 7.47 As for Figure 7.45. Data for US Whites, 1960–63

Secular trends

Over the period 1950 to 1963, the recorded crude death-rates from cancer of the larynx have remained virtually constant in US Whites. A very small decrease has occurred in Japan: 1·29 to 1·20 per 10^5 per year in males, and 0·44 to 0·34 (same units) in females. A marked fall has been recorded in England and Wales: from 3·72 (1950–51), to 2·77 (1962–63) in males (same units), and from 0·85 to 0·61 in females over the corresponding period.

Multicentricity: association with papilloma

Of 1100 patients with squamous cell carcinoma of the larynx studied by Moertel *et al.* (1961b), 18 had two discrete lesions, mainly one on each vocal cord. Another 22 patients in this series had associated (contiguous) squamous cell carcinoma involving the lips, oral cavity, pharynx or oesophagus.

In view of the suggestion that the mid-onset group requires three forbidden clones for initiation of malignancy, we can expect to find evidence for pre-malignant change promoted by one or two of these clones. This expectation is confirmed by the association in adults (but *not* in children) between papillomas and carcinoma (Willis, 1960). After repeated recurrences, initially non-invasive single or multiple papillomas have been observed to become carcinomatous; some papillae are malignant when first observed (Willis, 1960). Willis believes that all papillary growths in the larynx should be regarded as potentially malignant.

Malignant Neoplasms of the Small Intestine (7th ICD 152)

Cancers of the small intestine are much less common than those of the stomach, or of the large intestine and rectum. From Figures 7.48 to 7.50 we see that the numbers of deaths, even from four years of national mortality statistics, remain small. Below the age of 35 years in Japan, numbers are too small to define the early-onset group: the interpretation given in Table 7.15 for the other two populations must be regarded as provisional.

Values of k_1 and k_2 show no obvious sex-differential, but $S_{1,M} > S_{1,F}$ and $S_{2,M} > S_{2,F}$. These relations suggest that recessive-effect X-linked alleles contribute to both early- and late-onset predisposing genotypes. For the late-onset group, where the data are better defined, the frequency of the recessive X-linked allele suggested by the sex-ratio $S_{2,M}/S_{2,F}$ is 0·75 in England and Wales, 0·79 in Japan and 0·81 in US Whites.

Association with Peutz–Jeghers syndrome

Bearing in mind the association discussed above between familial intestinal polyposis and colorectal cancer, we need to inquire whether the early-onset

Table 7.15 Malignant Neoplasms of the Small Intestine (Tentative Analysis of Death-rates)

Population	Males				Females			
	Early-onset $(n=1, r=4)$		Late-onset $(n=1, r=7)$		Early-onset $(n=1, r=4)$		Late-onset $(n=1, r=7)$	
	k_1	S_1	k_2	S_2	k_1	S_1	k_2	S_2
England and Wales	$6·6 \times 10^{-8}$ yr^{-4}	$1·3 \times 10^{-4}$	$7·7 \times 10^{-14}$ yr^{-7}	$9·2 \times 10^{-4}$	$6·6 \times 10^{-8}$ yr^{-4}	$1·0 \times 10^{-4}$	$7·7 \times 10^{-14}$ yr^{-7}	$6·9 \times 10^{-4}$
Japan	?	small	$7·7 \times 10^{-14}$ yr^{-7}	$7·5 \times 10^{-4}$	?	small	$7·7 \times 10^{-14}$ yr^{-7}	$5·9 \times 10^{-4}$
US White	$6·6 \times 10^{-8}$ yr^{-4}	$1·5 \times 10^{-4}$	$4·1 \times 10^{-14}$ yr^{-7}	$1·23 \times 10^{-3}$	$6·6 \times 10^{-8}$ yr^{-4}	$7·5 \times 10^{-5}$	$4·1 \times 10^{-14}$ yr^{-7}	$1·0 \times 10^{-3}$

Latent period correction $= 5$ years.

form of cancer of the small intestine is associated with the Peutz–Jeghers syndrome. This syndrome is said to be inherited as an autosomal dominant (Jeghers, McKusick and Katz, 1949). The intestinal polyposis is associated with melanin pigmented spots on the oral mucosa, distal portions of the fingers and sometimes of the vaginal mucosa. Any part of the gastrointestinal tract, except the esophagus, can develop polyps, although the jejunum and ileum are most commonly affected.

Freeman and Ravdin (1959) reported that two polyps of the small intestine in a 35-year-old patient with Peutz–Jeghers syndrome became malignant and invaded the muscularis. Achord and Proctor (1963) documented a carcinoma of the stomach and metastasis in a 13-year-old Negro girl with Peutz–Jeghers syndrome. Horne, Payne and Fine (1963) described a girl with this syndrome who was first seen at the age of 12 years; she died at the age of 45 from a metastatic cancer in the region of the gastroduodenal junction. Reid (1965) described a 39-year-old woman with Peutz–Jeghers syndrome who died from carcinoma of the duodenum with metastasis; at autopsy, polyps were found throughout the remainder of the small and large intestine. Williams and Knudsen (1965) refer to a woman, age 52 years, who had carcinomatous change of a polyp, and a metastasis in a regional lymph node. (It should be remarked that malignant development in the Peutz–Jeghers syndrome is not confined to the small intestine: Humphries, Shepperd and Peters (1966) reported a case with colonic adenocarcinoma and an ovarian tumour.) The age at onset or death from cancer of the small intestine in these few cases suggests that patients with the Peutz–Jeghers syndrome contribute to the early-onset group.

Familial carcinoma of the duodenum, in association with polyposis, was reported by Ungar (1949). A girl aged 19 had multiple polyps of the colon, adenocarcinoma and papilliferous carcinoma of the duodenum. One brother died at 16 years with multiple polyps and carcinoma of the duodenum; another brother at 18 years had polyposis of the small intestine, single polyps of the colon and adenocarcinoma of the duodenum. In view of these many suggestions of progression from polyposis to carcinoma the tentative interpretation in Figures 7.48 to 7.50 of the early-onset group in terms of $n = 1$, $r = 4$ must be questioned: it seems more likely that $n > 1$. More extensive data, either for the onset of polyposis and/or for death-rates should eventually resolve this issue.

Association with Crohn's disease

Following the original description by Ginzburg, Schneider and Dreizin (1956), several reports have described the occurrence of carcinoma of the small bowel in patients with Crohn's disease—see the literature reviews and

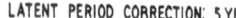

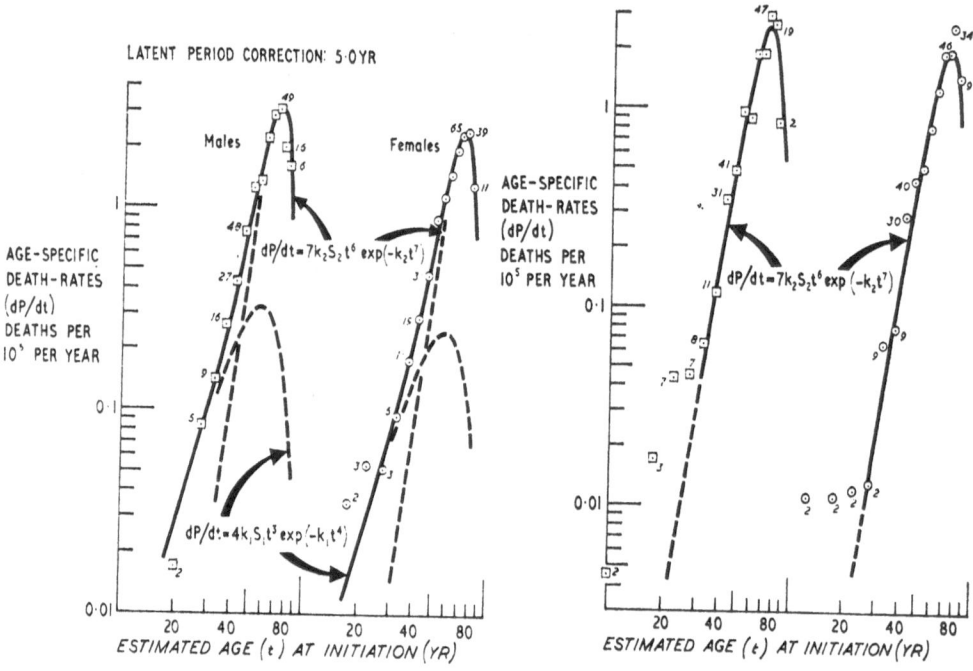

Figure 7.48

Figure 7.49

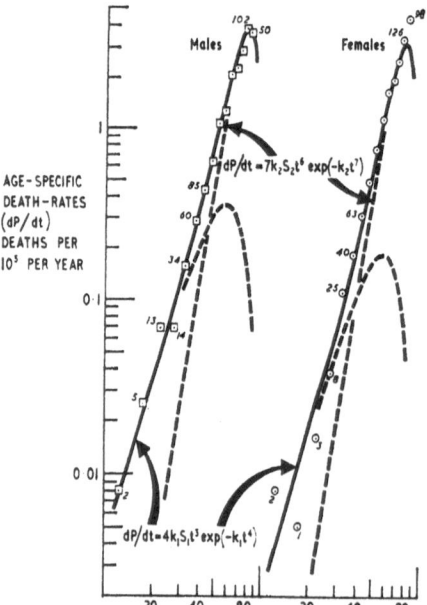

Figure 7.50

Figure 7.48 Sex-specific and age-specific death-rates from malignant neoplasms of the small intestine, England and Wales, 1960–63, in relation to estimated age at initiation (Segi and Kurihara, 1966). See Table 7.15

Figure 7.49 As for Figure 7.48. Data for Japan, 1960–63

Figure 7.50 As for Figure 7.48. Data for US Whites, 1960–63

case reports by Tyers, Steiger and Rudrick (1969) and by Bruni *et al.* (1971). Nevertheless, the association is a rare one. The mean age at diagnosis of the adenocarcinoma is 12 years earlier than in the general population (Tyers *et al.*, 1969). The difference in the modal ages for the two groups shown in Figures 7.48 and 7.50 is 15 to 20 years, and hence the malignancy associated with Crohn's disease may well belong to the early-onset group.

Tyers *et al.* (1969) reported that in seven out of 16 cases, the adeno-carcinoma of the small intestine in patients with Crohn's disease was multi-focal, or diffuse, in contrast to the usually localized carcinoma of the small intestine. The gross anatomical distribution also differs: the sites usually involved are the second part of the duodenum and the upper part of the jejunum, but in Crohn's disease, the ileum is most commonly affected (Tyers *et al.*, 1969).

Malignant Neoplasms of the Cervix Uteri (7th ICD 171) and the Corpus Uteri (7th ICD 172)

Survival from cancers of the neck and body of the uterus is often prolonged. Thus, over the geriod 1942–56, the average observed survival-rate in California at 15 years after diagnosis of cancer of the cervix, for all ages of onset, was 33 per cent; for cases with onset under the age of 45 years, the corresponding rate was 52 per cent (California Tumor Registry, 1963). A similarly good prognosis was recorded for malignant neoplasms at other uterine sites: the average survival at 15 years after diagnosis, for all ages of onset, was 38 per cent. For patients with onset under the age of 45 years, the corresponding rate was 66 per cent. Consequently, age-specific death-rates for these cancers are not suitable for estimating age-specific initiation-rates. I have therefore relied on the less numerous data from cancer registries to determine age-specific initiation-rates.

Cervix uteri

Willis (1960) divides carcinoma of the uterus into three groups: (a) epi-dermoid carcinoma of the cervix, with a relatively early onset; (b) endo-metrial adenocarcinoma of the corpus; and (c) adenocarcinoma of the cervix, which, like (b), has a relatively late onset. Malignancies of groups (a) and (b) are distinct in structure and behaviour, but (b) cannot always be separated from (c). These views of Willis are corroborated by the age-patterns.

Figure 7.51 shows the connection between the registry data for England and Wales (on the left) and mortality data (on the right) for cancer of the

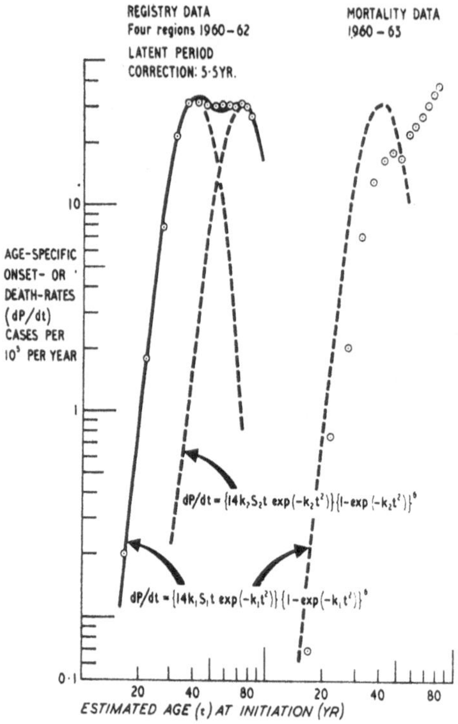

Figure 7.51

REGISTRY DATA
Four regions 1960–62
LATENT PERIOD
CORRECTION: 5·5 YR.

MORTALITY DATA
1960–63

AGE–SPECIFIC
ONSET– OR
DEATH–RATES
(dP/dt)
CASES PER
10^5 PER YEAR

10

1

0·1

$dP/dt = \{14k_2 S_2 t \exp(-k_2 t^2)\}\{1-\exp(-k_2 t^2)\}^5$

$dP/dt = \{14k_1 S_1 t \exp(-k_1 t^2)\}\{1-\exp(-k_1 t^2)\}^5$

20   40   80   20   40   80
ESTIMATED AGE (t) AT INITIATION (YR)

Figure 7.51

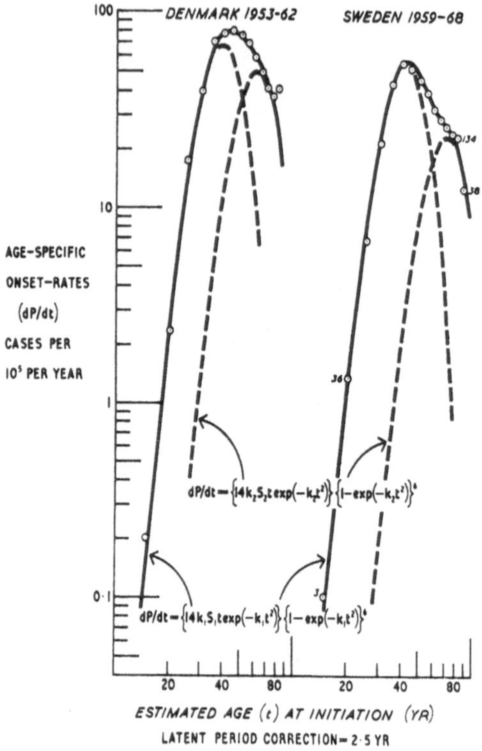

Figure 7.52

DENMARK 1953–62   SWEDEN 1959–68

100

AGE–SPECIFIC
ONSET–RATES
(dP/dt)
CASES PER
10^5 PER YEAR

10

1

0·1

$dP/dt = \{14k_2 S_2 t \exp(-k_2 t^2)\}\{1-\exp(-k_2 t^2)\}^4$

$dP/dt = \{14k_1 S_1 t \exp(-k_1 t^2)\}\{1-\exp(-k_1 t^2)\}^4$

20   40   80   20   40   80
ESTIMATED AGE (t) AT INITIATION (YR)
LATENT PERIOD CORRECTION= 2·5 YR

Figure 7.52

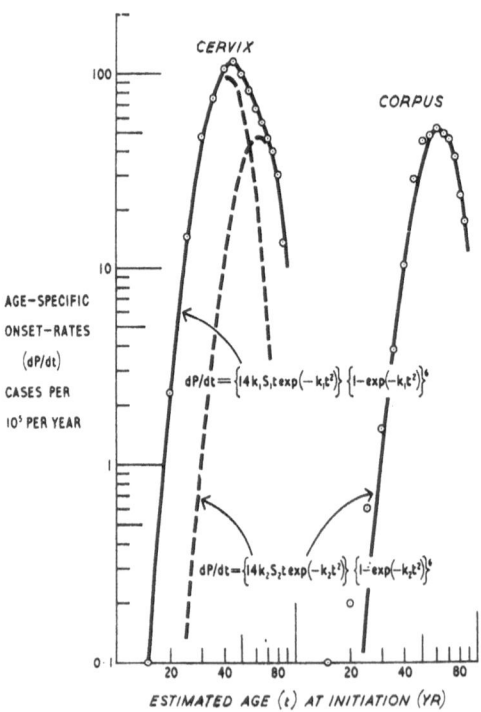

CERVIX

100

CORPUS

AGE–SPECIFIC
ONSET–RATES
(dP/dt)
CASES PER
10^5 PER YEAR

10

1

0·1

$dP/dt = \{14k_2 S_2 t \exp(-k_2 t^2)\}\{1-\exp(-k_2 t^2)\}^4$

$dP/dt = \{14k_1 S_1 t \exp(-k_1 t^2)\}\{1-\exp(-k_1 t^2)\}^4$

20   40   80   20   40   80
ESTIMATED AGE (t) AT INITIATION (YR)
LATENT PERIOD CORRECTION ~ 2·5 YR

Figure 7.53

Figure 7.51 Malignant neoplasms of the uterine cervix, Registry data for onset in four regions, England and Wales, 1960–62, left panel (Doll *et al.*, 1966); mortality data England and Wales, 1960–63, right panel (Segi and Kurihara, 1966), contrasted with the initiation curve for early-onset cases. See Table 7.16

Figure 7.52 Registry data for age-specific onset-rates, malignant neoplasms of the uterine cervix, Denmark, 1953–62, left panel (Doll *et al.*, 1966); and Sweden, 1959–68, right panel (Swedish Cancer Registry, 1971) in relation to estimated age at initiation. See Table 7.16

Figure 7.53 Registry data for age-specific onset-rates, German Democratic Republic, 1964–66, malignant neoplasms of the uterine cervix, left panel; and of the body of the uterus, right panel (Doll *et al.*, 1970), in relation to estimated age at initiation. See Tables 7.16 and 7.18

cervix uteri in similar populations, and over similar periods. The broken curve on the right of the figure is a replica of the one on the left, for the early-onset group. This curve is described by $n = 7$, $r = 2$.

Age-specific initiation-rates for the late-onset group are also interpreted in terms of the same form of equation ($n = 7$, $r = 2$) as the early-onset group, but with a much lower value of k and a different value of S. Needless to say, calculated values of S_1 and S_2 depend on the completeness of registration.

Figure 7.52 shows corresponding statistics from the Danish (1953–62) and Swedish (1959–68) cancer registries. Figure 7.53 presents data for cervical carcinoma (left panel) and for carcinoma of the corpus (right panel), from the German Democratic Republic registry, 1964–66.

Marked differences are seen in the values of S_1 (Table 7.16), ranging from a low of $7 \cdot 3 \times 10^{-3}$ (England and Wales, four regions, 1960–62), to a high of $2 \cdot 5 \times 10^{-3}$ (German Democratic Republic, 1964–66). This early-onset group corresponds to epidermoid carcinoma of the cervix, which is rarely seen under the age of 25 or after 65 (Willis, 1960). Differences in S_1 fail to correlate with the (closely similar) values of k_1.

Values of S_2 span a narrower range than S_1, from a low of $9 \cdot 5 \times 10^{-3}$ for Sweden, to a high of $1 \cdot 87 \times 10^{-2}$ for Denmark. However, k_2 shows a wider range of variation than k_1. The late-onset group corresponds to adenocarcinoma of the cervix (Willis, 1960).

Relation between dysplasia, intra-epithelial carcinoma and clinical invasive carcinoma of the cervix: further corroboration of theory

From cytological screening, Kashgarian and Dunn (1970) have determined the age-specific prevalence of women with intra-epithelial carcinoma (carcinoma *in situ*) in Memphis, Tennessee. They distinguished the following stages in the development of cervical cancer: no disease →intra-epithelial carcinoma →preclinical invasive cancer →clinical invasive cancer as recorded in cancer registries →death or cure.

The data of Kashgarian and Dunn (1970) can be used to test the hypotheses: (a) seven forbidden clones (as defined above) produce clinical invasive cancer; (b) six produce preclinical invasive cancer; and (c) five produce intra-epithelial carcinoma.

For this scheme of progression, the age-specific prevalence, $P_{t,\text{IE},1}$, of women of the early-onset group with initiated intra-epithelial cancer— which requires exactly five forbidden clones—should be described by $P_{t,5} - P_{t,6}$; that is by

$$P_{t,\text{IE},1} = S_1[\{1 - \exp(-k_1 t^2)\}^5 - \{1 - \exp(-k_1 t^2)\}^6] \qquad (7.1)$$

Similarly, the age-specific prevalence of women in the late-onset group with initiated intra-epithelial cancer, should be given by

$$P_{t,\text{IE},2} = S_2[\{1 - \exp(-k_2t^2)\}^5 - \{1 - \exp(-k_2t^2)\}^6] \qquad (7.2)$$

Figure 7.54 shows Kashgarian and Dunn's (1970) data for the age-specific prevalence of intra-epithelial cancer in 434 white women, and the theoretical curves based on equations (7.1) and (7.2). The closeness of fit, in view of the complexity of the data, the overall number of cases, and the problems of diagnosis, is remarkably satisfactory. Moreover, the value of k_1 ($1{\cdot}5 \times 10^{-3}$ year^{-2}) is almost the same as for the European countries (Table 7.16), and the value of k_2 ($4{\cdot}2 \times 10^{-4}$ year^{-2}) is the same as for England and Wales, 1960–62 (see Tables 7.16 and 7.17). S_1 is $9{\cdot}4 \times 10^{-2}$ and S_2 is $5{\cdot}5 \times 10^{-2}$. These high values, in comparison with those in Table 7.16, make it doubtful

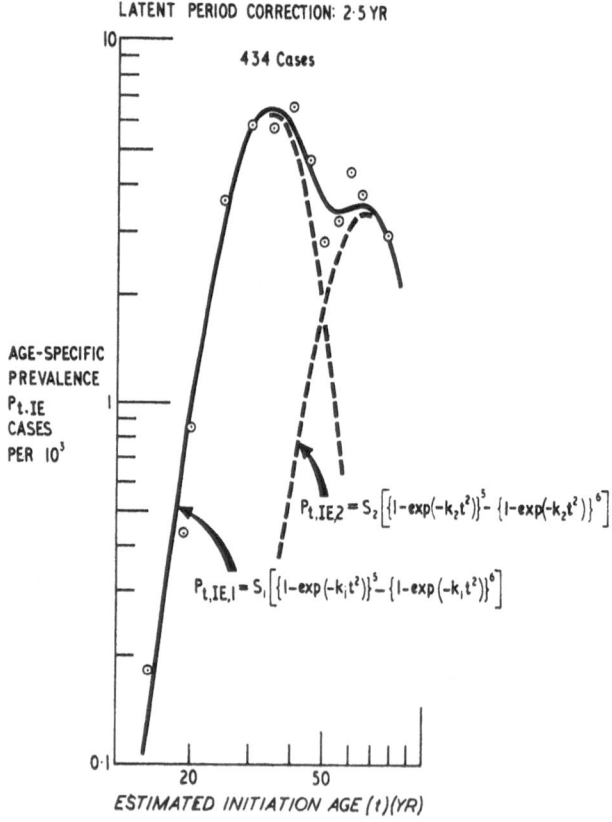

Figure 7.54 Age-specific prevalence of intra-epithelial carcinoma of the cervix (carcinoma *in situ*), white women, Memphis, in relation to estimated initiation age (Kashgarian and Dunn, 1970). See Table 7.17

Table 7.16 Malignant Neoplasms of the Cervix Uteri (Interpretation of Registry Data)

Population	Early-onset ($n=7$, $r=2$)		Late-onset ($n=7$, $r=2$)	
	k_1	S_1	k_2	S_2
England and Wales, four regions 1960–62	$1{\cdot}4 \times 10^{-3}$ yr^{-2}	$7{\cdot}3 \times 10^{-3}$	$4{\cdot}2 \times 10^{-4}$ yr^{-2}	$1{\cdot}31 \times 10^{-2}$
German Democratic Republic 1964–66	$1{\cdot}3 \times 10^{-3}$ yr^{-2}	$2{\cdot}47 \times 10^{-2}$	$5{\cdot}7 \times 10^{-4}$ yr^{-2}	$1{\cdot}79 \times 10^{-2}$
Denmark 1953–62	$1{\cdot}4 \times 10^{-3}$ yr^{-2}	$1{\cdot}81 \times 10^{-2}$	$5{\cdot}9 \times 10^{-4}$ yr^{-2}	$1{\cdot}87 \times 10^{-2}$
Sweden 1959–68	$1{\cdot}3 \times 10^{-3}$ yr^{-2}	$1{\cdot}36 \times 10^{-2}$	$4{\cdot}5 \times 10^{-4}$ yr^{-2}	$9{\cdot}5 \times 10^{-3}$

Latent period corrections $= 5{\cdot}5$ years England and Wales
$\qquad\qquad\qquad\qquad 2{\cdot}5$ years German Democratic Republic, Denmark and Sweden

Table 7.17 Intra-epithelial Carcinoma of the Uterine Cervix (Carcinoma in situ) (Interpretation of Kashgarian and Dunn's (1970) Data)

Population	Early-onset ($n=5$, $r=2$)		Late-onset ($n=5$, $r=2$)	
	k_1	S_1	k_2	S_2
Memphis, Tennessee (White)	$1{\cdot}5 \times 10^{-3}$ yr^{-2}	$9{\cdot}4 \times 10^{-2}$	$4{\cdot}2 \times 10^{-4}$ yr^{-2}	$5{\cdot}5 \times 10^{-2}$

whether all cases of intra-epithelial carcinoma progress to clinically invasive carcinoma.

The connection between atypical lesions, or dysplasia, and cervical carcinoma also has important clinical and theoretical implications. Although Kashgarian and Dunn (1970) do not give the age-specific prevalence of women with dysplasia, a large series based on a self-selected sample of 7000 women in Barbados, West Indies, has been reported by Barron and Richart (1971). Numbers of women above the age of 40 years with dysplasia are small, but below 40 years numbers are adequate to define the age-specific prevalence in the early-onset group (Figure 7.55). They are used to test the hypothesis: a single forbidden clone suffices to initiate dysplasia in both early- and late-onset groups; and five forbidden clones, as described above, initiate carcinoma in situ in both early- and late-onset groups.

On this scheme, the age-specific prevalence of women with initiated dysplasia who belong to the early-onset group should be given by

$$P_{t,D} = S_1[\{1 - \exp(-k_1 t^2)\} - \{1 - \exp(-k_1 t^2)\}^5] \qquad (7.3)$$

and for the late-onset group

$$P_{t,D} = S_2[\{1 - \exp(-k_2 t^2)\} - \{1 - \exp(-k_2 t^2)\}^5] \qquad (7.4)$$

Figure 7.55 shows the good fit of Barron and Richart's (1971) data to the sum of equations (7.3) and (7.4.) The value of k_1 is $2 \cdot 0 \times 10^{-3}$ year^{-2} and

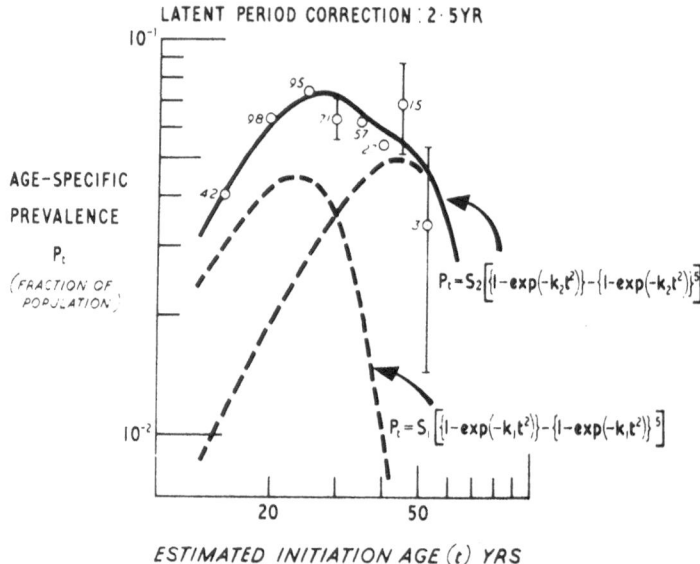

Figure 7.55 Age-specific prevalence of cervical dysplasia, Barbados, in relation to estimated initiation age (Barron and Richart, 1971)

that of k_2 about $5 \cdot 7 \times 10^{-4}$ year^{-2}, which is within the range found for the European countries. The value of S_1 is $1 \cdot 8 \times 10^{-1}$ and of S_2 is $2 \cdot 1 \times 10^{-1}$. These values for the proportion of the population predisposed to cervical dysplasia are much higher than those in Table 7.16 that relate to carcinoma. They raise the question as to whether dysplasia, given time, would always progress to carcinoma in situ. Successive screenings of women in a large population could answer this question and the related one concerning progression from intra-epithelial to clinically invasive carcinoma.

Thomas (1973) found that women with carcinoma in situ are epidemiologically similar to those with invasive carcinoma of the cervix, but that only a portion of women with dysplasia are epidemiologically similar to those with carcinoma in situ. This study suggests that only certain women with dysplasia are genetically predisposed to carcinoma in situ and invasive carcinoma. Equations (7.3) and (7.4) assume, however, that all women with initiated dysplasia progress to carcinoma in situ. The agreement (Figure 7.55) with these equations could be explained if dysplasia regresses with kinetics similar to those that describe progression to carcinoma *in situ*. However, the numbers of cases in Figure 7.55 are inadequate to resolve the problem.

When we consider the age-specific prevalence of dysplasia at low *t*, we cannot easily avoid the implication that it is initiated by two random events —for example, two somatic gene mutations in a single cell. We encounter analogous situations in numerous other diseases that have no connection with neoplastic change, but whose lesions have a multifocal or widespread anatomical distribution in the body (Burch, 1968(a)).

Essentially, we have to explain how, in non-neoplastic and pre-neoplastic disorders, a small number of random events, or only one, can change an astronomical number of target cells. The remarkable properties of these events indicate that they are gene mutations in somatic cells whose number remains constant throughout postnatal life. So far as I can discern, only hypotheses along the broad lines of Burnet's forbidden clone theory can cope plausibly with this type of evidence. Following Burnet, the effects of somatic mutation in, say, a single stem cell, are 'amplified' first by the growth of a clone of cells from the mutant stem cell, and then, when the target tissue lies behind a blood-tissue barrier, by the synthesis and secretion of mutant humoral factors.

A carcinoma—almost by definition—is the consequence of a breakdown in the normal control of growth and tissue size. The mathematics of the age-distributions of malignant and pre-malignant states, together with findings from pathology (see below), both imply that the breakdown of growth-control is initiated in the central part of the homeostatic system. As Orr (1958) has emphasized, carcinoma *in situ* cannot be explained on the basis of multiplication from a single epithelial cell. Similar or even more cogent arguments apply to cervical dysplasia.

Corpus uteri

Registry data from Denmark, the German Democratic Republic and Sweden are shown relative to the curve for which $n = 7$, $r = 2$ (Figures 7.53 and 7.56): the k values are the same as those used to fit the late-onset group of cervical carcinoma (Figures 7.52 and 7.53).

Fascinating connections between the registry data and the theoretical curves emerge. The Swedish and German Democratic Republic data at $t < 60$ years show somewhat erratic deviations above the theoretical curve, but the Danish data deviate below it. (Large deviations are seen in the data for England and Wales—not illustrated here.) In view of the difficulty of distinguishing between borderline endometrial adenocarcinoma of the corpus, and adenocarcinoma of the cervix (Willis, 1960), it is likely that

these deviations arise principally from diagnostic ambiguity. In the data
from Denmark (Figure 7.52), we see a wild high point for the rates of
cervical carcinoma in the highest age-group (80+ year) complemented by
a wild low point for carcinoma of the corpus in the corresponding age-group
(Figure 7.56).

Table 7.18 Malignant Neoplasms of Corpus Uteri (Analysis of Registry
Data for Onset)

Population	$(n=7, r=2)$	
	k (yr^{-2})	S
Denmark 1953–62	$5 \cdot 9 \times 10^{-4}$	$1 \cdot 93 \times 10^{-2}$
German Democratic Republic 1964–66	$5 \cdot 7 \times 10^{-4}$	$1 \cdot 98 \times 10^{-2}$
Sweden 1959–68	$4 \cdot 5 \times 10^{-4}$	$2 \cdot 43 \times 10^{-2}$

Latent period correction $= 2 \cdot 5$ years

Overall, the data suggest that the kinetics of initiation of adenocarcinoma
of the cervix ($n=7$, $r=2$, k as in the Table 7.16) are identical with those
for the initiation of adenocarcinoma of the corpus. In all the data we find
a suggestion of a small early-onset group of cancer of the corpus below
$t = 30$ years.

Secular trends

Crude death-rates for malignant neoplasms of all parts of the uterus declined
steadily over the period 1950 to 1963 in US Whites, Japan, England and
Wales, and Norway, but increased steadily in Denmark and Sweden (Segi
and Kurihara, 1966). Comparisons between reliable onset-, and death-rates,
could afford valuable pointers to the trends in survival-rates.

Cancer families and endometrial cancer: multiple primaries

Evidence for the occurrence of uterine cancer in cancer families has been
reviewed by Koller (1957) and Lynch (1967). In the famous Family 'G' of
Warthin (1913), a follow-up showed that 15 out of the 23 cancers in females
were endometrial; no case of cervical carcinoma has been reported (see the
reviews of Koller (1957) and Willis (1960)). In Lynch's (1967) Family '1',
12 out of 26 females with cancer had endometrial cancer, and only one had
cervical cancer. Out of 11 affected females in Family '2', five had endometrial cancer and no cervical cases were found (Lynch, 1967). Summarizing
his findings for six cancer families with a total of 201 cancers in both sexes,

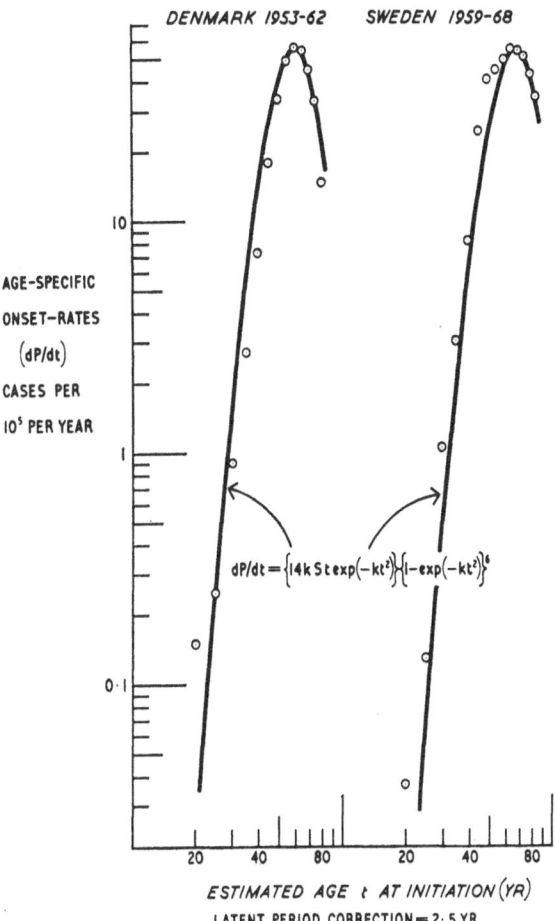

Figure 7.56 Age-specific onset-rates, malignant neoplasms of the corpus uteri, Denmark, 1953–62, left panel; Sweden 1959–68, right panel, in relation to estimated age at initiation (Doll *et al.*, 1966; Swedish Cancer Registry, 1971). See Table 7.18

Lynch (1967) recorded 45 cases of endometrial cancer, but only two of cancer of the cervix.

Schottenfeld *et al.* (1971) found a significant positive association between carcinoma of the corpus uteri and subsequent cancer of the thyroid (based on only three cases, however); the frequencies of second cancers of the breast and ovary were double the expected values but because of small numbers (10 and 2 respectively) the increases were not significant. No significant associations with second cancers at other sites were found in women with epidermoid carcinomas of the uterine cervix, vagina or vulva (Schottenfeld and Berg, 1971).

Pre-malignant change

The interpretations shown in Figures 7.51 to 7.56 indicate that seven forbidden clones are needed to initiate any one of the three types of fatal
clinical uterine cancer. Some of the epidemiological evidence for pre-
malignant change in the progression to cervical cancer has been described
above. The pathological evidence has been reviewed by Willis (1960).

Endometrial hyperplasias form a large and diverse group, some of which
progress simply to carcinoma. No clearcut dividing line can be drawn
between hyperplasia and carcinoma; indeed, hyperplasia and carcinoma
may co-exist, with apparent transitions from one to the other (Willis, 1960).
Occasionally, endometrial polyps give rise to carcinomas. Willis (1960)
claims that endometrial carcinoma often develops from a large field of
tissue and sometimes, perhaps, from the entire endometrium. At other
times, a multifocal origin is observed.

The literature of epidermoid carcinomas of the cervix abounds with
descriptions of various pre-cancerous hyperplastic and metaplastic changes
(Willis, 1960). Nevertheless, Willis and others consider that many of the
so-called pre-cancerous lesions of the cervical epithelia are benign and that
carcinoma *in situ* is often diagnosed when simple metaplasia only is present.
When we consider that five forbidden clones initiate carcinoma *in situ*—as
diagnosed in Kashgarian and Dunr's (1970) study—this view could well be
correct, for it is clear that metaplasia precedes hyperplasia and is produced
by fewer than five forbidden clones. Dysplasia, as diagnosed by Barron and
Richart (1971), results from a single forbidden clone.

Willis's (1960) Figure 249 indicates that a cervical carcinoma has arisen
from an extensive field of epithelium rather than from a single focus. Other
studies are cited that reveal a widespread and often multicentric origin for
cervical carcinoma (Willis, 1960). Again, theory and pathology agree
excellently.

Malignant Neoplasms of the Skin (7th ICD 190 and 191)

Because of their heterogeneity—of both site and histological type—skin
tumours present, on the basis of available statistics, an almost insuperable
problem of interpretation. National mortality statistics fail to reveal the
numerous non-fatal skin tumours. Prognosis is often excellent. In Calfornia,
1942-56, the observed survival for patients (both sexes) in whom the
diagnosis of skin tumour (other than melanoma) had been made under
45 years of age, was 85 per cent at 15 years after diagnosis. For the same
age-group, observed survival from malignant melanoma was 50 per cent
at 15 years after diagnosis (California Tumour Registry, 1963). A proper

analysis of the genetics and initiation of the many types of skin cancer would require adequate statistics for the age at onset, by cell type and anatomical site.

Despite these complications I have found that mortality statistics for all types of skin tumours combined, from England and Wales, US Whites and Japan show remarkably similar age-patterns. However, the heterogeneity and long latent period preclude unambiguous analysis and the data are not illustrated here.

Malignant melanoma

Mihm, Clark and From (1971) describe three main types of melanoma: lentigomaligna melanoma of exposed cutaneous surfaces, with median age at onset of 70 years; superficial spreading melanoma, occurring anywhere on the body surface, with median age of onset 56; and nodular melanoma, median age 46 years. Veronesi, Cascinelli and Preda (1971) distinguish three types of malignant melanoma with a relatively good prognosis, and four types with a relatively bad prognosis. In view of this multiplicity of types, the complexities in the age-distributions are not surprising.

The Swedish Cancer Registry has published details of the onset of malignant melanoma of the skin, by anatomical site, for eight separate categories. Numbers are generally small and the only category for which they are large enough, and the age-pattern is simple enough, to allow reasonably confident analysis is malignant melanoma of trunk skin in males (7th ICD 190.5). Data for 1959–68 are illustrated in Figure 7.57. They are interpreted in terms of the equation in which $n=3$, $r=2$, $k=5\cdot4\times10^{-4}$ year^{-2} and $S=1\cdot7\times10^{-3}$. Because many malignant melanomas arise in pigmented moles, the epidemiological relation of the benign to the malignant conditions would merit study.

Exposure to sunshine is widely believed to be an important causal factor, although in Japan the overall incidence of malignant melanoma is higher in the less sunny part of the country (Mori, 1971). Elwood and Lee (1974) point out that, if sunshine has the importance claimed for it: (a) tumours should arise mainly on exposed sites; and (b) in geographical regions where the incidence of malignant melanoma is high, the concentration of tumours should be greatest on exposed sites. Neither expectation is realised. Elwood and Lee conclude that factors other than sunshine must play a large part in the aetiology of malignant melanoma.

In this context it is interesting to note that, although basal cell epitheliomas in Kentucky have a raised incidence from July to September, there is no seasonal change in the proportion of tumours at exposed to unexposed sites, or in the male/female ratio (Owen et al., 1974).

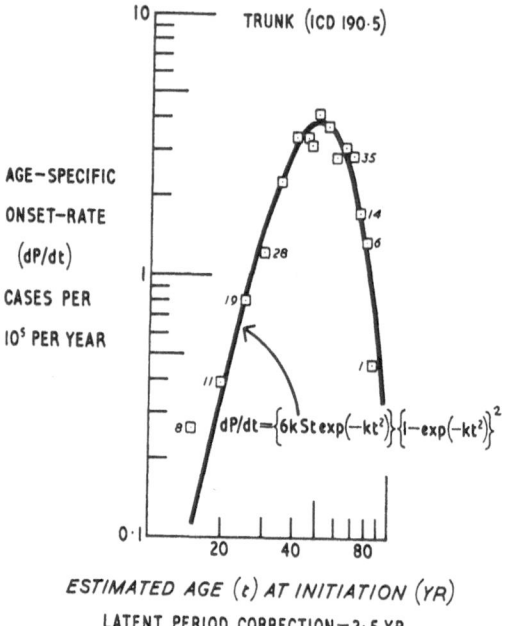

$$dP/dt = \left\{6kSt\exp(-kt^2)\right\}\left\{1-\exp(-kt^2)\right\}^2$$

ESTIMATED AGE (t) AT INITIATION (YR)
LATENT PERIOD CORRECTION = 2·5 YR

Figure 7.57 Age-specific onset-rates, males, malignant melanoma of the skin, trunk region, Sweden, 1959–68, in relation to estimated age at initiation (Swedish Cancer Registry, 1971)

Squamous cell skin carcinomas

Swanbeck and Hillstrom (1971) published age-specific onset-rates, taken from the Swedish Cancer Registry, for squamous cell skin cancers of the genitals and of the head. These data combine specificity by cell type and anatomical site on the one hand, with fairly large numbers on the other (Figure 7.58). For squamous cell skin cancer of the genitals, the age-distribution of all except a few early-onset cases is described by the equation in which $n=1$, $r=6$ and $k \simeq 1\cdot0 \times 10^{-12}$ year^{-6}.

A similar early-onset group contributes to cancers of the head, but the age-distribution for most cases at this site is adequately described by the sum of two functions: one with $n=1$, $r=6$, $k=6\cdot0 \times 10^{-12}$ year^{-6}; and the other with $n=1$, $r=12$, $k=2\cdot5 \times 10^{-24}$ year^{-12}.

Values of S cannot be calculated because some of the data apply to the period 1958 to 1963, but others, from certain areas, extend to 1965.

A virtue of these data of Swanbeck and Hillstrom (1971) and of Swanbeck (1971) is the detail at the upper end of the lifespan. Quinquennial age-groups up to 94 years have been studied and the highest age-group for which data are presented is 95 years and above, in place of the more familiar 85 years

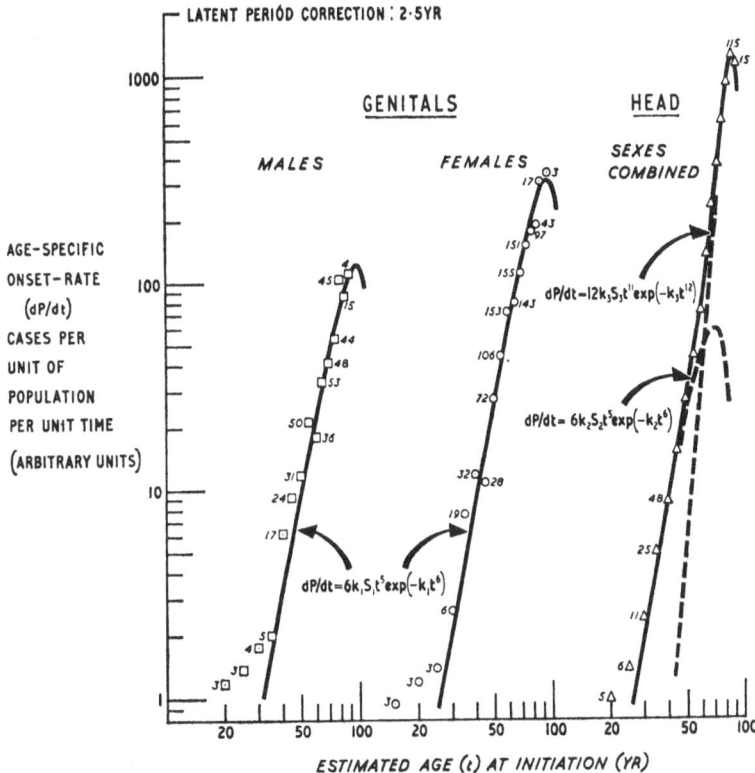

Figure 7.58 Age-specific onset-rates, squamous cell skin carcinoma, genital region, males (left curve), females (centre curve) and head region, sexes combined (right curve), in relation to estimated age at initiation (Swanbeck and Hillström, 1971)

and above, or the thoroughly reprehensible 75 years and above. To recover statistical detail once it has been pooled is like unscrambling eggs.

Unfortunately, numbers of cases of squamous cell skin cancer of the lower limbs (Swanbeck and Hillstrom, 1969), and of the arm and hand (Swanbeck and Hillstrom, 1970), are too small for unambiguous analysis.

This section shows the need for further statistics of the onset of squamous cell skin cancers, by anatomical site, from other countries. Particularly interesting would be a detailed comparison of the age-distributions for geographical areas with widely differing amounts and intensities of sunshine. Similar details would also be welcome for basal cell carcinoma of the skin. In Sweden squamous cell skin carcinoma affects the external ear of men about nine times more frequently than that of women; this tumour also shows a higher incidence at the exposed parts of the skin in the southern part of Sweden than in the northern part (Swanbeck, 1971). This Swedish evidence, therefore, is consistent with (but does not prove) the hypothesis that solar radiation enhances the incidence of squamous cell carcinomas.

Swanbeck and Hillstrom found about the same frequency of psoriasis and eczema in the non-cancer population as in those with squamous cell skin cancer (Swanbeck, 1971). Patients in Sweden with psoriasis or eczema have been extensively treated with coal tar, while psoriatic patients are often treated with ultraviolet light and soft x-rays. Apparently, these treatments with known carcinogenic agents have had little effect on the incidence of skin cancer. Swanbeck (1971) suggested that man may be a species that is not particularly susceptible to agents such as coal tar.

Heredity: multicentricity

The heredity of skin cancer has been reviewed by Lynch (1969). Berendes (1974) has reviewed the genetics and pathology of benign and malignant multiple tumours of the skin.

Classical examples of the heredity of cancer have: (a) a simple scheme of inheritance, such as autosomal dominance or recessiveness; and (b) a high penetrance, generally during childhood, adolescence or early adulthood. At least two types of skin cancer meet these criteria (Lynch, 1967). Predisposition to the multiple naevoid basal cell carcinoma syndrome is believed to require a simple autosomal dominant gene: 80 to 90 per cent of predisposed individuals have basal cell lesions before 50 years of age (Anderson *et al.*, 1967). An autosomal recessive gene probably predisposes to xeroderma pigmentosum. The onset of freckling occurs generally before 12 years of age and this condition is followed by various skin changes, including malignant epitheliomas. Neoplastic change usually takes the form of basal cell and squamous cell carcinomas although malignant melanoma may also develop (El-Hefnawi, Maynard Smith and Penrose, 1965; Lynch, 1967). It would be interesting to determine from age-distributions how many forbidden clones initiate freckling and whether additional clones, characterized by the same values of k and r, initiate malignant development. The analogy with other pre-malignant conditions such as familial intestinal polyposis and cervical dysplasia might or might not be relevant, but analysis of well-defined age-distributions could provide illumination.

Both the naevoid basal cell carcinoma syndrome and xeroderma pigmentosum, represent outstanding examples of disorders with a simple inheritance, in which cancer development is also undeniably multicentric. Although the age-distribution of the onset of naevoid basal cell carcinoma is not very accurately defined (Anderson *et al.*, 1967), it suggests that the first malignant lesions are initiated as the result of a single somatic mutation. In addition to the basal cell carcinomas, this syndrome generally includes jaw cysts, skeletal anomalies, pits of hands and feet, and sometimes, medulloblastoma (Gorlin *et al.*, 1965; Anderson *et al.*, 1976).

Bart and Schnall (1973) found that darkly pigmented basal cell carcinoma is uncommon in patients with light-coloured eyes. Out of 40 cases, 36 appeared in patients with dark brown eyes, four in association with light brown and none in patients with blue, grey or green eyes. They confirmed the absence of association between malignant melanomas and eye colour; 20 melanomas appeared in patients with dark brown eyes, eight in light brown and 22 in blue-, grey-, or green-eyed patients.

Careful investigation of squamous cell carcinomas of the oral stratified epithelium has revealed the multifocal origin of these tumours (Slaughter, Southwick and Smejkal, 1953). Gross and microscopic examinations were made of tumours of the lip, oral cavity and pharynx in 783 patients. Independent multiple tumours were found in 88 patients, an incidence that was far in excess of chance occurrence. Furthermore, microscopic evidence of multicentric origin was demonstrated by serial section in all excised tumours less than 1 cm in diameter. Also, hyperplastic, often atypical epithelium, surrounded all oral cancers for varying distances (Slaughter *et al.*, 1953).

Although the heredity of the common skin cancers is probably polygenic, many reports describe aggregations of malignant melanoma of the skin in families and twins—see for example, Cawley (1953); Schoch (1963); Turkington (1965); Katzenellenbogen and Sandbank (1966); Smith *et al.* (1966); Andrews (1968); Lynch and Krush (1968); Anderson, Smith and McBride (1967); St.-Arneault *et al.* (1970); Anderson (1971(a)); and Wallace, Exton and McLeod (1971).

The paper of St.-Arneault *et al.* (1970) warrants special mention. They studied a set of triplets consisting of monozygotic male twins and a fraternal brother. The monozygotic twins both developed malignant melanoma at 53 years of age. In each twin, the malignancy developed from a pre-existing mole at an almost identical position on the left chest. Histological findings were identical for both tumours. Although the near-concordance for age at onset should probably be regarded as somewhat coincidental, the congruence of cancer type, mode of development, and anatomical siting in these monozygotic twins, points to the powerful role of genetic factors (St.-Arneault *et al.*, 1970). In contrast to these solitary foci, Kahn and Donaldson (1970) describe a patient with multiple primary melanoma in whom more than 100 widely separated nevi developed over a three-year period.

'Turban tumours', or Brooke's, or Fordyce's disease, is another striking example of a skin tumour with multicentric origin that is often familial. The disease is more common in women than in men (Willis, 1960), hence predisposition is probably polygenic, with an X-linked dominant, as well as an autosomal factor. Berendes (1974), however, follows Guggenheim in regarding the predisposition as autosomal dominant.

Tumours of sebaceous glands are rare in man. According to Bakker and Tjon A Joe (1971), only about 80 cases had been reported in the literature. Apart from two cases, the remainder had all been described as solitary. However, the male patient described by Bakker and Tjon A Joe (1971) developed over the course of twelve years, 18 almost identical sebaceous gland tumours, at several different sites. Nine were widely spaced on the back, three on the breast, two on the face and four at the extremities. This patient was also treated twice for a carcinoma of the colon and once for a carcinoma of the stomach. His father died at a rather young age, probably from carcinoma of the colon.

Torre (1968) described a patient in whom more than 100 sebaceous tumours were treated cryosurgically. A primary carcinoma of Vater's ampulla and a carcinoma of the colon were also included in this patient's history. Biopsies of the sebaceous tumours were variously described as 'sebaceous adenoma', 'sebaceous carcinoma' and 'basal cell epitheliomata with sebaceous differentation'. The rarity of the association of multiple sebaceous tumours with carcinoma at other sites, together with the absence of a simple family history, points to the rare aggregation in Torre's patient of two or more predisposing genes.

Where skin cancers in general are concerned, Silverstone and Searle (1970) tried to assess the influence of several factors in the aetiology and pathogenesis of skin cancer and solar keratosis, in Queensland, Australia. For both sexes, both diseases, and all age-groups, the most powerful single discriminant proved to be susceptibility to sunburn. Silverstone and Searle found that genetically based factors as a group were of greater prognostic importance than environmental factors. However, Wooldridge and Frerichs (1971) described a patient with multiple actinic keratoses that developed into clinical carcinoma on prominently sun-damaged skin.

Again in Australia, Lane Brown et al. (1971) tested the general impression that persons of Celtic origin are particularly susceptible to skin cancer. They used the surname as a genetic marker although subjects and controls were also questioned about their ancestry. A disproportionate representation of persons with a Celtic genetic heritage was found among patients with skin cancer. Lane Brown et al. (1971) concluded that the Celtic component of the Australian population is unusually susceptible to skin cancer, including melanoma, basal-cell carcinoma and squamous-cell carcinoma. Lane Brown and Melia (1973) made a similar finding in Boston, Massachusetts: the incidence of skin cancer is relatively high among persons with Celtic surnames. Skin cancer, they claim, associates with 'Celticity'.

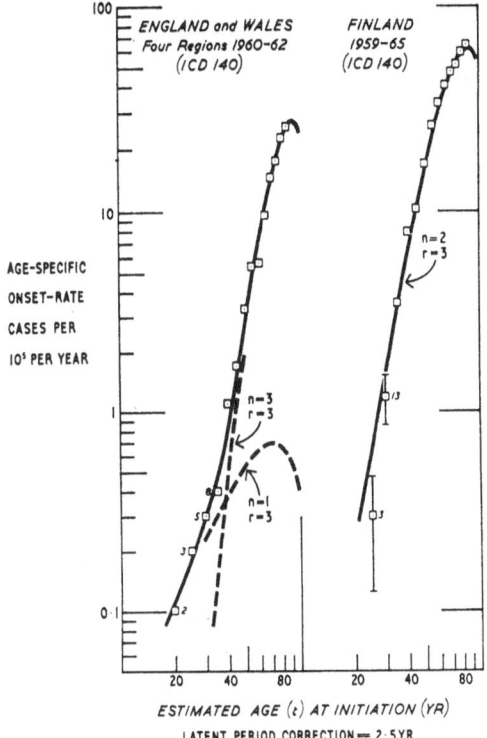

Figure 7.59 Age-specific onset-rates, malignant neoplasms of lip, males, four regions of England and Wales, 1960–62 (left), and Finland, 1959–65 (right), in relation to estimated age at initiation (Doll *et al.*, 1966)

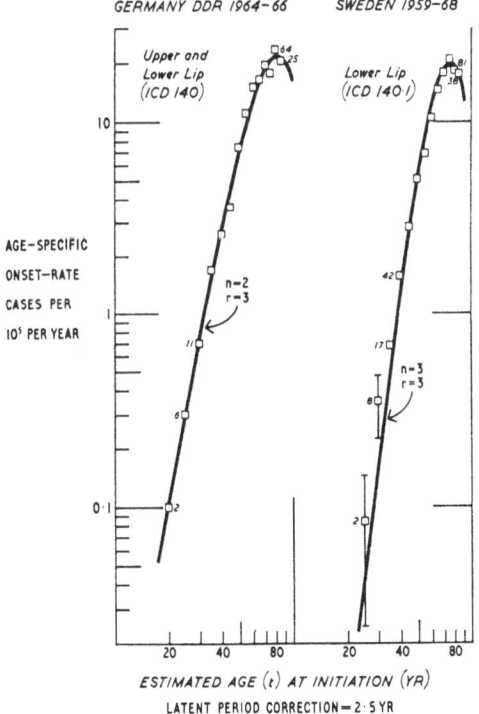

Figure 7.60 As for Figure 7.59. Data for German Democratic Republic, 1964–66 (left), and Sweden, 1959–68 (right) (Doll *et al.*, 1970; Swedish Cancer Registry, 1971)

Malignant Neoplasms of the Buccal Cavity and Pharynx (7th ICD 140–148)

Data for this group of malignancies, pooled by Segi and Kurihara (1966), are far too heterogeneous for satisfactory age-analysis. Numbers of deaths, moreover, are rather small. Easily the most common member of the group is cancer of the lip in males (ICD 140), but survival from this malignancy is high. Thus, for males in all age groups, 1942–56, the average relative survival recorded by the California Tumor Registry (1963), at 13 years from registration was 67 per cent. Consequently, I have had to rely primarily on registry data for onset. These are of unusual interest, however, because they reveal some distinct intercountry differences in age-patterns (Figures 7.59 and 7.60).

Malignant neoplasms of lip (7th ICD 140)

This cancer is much more common in males than females. Data for males, in four regions of England and Wales, 1960–62, are analysed in terms of a late-onset group characterized by $n = 3$, $r = 3$ and a small, early-onset group ($n = 1$, $r = 3$). The same values of k (2.0×10^{-6} year^{-3}) are used to fit the contributions from the two groups (Table 7.19). Finnish registry data for

Table 7.19 Malignant Neoplasms of the Lip (ICD 140) in Males (Interpretation of Registry Statistics for Onset)

Population and group		n	r	k (10^{-6} yr^{-3})	S
England and Wales four regions 1960–62	Early-onset	1	3	2·0	4.7×10^{-4}
	Late-onset	3	3	2·0	1.34×10^{-2}
Finland 1959–65		2	3	1·8	3.6×10^{-2}
German Democratic Republic 1964–66		2	3	2·1	1.17×10^{-2}
Sweden 1959–68 lower lip only (ICD 140·1)		3	3	3·5	8.3×10^{-3}

Latent period correction = 2·5 years

males, 1959–65, show a high incidence, but the age-dependence above $t = 40$ year is much less steep than in England and Wales (Figure 7.59), or Sweden (Figure 7.60), and the data are fitted by the single equation in which $n = 2$, $r = 3$. The data from the German Democratic Republic can also be fitted by the same equation although the incidence is much lower than in Finland (see Figure 7.60) but statistics from Sweden, 1959–68, for the lower lip only, can be fitted to the single function in which $n = 3$, $r = 3$. (There is a slight, but not statistically significant suggestion of a small early-onset group in Sweden, resembling that in England and Wales.)

Cancers of the upper lip are relatively rare. In her survey of the literature of Western countries Lane-Claypon (1930) found that, among patients with cancer of the lip, the lower lip was reported affected in 96·4 per cent of males and in 76·2 per cent of females. In Swedish males, 1959–68, the lower lip was affected in 1399 cases, but the upper lip in only 74 cases, or 5 per cent. The corresponding numbers for females were 97 lower lip, and 41 upper lip. The proportion of female cases with an affected lower lip (70 per cent), conforms well to Lane-Claypon's (1930) survey data. Above the age of 70, some 504 male cases were of the lower lip, and 42, or 7·7 per cent, were of the upper lip. Hence, cancers of the upper lip tend to be of slightly later onset than those of the lower lip. The high value of k in Sweden (Figure 7.60, Table 7.19) might be explained, in part, by the exclusion of statistics for the upper lip. However, cancers of the upper lip cannot be held responsible for the larger differences in the age-patterns between Finland and Germany on the one hand, and England and Wales and Sweden on the other.

The source of these very unusual differences that reside in the value of n, the number of initiated forbidden clones, calls for discussion. At least three hypotheses should be considered: (a) diagnosis of onset is made at different levels of progression—minimal in Finland and East Germany, and at a more advanced level in England and Wales, and Sweden; (b) genetic differences—correlated with nationality—modify the degree of progression associated with one, two or three forbidden clones; and (c) environmental factors facilitate, or inhibit, the degree of progression. Despite the good survival from cancer of the lip, mortality data shed some light on these possibilities.

The World Health Organization (1970) compilation does not include mortality statistics for East Germany and I have therefore used those for West Germany (Figure 7.61). Numbers of deaths from cancer of the lip in Sweden, 1955–65, were too small to define the age-dependence reliably, but those for England and Wales, and Finland, are sufficient for this purpose. In Figure 7.61 the mortality data for the three populations are seen in relation to the curve of the equation: $dP/dt \propto t^8$. In contrast to the differences between the registry statistics for onset, all the mortality data show a similar age-dependence. Absolute death-rates for Finland (as for the onset-rates) are much higher than in England and Wales. However, the similarities in the age-dependence for death-rates tend to favour hypothesis (a) over the other two.

Pathology—Many authors have reported pre-cancerous lesions of the lips, the commonest of which appears to be a bleb or ulcer; later authors refer to

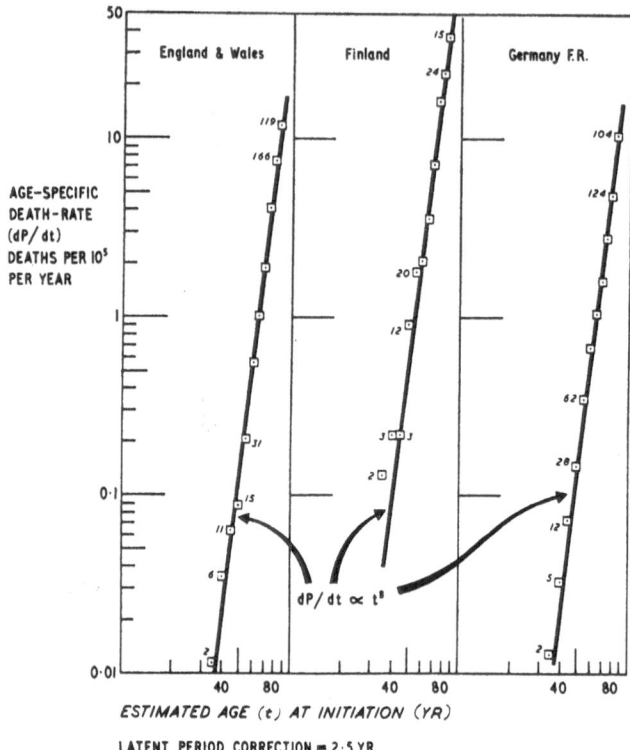

Figure 7.61 Age-specific death-rates, malignant neoplasms of lip, males, 1955–65, England and Wales (left panel), Finland (centre panel) and German Federal Republic (right panel), in relation to estimated age at initiation (World Health Organization, 1970)

leucoplakia. Bloodgood (1914) believed that all cancers of the lip are preceded by a benign condition; the first change observed by patients is a scab that can be pulled off. The occasional early-onset case recorded in registries in England and Wales ($n = 1$, $r = 3$, Figure 7.59) might constitute an exception to Bloodgood's generalization. According to Willis (1960), early tumours can be seen to arise from fields of predisposed tissue that include both epidermis and mucosa.

The pathology, therefore, bears out the implication from age-pattern analysis of multiple forbidden clones and pre-malignant change. Age-specific statistics for cancer of the lip in smokers of clay pipes could be used to test the hypothesis that the onset of a diagnosable neoplastic condition in such smokers requires fewer forbidden clones than in non-pipesmokers.

Table 7.20 Malignant Neoplasms of the Tongue (7th ICD 141) (Interpretation of Mortality Statistics)

Population	Males				Females			
	Early-onset $(n=1, r=5)$		Late-onset $(n=1, r=8)$		Early-onset $(n=1, r=5)$		Late-onset $(n=1, r=8)$	
	k_1	S_1	k_2	S_2	k_1	S_1	k_2	S_2
England and Wales 1955–65	1.8×10^{-9} yr^{-5}	5.2×10^{-5}	1×10^{-16} yr^{-8}	1.2×10^{-2}	1.8×10^{-9} yr^{-5}	4.4×10^{-5}	1×10^{-16} yr^{-8}	3.3×10^{-3}
Japan 1955–65	1.8×10^{-9} yr^{-5}	1.5×10^{-4}	7×10^{-16} yr^{-8}	1.4×10^{-3}	1.8×10^{-9} yr^{-5}	1.0×10^{-4}	3×10^{-16} yr^{-8}	1.2×10^{-3}

Latent period correction=2·5 years.

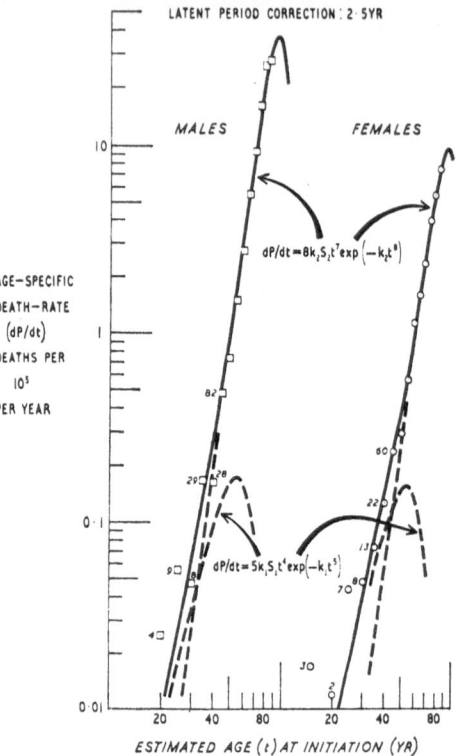

Figure 7.62 Sex-specific and age-specific death-rates from malignant neoplasms of the tongue, England and Wales, 1955–65, in relation to estimated age at initiation (World Health Organization, 1970). See Table 7.20.

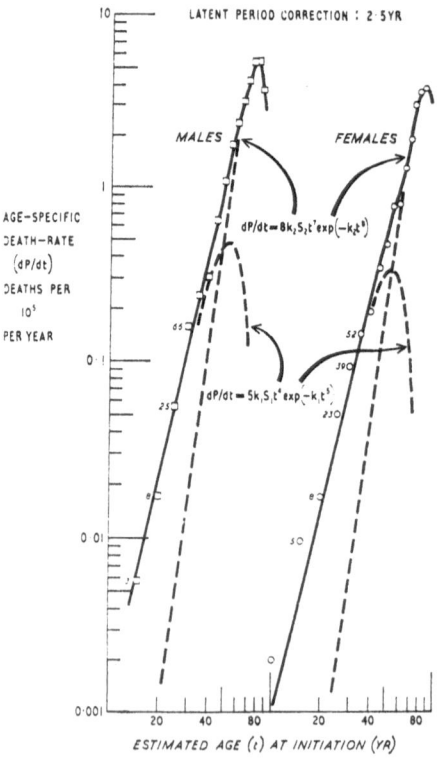

Figure 7.63 As for Figure 7.62. Data for Japan, 1955–65

Malignant neoplasms of tongue (7th ICD 141)

Although this is a fairly rare condition, survival is much poorer than for cancer of the lip and I have analysed mortality statistics for England and Wales (Figure 7.62) and Japan (Figure 7.63) for the years 1955–65 inclusive (WHO, 1970).

The data are analysed in terms of an early-onset group ($n = 1$, $r = 5$) and a late-onset group ($n = 1$, $r = 8$). For the early-onset group, k values do not differ appreciably, either between males or females, or between the two populations (Table 7.20): however, values of S in Japan are markedly higher. In the late-onset group, values of S in Japan are very much lower than in England and Wales, and k values are markedly higher (Table 7.20). In the England and Wales population, $S_{2,M}/S_{2,F} \simeq 4$, but in Japan, the corresponding ratio only just exceeds unity.

The genotypes that predispose to cancer of the tongue and to lip cancer probably involve sex-linked, as well as autosomal factors.

Malignant Neoplasms of the Kidney (7th ICD 180) Adult Onset

Segi and Kurihara (1966) do not abstract statistics for cancer of the kidney. Accordingly, mortality statistics for England and Wales (1955–65), Japan (1960–65) and US all races (1960–65) are taken from the World Health Organization (1970)—see Figures 7.64 to 7.66. Statistics for the onset of malignant neoplasms of the renal parenchyma (7th ICD 180·0), which is much more commonly affected than the renal pelvis, are taken from the Swedish Cancer Registry (1970(a), (b); 1971(a), (b))—see Figure 7.67. British statistics for Wilms's tumour are illustrated in Chapter 9.

All statistics for kidney cancer of adult onset are fitted to the equation in which $n = 1$, $r = 6$ (Figures 7.64 to 7.67 and Table 7.21). To judge from the Japanese statistics, in which the mode is well defined (Figure 7.65), and from the Swedish registry statistics, which are uncomplicated by differential survival at high t, $k_M = k_F$. Suggestions to the contrary (Figures 7.64 and 7.66) probably arise from artefacts and/or the slightly better survival of women at high t (California Tumor Registry, 1963).

The sex-ratio, S_M/S_F, for all cancers of the kidney ranges from 1·4 to 1·7 and that for cancers of the renal pelvis is about 2·0 (Swedish Cancer Registry, 1970(a), (b); 1971(a), (b)). These sex-ratios could be explained if a recessive-effect X-linked allele, of rather high frequency, predisposes to cancer of the kidney. Cancer of the renal pelvis probably involves a different X-linked gene from cancer of the parenchyma. To account for the rather low frequency of predisposed persons, autosomal, as well as X-linked predisposing factors, need to be postulated.

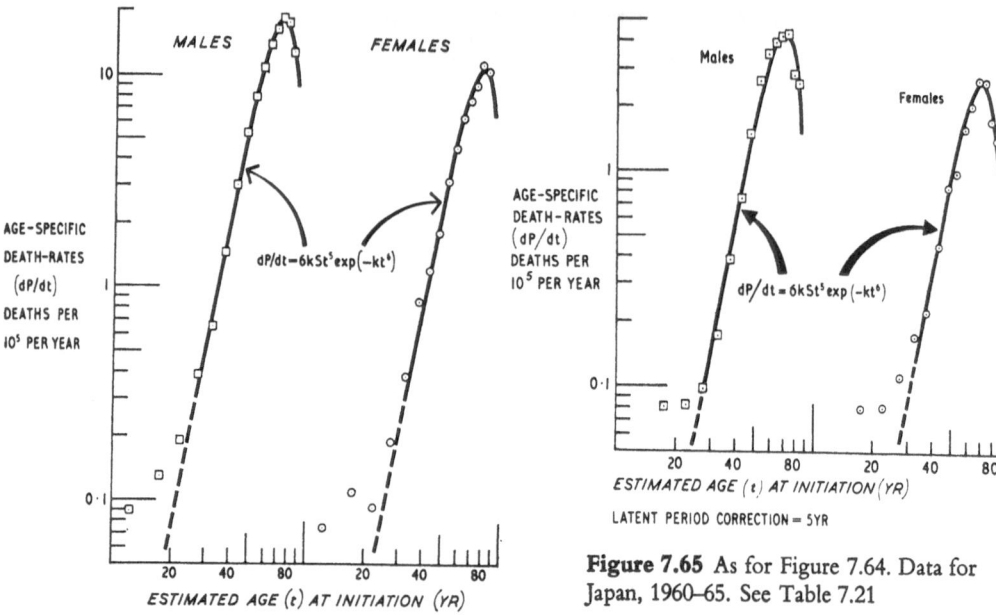

Figure 7.64 Sex-specific and age-specific death-rates from malignant neoplasms of the kidney, England and Wales, 1955–65, in relation to estimated age at initiation (World Health Organization, 1970)

Figure 7.65 As for Figure 7.64. Data for Japan, 1960–65. See Table 7.21

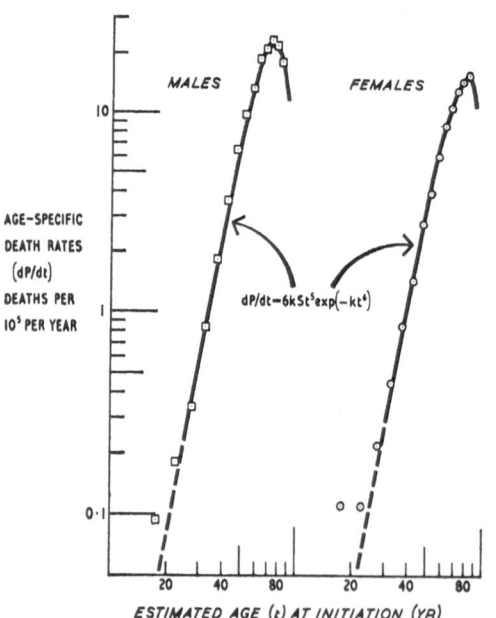

Figure 7.66 As for Figure 7.64. Data for US (all races), 1960–65

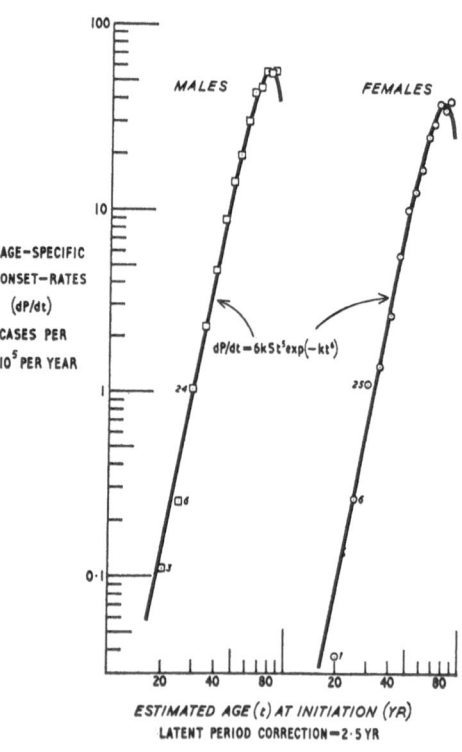

Figure 7.67 Sex-specific and age-specific onset-rates, malignant neoplasms of the renal parenchyma, Sweden, 1959–68, in relation to estimated age at initiation (Swedish Cancer Registry, 1971)

Table 7.21 Malignant Neoplasms of the Kidney, Adult Onset (ICD 180)
(Interpretation of Mortality and Onset Statistics)

Population	Males		Females		S_M/S_F
	k (10^{-12} yr^{-6})	S	k (10^{-12} yr^{-6})	S	
England and Wales mortality 1955–65	6·1	$6·3 \times 10^{-3}$	3·8	$4·0 \times 10^{-3}$	1·6
Japan, mortality 1960–65	7·2	$1·4 \times 10^{-3}$	7·2	$8·3 \times 10^{-4}$	1·7
United States, all races, mortality 1960–65	5·2	$8·0 \times 10^{-2}$	3·3	$5·9 \times 10^{-3}$	1·4
Sweden, onset of cancer of renal parenchyma (ICD 180·1) 1959–68	3·8	$2·0 \times 10^{-2}$	3·8	$1·4 \times 10^{-2}$	1·5

Latent period corrections: 5 years, mortality statistics
2·5 years, onset statistics

Cancer of the kidney is relatively common in Sweden (parenchymal cases—Table 7.21—account for 84 per cent of the total male incidence for that organ and 87 per cent of the total female incidence), and relatively uncommon in Japan (Table 7.21).

Although about 3·6 per cent of cases of Wilms's tumour are bilateral (Scott, 1955), only 20 cases of non-metastatic bilateral renal cell carcinoma had been reported in the English-language literature up to 1973 (Hyman, Voges and Finlay, 1973). This low frequency may, in part, be a consequence of the strictness of the criteria for establishing bilaterality and excluding metastasis.

Malignant Neoplasms of the Testis (7th ICD 178)

Because of: (a) the relatively good average survival from cancers of the testis; (b) the complexity of the age-pattern; and (c) small numbers in any one series, I have analysed pooled registry statistics from Denmark, England and Wales, the German Democratic Republic, Norway, Scotland and Sweden (Figure 7.68 and Table 7.22). But in view of the complexity of the age-pattern and the possibility that values of the kinetic constants (k) might differ slightly from country to country, the interpretation should be regarded as highly tentative.

Table 7.22 Malignant Neoplasms of the Testis (7th ICD 178) (Weighted Averages for Registry Data: Denmark 1953–62; England and Wales, Four Regions 1960–62; Birmingham Region 1963–66; German Democratic Republic 1964–66; Norway 1959–66; Scotland 1963–66; Sweden 1959–65)

Type of cancer	Characteristics of age-dependence		k	S
	n	r		
Adenocarcinoma, infant	1	1	$3 \cdot 6 \times 10^{-1}$ yr^{-1}	$2 \cdot 9 \times 10^{-5}$
Teratoma	4	2	$1 \cdot 9 \times 10^{-3}$ yr^{-2}	$1 \cdot 8 \times 10^{-3}$
Seminoma	1 ?	7	$5 \cdot 8 \times 10^{-13}$ yr^{-7}	$3 \cdot 1 \times 10^{-4}$
?	1 ?	9	$7 \cdot 4 \times 10^{-18}$ yr^{-9}	$6 \cdot 8 \times 10^{-4}$

The small early-onset group, described in terms of $n = 1$, $r = 1$, requires data by each year of age for confirmation. In Chevason's (1906) series, five infants were recorded with teratomas. Willis (1960) refers to a 'distinctive tubular and papillary carcinoma with vacuolated, sometimes mucinous, cells' that occurs in infants, usually under 2 years of age. In Swedish Cancer Registry statistics, 1959–65, 17 cases of malignant teratoma were recorded with onset before 15 years of age and none of seminoma. The same source of statistics also indicates that most cases of teratoma are initiated with kinetics described by $n = 4$, $r = 2$, and a modal age at about $t = 25$ years. Willis (1960) states that the average age of onset of seminomas is more than a decade later than that of teratomas and this is borne out by the Swedish statistics. Late-onset cases comprise both seminomas and malignant teratomas, the former predominating.

If it should be confirmed that most cases of teratoma are initiated by four forbidden clones ($n = 4$), it would be interesting to determine whether each clone promotes a distinctive differentiation in target cells. In this connection it is worth noting that benign teratomas of the ovary result from three forbidden clones ($n = 3$, $r = 1$)—see Figure 7.69. Plattner and Oxern (1973) have reviewed the literature of familial aggregations of dermoid cysts and describe a mother and two daughters, each with bilateral ovarian cystic teratomas.

The idea that teratomas 'originate' during early embryonic life, is not supported by Figures 7.68 and 7.69.

Teratomas and carcinomas of the testis may be bilateral (Willis, 1960). In most series, unilateral teratomas (the great majority) show a right-sided, roughly two to one, predominance (Willis, 1960). To explain the consistent bias to the right testicle, we can scarcely avoid a biological theory, which

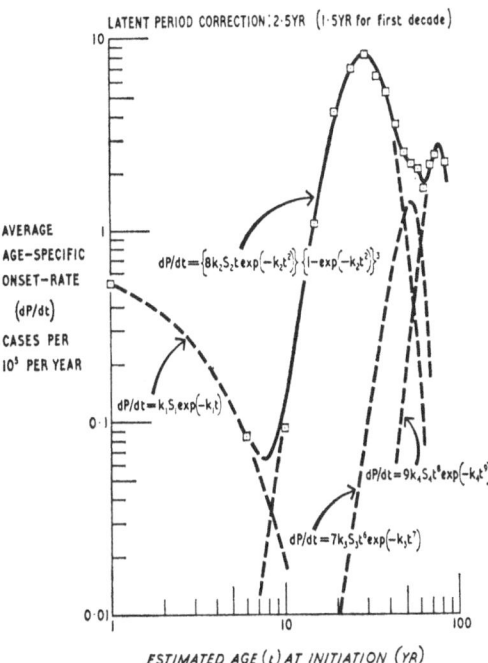

Figure 7.68 Age-specific onset-rate, from pooled registry data (Denmark, England and Wales, German Democratic Republic, Norway, Scotland and Sweden), for malignant neoplasms of the testis, in relation to estimated age at initiation (Doll *et al.*, 1966, 1970). See Table 7.22

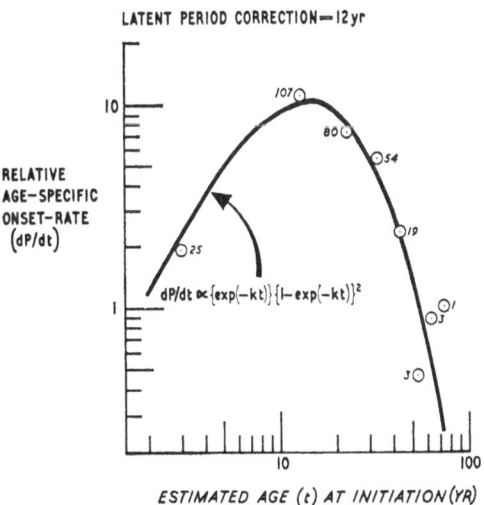

Figure 7.69 Relative age-specific onset-rates, benign teratomas of the ovary, in relation to estimated age at initiation (Caruso *et al.*, 1971)

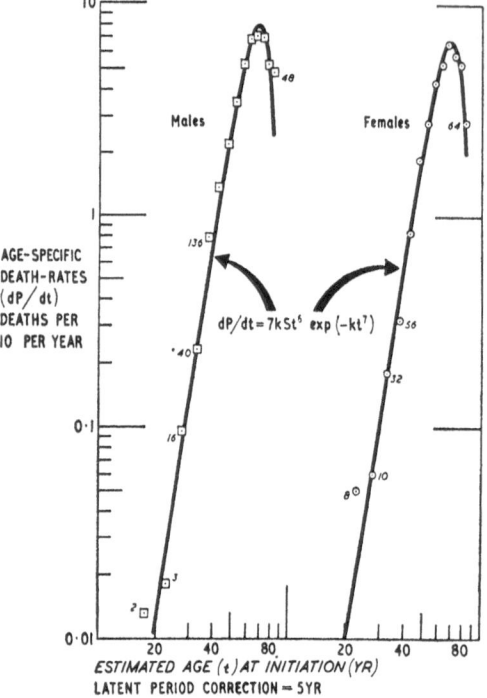

Figure 7.70

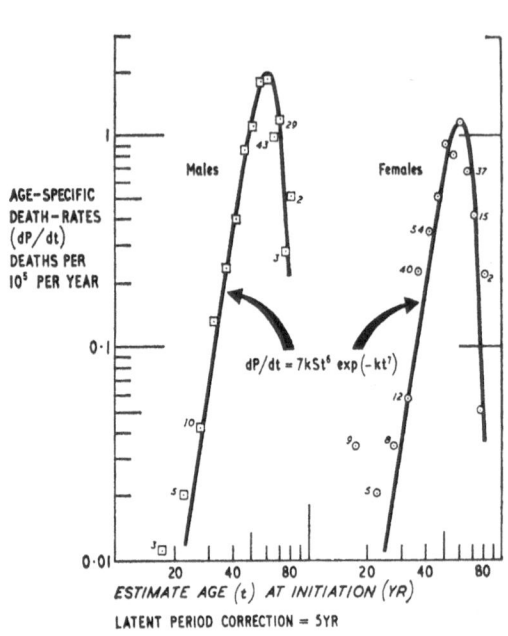

Figure 7.71

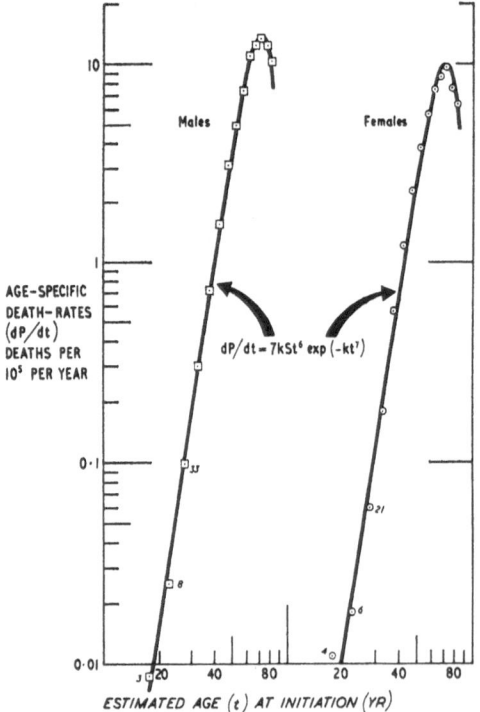

Figure 7.72

Figure 7.70 Sex-specific and age-specific death-rates, multiple myeloma, England and Wales, 1955–65, in relation to estimated age at initiation (World Health Organization, 1970). See Table 7.23

Figure 7.71 As for Figure 7.70. Data for Japan, 1960–65

Figure 7.72 As for Figure 7.70. Data for US (all races), 1960–65

emphasizes the distinction between left and right among paired organs. In my theory, laterality, as well as more conventional tissue specificity, is genetically determined. Distinctions between left and right are merely one aspect of morphology and, as such, they are determined by the MCP–TCF growth-control system.

Various instances of the familial occurrence of testicular teratomas and seminomas have been reported—see Willis (1960).

Multiple Myeloma, Plasmocytoma (7th ICD 203)

Mortality statistics for England and Wales, Japan, United States (all races), and Sweden; and registry statistics for the onset of multiple myeloma in Sweden, are analysed in Figures 7.70 to 7.74. The age-patterns appear reasonably homogeneous, apart from small surpluses in the lowest age-groups in the Japanese data.

For each set of data: k_M appears to be equal to k_F; and $S_M > S_F$ (Table 7.23). The highest value of k and the lowest values of S_M and S_F are obtained from the Japanese data. The apparent secular increases of S_M and S_F deduced from Swedish Registry statistics may be due, in part, to increasing levels of diagnosis.

Because $S_M > S_F$, a recessive effect X-linked allele (of frequency about 0·6 to 0·9) probably contributes to the polygenic predisposition. Some ten instances of familial multiple myeloma, including one family with affected father, son and daughter, and others involving two or three siblings, were reviewed by Robbins (1967). McKusick (1966) regards multiple myeloma as an autosomal recessive disorder, but in view of the sex ratios in four populations (Table 7.23), so simple a scheme must be doubted.

Relation between benign and malignant plasma cell tumours

Fifty-two subjects with the benign disease were followed for two-and-a-half years and the plasma protein M-components present originally remained demonstrable in all of them, and at similar concentrations (Axelsson and Hallen, 1968). However, Norgaard (1971) reported three patients diagnosed with M-components between 1950 and 1952; at intervals ranging from 15 to 24 years after the initial diagnosis, all three patients presented with symptoms of multiple myeloma and died within one year of this diagnosis. Norgaard (1971) reviewed various other reports in the literature in which multiple myeloma developed 5–16 years after the discovery of paraprotein-aemia. We also have to remember that benign monoclonal gammopathy is about 40 to 50 times more common than multiple myeloma (Axelsson and Hallen, 1968). Another feature concerning latency needs to be pointed out.

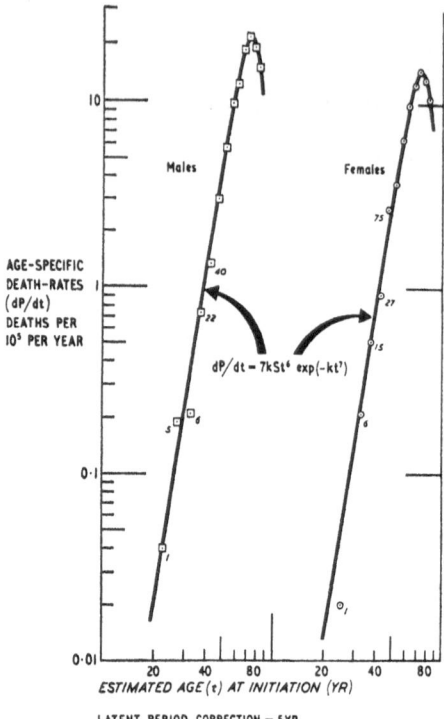

Figure 7.73 As for Figure 7.70. Data for Sweden, 1955–65

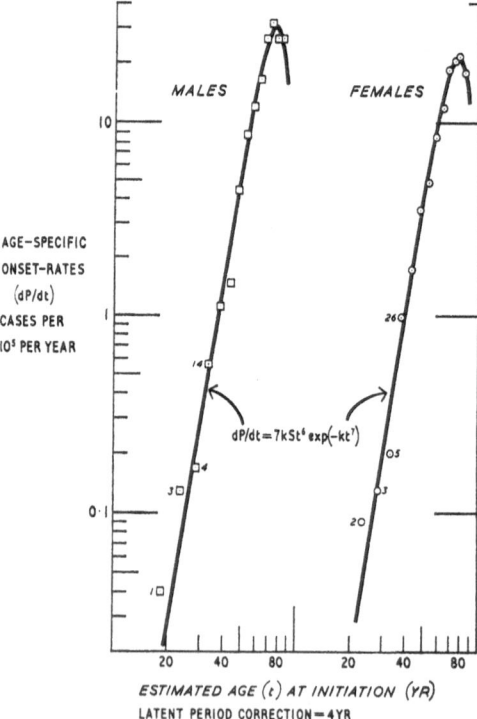

Figure 7.74 Sex-specific and age-specific onset-rates multiple myeloma, Sweden 1959–1968, in relation to estimated age at initiation (Swedish Cancer Registry, 1971). See Table 7.23

Table 7.23 Multiple Myeloma, Plasmocytoma (7th ICD 203) (Interpretation of Mortality and Onset Statistics)

Population	$(n = 1, r = 7)$				S_M/S_F
	Males		Females		
	k (yr^{-7})	S	k (yr^{-7})	S	
England and Wales mortality 1955–65	$1 \cdot 2 \times 10^{-13}$	$2 \cdot 1 \times 10^{-13}$	$1 \cdot 2 \times 10^{-13}$	$1 \cdot 8 \times 10^{-3}$	$1 \cdot 15$
Japan, mortality 1960–65	$2 \cdot 3 \times 10^{-13}$	$4 \cdot 8 \times 10^{-4}$	$2 \cdot 3 \times 10^{-13}$	$2 \cdot 8 \times 10^{-4}$	$1 \cdot 70$
US, all races, mortality 1960–65	$8 \cdot 2 \times 10^{-14}$	$4 \cdot 1 \times 10^{-3}$	$8 \cdot 2 \times 10^{-14}$	$2 \cdot 8 \times 10^{-3}$	$1 \cdot 46$
Sweden, mortality 1955–65	$6 \cdot 8 \times 10^{-14}$	$6 \cdot 2 \times 10^{-3}$	$6 \cdot 8 \times 10^{-14}$	$4 \cdot 2 \times 10^{-3}$	$1 \cdot 48$
Sweden, onset 1959–68	$5 \cdot 7 \times 10^{-14}$	$9 \cdot 2 \times 10^{-3}$	$5 \cdot 7 \times 10^{-14}$	$6 \cdot 5 \times 10^{-3}$	$1 \cdot 42$

Latent period corrections: mortality statistics, 5 years
onset statistics, 4 years

Prognosis for multiple myeloma is very poor; about one-half of all patients die within nine months of diagnosis (Norgaard, 1971). Nevertheless, the latent period correction adopted in Figures 7.70 to 7.73 to allow for the interval between initiation and death is 5 years, and the correction for the interval between initiation and diagnosis used in Figure 7.74 is 4 years. In this type of situation we might expect that multiple myeloma arises from a benign gammopathy through progression. Hence we would expect to find $n > 1$ for the initiation of multiple myeloma.

We have, therefore, to consider that the interpretation of the age-patterns in terms of $n = 1$, $r = 7$ is incorrect, despite the excellence of the fits in Figures 7.70 and 7.74. Two groups might be involved: a main (late-onset) group with, say, $n = 2$, $r = 5$; and an early-onset group which fills in what would otherwise be a gap, between the observed and theoretical dP/dt at low t. On this view, benign gammopathy would be initiated by a single forbidden clone, and the small proportion of cases that become malignant would require two forbidden clones. The difficulty about this interpretation is that most cases of malignant myeloma (excepting only those with near-simultaneous initiation of two forbidden clones) would be preceded by a stage of benign gammopathy. This hypothesis is difficult to disprove and equally difficult to verify.

Alternatively, a small proportion of persons are predisposed both to benign gammopathy and to multiple myeloma, which should be regarded as separate diseases. Generally, but not invariably, the onset of benign gammopathy precedes that of multiple myeloma.

Accurate data for the age-dependence of benign gammopathy—although difficult to obtain—could, in principle, distinguish between these alternatives.

Plasma cell tumours: problems of pathogenesis

Aspects of multiple myeloma, and indeed benign gammopathies, that particularly concern us, are the nature of the cells of origin and its unicellular (or unifocal), versus multicellular (or multifocal), origin. Most myeloma paraproteins at the time of diagnosis appear to be homogeneous, although occasionally, patients are found with two serum M-components. (See case reports and literature reviews by Rosen, Smith and Block (1967); Dammacco, Trizio and Bonomz (1969); and Wang *et al.* (1969).) However, the degree of homogeneity of myeloma proteins at the first onset of the disease cannot be assessed.

The plasma cell series raises interesting problems in the context of growth-control. Normally, any particular clone develops in response to a particular antigenic stimulus and hence the number of cells in an elicited clone is not regulated by the central system of growth-control. The central system regulates symmetrical mitosis, whereas the development of plasma cell clones from B-lymphocytes involves some degree of asymmetrical mitosis. Hence, under normal physiological conditions, some mechanism other than that of central growth-control is needed to regulate the number of plasma cells. Myeloma may result, therefore, from an autoaggressive attack on cells (perhaps neither B-lymphocytes nor plasma cells) that regulate and limit the normal formation of clones of antibody-producing cells.

A remarkable property of myeloma proteins that needs to be accounted for in any satisfactory theory of their pathogenesis is the non-random specificity of their antibody activity (Grey *et al.*, 1968; Metzger, 1969; Schubert, Ramon and Cohn, 1970; and Warner, MacKenzie and Fudenberg, 1971). A high proportion of such proteins show autoantibody activity (antiglobulin, antilipoprotein, antinucleic acid). The resolution of the problem of pathogenesis will probably have to await a better understanding of the mechanism and regulation of the normal immune response. I have proposed that a negative-feedback control normally governs the level of synthesis of a specific antibody (Burch, 1968(a)). This mechanism postulates receptor cells (perhaps specialized macrophages) that respond to antibody uncombined with antigen to limit the proliferation of plasma cells. Among the many possibilities, we should consider that an autoaggressive attack on feedback receptor cells leads indirectly to multiple myeloma.

Leukaemia (7th ICD 204)

Most of the earlier statistics published for the onset of, or death from, leukaemia do not detail the many distinctive forms of the disease. However, Swedish Registry statistics, two special studies in the United States, and recent statistics of the Registrar General of England and Wales provide sufficient detail, and large enough numbers, to permit analyses of the age-dependence of the main types of leukaemia.

Chronic lymphocytic leukaemia (7th ICD 204·0)

Figure 7.75 shows age-specific onset-rates, Sweden 1959–68; and Figure 7.76 shows relative age-specific onset-rates recorded for White patients in 98 US hospitals, 1940–62 (Cutler *et al.*, 1967). The main, late-onset group, is represented in both instances by the equation in which $n=1$, $r=7$. With a sex ratio (S_M/S_F) of 2·02 (Sweden) and 1·85 (US hospital series), an X-linked recessive factor of frequency around 0·5, and one or more autosomal factors, are likely to feature in the predisposing genotype.

By assuming an average latent period of 10 years between initiation and death (in contrast to 2·5 years for onset), age-specific mortality statistics for chronic lymphocytic leukaemia in England and Wales, 1968–71, can also be described by the same equation ($n=1$, $r=7$) (Figure 7.77). The sex-ratio S_M/S_F of 1·88 is close to that for the US hospital series (Table 7.24).

Most cases of chronic lymphocytic leukaemia appear to involve B-lymphocytes and hence they do not correspond to the proliferation of forbidden clones of growth-control (T) lymphocytes.

Chronic myeloid leukaemia (7th ICD 204·1)

From about 15 years and upwards, the age-pattern of chronic myeloid leukaemia can be represented in terms of two distinctive groups—see Figures 7.78 to 7.80 and Table 7.24. Numbers are small and the interpretation might need to be modified when more abundant data become available. In both early- and late-onset groups, from Sweden, USA and England and Wales, the sex ratio, S_M/S_F, exceeds unity. Again, both X-linked and autosomal predisposing factors appear to be implicated.

The latent period correction for the onset statistics is 2·5 years (as for chronic lymphocytic leukaemia), but for death-rates in England and Wales the correction is 5 years, which is half the value for chronic lymphocytic leukaemia.

Chromosomal abnormality and clonal origin—Chronic myeloid leukaemia holds a special interest, inasmuch as most cases are characterized by an abnormal

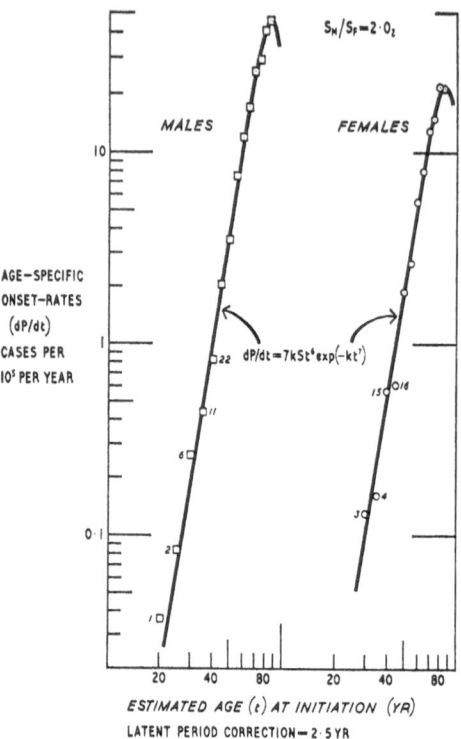

Figure 7.75 Sex-specific and age-specific onset-rates, chronic lymphocytic leukaemia, Sweden 1959–68, in relation to estimated age at initiation (Swedish Cancer Registry, 1971). See Table 7.24

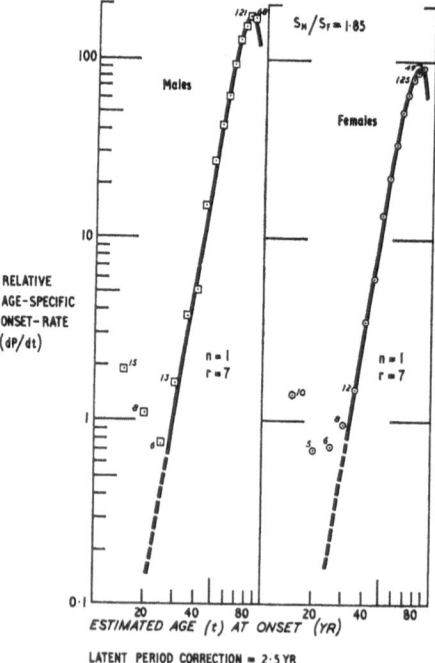

Figure 7.76 Relative sex-specific and age-specific onset-rates, chronic lymphocytic leukaemia. white patients in 98 US hospitals, 1940–62, in relation to estimated age at initiation (Cutler *et al.*, 1967). See Table 7.24

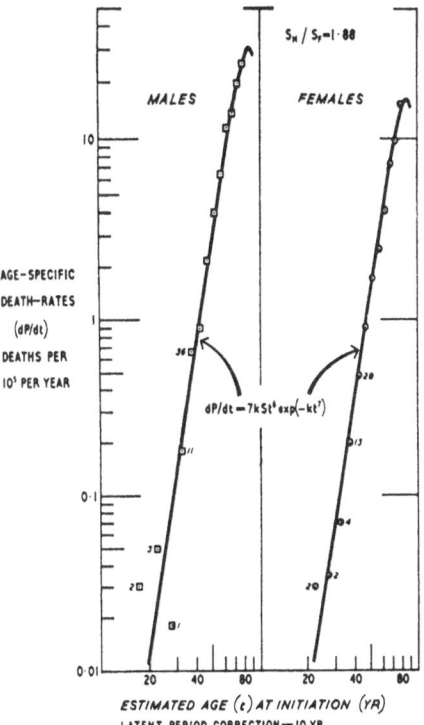

Figure 7.77 Sex-specific and age-specific death-rates, chronic lymphocytic leukaemia, England and Wales, 1968–71, in relation to estimated age at initiation (Registrar General, Annual Medical Reports. See Table 7.24

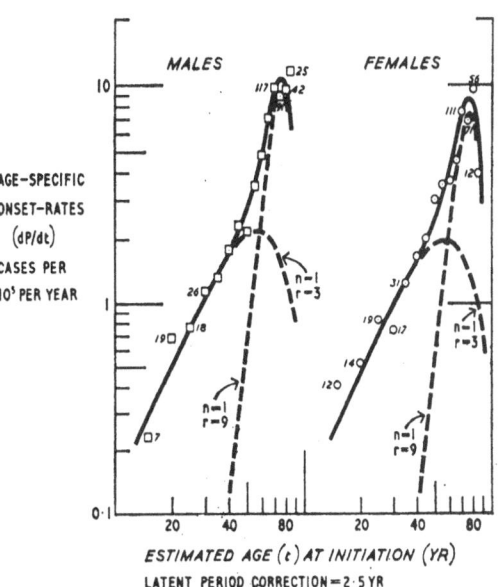

Figure 7.78 Sex-specific and age-specific onset-rates, chronic myeloid leukaemia, Sweden, 1959–68, in relation to estimated age at initiation (Swedish Cancer Registry, 1971)

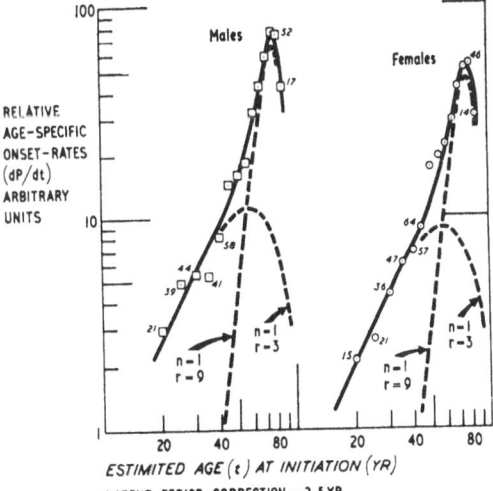

Figure 7.79 Relative sex-specific and age-specific onset-rates, chronic myeloid leukaemia, white patients in 98 US hospitals, 1940–62, in relation to estimated age at initiation (Cutler *et al.*, 1967). See Table 7.24

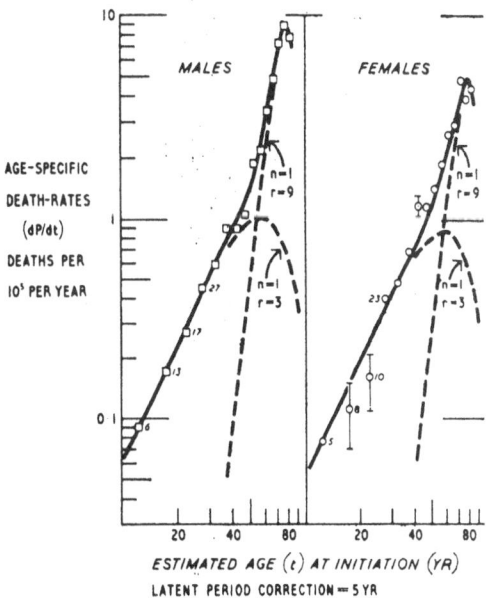

Figure 7.80 Sex-specific and age-specific death-rates, chronic myeloid leukaemia, England and Wales, 1968–71, in relation to estimated age at initiation (Registrar General, Annual Medical Reports). See Table 7.24

Table 7.24 Chronic Leukaemias: Interpretation of Registry, Hospital and Mortality Statistics

Source of statistics	Leukaemia type	n	r	k	S_M	S_F	S_M/S_F
Swedish Registry 1959–68	Chronic lymphocytic	1	7	2.4×10^{-14} yr^{-7}	1.54×10^{-2}	7.6×10^{-3}	2·02
98 US hospitals (onset, relative rates)	,,	1	7	4.0×10^{-14} yr^{-7}	?	?	1·85
England and Wales Mortality 1968–71	,,	1	7	2.4×10^{-14} yr^{-7}	1.04×10^{-2}	5.5×10^{-3}	1·88
Swedish Registry 1959–68	Chronic myeloid (early-onset)	1	3	3.5×10^{-6} yr^{-3}	1.21×10^{-3}	1.10×10^{-3}	1·10
98 US hospitals (onset, relative rates)	,,	1	3	3.5×10^{-6} yr^{-3}	?	?	1·28
England and Wales Mortality 1968–71	,,	1	3	3.5×10^{-6} yr^{-3}	5.7×10^{-4}	4.9×10^{-4}	1·16
Swedish Registry 1959–68	Chronic myeloid (late-onset)	1	9	9.4×10^{-18} yr^{-9}	2.17×10^{-3}	1.77×10^{-3}	1·23
98 US hospitals (onset, relative rates)	,,	1	9	9.4×10^{-18} yr^{-9}	?	?	1·43
England and Wales Mortality 1968–71	,,	1	9	7.4×10^{-18} yr^{-9}	1.9×10^{-3}	1.06×10^{-3}	1·8

G-group chromosome, the Philadelphia-1 chromosome (Ph[1]), first discovered by Nowell and Hungerford (1961) in cells of the bone marrow. Once believed to be a deletion from the long arm of chromosome 21, the use of the latest fluorescent staining techniques indicates that the abnormality probably results from a translocation. Rowley (1973), and Petit and Cauchie (1973) have observed a translocation from the long arm of 22 to the long arm of 9. Hayata, Kakati and Sandberg (1973) confirmed this observation in their study of a series of patients with chronic myeloid leukaemia, but found one patient (male, 52 years) with a translocation from the long arm of 22 to the long arm of 2.

The pathogenesis of the chromosomal abnormality and its connection with the leukaemic condition remain unresolved. Indeed, as Figures 7.78 to 7.80 might lead us to expect, not all cases of chronic myeloid leukaemia exhibit the Ph[1] chromosome. Ezdinli et al. (1970) examined 61 adult patients with typical chronic myelocytic leukaemia. The median age of the 43 patients with the Ph[1] chromosome was 48 years, whereas that of the 18 Ph[1]-negative patients was 66 years. Evidently, the Ph[1]-positive cases belong largely or wholly to the early-onset group ($n = 1$, $r = 3$) and the Ph[1]-negative cases belong largely or wholly to the late-onset group ($n = 1$, $r = 9$).

Does the chromosomal abnormality correspond to any one or more of the three initiating events, or does it result from them, or is it independent of them? According to my theory, the random events that initiate auto-aggressive disease are somatic gene mutations, perhaps DNA strand-switching mutations. A chromosomal translocation could only constitute an initiating event if it were accompanied by one or more changes in MCP synthesis.

If the chromosomal translocation is a consequence, rather than a cause, of initiating events it could arise: (a) as the result of an attack by a mutant MCP on a target cell; or (b) from the attack of a defence immunoglobulin antibody on a mutant growth-control, or target, stem cell. Mechanism (a) might, or might not, be causally related to the development of leukaemia.

If it could be shown that the first appearance of the Ph[1] chromosome consistently preceded the first onset of leukaemia by an interval well in excess of the average latent period (about two to three years), a non-causal connection would be the more plausible interpretation.

Canellos and Whang-Peng (1972) described an untreated patient in whom a low percentage of Ph[1]-positive cells was present for nearly $5\frac{1}{2}$ years before the onset of a subacute leukaemia. Baccarani, Zaccaria and Tura (1973) examined a patient (female, 33 years) on March 30, 1972 with a white cell count of 28400 per mm[3] and with the Ph[1] chromosome in all metaphases scored. The bone marrow was hypercellular with increased granulopoiesis but the clinical findings were normal and had remained so until March 1973 when the white cell count had decreased to 16000 per mm³. They considered that their patient, and the one studied by Canellos and Whang-Peng, were borderline cases of 'smouldering' chronic myeloid leukaemia and that the significance of the Ph¹-positive state is its ability to develop into an acute blastic leukaemia. However, Verhest and van Schoubroeck (1973) described a patient with polycythaemia vera, first examined and treated in June 1966, when a Ph¹ chromosome was found in 10 per cent of mitoses analysed. In July 1972, 150 mitoses were scrutinized and no Ph¹-positive cell could be identified. In 1973, the polycythaemia vera remained quiescent and no leukaemia had developed.

These isolated observations tend to favour the view that the Ph¹ chromosome is not causally related to chronic myeloid leukaemia. The Ph¹ state may be induced—mainly in those predisposed to early-onset chronic myeloid leukaemia—by an independent forbidden clone. Its disappearance follows the spontaneous or therapeutic suppression of the inducing forbidden clone. More intensive observations should resolve this problem.

It has been argued that studies of the biochemical or chromosomal characteristics of lines of neoplastic cells should be able to decide between the hypotheses of unicellular, or multicellular, origin. But where should the origin of a neoplasm be located? Without going too deeply into semantics, my theory may be said to locate it in one, or more (n), mutant growth-control stem cells. Leukaemias introduce a special ambiguity because those types involving T-lymphocytes, and others involving cells of the humoral growth-control system (other specialized lymphocytes and/or basophilic granulocytes?), can be regarded as neoplastic proliferations of mutant growth-control cells (Burch, 1968(a)). But even in such instances, the logic of the age-distributions illustrated in this section still demands that the mutant MCP should attack cells of a target tissue (see Chapter 4). Target cells could well be receptor cells for affector TCFs located centrally in the afferent limb of the negative-feedback control system (Burch, 1968(a)). Normally, these central receptor cells respond to affector TCFs so that, when the target tissue has reached its equilibrium size, they prevent the release of effector MCPs. Impairment of this inhibitory function of specific receptor cells could lead, in theory, to the excessive proliferation of a clone of growth-control cells, that is, to leukaemic change. Such a leukaemia results from an autoaggressive attack by a forbidden clone on its own control system.

These several considerations emphasize the caution needed when interpreting biochemical or chromosomal studies of neoplastic cells. When $n = 1$, I conclude that a single forbidden clone attacks a specific set of target cells carrying a specific TCF. Although in the limiting case this 'set' may comprise a single cell only, it may also comprise numerous cells, with identical TCFs, at various anatomical sites. But even in this latter instance of multifocal transformation, the forbidden clone may well induce characteristic biochemical, chromosomal, immunological, or other abnormalities, common to all transformed target cells (Burch et al., 1973).

My theory poses, therefore, a new investigational problem: When age-analysis implies, say, that $n = 3$, can we identify experimentally three distinctive mutant MCPs and three distinctive complementary TCFs? Such questions will not be easy to answer, but at least they are answerable in principle.

Cyclic leucocytosis—Cyclic, or periodic, changes are seen in various non-malignant autoaggressive diseases and hence it is of interest that cyclic leucocytosis—and thrombocytosis—have been observed in patients with chronic myeloid leukaemia (Morley, Baikie and Galton, 1967; Vodopick et al., 1972). Under certain conditions, a homeostatic or negative-feedback control system incorporating a time-delay will oscillate. Morley (1966) has found that healthy individuals show an oscillating neutrophil count, with a period of 14 to 24 days. Hence, the oscillation of leucocyte and platelet counts observed in patients with chronic myeloid leukaemia might reflect the partial retention of a normal homeostatic control (Morley et al., 1967). Leucocyte and platelet counts showed a similar period of oscillation (30 to about 110 days), but a slightly different phase, leucocytes lagging several days behind platelets (Morley et al., 1972). The similarity of the periods points to a control common to the two systems. From the fundamental point of view, the most significant feature of these investigations is the demonstration of a control over the level of a neoplastic (leukaemic) process. The idea—held by some—that neoplastic growth is always unrestrained needs to be abandoned.

Acute lymphocytic leukaemia (7th ICD 204·3)

Acute lymphocytic leukaemia has a highly complicated age-distribution, which, combined with rather small numbers and diagnostic difficulties, renders elusive a comprehensive analysis. For the pre-adolescent phase, statistics are required for each year of age. Data from the Oxford Survey (England and Wales) for the age-range 0 to nine years are analysed in Chapter 9; those for 20 US hospitals, 1955 to 1964, covering the entire age-range (Zippin et al., 1971), receive a tentative analysis in Figure 7.81. Because these are relative rates, and in view of the somewhat uncertain nature of the age-pattern above $t = 10$ years, no table of parameters is given. A minimum

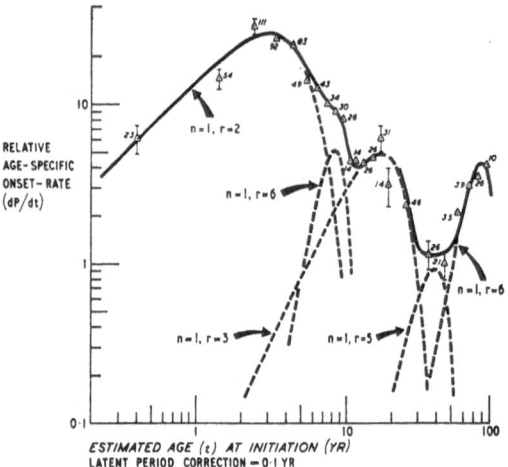

Figure 7.81 Relative age-specific onset-rates, sexes combined, acute lymphocytic leukaemia, 20 US hospitals, 1955–64, in relation to estimated age at initiation (Zippin *et al.*, 1971)

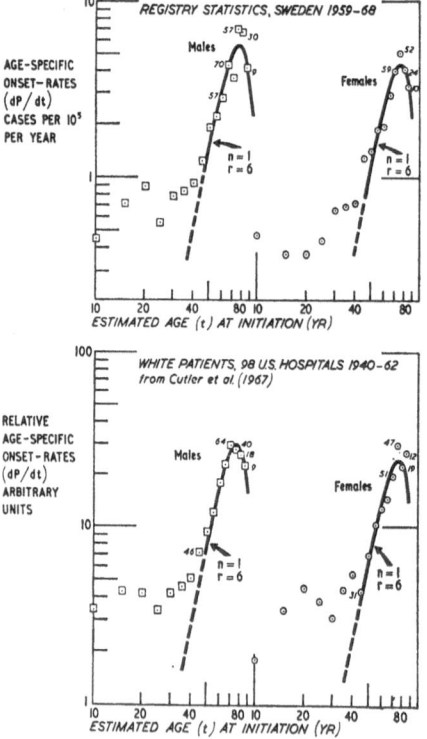

Figure 7.82 Upper panel: Sex-specific and age-specific onset-rates, acute myeloid leukaemia, Sweden, 1959–68, in relation to estimated age at initiation (Swedish Cancer Registry, 1971). Lower panel: Relative sex-specific and age-specific onset-rates, acute myeloid leukaemia, white patients in 98 US hospitals, 1940–62, in relation to estimated age at initiation (Cutler *et al.*, 1967). Latent period correction = 2.5 years throughout

of five stochastic functions is needed to fit this unusually complicated age-distribution. Mortality statistics for England and Wales, 1968–71, (not illustrated) show a similar pattern and complexity, although the late-onset group ($n = 1$, $r = 6$?) is relatively more conspicuous than in the US data of Zippin et al. (1971) shown in Figure 7.81.

Acute myeloid leukaemia (7th ICD 204·6)

Statistics for the onset of this type of leukaemia show a somewhat indefinite pattern below $t = 45$ years, although late-onset cases in Sweden and the USA give a reasonably good fit to the equation in which $n = 1$, $r = 6$ (Figure 7.82). For this late-onset group, the Swedish statistics for absolute rates yield: $k_M = k_F = 4·4 \times 10^{-12}$ year^{-6}; $S_M = 1·9 \times 10^{-3}$; $S_F = 1·5 \times 10^{-3}$. Acute myeloid leukaemia makes a substantial contribution to the overall mortality from leukaemia during the first year or two of life (see Chapter 9).

Leukaemia: twins and familial studies

The numerous reports of leukaemia among twins, 1928 to 1969, have been reviewed by Keith and Brown (1971). Concordance for monozygotic (MZ) twin pairs is of particular interest. For perinatal–congenital leukaemia, the reported average concordance is 91 per cent; for early childhood 17 per cent (only one concordant pair and five discordant); and for adult cases 40 per cent. If predisposition is determined entirely by the genotype and no extrinsic factors are needed to precipitate a disease then, making proper allowance for penetrance and intercurrent mortality from other diseases, the corrected concordance in monozygotic twin pairs would normally be expected to be 100 per cent. In the complex group of diseases described by the term 'leukaemia', it is doubtful whether proper correction for penetrance could in general be achieved, because it would seldom be possible to allocate the first affected twin unambiguously to a specific group, except perhaps, for cases of Ph^1-positive and Ph^1-negative chronic myeloid leukaemia.

The concordance values derived from Keith and Brown's (1971) literature survey will all be minimum values; inadequate periods of follow-up and the absence of a correction for intercurrent mortality, will both reduce concordance below the theoretical 100 per cent. (Somatic mutation during embryogenesis and foetal life might also produce discordance between monozygotic twins.) However, because concordance for monozygotic twin pairs is higher than for dizygotic twin pairs in all age-groups (Keith and Brown, 1971), and taking into account the numerous reports of familial aggregations of leukaemia (including one by McPhedran, Heath and Lee (1969) of ten cases in two interrelated families), together with the associations of leukaemia with trisomy 21 and the Christchurch chromosome (Fitzgerald and Hamer, 1969; Juberg and Jones, 1970), there can be little doubt that genetic factors are important to the aetiology of many, if not all, cases of natural leukaemia. The age-patterns of the several forms of natural leukaemia illustrated here suggest that a specific genetic predisposition is present in all instances.

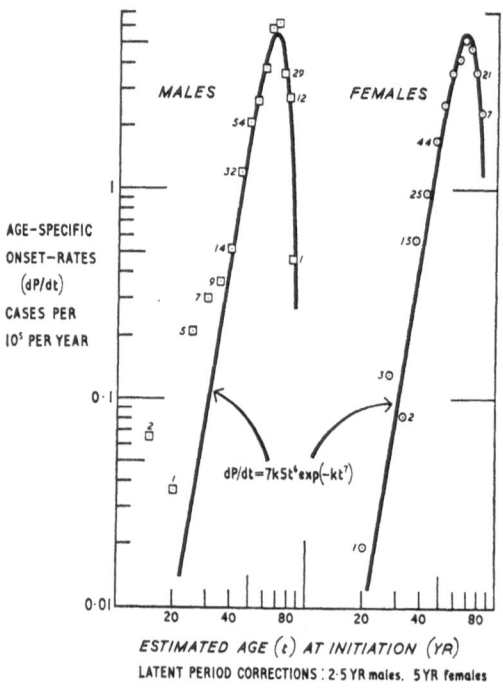

Figure 7.83 Sex-specific and age-specific onset-rates, polycythaemia vera, Sweden, 1959–68, in relation to estimated age at initiation (Swedish Cancer Registry, 1971)

Polycythaemia vera (7th ICD 204·5)

Figure 7.83 shows the age-specific onset-rates of polycythaemia vera as recorded by the Swedish Cancer Registry, 1959–68. Numbers of cases are small and onset is difficult to assess but most of the data, apart from some early-onset male cases, can be fitted adequately to the equation with $n = 1$, $r = 7$. Latent period corrections show a fairly clearcut sex-difference: 2·5 years for males and 5 years for females. This is an unusual difference where neoplastic disorders are concerned although it is commonplace among non-neoplastic so-called 'autoimmune' diseases. We find that this sex-difference characterizes those diseases, of which systemic lupus erythematosus is the classical example, in which the primary pathogenic agents are believed to be T-lymphocytes carrying cell-bound mutant MCPs (Burch, 1968(a);

Burch and Rowell, 1968, 1970). If the target cells in polycythaemia vera belong to the erythrocytic series itself (and that is not self-evident), the forbidden clone would be expected to show the observed 2:1 (F/M) sex ratio.

In these Swedish data, $S_M \simeq S_F \simeq 1 \cdot 5 \times 10^{-3}$. In other series reviewed by Modan (1965), the sex-ratio, M/F, of the *numbers* of cases has ranged from 0·7 to two.

The many reports of the co-existence of polycythaemia vera and multiple myeloma have been reviewed by Dittmar *et al.* (1968). These authors described a male patient with longstanding polycythaemia vera who developed a myeloma-like disease with two paraproteins (γG type K and γA type L) in the serum and two Bence Jones proteins (kappa and lambda) in the urine. The patient had been treated with ^{32}P, chemotherapy and phlebotomies. Modan (1965) suggests that the association between polycythaemia vera and leukaemia—or, at least, part of it—should be attributed to the therapeutic use of ^{32}P or x-rays.

Various reports of the familial aggregation of polycythaemia vera have appeared, some of which have been criticized by subsequent authors. Modan (1965) reviewed this controversial literature and pointed out that no case-control study had been undertaken. However, Figure 7.83 indicates that most late-onset cases of polycythaemia vera are restricted to a particular subpopulation. I am unaware of any realistic alternatives to the view that the specificity of the subpopulation is determined by genetic factors.

Levin, Houston and Ritzman (1967) reported two brothers with polycythaemia vera and the presence of the Ph^1 chromosome in marrow aspirates. The disease had been diagnosed in one brother 22 years prior to the report and he had been treated with ^{32}P on several occasions. Diagnosis of polycythaemia vera and cytogenetic examination of the second brother had been made just prior to the report and before commencing therapy. Modan *et al.* (1971) investigated the high incidence of polycythaemia vera among Jews in Baltimore City, US and Israel. They found no appreciable difference in incidence between European-born Israelis and Baltimore Jews. Thus, incidence in a fairly well-defined racial group appears to be largely independent of residence and to that extent the genetic hypothesis is supported.

Hodgkin's Disease (7th ICD 201)

On the basis of its age-pattern, MacMahon has proposed that Hodgkin's disease is a combination of at least two, and perhaps three, aetiologically distinct entities (MacMahon, 1966; Cole, MacMahon and Aisenberg, 1968). I have supported this proposal and have shown that, in addition to the two main modes, a very small group, with onset predominantly during

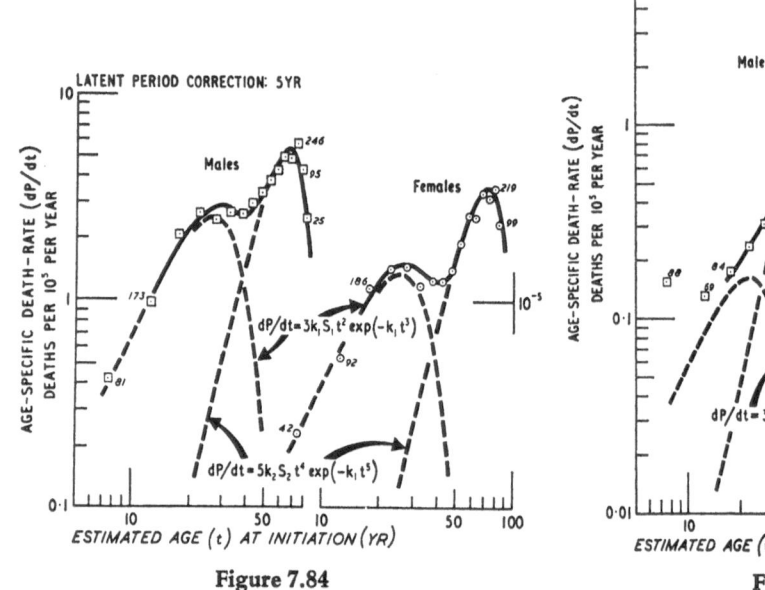

Figure 7.84

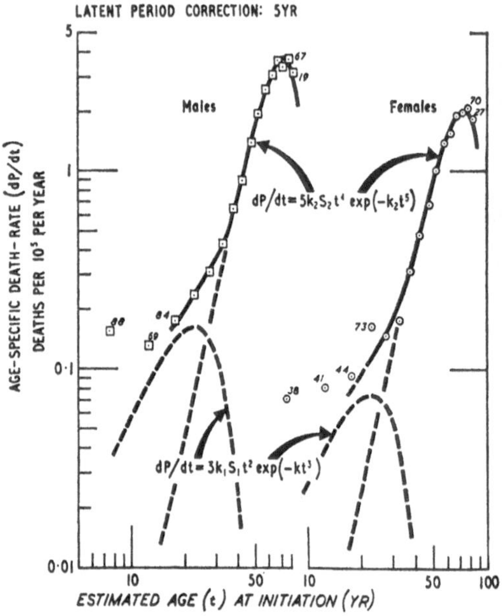

Figure 7.85

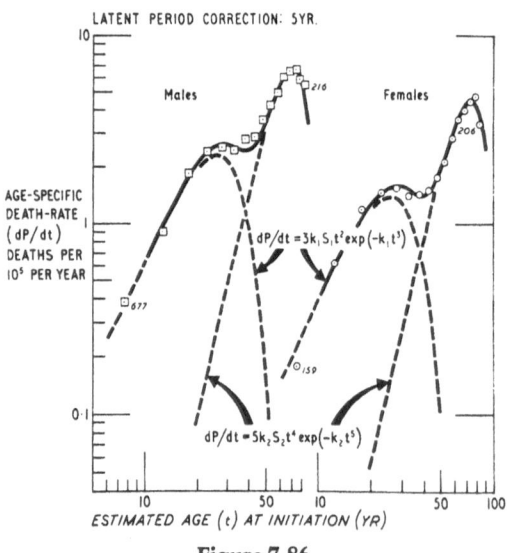

Figure 7.86

Figure 7.84 Sex-specific and age-specific death-rates, Hodgkin's disease, England and Wales, 1955–65, in relation to estimated age at initiation (World Health Organization, 1970). See Table 7.25

Figure 7.85 As for Figure 7.84. Data for Japan, 1955–65

Figure 7.86 As for Figure 7.84. Data for US (all races), 1955–65

Table 7.25 Hodgkin's Disease (7th ICD 201) (Tentative Analysis of Mortality Data for Two Main Groups ($t > 10$ years))

Population	Males				Females			
	$(n=1, r=3)$		$(n=1, r=5)$		$(n=1, r=3)$		$(n=1, r=5)$	
	k_1 (yr^{-3})	S_1	k_2 (yr^{-5})	S_2	k_1 (yr^{-3})	S_1	k_2 (yr^{-5})	S_2
England and Wales 1955–65	3.7×10^{-5}	6.4×10^{-4}	6.9×10^{-10}	2.0×10^{-3}	3.7×10^{-5}	3.3×10^{-4}	4.5×10^{-10}	1.4×10^{-3}
Japan 1955–65	5.4×10^{-5}	3.6×10^{-5}	3.9×10^{-10}	1.5×10^{-3}	5.4×10^{-5}	1.6×10^{-5}	3.9×10^{-10}	8.4×10^{-4}
US (all races) 1955–65	3.7×10^{-5}	5.8×10^{-4}	4.5×10^{-10}	2.7×10^{-3}	3.7×10^{-5}	3.5×10^{-5}	3.9×10^{-4}	1.8×10^{-3}

Latent period correction $= 5$ years.

childhood, has an age-distribution in the USA (Fraumeni and Li, 1969), described by: $dP/dt = 2kSt \exp(-kt^2)$. The initiation mode occurs at about $t =$ seven years; $S_M \simeq 1.3 \times 10^{-5}$; $S_F \simeq 4 \times 10^{-6}$ (Burch, 1970(b)).

Mortality statistics (WHO, 1970) for England and Wales, Japan and the USA (all races), covering the period 1955–65, are analysed in Figures 7.84 to 7.86. They are fitted to two stochastic functions: $n = 1$, $r = 3$; and $n = 1$, $r = 5$, but because the data do not contain sufficient detail to define the early-onset group, the interpretation $n = 1$, $r = 3$ for the mid-onset group should be regarded as tentative.

Davidson and Clarke (1970) classified Hodgkin's disease into two main types by histological and anatomical criteria. They defined Type I in terms of 'lymphocyte predominance, mixed cellularity, retroperitoneal glands, superficial'; cases of this type have a peak age of onset above 50 years. Type II was defined in terms of 'nodular sclerosis, mixed cellularity, and central glands'; the peak age of onset is between 15 and 25 years. These types appear to correspond with the two main groups implied by the analysis in Figures 7.84 to 7.86. However, they do not exhaust the heterogeneity of the disease. Neiman, Rosen and Lukes (1973) described 13 cases of lymphocyte-depletion Hodgkin's disease, which disseminates widely and progresses rapidly: survival from initial presentation ranged from five to ten months. Age of onset ranged from 18 to 73 years with a median of 51 years; it remains to be determined whether the kinetics of initiation resemble those of the main late-onset group, with $n = 1$, $r = 5$.

Rosenberg and Kaplan (1966) favour the idea of a unifocal origin followed by spread along adjacent lymphoid channels, but Smithers (1967) argues (more persuasively in my view) in favour of multifocal origin for Hodgkin's disease. Not one of the 100 untreated patients examined by Rosenberg and Kaplan (1966) had only one affected lymph node at presentation; bilateral symmetry of neck gland involvement was found in 56 of these patients. Willis (1960) believes that the disease arises multifocally, or diffusely, in at least some patients, but that metastatic spread contributes to its dissemination.

Genetic factor

According to Halazun, Kerr and Lukens (1972), the occurrence of Hodgkin's disease in more than one member of a family had been reported in about 80 families. They described the disease in three cousins (5, 11 and 12 years of age at onset) from an ethnic group (Amish) which has a high degree of inbreeding. An even larger aggregation, with no fewer than seven cases in a single Newfoundland family, has been described by Buehler et al. (1975) and attributed by them to genetic factors. In several reports, the same localization of the primary disease has been described in relatives of probands

(Thorling, 1973), indicating that the anatomical distribution of the primary lesions in spontaneous malignant disease is genetically determined (Burch, 1968a). From his review of familial studies of Hodgkin's disease Fraumeni (1974) estimated that first-degree relatives of probands have about a threefold excess risk of the disease.

Statistically significant associations between one or more histocompatibility antigens and a disease provide direct evidence for genetic predisposition. Several groups have found an apparently significant association between Hodgkin's disease and the HL-A5 antigen, but others have failed to confirm it. The specificity of the test antisera used by different workers has not always been the same and the extent of the association may differ from one population to another, and between the different types of Hodgkin's disease.

In small-scale studies, Kissmeyer-Nielson (1971) and Sybesma et al. (1972) found no association between Hodgkin's disease and HL-A5 but a positive association with HL-A8. In a fairly large study (112 patients, 122 controls) Falk and Osoba (1971) found that HL-A8 was increased in frequency only in patients who had had the disease for more than 5 years; however, the frequencies of HL-A1 and HL-A5 were found to be high, regardless of the duration of the disease. Of special importance from the present point of view is the finding that HL-A8 is more frequent in patients with mixed cellularity and lymphocytic predominance than in those with nodular sclerosis (Falk and Osoba, 1971). Careful attention to age of onset and histology—recognizing that Hodgkin's disease is not a homogeneous entity—might resolve some of the apparent discrepancies in the investigations of histocompatibility antigens.

An infectious disease?

Vianna, Greenwald and Davies (1971) described a remarkable aggregation of cases of Hodgkin's disease. From a student group at an Albany, New York, high school, they traced among the students, their contacts, and their contacts' contacts, 31 cases of Hodgkin's disease and three cases of other lymphomas diagnosed between 1948 and 1971. In a critical review, Heath (1972) attempted to answer the questions: Does the aggregation reflect person-to-person spread of an infectious agent, or does it represent a chance episode? Although unable to reach an answer, Heath (1972) pointed out: (a) epidemics of Hodgkin's disease are certainly uncommon; (b) Vianna et al. (1971) found no indication of specific latency among the time intervals between contact and diagnosis; (c) they found only one instance of familial disease; (d) the disease is not markedly seasonal; and (e) it does not regularly occur in clusters.

Five connubial instances (husband and wife) of the disease have been reported, but this incidence probably does not exceed chance expectation (Fraumeni, 1974).

Rosdahl, Larsen and Clemmesen (1974) have reported a positive association between infectious mononucleosis and the onset of Hodgkin's disease after an interval of at least one year. As these authors point out, such associations do not constitute proof of a causal relation. A positive association between predisposing genetic factors could well account for this type of association between two diseases.

The overall epidemiological evidence for an infectious aetiology is, therefore, unimpressive.

Burkitt's Lymphoma

Because of its peculiar geographical distribution, the human malignancy with the strongest claim to an infectious aetiology is, perhaps, Burkitt's lymphoma (Burkitt, 1962; Burkitt and Wright, 1966).

Elsewhere, I have analysed the age-dependence of Adatia's (1966) series for lymphoma of the jaws, Uganda, 1953 to 1965 (Burch, 1968(a)). Below the age of 20 years, two main groups can be distinguished with the following characteristics: The early-onset group ($n = 1$, $r = 3$) shows an initiation mode of 3·8 years (females) and 4·8 years (males) for a latent period correction of 1·5 years; $k_M = 6 \times 10^{-3}$ year^{-3}, $k_F = 2k_M = 1·2 \times 10^{-2}$ year^{-3},—indicating that one of the three initiating somatic mutations affects an X-linked gene; the disease is commoner in males and $S_M/S_F \simeq 3·4$. Initiation modes for the late-onset group are about 8·1 years (females) and 10·2 years (males); probably, $n = 3$, $r = 3$; $k_M = 1·35 \times 10^{-3}$ year^{-3}, $k_F = 2k_M = 2·7 \times 10^{-3}$ year^{-3} again pointing to the somatic mutation of an X-linked gene—and $S_M/S_F \simeq$ 1·9. Absolute values of S cannot be derived because the size of the population from which cases were drawn was not given.

The anatomical distribution of tumours among the four quadrants of the jaws was found to be extremely non-random (Adatia, 1966). In 163 patients, only one side of the mandible or maxilla was affected; in 39 patients two quadrants were affected; in seven patients, three were; but in 41 patients all four quadrants were involved. Siting will therefore be determined by multiple MCP–TCF genes (Burch, 1968(a)).

Although the age-dependence and anatomical distribution of Burkitt's lymphoma suggest a classical autoaggressive disease, these data do not bear on the question as to whether an infective agent is essential to the proliferation of forbidden clones and the precipitation of the disease (Burch, 1968(a) and Chapter 8). Evidence for space–time clustering and/or marked seasonal onset is helpful in this respect.

Pike, Williams and Wright (1967) reported significant space–time clustering of patients with Burkitt's tumour in the West Nile district of Uganda, 1961–66, but because the statistical tests assume a uniform distribution of genetically predisposed persons among the general population, such claims have to be approached with caution (Burch, 1968(a)). A more recent study of space–time clustering of Burkitt's lymphoma in the North Mara district of Tanzania, 1964–70, by Brubaker, Geser and Pike (1973) has failed to yield any results even remotely approaching statistical significance. The authors believe their negative findings cast doubt on the validity of the clustering reported earlier (Pike *et al.*, 1967) for the West Nile district of Uganda.

Williams, Day and Geser (1974) found a significant seasonal variation in the onset of Burkitt's lymphoma in the West Nile district of Uganda. During the first 6 months of each year (over the period, 1961 to 1973), a total of 69 cases presented and during the last 6 months of each year some 102 new cases were seen in all. In view of the estimated average latent period between initiation and onset of about 1·5 year (Burch, 1968(a)), one or more seasonal factors (infectious and/or allergic) might well provoke the growth of a latent tumour to the overt phase. If a seasonal factor, such as a virus, were essential to the precipitation of the growth of forbidden clones, clearcut space–time clustering should be observed.

The Epstein–Barr (EB) virus has been strongly fancied as an aetiological agent (Klein, 1971). However, one-third of Burkitt's lymphoma patients studied in the USA had no detectable levels of antibody to the EB virus (Hirshaut, Cohen and Stevens, 1973). Antibody titres in American cases did not differ significantly from those found in an age-, sex- and race-matched control group.

Overall, the evidence for an *essential* infective agent in the pathogenesis of Burkitt's lymphoma remains unconvincing.

Bone Sarcoma

Most published statistics for malignant tumours of the bone (7th ICD 196) fail to distinguish the type of tumour. However, the Registrar General (1958) gave the details of sex-specific and age-specific death-rates for malignant neoplasms of bone (except the jaw) described as sarcoma, for the years 1945–47 and 1954–56. This is the most common primary malignancy of bone. Mean values for the two periods are graphed in Figure 7.87. The age-pattern for a distinctive group with onset predominantly before 5 years of age is not defined (because of the use of 5-year age-ranges) and hence the equation for the group with the mode at about $t = 15$ years might need to be revised when more detailed data become available. Table 7.26 gives the

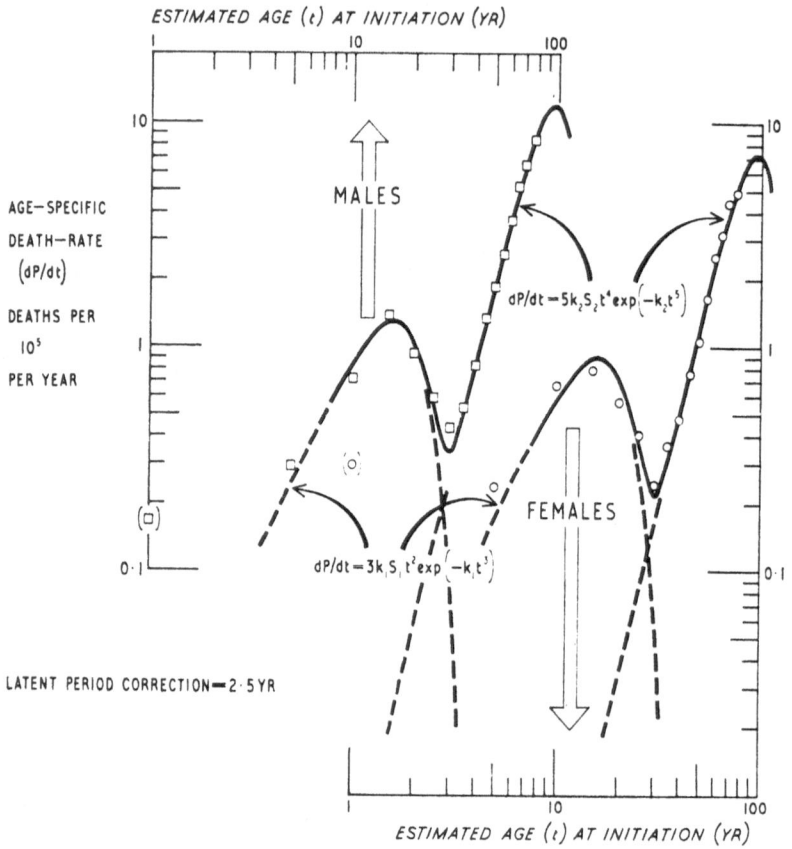

Figure 7.87 Sex-specific and age-specific death-rates, sarcoma of bone (excluding jaw), England and Wales, 1945–47 and 1954–56, in relation to estimated age at initiation (Registrar General, 1958). See Table 7.26

parameters that describe the tentative analysis in Figure 7.87.

There is a strong association between Paget's disease of the bone—a recognized inherited disorder—and late-onset bone sarcoma, which has not usually been regarded as genetically based (Price, 1961; Boyd et al., 1969). However, Price (1961) reports that familial cases of osteogenic sarcoma are somewhat more common than those of Paget's disease.

Malignant Neoplasms of the Eye (7th ICD 192)

Malignant melanoma

Most cancers of the eye are malignant melanomas, although below the age of ten, almost all are retinoblastomas. Statistics for the onset of malignant

Table 7.26 Sarcoma of Bone, except Jaw (Tentative Interpretation of Mortality Statistics)

Population	Males				Females			
	Early-onset $(n=1, r=3)$		Late-onset $(n=1, r=5)$		Early-onset $(n=1, r=3)$		Late-onset $(n=1, r=5)$	
	k_1 (yr^{-3})	S_1	k_2 (yr^{-5})	S_2	k_1 (yr^{-3})	S_1	k_2 (yr^{-5})	S_2
England and Wales 1945–47 and 1954–56	$1 \cdot 7 \times 10^{-4}$	$1 \cdot 9 \times 10^{-4}$	10^{-10}	$6 \cdot 2 \times 10^{-3}$	$1 \cdot 7 \times 10^{-4}$	$1 \cdot 3 \times 10^{-4}$	10^{-10}	$3 \cdot 9 \times 10^{-3}$

Latent period correction = 2·5 years

melanoma of the eye in Sweden, 1959–65 (Swedish Cancer Registry, 1971) are analysed in Figure 7.88.

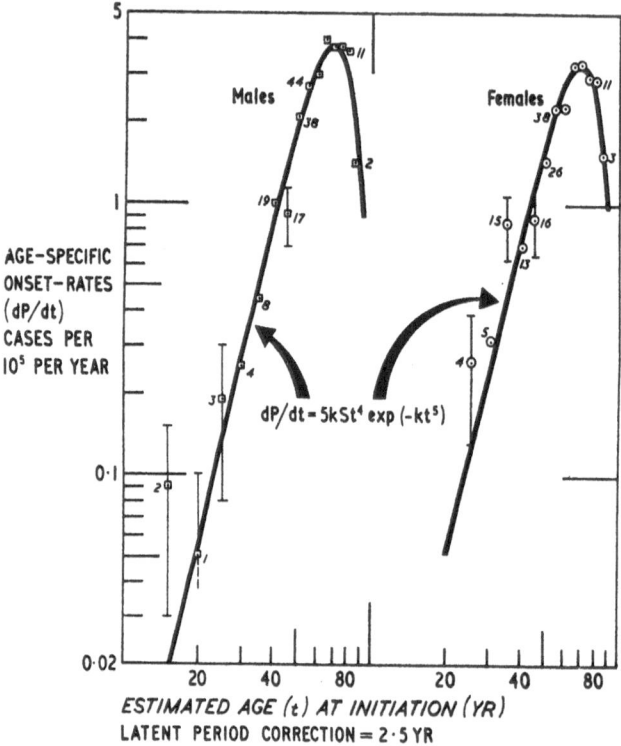

Figure 7.88 Sex-specific and age-specific onset rates, malignant melanoma of the eye, Sweden, 1959–65, in relation to estimated age at initiation (Swedish Cancer Registry, 1971). See Table 7.27

Numbers are small, but the graph suggests that malignant melanoma of the eye is largely or wholly confined (in Sweden at least) to a single genetic group. Probably, five somatic mutations in a single growth-control stem cell initiate this malignancy ($n = 1$, $r = 5$). Table 7.27 lists the parameters used to fit the data in Figure 7.88.

Assuming that a recessive-effect X-linked gene accounts for the sex-ratio, its frequency in the Swedish population is about 0·85. Additional (auto-somal) predisposing factors are needed to account for the low values of S_M and S_F. Not surprisingly in view of the polygenic inheritance, familial cases are rare, but an hereditary predisposition has been suggested (Duke-Elder and Perkins, 1966). In their literature review, Duke-Elder and Perkins (1966) refer to one report of transmission from grandfather to mother to

Table 7.27 Malignant Melanoma of the Eye

Population	k $(n=1, r=5)$ yr^{-5}	S_M	S_F	S_M/S_F
Sweden 1959–65	$5\cdot2\times10^{-10}$	$1\cdot45\times10^{-3}$	$1\cdot23\times10^{-3}$	$1\cdot18$

Latent period correction $=2\cdot5$ years

daughter; another of mother to daughter; and, even more impressively, of seven affected individuals in four generations of one family.

The laterality of malignant melanomas of the eye, with predilection for the left eye, holds much interest. In the recent series of males from US Veteran's Administration hospitals studied by Keller (1973), malignant melanomas affected the right eye in 74 patients and the left in 122 patients. The ratio (L/R) of 1·65 departs very significantly from unity ($P=0\cdot0003$). Carcinomas *in situ* (20R; 17L) showed no significant predilection for either eye (Keller, 1973).

Unlike retinoblastomas (see below), malignant melanomas of the eye are seldom bilateral. At the time of the review by Duke-Elder and Perkins (1966), only two cases of simultaneous bilaterality had been reported. The interval between the involvement of the first and second eyes usually ranges from six months to 8 years. These scanty data suggest that a single forbidden clone might be responsible for simultaneous or near-simultaneous bilateral cases, but that metastases, or two independent forbidden clones, are involved when the interval is more than a few years.

Retinoblastoma

Data for age at first treatment obtained from the Oxford Survey of Childhood Cancers, mainly for the period 1953–65 (Stewart, 1969), are analysed in Figure 7.89. These comprise 144 male and 135 female cases.

Jenson and Miller (1971) discussed mortality-rates from retinoblastoma in United States children, 1960–67, by race. They pointed out that the peak at 2 to 3 years of age is more prominent in statistics for Negroes than in those for Whites. Their data for age at diagnosis in hospital series are shown in Figures 7.90 and 7.91. The age-distribution of the population from which these cases were drawn is unknown and the use of numbers of cases instead of dP/dt will not seriously distort analysis, the results of which are shown in Table 7.28. None of the data graphed in Figures 7.89 to 7.91 are absolute rates and hence they do not enable values of S to be calculated.

From registry statistics for the German Democratic Republic, 1964–66

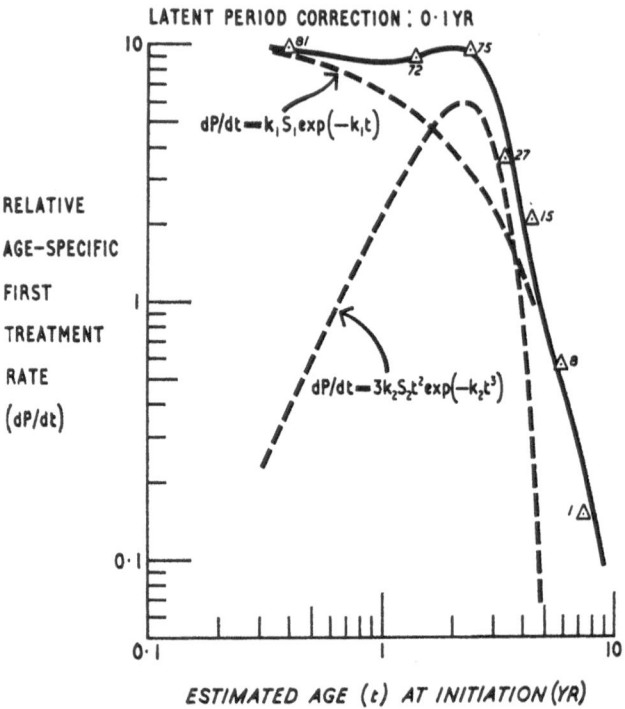

Figure 7.89 Relative age-specific first treatment rate, sexes combined, retinoblastoma, England and Wales, mainly 1953–65, in relation to estimated age at initiation (Stewart, 1969). See Table 7.28

Table 7.28 Retinoblastoma

Population	Sexes combined		
	$(n=1, r=1)$ k_1 (yr^{-1})	$(n=1, r=3)$ k_2 (yr^{-3})	S_1/S_2
England and Wales (mainly 1953–65) Oxford Survey (Stewart, 1969)	0·52	$5·7 \times 10^{-2}$	1·6
US Whites, hospital series (Jensen and Miller, 1971)	0·52	$6·8 \times 10^{-2}$	2·7
US Negroes, hospital series (Jensen and Miller, 1971)	0·42	$6·4 \times 10^{-2}$	1·3

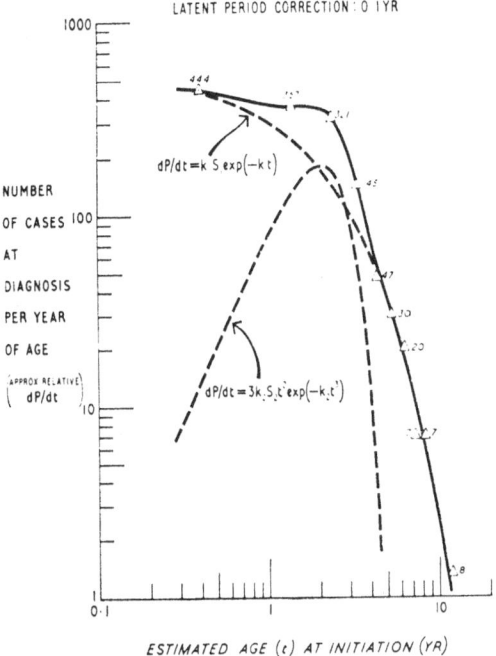

Figure 7.90 Number of cases of retinoblastoma at diagnosis, by age, US White children 1960–67 (sexes combined), in relation to estimated age at initiation (Jensen and Miller, 1971). See Table 7.28

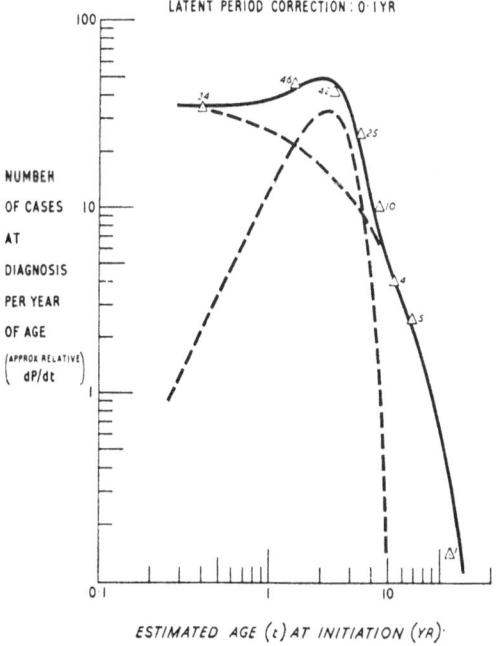

Figure 7.91 As for Figure 7.90. Data for US Negroes

(Doll *et al.*, 1970), I have been able to estimate, very approximately, that $S_1 = 4 \times 10^{-5}$ and $S_2 = 1 \cdot 6 \times 10^{-5}$ (sexes combined). The frequency of the disease is increasing throughout the world. In Holland it was estimated to be about 3×10^{-5} (per live birth) in 1927–29, but by 1950–69, it had increased to $6 \cdot 6 \times 10^{-5}$ (Schappert-Kimmijser, Hemmes, and Nijland, 1966).

From the age of diagnosis of 23 bilateral and 25 unilateral cases given by Knudson (1971), it is clear, despite the small numbers, that bilateral cases belong mainly to group 1 ($n = 1$, $r = 1$) and that unilateral cases belong mainly to group 2 ($n = 1$, $r = 3$). However, the occurrence of three unilateral cases in the first year of life—as against $0 \cdot 5$ expected—suggests that some unilateral cases might belong to group 1. Familial evidence (see below) supports this suggestion.

Retinoblastoma constitutes an important example, therefore, of a disease in which bilateral growths may be initiated by a single random event ($n = 1$, $r = 1$). Out of a total of 20 bilateral cases studied by Leelawongs and Regan (1968), some 18 were seen to be bilateral at the first examination. The near-simultaneity of appearance of most bilateral cases refutes Knudson's (1971) theory, in which somatic mutations are assumed to occur in retinoblasts. The chance of random somatic mutations occurring almost simultaneously in both eyes will be small. Occasionally, the interval between the appearance of a tumour in one eye, and the other, may extend to several years. Such instances could be explained if two independent forbidden clones in either a group 1 or a group 2 person are implicated, one specific for the left eye and the other for the right eye. Duke-Elder (1940) and Willis (1960) emphasize that bilateral retinoblastomas are *not* due to spread from one eye to the other. Moreover, even at an early stage, the tumours are often multiple and sometimes the whole retina is seen to be sprinkled with miliary growths of various sizes. Duke-Elder (1940) argued that many of these represent independent foci, as opposed to metastases.

Genetics

Until recently, it was believed that familial cases of retinoblastoma are due to an autosomal dominant gene and that all non-familial, or sporadic, cases should be attributed to the same, newly mutant, gene. From their own studies and a survey of the literature, Nielsen and Goldschmidt (1968) found that 81 patients who survived a sporadic retinoblastoma had a total of 159 children; of these, only seven (4·4 per cent) developed retinoblastoma. Hence the great majority of sporadic cases cannot be attributed to a new germ cell mutation. That there are (at least) two genetically distinctive forms of the disease, as implied by Figures 7.89 to 7.91, has not been widely appreciated.

The attribution of all familial cases to a single autosomal dominant gene must also be treated with reserve, because the phenomenon of the 'skipped generation' (transmission via a non-affected parent) is sometimes manifested (Weller, 1941; Schappert-Kimmijser et al., 1966) and the 'penetrance' of the gene is estimated to range from 80 per cent (Schappert-Kimmijser et al., 1966) to 95 per cent (Falls and Neel, 1951). Familial cases are often, but not always, bilateral (Fraser and Friedmann, 1967), and hence they belong in the main to group 1. Nevertheless, many sporadic bilateral cases have been reported (Schappert-Kimmijser et al., 1966; Pellié et al., 1973). In a remarkable Australian family reported by Newton (1902), ten out of 16 siblings developed retinoblastoma, seven bilaterally. Neither parent was affected, although a brother of the father had died at the age of 1 year of 'some eye complaint'.

Inheritance for cases in group 2 is probably polygenic; evidence reviewed by Weller (1941) renders improbable a simple autosomal recessive scheme.

The problem of the 'skipped generation' and 'incomplete penetrance' calls for discussion. Perhaps the simplest hypothesis invokes a polygenic scheme in which the predisposing genotype consists of the 'main' (rare) autosomal dominant gene, together with one or more other genes whose frequency in the population is high, but less than unity. However, incomplete penetrance, as well as possible occasional discordance in monozygotic twins (Schappert-Kimmijser et al., 1960), could both be accounted for by invoking somatic gene mutation during embryogenesis. If at an early stage of embryogenesis, DNA strand-switching occurred at the predisposing autosomal gene in an appropriate precursor growth-control cell, then the gene would be converted to a 'harmless' form. The eventual growth-control stem cells would synthesize a 'harmless' MCP which, in turn, would induce a corresponding TCF in presumptive retinal target cells. Subsequent somatic mutation of the 'harmless' gene during postnatal life would not lead to the formation of a pathogenic forbidden clone.

Another possibility concerns an essential extrinsic factor. If a specific factor such as an infective agent—for example, a virus, or an allergen—is needed to precipitate the growth of a forbidden clone, then the degree of penetrance of the disease will depend on the presence in the environment of the precipitating factor. The consistently high level of penetrance of group 1 retinoblastoma demands an almost ubiquitous factor: this renders the hypothesis unlikely without completely disposing of it. Only intensive systematic study will resolve this kind of problem.

To summarize the conclusions of this section:

(1) two distinctive genotypes are at risk with respect to retinoblastoma;
(2) most familial cases belong to genotype 1, which might be characterized

by a single autosomal dominant gene although a more complicated scheme, in which the main autosomal dominant gene is supplemented by another gene (or genes) of high frequency, cannot be completely eliminated;

(3) most group 1 cases are bilateral and are initiated by a single (postnatal) somatic gene mutation ($n=1$, $r=1$) in a growth-control stem cell;

(4) genetic factors determine whether the left, right, or both eyes are affected, both in group 1 and group 2 cases;

(5) predisposition in group 2 is almost certainly polygenic;

(6) the initiation of the disease in this genotype requires three somatic mutations, in a single growth-control stem cell ($n=1$, $r=3$); and

(7) most cases in group 2 are unilateral.

Malignant Neoplasms of the Brain and Cerebral Meninges (7th ICD 193.0)

Although cancers of the brain are not rare, they comprise many distinctive histological types. The Swedish Cancer Registry (1971) gives the age of onset for 18 histological categories of brain cancer, for the period 1959–65. The only category that has large enough numbers and a simple enough age-pattern for plausible (partial) analysis, is the commonest one, glioblastoma. Some 1790 cases, out of a total of 4868 cases of brain cancer, were put in this category. Figure 7.92 shows the age-distribution of onset. At least two early-onset groups can be distinguished in the overall data, but the numbers at low t are too small to define their age-distribution accurately.

Above $t=25$ years, the data for men and women give a good fit to the equation in which $n=1$, $r=5$. For both sexes $k=9{\cdot}3\times10^{-10}$ year^{-5}. The proportions of the Swedish population predisposed are: $S_M=3{\cdot}6\times10^{-3}$ and $S_F=2{\cdot}8\times10^{-3}$, giving a sex-ratio, S_M/S_F, of $1{\cdot}3$. If this male predominance results from a recessive-effect X-linked allele, its frequency in Sweden is about 0·77. Hence the frequency of predisposing autosomal factors is expected to be in the region of 5×10^{-3}.

The literature (up to 1966) of the genetic aspects of tumours of the central and peripheral nervous systems has been reviewed by Aita (1967). As would be expected, brain tumours in concordant monozygotic twins are commonly identical for histological type and even for anatomical location.

Multiple gliomas are fairly common. Glioblastoma multiforme occurs as a multiple growth in about 10 per cent of cases (Courville, 1950). From his own series of multiple gliomas, Willis (1960) concluded that, with rare exceptions, multiplicity cannot be explained by metastasis and must be attributed to a multifocal origin. Certain astrocytomas affect large areas of the brain, such as a large part of one or both hemispheres, in a diffuse manner.

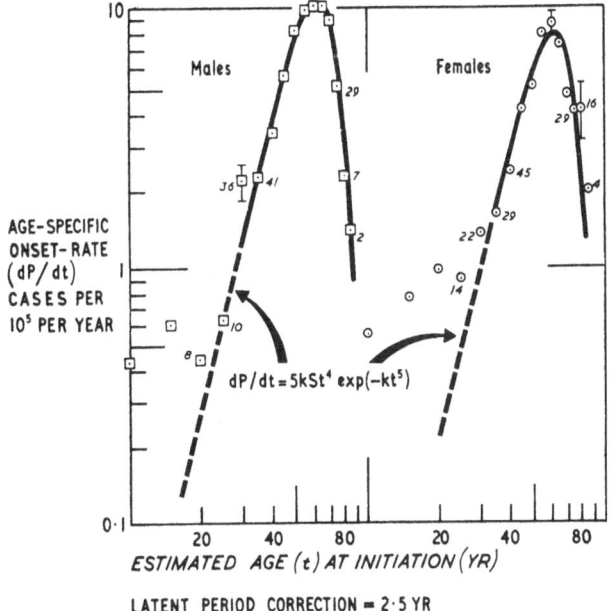

Figure 7.92 Sex-specific and age-specific onset-rates, glioblastoma, Sweden, 1959–65, in relation to estimated age at initiation (Swedish Cancer Registry, 1971)

Willis (1960) concurs with Scherer (1940) in the view that these diffuse tumours cannot be wholly explained as a proliferative invasion of surrounding tissues; they are diffuse in origin.

General Discussion

Perhaps the outstanding feature of this chapter is the high degree of reproducibility in the age-patterns of well-defined cancers, from country to country and from continent to continent. With rare exceptions, the age-dependence of a genetically specific cancer can be accurately described in terms of a simple stochastic equation, based on a simple biological model. According to the model, any given 'natural' cancer is confined to genetically predisposed persons who constitute a proportion, S, of the general population; initiation follows the random occurrence of r specific somatic gene mutations, in each of n specific growth-control stem cells.

Calculated values of S for a defined cancer sometimes differ widely from country to country, and especially between Japan and Western countries. Non-uniformity of diagnostic standards might sometimes account for at least a portion of such differences, but there is no reason to doubt that genes may differ in frequency from one population to another, both within and between countries. In the next chapter I shall consider whether environmental factors—other than diagnosis—can affect the apparent value of S.

The average rate at which initiating somatic mutations occur often shows marked differences between Japanese and Western populations, but only small differences, generally, among Western countries. Although Japan often shows the highest rates of somatic mutation this ranking is not always found and hence it is unlikely that a general environmental carcinogen in Japan can be held responsible for the high rates. Subtle differences in the base-sequence of MCP–TCF genes between populations could account more plausibly for contrasting rates.

The largely invariant properties of cancers reside neither in S nor in the average rate of somatic mutation (as reflected in the kinetic constant k), but in the *shapes* of the age-distributions of onset- and death-rates. These are described by the parameters n and r. Among the many sites considered, only the registry data for the onset of cancer of the lip show reasonably clearcut differences between different populations. For late-onset cases in England and Wales, and Sweden, $n = 3$, $r = 3$; but in Finland and the German Democratic Republic, $n = 2$, $r = 3$. However, mortality statistics from England and Wales, Finland and the German Federal Republic show no appreciable differences in age-pattern; age-specific death-rates for cancer of the lip are closely proportional to t^8 in all three populations. It seems likely, therefore, that the onset of malignancy is diagnosed at an earlier stage in Finland and the German Democratic Republic than in the other two countries. Substantial biological differences are probably absent. (I have been unable to obtain adequate statistics for those cancers of exposed skin that are believed to depend on ultraviolet light. It would not be altogether surprising if severe exposure to sunshine produced a repair reaction that reduced the requirement for the number, n, of initiating forbidden clones.)

The large measure of invariance observed in n and r implies not only a high degree of biological reproducibility, but also a satisfactory consistency in diagnosis with respect to age. That is to say, diagnosis is either accurate, or, if it is inaccurate, it usually entails underdiagnosis to an extent that is fairly independent of age. Overdiagnosis—including false-positive diagnoses —will generally distort the age-pattern because the age-dependence of one cancer usually differs from that of another. (The rather special example of lung cancer which has involved large errors of diagnosis—and probably still does—is discussed at length in Chapter 10.) If environmental factors contribute to the pathogenesis of the bulk of cancers recorded in national statistics, then they very seldom influence n or r. Occasional occupational cancers, involving 'unnatural' values of n and/or r, would not be revealed by pooled national statistics.

Where national mortality statistics are expected to describe a homogeneous cancer at a given site, then of the examples analysed in this chapter, only those for cancer of the esophagus show conspicuous and irregular discrepancies from country to country that also violate theory. Willis (1960) gives good reasons for believing that diagnostic error—particularly confusion between cancers of the esophagus and stomach—can be held largely, or wholly, responsible for these discrepancies. In a study of diagnostic reliability, Willis found two false positives for every three true diagnoses of carcinoma of the esophagus.

The general findings from this chapter remind us that great caution must be exercised when we seek to interpret the incidence of cancer in migrant populations. A few exceptions apart, death-rates from specific cancers in Japanese immigrants to the United States tend to lie between the national levels for Japan and the United States (Haenszel and Kurihara, 1968). We are tempted to interpret such data in terms of the differential levels of extrinsic carcinogens. However, emigrants cannot be regarded as a random sample of their community of origin and hence, in a rigorous analysis, the possibility of associations (positive or negative) between the 'genetic predisposition to emigration' and the predisposition to a specific cancer, must always be entertained until disproved. Furthermore, levels of diagnosis, therapy and reporting all need to be compared before differences in incidence can be accepted as genuine.

In contrast to the findings of Haenszel and Kurihara (1968), Staszewski (1974) found that mortality from cancers of the buccal cavity and pharynx, esophagus and larynx, was markedly higher in male Polish-born migrants to the USA, than in non-migrant Polish males or US native white males. Rates for female Polish-born migrants differed little from non-migrant Polish females, or US native white females. However, male Polish-born migrants to the USA are not a random sample of Polish males. On the simplest interpretation, the constitutional tendency to migrate associates with an above-average risk of cancers of the buccal cavity and pharynx, esophagus and larynx.

Initiation

In many instances, the evidence for the age-dependence of a malignancy, when combined with the indications from pathology for multifocal origin, leave no doubt that initiating events occur in a central location. Such implications are particularly impressive when invasive growth is preceded by recognizable pre-malignant changes, as in carcinoma of the uterine cervix and colorectal cancer associated with familial intestinal polyposis. Moreover, whenever the statistics for the age-dependence of a malignancy are adequate to assess the behaviour of k from $t=0$ to $t=20$ years, they are always consistent with the hypothesis that k remains constant during post-natal growth.

In this respect, as in many others, the initiation of malignant diseases resembles that of non-malignant diseases (Burch, 1968(a)). We have little alternative but to conclude that the number (L) of central cells at somatic mutational risk remains constant during postnatal growth. For reasons given in Chapter 4 and elsewhere (Burch and Burwell, 1965; Burch, 1968(a)), we infer that the fixed number of central stem cells act as the comparator in the central control of growth.

However, the most important implication of the age dependence of the malignant diseases (as well as of non-malignant diseases), concerns the role of predisposing genes. These serve a double function: they code for re-cognition proteins both in central growth-control cells and in target cells (Burch and Burwell, 1965; Burch, 1968(a)). In malignant diseases, neoplastic growth develops as the result of an attack on target cells, which may be located at one, or multiple, anatomical sites. (In certain instances, the attacked target cells may not proliferate: they may release other cells from pro-liferative restraints.) The identity recognition relations that form the basis for the normal control of growth give way, in autoaggressive disease, to pathogenic recognition relations between mutant MCPs and complementary target TCFs. In Chapter 9, I shall argue that, during the *promotion* phase, genes that code for TCFs in target cells also undergo DNA strand-switching mutation.

The idea that initiation occurs in central growth-control cells, which to me seems to be inescapable, nevertheless runs counter to the assumptions adopted by most experimental oncologists. It is widely assumed that the changes that *initiate* natural neoplastic growth occur in the target tissue itself. Although Smithers (1962) has vigorously attacked this assumption, it still predominates. When experts in different branches of oncology fail to agree over so basic an issue, the wisdom of 'crash programmes to eliminate cancer' must be queried.

In the light of the above conclusions it is scarcely surprising that *in vitro* cultures, both of normal and malignant cells, show better outgrowths in a medium containing autologous serum than in a medium containing pooled human serum (Cobb and Walker, 1961; Kahn and Donaldson, 1970). Cobb and Walker (1961) found that implants from leiomysarcomas and breast carcinomas required as much as 50 per cent autologous serum to be added to Eagle's medium before even limited growth could be promoted *in vitro*. Flaxman (1972) found that non-keratinizing basal cell cancers excised from patients could be made to synthesize keratin, and to show some degree of contact inhibition, when held on a clot of chick plasma and embryo extract immersed in Eagle's minimal essential medium containing 10 per cent fetal calf serum and antibodies. He concluded that the *in vivo* environment—rather than a permanent genetic change—is responsible for the suspension of keratinization in cancer cells.

Heredity and studies of cancer in twins

According to theory, the true value of S, the proportion of the population prediposed to a specific cancer, is determined by genetic factors. Generally, values of S calculated from onset or mortality statistics are very substantially less than unity. It follows that, in twins studies, the average age-corrected concordance of such a cancer in monozygotic twins should generally be higher than that in dizygotic twins. (In view of the frequent differences in the genetic predisposition between the sexes, it will often be necessary to compare monozygotic twin pairs of a given sex with dizygotic twin pairs of the same sex.)

The significance of the ratio of the average concordance in monozygotic twins to that in dizygotic twins appears to be so widely misunderstood that a brief outline of the problem will be given here.

Suppose predisposition to an age-dependent disease involves an autosomal dominant gene of low frequency. For simplicity, suppose the disease is a chronic one with no associated mortality and that the duration of the latent period between initiation and onset is very short. Suppose the age-specific prevalence of the disease in the general population (both sexes) is given by: $P_t = S\{1 - \exp(-kt^r)\}$. Suppose we examine all twins in the population and determine the prevalence of the disease at age t_1 years. The average concordance of the disease among predisposed monozygotic twin pairs will be the probability that both have developed the disease at age t_1, that is, $\{1 - \exp(-kt_1^r)\}^2$, while that among dizygotic twin pairs, at least one member of which is predisposed, will be $0 \cdot 5\{1 - \exp(-kt_1^r)\}^2$. (The average penetrance, which is equal to P_{t_1}/S, will in this example be the same for all groups of predisposed persons. If one twin of a monozygotic pair is predisposed, we assume the co-twin will also be predisposed. If one twin of a dizygotic pair is predisposed then, for a low-frequency autosomal gene, we assume that the chance of the co-twin being predisposed is $0 \cdot 5$.) Hence, in this simple example, the ratio of concordance at age t_1 in monozygotic twins, to that in dizygotic twins, will be two.

If the frequency of the predisposing autosomal dominant gene is not low, the ratio will be less than 2. In the limiting case, when the frequency of the predisposing gene is unity, the ratio of concordances will also be unity.

It is sometimes supposed that the importance of genetic factors is related to the *magnitude* of this ratio of concordances. The larger the ratio, it is said, the more important the role of inheritance. However, in this very simple, but not unrealistic example, in which a disease will arise *only* in genetically predisposed individuals, we find that the ratio of age-corrected concordances (monozygotic/dizygotic) will lie between 1 and 2, depending on the frequency of the predisposing autosomal dominant gene. It is easily shown that if predisposition involves autosomal recessive inheritance, then for an allele of low frequency, the ratio of concordances (monozygotic/dizygotic) will be 4. For polygenic predisposition, involving alleles of low frequency, large ratios can readily arise. Hence the magnitude of the concordance ratio depends on the mode of inheritance: low values (between 1 and 2) can be fully consistent with the hypothesis of an *essential* role for predisposing genes.

From this elementary analysis, and the complexities of inheritance revealed throughout the chapter, we can begin to appreciate the numerous pitfalls that await the investigator of cancer in twins. The following complications require special emphasis.

(1) Meaningful concordance ratios for a cancer can only be obtained if we compare like with like. Even when errors of diagnosis and selection can be reduced to a minimum, we often find genetic heterogeneity within a given ICD site category. Thus malignant neoplasms of the stomach (ICD 151) are genetically heterogeneous in women (and probably in Japanese men), consisting of at least two distinctive groups. Both female genotypes differ from the (main) predisposing genotypes in males. When two or more genotypes predispose to cancer at the same site, seriously misleading concordance ratios might result if a positive or negative association exists between one genotype, and one or more of the others.

(2) In all circumstances, including that of homogeneous inheritance—see below—the importance of correcting concordances to a standard age cannot be overemphasized. With the typically steep age-dependence of cancers, penetrance changes rapidly with age. For example, when the penetrance P_t/S is proportional to t^6, then at $t = 60$ years, P_t is three times higher than at $t = 50$ years.

The term 'homogeneous' in the above context needs clarification. The age-distributions of, for example, cancer of the pancreas and cancer of the bladder suggest that in the great majority of cases (and possibly all) the mechanism of initiation is homogeneous. It still does not follow that all individuals affected by the same type of cancer will have identical predisposing genes. The precise location of potential target cells within, say, the bladder epithelium, will be determined by genetic factors, which, in general, will differ from person to person. However, the genes determining the 'microsite' may not be essential to cancer predisposition as such. Different combinations of alleles at loci determining the 'microsite' will alter the anatomical location of potential target cells. Here, the term 'homogeneity' is intended to apply to those genes that are *essential* to the specific cancer diathesis. If, however, at the 'essential' *a* locus, homozygous alleles a_1/a_1 contribute to one predisposing genotype, and a_2/a_2 contribute to another, while the heterozygote a_1/a_2 is *not* predisposed, then the genotype involving a_1/a_1 and the one involving a_2/a_2 would, of course, be classed as heterogeneous.

The large study of twins by Harvald and Hauge (1963) needs to be reviewed in the light of the above analysis. These authors attempted to trace all twins born in Denmark between 1870 and 1910 and to record all cases of cancer occurring in the series from 1921 onwards. Deaths occurring before 1921 were ignored. They estimated that about 15 000 pairs of twins should have survived five years of age: some 6893 pairs were actually traced and hence the risk of bias is substantial. I quote their conclusions in full:

> The finding that the rate of concordance of cancer in general does not differ significantly between monozygous and dizygous twins implies that the diversity in the population with regard to the development of cancer in general is not to any significant extent determined by genes. Concordance as to site is obviously exceptional. The observed specific concordance rates, 8/164 in monozygous twins and 9/340 in dizygous same-sexed twins, justify the conclusion that the genetic influence, also with respect to tumour localization, is negligible compared to the effect of other factors constituting the aetiology of malignant growths, even if larger materials would show a statistically significant difference. As far as comparison with the vital statistics in Denmark is possible, no discrepancies have been found between the general population and the present twin material with regard to the relative cancer mortality.

My discussion has shown the formidable difficulty of drawing reliable conclusions from studies of the concordance of *genetically homogeneous* cancers in twins; when all cancers are considered, difficulties are compounded. Negative associations between cancers at different sites are commonplace. Concordances for negatively associated cancers will be more frequent in dizygotic than in monozygotic twin pairs. Harvald and Hauge's (1963) findings for the concordance of cancer in general show that the same gene, or genes, do not predispose to all cancers; many other considerations also testify to this conclusion. Their findings for site-concordance relate to less heterogeneous (but still far from homogeneous) categories. Site-concordances in monozygotic twins were reported for carcinoma of the stomach (one pair), carcinoma of the intestine (one pair), and carcinoma of the breast (two pairs). Site concordances in like-sexed dizygotic twins were recorded for carcinoma of the stomach (one possible pair—diagnosis in one twin not verified histologically), carcinoma of the intestine (one pair), and carcinoma of the breast (two pairs).

From their age-dependence, we have seen that cancers at all these sites probably involve genetic heterogeneity, and, quite apart from the limitations of small numbers and the problems of penetrance, the meaning of the nominally higher site concordance in monozygotic over that in dizygotic twins, cannot be interpreted in terms of a specific scheme of inheritance. As I showed at the beginning of this section, a concordance ratio (monozygotic/dizygotic) of between 1 and 2 can be consistent with the hypothesis that an autosomal dominant gene plays an essential predisposing role. Future studies of cancer in twins should concentrate, as far as possible on those specific malignancies that might be presumed to be genetically homogeneous. Sometimes, age at onset can be used to effect a partial separation between genetically distinctive, early- and late-onset groups. But to correct for inter-current mortality and the dependence of penetrance on age, and to obtain adequate numbers, very large and sophisticated surveys will be needed.

The direct investigation of antigenic determinants on MCPs and TCFs in non-twins might eventually contribute more to the understanding of the genetics of cancers than large-scale epidemiological studies. Those numerous studies already carried out that show associations between major histo-compatibility antigens on the one hand, and malignant and non-malignant diseases on the other, illustrate the potential power of this type of investigation. However, the major histocompatibility antigens represent the lowest level of specificity in the hierarchical structure of MCPs and TCFs. When investigations of minor histocompatibility antigens, and tissue-specific antigens become possible, they should prove even more rewarding.

Ideally, the evidence described and analysed in this chapter should be used to test other theories of carcinogenesis. I am unaware of any other theories, apart from those mentioned in Chapter 6, that are sufficiently detailed to lend themselves to this kind of test. Unfortunately, the earlier theories described in Chapter 6 were not intended to interpret age-dependencies that depart at high t from a simple power law of the form : $dP/dt \propto t^r$. Hirsch's (1974) generalization of Curtis's (1967, 1969) theory leads, with certain assumptions, to the same mathematical formulation as mine, but it fails to explain the multicentric origin of many tumours and the constancy of k during the growth phase.

CHAPTER 8

Infectious Diseases and Oncogenic Viruses

Many oncologists, especially among those on the Western side of the Atlantic, believe that viruses are the *essential* cause of cancers (Huebner, 1961). It has not yet been established, however, that a virus is causally related to any malignancy in man. The high degree of reproducibility of the age-patterns of cancers in different populations (see Chapter 7) renders it highly improbable that infective agents can contribute to the *initiation* phase of carcinogenesis. But this by no means eliminates other hypotheses of viral involvement as this chapter will demonstrate.

Faith in oncogenic viruses stems partly from the enormous success of the microbial theory of disease and partly from the prospects for prophylaxis that effective immunization would bring. In its simplest form, the microbial theory states that infectious disease is caused primarily by the transmission of a micro-organism from one host to another. Although this simple idea of unrestricted host-to-host transmission has been discarded in Gross's (1951, 1970, 1974) theory of 'vertical' transmission (from one generation to the next), and in the latest theories of 'oncogenes' (Huebner and Todaro, 1969), and 'protoviruses' (Temin, 1971, 1972), no other concept has had such profound influence on twentieth-century medicine.

In my view, Sir Macfarlane Burnet's concept of 'forbidden clones' rates as the most profound *intellectual* contribution to the understanding of disease, although few, I suspect—including Burnet—would share that assessment. Indeed, many avoid the idea altogether and some are baffled by it. Forbidden clones, with their origins in *random* and seemingly non-preventable somatic mutations, offend against the prevailing ethos of environmental determinism. The empirically minded prefer to 'see' the causal agent—if not with the unaided eye then with the optical or electron microscope. Still more important, optimistic environmentalists hope to *control* the causal agent. The microbial theory, boosted by spectacular success, belongs to the *zeitgeist*. If medical research were rationally planned (heaven forbid!) our main prophylactic efforts would be devoted to the eradication of those obviously infectious diseases that still plague us. I venture to predict that many years will elapse before we gain effective control (if ever we do) of non-infectious malignant and degenerative diseases.

Whatever relevance the microbial theory may have to oncology—and I agree with Stewart (1968) who describes the theory as a 'gross oversimplification'—no book on the biology of cancer can afford to ignore totally the current preoccupation with oncogenic viruses. Bearing in mind the previous chapter, the sex- and age-dependence of recognized infectious diseases assume special importance.

Age-dependence of Acute Infectious Diseases

As with non-malignant non-infectious diseases, the age-dependence of infectious diseases has aroused almost no theoretical interest. We are, perhaps, so familiar with the characteristic impact of acute infectious diseases in infancy and childhood that we feel it requires no explanation. We may incline to the view that the age of contracting an infectious disease depends only on the chance of being infected. Special circumstances apart, we would expect the chance of being infected through host-to-host transmission to be more or less independent of age.

I have previously shown that, in non-immunized populations, the age-patterns of poliomyelitis, mumps, and early- and late-onset infectious hepatitis, all conform to the simple stochastic model described in Chapter 6 and illustrated in Chapter 7 (Burch, 1968(a)). Further examples of the age-patterns of infectious diseases are shown in Figures 8.1 to 8.10. In every instance the latent period between initiation and onset appears to be very short—much less than one year. (Because of the uncertainty regarding the age at which $t = 0$, the exact duration of the latent period between the end of initiation and the onset of disease cannot be estimated from mathematical analysis of age-patterns.)

Unfortunately, suitably detailed statistics for analysis are scarce. From Figures 8.1, 8.2 and 8.4 to 8.10, we see that age-patterns often contain considerable structure during the early years of life. In the examples of German measles and whooping cough it would be helpful to have statistics for onset by each month of age over the first year of life. Since 1969, the Registrar-General has published notifications for whooping cough by

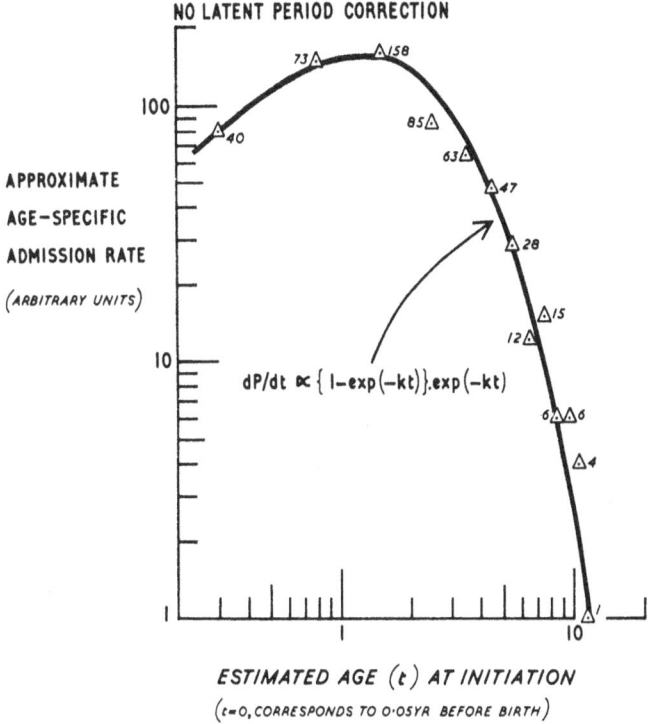

NO LATENT PERIOD CORRECTION

APPROXIMATE

AGE-SPECIFIC

ADMISSION RATE

(*ARBITRARY UNITS*)

$$dP/dt \propto \{ 1-\exp(-kt) \}.\exp(-kt)$$

ESTIMATED AGE (*t*) AT INITIATION

(*t=0, CORRESPONDS TO 0·05YR BEFORE BIRTH*)

Figure 8.1 Relative age-specific admission rate, sexes combined, for cases of acute respiratory disease associated with para-influenza viruses, Port of Spain General Hospital, October–December 1967, as a function of estimated initiation age (Bisno *et al.*, 1970). Assuming no latent period correction, the zero of the age scale is deduced to be about 0·05 years before birth: the theoretical curve has the parameters $n=2$, $r=1$

three-month intervals for the first year of life, but for higher ages the intervals are too crude for precise analysis (Figures 8.9 and 8.10). In spite of these limitations, Figures 8.6 to 8.10 enable some interesting comparisons to be made.

The statistics of Collins, Wheeler and Shannon (1942) for cases of whooping cough in 28 large US cities, 1935–36, show two clearcut groups below ten years of age (Figure 8.6). Although the number of points is insufficient to define reliably the early-onset group (tentatively represented by $n=1$, $r=2$, $k \simeq 0.76$ year^{-2}), the main group, with a mode at about four years, is well defined by $n=1$, $r=2$, $k \simeq 3.2 \times 10^{-2}$ year^{-2}. Statistics for England and Wales, 1944 and 1945, are shown in Figure 8.7 and for 1946 and 1950 in Figure 8.8. These cover a period before the general introduction of anti-pertussis vaccine. With only one available point, the early-onset group cannot be defined in Figures 8.7 and 8.8, but the main group (mode at

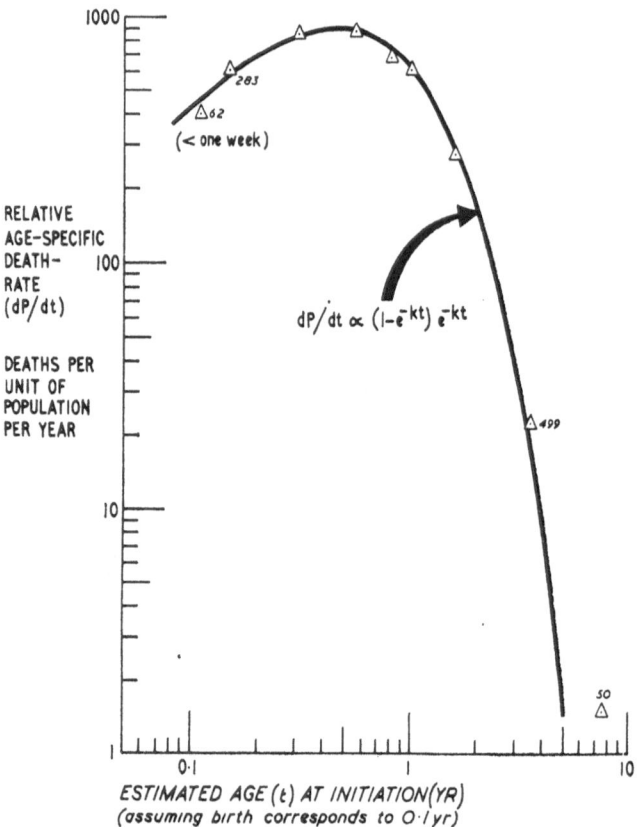

Figure 8.2 Relative age-specific death rate, sexes combined, from gastro-enteritis in Bantu children, 1955–66, as a function of estimated initiation age (Spencer and Coster, 1969). Assuming no latent period correction, the zero of the age scale is deduced to be about 0·1 year before birth: the theoretical curve has the parameters $n=2$, $r=1$

four years) has the same pattern as in the US data and remains virtually invariant in shape ($n=1$, $r=2$) and modal age (constant $k=3\cdot2\times10^{-2}$ year^{-2}), despite large changes in the level of infection from year to year. (In 1950, the mode at four years was 2·3 times higher than in 1945.) The single point for the first year of life suffices to show that the relative levels of the early- and main-onset groups changed little over the years 1944, 1945, 1946 and 1950.

Data graphed in Figures 8.9 and 8.10 for the years 1969 and 1971 relate to the period after the general introduction of antipertussis vaccine. Incidence levels are very much lower—by up to a factor of about 40 at $t=$ four years— than those for the pre-vaccine era illustrated in Figures 8.7 and 8.8. (But note

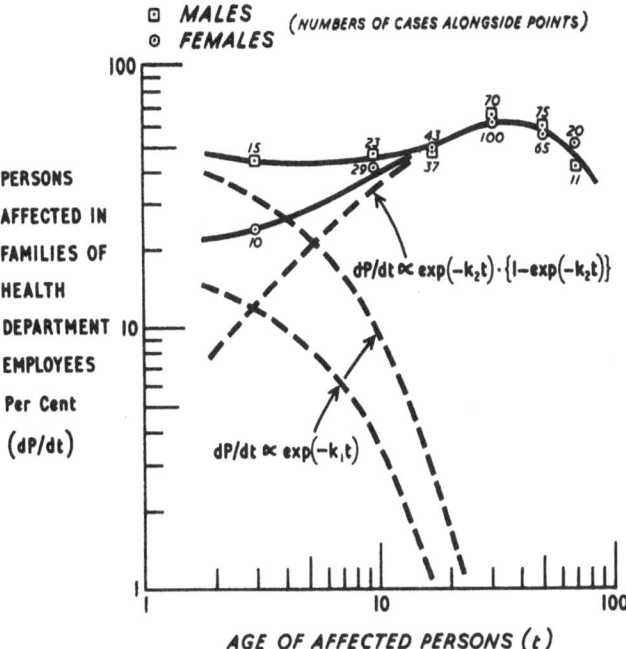

Figure 8.3 Relative age-specific and sex-specific frequency of clinical infection among families of Health Department employees (per cent) with Hong Kong influenza, Milwaukee, winter 1968–69, as a function of age (Piraino, Brown and Krumbiegel, 1970). Two genetically distinctive groups of affected persons can be discerned. The (poorly-defined) early-onset group, males predominating, is described by the curve with parameters $n = 1$, $r = 1$; the late-onset group, with a sex ratio of approximately unity, is described by the curve with parameters, $n = 2$, $r = 1$; no latent period correction is applied

a disturbing increase in the level of notification—a factor of three at $t = $ four years—from 1969 to 1971.) Despite these vastly lower levels and the widespread use of a fairly effective vaccine, we see that the shape of the age-pattern for the main group remains almost unaltered. (Curiously, the modal age for 1971 appears to be slightly raised, by about 0·4 years, over all other years. This might result from a declining proportion of effectively vaccine-immunized children with increasing age, above $t \simeq $ three years.)

The most interesting comparison concerns the age-pattern during the first year of life. In Figures 8.9 and 8.10, I have fitted the points at $t = 0·875$ years and 1·5 years to the curve: $n = 1$, $r = 2$, $k \simeq 0·91$ years, which is similar to the corresponding curve for the 1935–36 US data in Figure 8.6. We see that below $t = 0·8$ years, notifications lie well above the theoretical curve and more conspicuously in 1971 than in 1969. This is a consequence of the

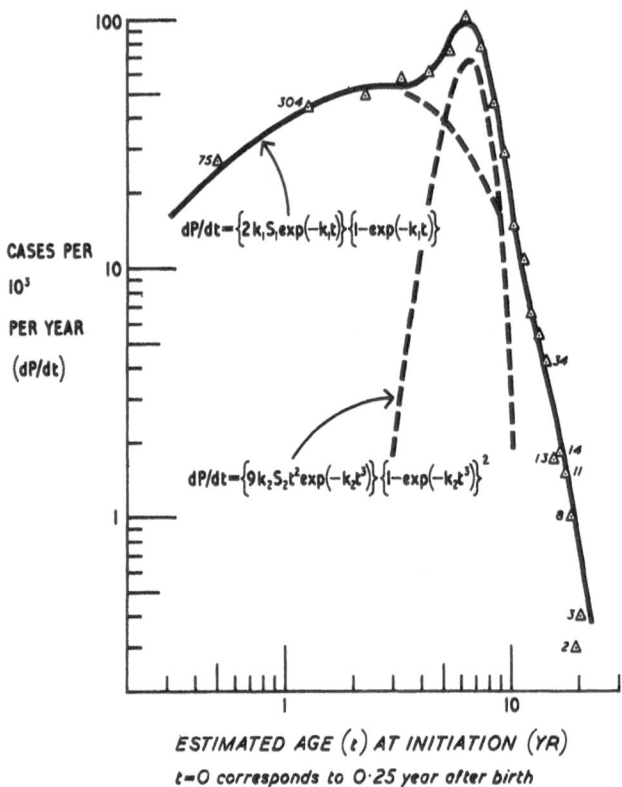

CASES PER
10^5
PER YEAR
(dP/dt)

$$dP/dt = \left\{2k_1S_1\exp(-k_1t)\right\}\left\{1-\exp(-k_1t)\right\}$$

$$dP/dt = \left\{9k_2S_2t^2\exp(-k_2t^3)\right\}\left\{1-\exp(-k_2t^3)\right\}^2$$

ESTIMATED AGE (t) AT INITIATION (YR)

$t=0$ corresponds to 0·25 year after birth

Figure 8.4 Age-specific onset rate, sexes combined, for cases of chickenpox in 28 large US cities, 1935–36, as a function of estimated age at initiation (Collins, Wheeler and Shannon, 1942). Assuming no latent period correction, the zero of the initiation age scale is deduced to be about 0·25 years after birth. The curve for the predominantly early onset group is described by the parameters $n=2$, $r=1$; the curve with mode at 6 to 7 years is described by $n=3$, $r=3$

age at which vaccination was carried out: six months to ten months. Nevertheless, although babies less than six months of age receive no direct protection, levels of whooping cough have been greatly reduced in this age-range relative to those seen prior to the use of vaccines (compare Figures 8.7 and 8.8 with 8.9 and 8.10). This suggests that transmission of the pertussis and parapertussis bacteria has diminished because of immunization in the higher age-groups.

I have not calculated the values of S that are implicit in the data graphed in Figures 8.1 to 8.10 for reasons that will become apparent. It may be helpful at this juncture to consider the overall interpretation that these age-patterns of acute infectious, self-terminating, diseases dictate.

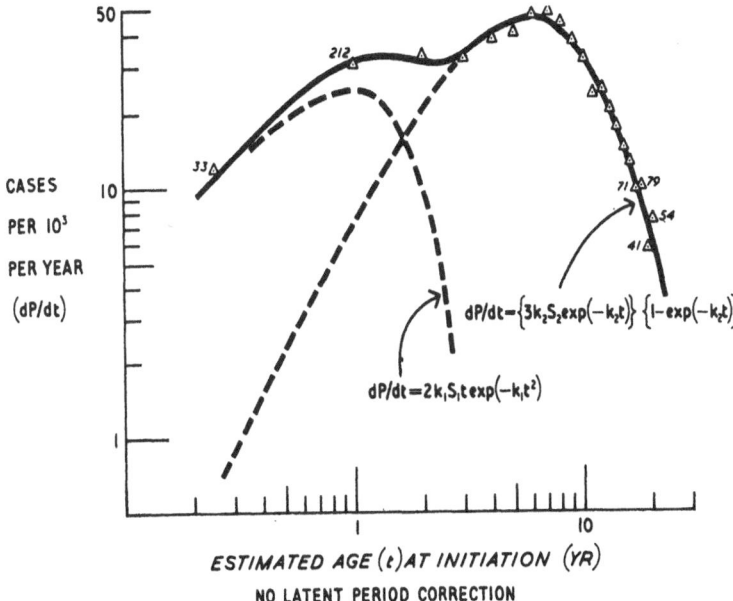

Figure 8.5 Age-specific onset rate, sexes combined, for cases of German measles in 28 large US cities, 1935–36, as a function of estimated age at initiation (Collins *et al.*, 1942). Assuming no latent period correction, $t=0$ corresponds to birth. The early-onset group is described by the curve with parameters, $n=1$, $r=2$; and the late-onset group by the curve with parameters $n=3$, $r=1$

Implications of age-patterns of acute infectious diseases

We should, perhaps, start from scratch and ask the question: Are the random events that initiate age-dependent disease not somatic mutations at all, but infective episodes? The following features dispose of any such suggestion.

(1) The shapes and modal age of the age-patterns for a defined disease such as whooping cough, when these are not distorted by artificial immunization procedures or other artefacts, remain effectively invariant from country to country, and from year to year, even when the level of infection changes by more than an order of magnitude.

(2) Generally, no two infectious diseases have the same age-patterns, as defined by the values of n, r and k; we would expect host-to-host transmission to show similar characteristics for similar micro-organisms.

(3) The average rate of the implied initiating events is effectively independent both of age and calendar time; the rate of infection, however, can vary widely from season to season and from year to year.

(4) The conformity of some age-patterns to Yule statistics ($n>1$, $r=1$) would be compatible with the idea that n independent random infective

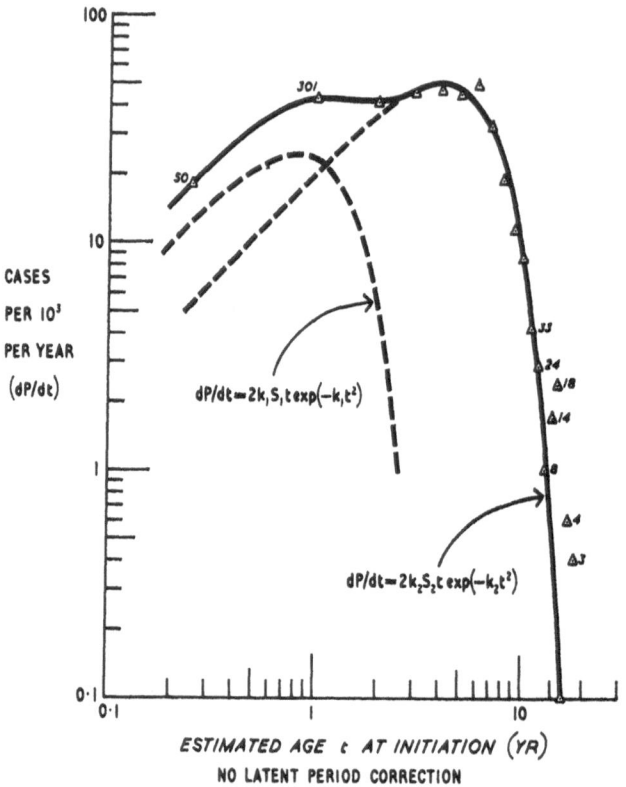

Figure 8.6 Age-specific onset rate, sexes combined, for cases of whooping cough in 28 large US cities, 1935–36, as a function of estimated age at initiation (Collins *et al.* 1942). Assuming no latent period correction, $t=0$ corresponds to birth. The age-distributions in both early and late onset groups are represented by the equation with $n=1$, $r=2$, but $k_1 \simeq 0.76$ year^{-2} and $k_2 \simeq 3.2 \times 10^{-2}$ year^{-2}

episodes initiate disease; however, the requirement that the average rate of such random episodes is independent of age and secular time—point (3)—cannot be reconciled with observation.

(5) In attempting to use the infective episode hypothesis to explain the conformity of some age-patterns to Weibull statistics ($n=1$, $r>1$), we would have to cope not only with the (insurmountable) difficulties of (4), but with the additional requirement for 'dependency', such as the random infection by multiple (r) agents, of one single cell, out of many at risk.

Features (1) to (5) force us to conclude that the age-patterns of acute infectious diseases, and the kinetics of the random initiating events, are largely or wholly determined *not by the infective agent, but by the host*. That is to say, the onset of an acute infectious disease such as whooping cough

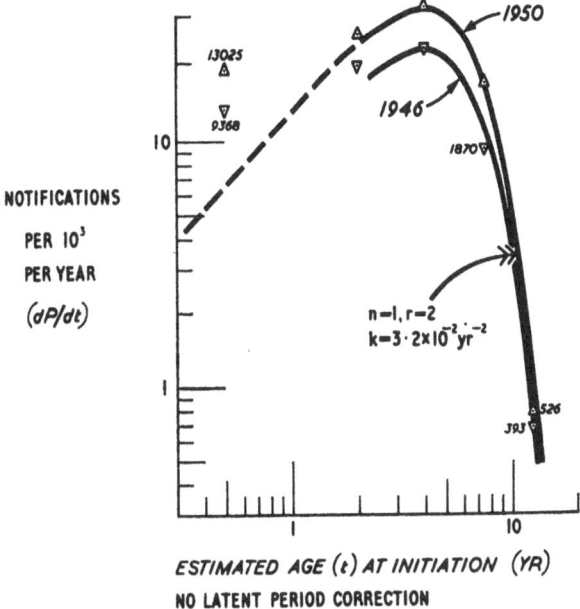

Figure 8.7 Registrar-General's statistics for age-specific notifications of whooping cough, sexes combined, England and Wales, 1944 (triangles) and 1945 (inverted triangles), in relation to estimated age at initiation. Compare with Figure 8.6. The value of k for the late onset group is approximately $3 \cdot 2 \times 10^{-2}$ year^{-2} in both countries

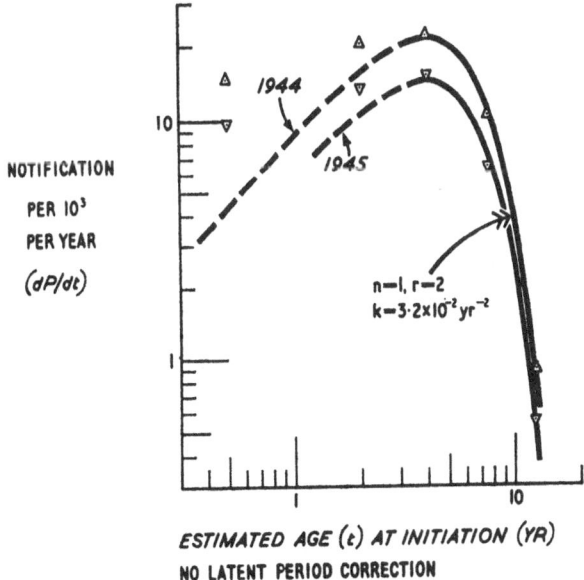

Figure 8.8 As for Figure 8.7. Data for 1950 (triangles) and for 1946 (inverted triangles)

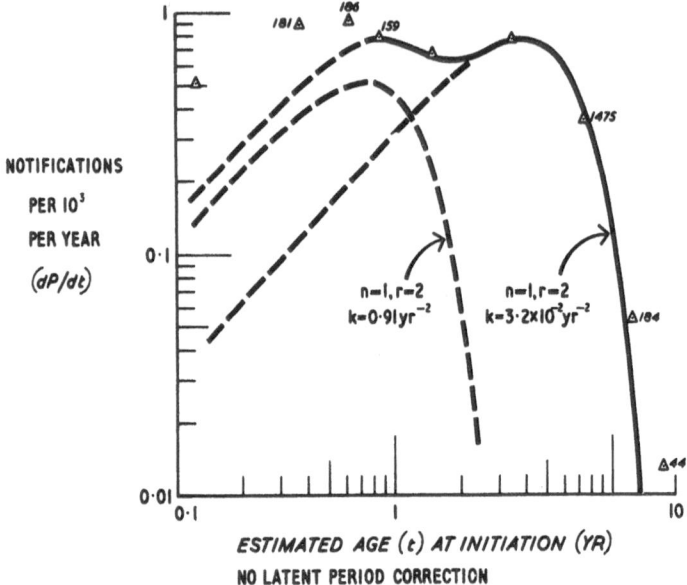

Figure 8.9 As for Figure 8.7. Data for 1969—see text, page 249

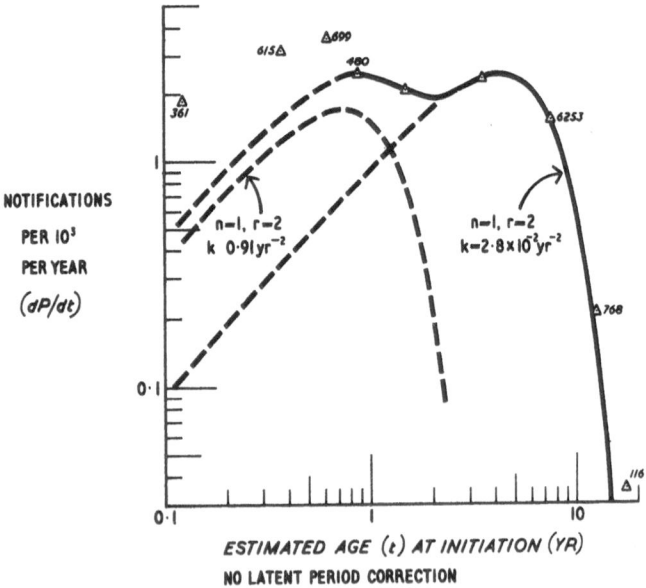

Figure 8.10 As for Figure 8.7. Data for 1971—see text, page 249

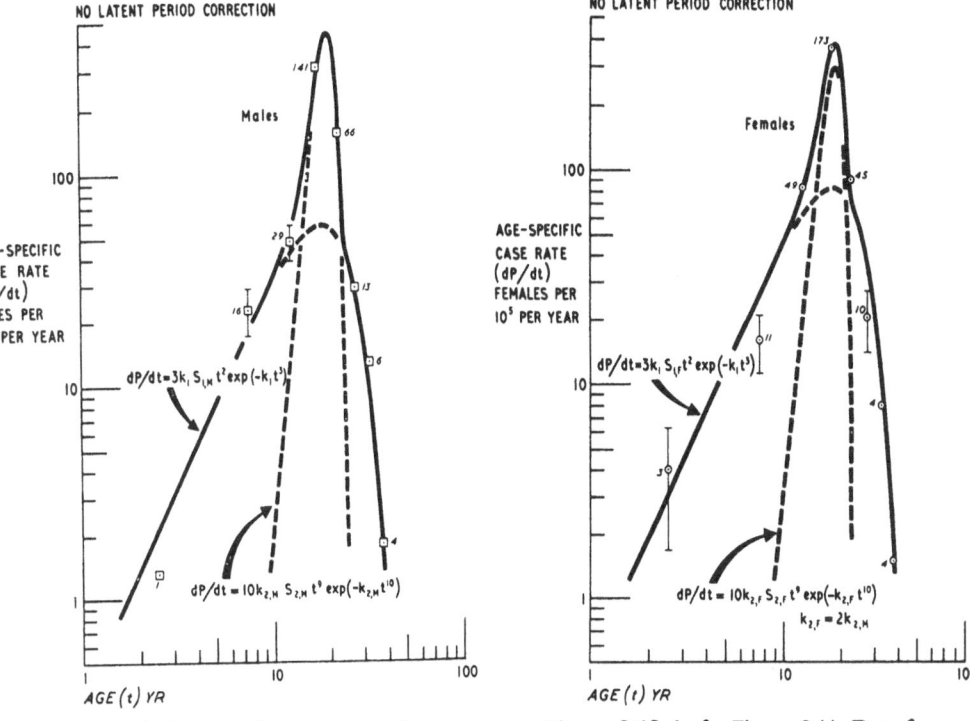

Figure 8.11 Age-specific onset rate for male cases of infectious mononucleosis, metropolitan Atlanta, 1968, in relation to estimated age at initiation (Heath, Brodsky and Potolsky, 1972). For the broad distribution, $n=1$, $r=3$, $k_1 \simeq 1\cdot1 \times 10^{-4}$, year^{-3}, $S_{1,M} = 1\cdot0 \times 10^{-2}$; for the narrow distribution, $n=1$, $r=10$, $k_2 \simeq 1\cdot0 \times 10^{-14}$ year^{-10}, and $S_{2,M} = 2\cdot2 \times 10^{-2}$

Figure 8.12 As for Figure 8.11. Data for females: for the broad distribution, $n=1$, $r=3$, $k_1 \simeq 1\cdot1 \times 10^{-4}$ year, $S_{1,F} = 1\cdot5 \times 10^{-2}$; for the narrow distribution, $n=1$, $r=10$, $k_{2,F} = 2k_{2,M} = 2\cdot0 \times 10^{-14}$ year^{-10} and $S_{2,F} = 1\cdot5 \times 10^{-2}$

requires two factors: (a) an *extrinsic* contribution—the presence in the non-immunized host of the infective microorganism; and (b) an *intrinsic* contribution—the simultaneous presence in the non-immunized, genetically predisposed host, of a recently initiated specific mutant growth-control stem cell (Burch 1968(a)). Surprisingly, the main rate-determining factor with respect to age is (b), rather than (a), although the *level* of an epidemic will depend on, first, the proportion of susceptibles in the population and, second, the proportion of those susceptibles that become infected.

Basis of natural immunity

In the absence of the infective agent, the endogenous defence mechanism prevents the mutant growth-control stem cell from propagating a pathogenically effective forbidden clone. Moreover, because the kinetics (as defined by k) remain constant from year to year, it follows (for $n = 1$, $r > 1$) that only 'first' forbidden clones produce disease in the infected host. In other words, if a 'first' forbidden clone arises in the absence of the precipitating infective agent, the host becomes immunized by his own mutant clonal cells against further identical forbidden clones that might arise in the presence of the infective agent. This new interpretation differs from the conventional view which holds that natural immunity arises from a subclinical infection.

In the absence of the appropriately mutant growth-control stem cell, the infective agent merely elicits an immune response and establishes (usually temporarily) the *carrier state* in which the micro-organism is present in the host, although the characteristic signs and symptoms of the associated disease are absent. Such an infection, in the absence of the pathogenic forbidden clone, fails to produce long-term natural immunity in the host.

When the age-distribution of an acute infectious disease conforms closely with the differentiated versions of the stochastic equations described in Chapter 6, we can infer that the risk of infection is virtually independent of age. When the risk of infection (for example, venereal) depends on age, then departures from the simple stochastic model must be anticipated. Figures 8.9 and 8.10 show, not surprisingly, that the risk of whooping cough depends on the age of vaccination and that prior to vaccination the risk is enhanced. This enhanced risk will depend on the extent of immunity among other members of the population.

It is especially important to observe that the age-distribution of onset of the acute infectious diseases conforms to the differentiated (dP/dt) rather than the prevalence (P_t) versions of the standard stochastic equations. This implies, as argued above, that if a potentially pathogenic forbidden clone is initiated in the absence of the infectious agent it fails to produce disease when the host is subsequently infected. On the contrary, it produces relative and, perhaps, permanent long-term immunity. However, *natural infection before the initiation of a potentially pathogenic forbidden clone seldom, if ever, establishes long-term natural immunity*. Fortunately, appropriate vaccines can confer a high degree of immunity. Presumably the high intensity of the antigenic challenge stimulates an adequate immune response. When a person suffers a second clinical attack of an acute infectious disease, years after a first attack, he might be genetically predisposed to both early- and late-onset forms of the disease. Alternatively, if only one genetically predisposed group is at risk, then we would need to postulate that the first disease episode fails to confer permanent immunity.

In the case of recurrent infectious diseases such as the common cold, and allergic diseases such as hay fever, we must presume that the forbidden clone, or clones, fail to produce immunity. A new infection, or a seasonal allergen, reactivates a pre-existing forbidden clone or clones by competing for limited defence resources.

Infectious Disease as Precipitated Autoaggressive Disease

To summarize: within my unified theory an acute infectious disease is a particular form of autoaggressive disease in which the *primary* and *essential* role of the invading micro-organism—but not necessarily the only one—is the successful monopolization of those defence resources that otherwise would be efficiently directed against specific mutant growth-control cells. One or more antigenic determinants of the micro-organism compete with one or more antigens of the specific mutant growth-control cells for the same immunoglobulin antibodies. This accounts for the specificity of the acute infectious diseases including the anatomical specificity of the lesions. The theory also defines the nature of the genetic predisposition to infectious disease, which is essentially similar to that for other non-infectious auto-aggressive diseases.

It follows that, if the concentration of specific defence antibodies can be raised adequately prior to an infection, then the host should be able to cope both with the extrinsic infective agent and the intrinsic mutant growth-control stem cell. In other words, and as we know already, suitable passive or active immunization will prevent, or greatly diminish, the incidence of an infectious disease.

Where the age-distribution for a disease obeys Yule $(n > 1, r = 1)$, or combined Yule–Weibull $(n > 1, r > 1)$ statistics, we can infer that defence antibodies fail to *eliminate* the $(n - 1)$ specifically mutant growth-control stem cells that contribute forbidden clones—together with the final $(n$th$)$ mutant stem cell—to cause the development of disease in the infected person. In some way, the $(n - 1)$ forbidden clones fail to produce detectable disease, either because the cooperative action of n forbidden clones is biologically essential, or because the defence mechanism curbs the proliferation of $(n - 1)$ clones. However, if the nth forbidden clone arises in the absence of the precipitating micro-organism, then long-term immunity is induced.

Another theoretical consequence calls for special mention here. If malignant and infectious diseases are both forms of autoaggressive disease, then in principle, there would seem to be no reason why some malignant diseases should not be infectious. Although this expectation is clearly realized for certain malignancies in experimental animals it is surprising and puzzling why the same is not obviously true of man. Burkitt's lymphoma, for example, may prove to be precipitated by an oncogenic virus but the evidence available so far (see Chapter 7) is not wholly propitious. Burkitt himself has abandoned the idea of a simple viral aetiology and believes that chronic malaria *and* an oncogenic virus are together implicated in the pathogenesis of the disease (Burkitt, 1969; Kafuko and Burkitt, 1970).

Problems of Establishing a Viral Aetiology

How might we establish that a host-to-host (non-vertical) transmitted virus is essential to the pathogenesis of a cancer in man? Before attempting to answer this question we need to consider a critique of the germ theory of disease. In a devastating attack on conventional germ theory, Stewart (1968) criticized each of Koch's four postulates. I shall illustrate and amplify his arguments.

Koch's postulates

(1) *A given pathogenic germ is invariably associated with a given disease.*

At the outset, we need to bear in mind that not all influenza viruses, for example, are identical. Furthermore, a disease that is broadly described as 'influenza' or 'poliomyelitis' etc., may affect more than one distinctive genotype and the clinical features of the disease may well differ in detail from genotype to genotype. When more than one genotype is at risk, the relative proportions of affected genotypes might differ from one epidemic to another, and from one population to another. Hence, the overall age-patterns (but, in the absence of complications, not the shapes of the separate components) might differ from epidemic to epidemic. In principle, an antigenic determinant on a micro-organism might cross-react with antigens on more than one type of forbidden clone. The same micro-organism could then cause different diseases. Koch's first postulate will be valid only when we can demonstrate the homogeneity, both of the susceptible host genotype and of the invading micro-organism. The definition of 'a given disease' is far from clear; it raises fundamental and unsettled nosological issues.

Stewart reminds us that a given pathogenic germ does not invariably produce the 'associated disease'; the poliovirus, or other enteroviruses, pneumococci, or streptococci etc., can be present in a host without any signs of the 'associated disease' being apparent. Heston *et al.* (1970) found that only 39 per cent of strain A female mice exhibiting the mammary tumour virus antigen at the second lactation developed mammary tumours. Lautrop (1971) calculated that only about 3·3 per cent of children infected with *Bordetella parapertussis* in Denmark developed clinically typical whooping cough. This widespread phenomenon of the *carrier state*, which is not acknowledged in Koch's postulates, forms an essential part of my theory; the appropriate newly initiated forbidden clone has also to be present in the non-immunized person if symptoms and signs of acute infectious disease are to manifest.

(2) *It must be possible to isolate the pathogenic germ in pure culture from the characteristic lesions of the disease.*

Stewart points out that this postulate will necessarily be valid if the disease is defined exclusively in terms of the anticipated isolate, as for example, for gonorrhoea, anthrax and tuberculosis. However, in the case of pneumonia, the isolate might be a pneumoccocus, mycoplasma or any one of several viruses. Furthermore, the prevalence of any one of these micro-organisms in the carrier state might be far greater than the prevalence of morbidity.

In terms of my theory, the proliferation of a given forbidden clone might well be precipitated by a variety of micro-organisms. The essential requirement is that the infective agent shall compete effectively for one or more specific defence antibodies. This does not necessarily entail that the different micro-organisms should bear the same, or cross-reacting, antigens because when several somatic mutations are needed to initiate a forbidden clone, the mutant MCPs synthesized by that clone might well display several distinctive 'not-self' antigens.

If the 'characteristic lesion' of a cancer is taken to be the malignant growth itself, then according to my theory, there is no necessity to demonstrate the existence of the putative oncogenic virus in the cells of the cancer. Failure to demonstrate the virus in tumour tissue could still be consistent with the hypothesis that the virus allowed the initiating forbidden clone to proliferate. The mutant MCPs of the forbidden clone might well transform cells in the target tissue without any direct help from the infective agent. In any case, an interval of several years can elapse between the initiation of a forbidden clone and diagnosis of the associated cancer. If, in contrast to the acute infectious non-malignant diseases, a forbidden clone can continue active once the precipitating virus has been eliminated, or alternatively, if a cancer can acquire autonomy and grow in the absence of the promoting forbidden clone, then, by the time cancer has been diagnosed, the virus might have disappeared from the host.

(3) *The pathogenic germ should reproduce the disease when inoculated into animals.*

For certain germs and a few species this postulate holds. But as Stewart remarks, for the majority of micro-organisms, including most viruses, this postulate simply cannot be fulfilled even when massive inocula are used. According to my theory, this postulate will hold only when a substantial

degree of cross-reactivity obtains between one or more of the antigens of a
mutant MCP of one species, and one or more of the antigens of a corresponding mutant MCP of another species. Although on evolutionary and
functional considerations we must expect *similarity* between corresponding
MCPs—normal and mutant—of different mammalian species, we must also
expect significant differences. Such differences lie at the very basis of
speciation. Hence, the inability to satisfy Koch's third postulate does not
constitute a valid reason for rejecting the hypothesis that a specific micro-
organism is essential to the development of a particular disease, in a given
species.

(4) *The pathogenic germ should be isolated in pure culture from the experimental
lesion.*

Stewart observes that this postulate is merely a corollary of (2) and (3)
and not an independent requirement. When (2) and (3) fail, so must (4).

From the above arguments I conclude that the onset of a cancer could well
be precipitated by an oncogenic virus despite an inability to fulfill Koch's
postulates. Bryan (1962) has stressed the extreme difficulty of satisfying even
the first of Koch's postulates where tumorigenic viruses are concerned.
Rowe (1965) has concluded that, in testing hypotheses of viral aetiology,
we are not bound by Koch's postulates. A revision of these postulates would
appear to be overdue.

Epidemiology and the quest for oncogenic viruses

In Chapter 7 we saw that the age-patterns of many malignant diseases
conform to certain simple stochastic rules. Where diagnosis is reliable I
have not yet discovered a clearcut exception. Such evidence supports the
hypothesis that in large general populations most, if not all, cases of malignant
disease entail an autoaggressive mechanism. But it does not answer the
question: Is a host-to-host transmitted oncogenic virus necessary to one or
more of the several phases of malignant development?

If we were to find that the onset of a specific malignancy exhibited large
seasonal and/or annual fluctuations, then we would be able to conclude,
with some confidence, that onset is precipitated by some form of 'antigenic
agent' with large seasonal and/or annual fluctuations of epidemicity. We
would then have to decide—on the basis of epidemiological and experimental
observations—whether the antigenic agent is a micro-organism or an
allergen.

But suppose we were unable to find large-scale fluctuations of onset?
Would that constitute decisive evidence against a classical viral aetiology? I
believe not. For, consider the case of an endemic virus. We can readily
imagine a situation in which everyone, or almost everyone, in a population

is being infected and reinfected with an oncogenic virus, but only those people with the necessary forbidden clone(s) will develop the associated malignancy. Even if marked seasonal or annual fluctuations in the prevalence of the virus were to occur, a long and randomly variable latent period between the initiation of a forbidden clone and the diagnosis of, or death from, the associated cancer would tend to mask such fluctuations. If populations could be investigated in which the putative oncogenic virus were non-endemic, they might furnish critical evidence for temporal fluctuations. It would then be important to show that *every* affected person in such a population had been infected with the suspected virus. To take the example of Burkitt's lymphoma, the occasional case that arises in non-endemic areas is, in some ways, of greater epidemiological interest than those that arise in the tumour endemic areas of East Africa. Do all such sporadic cases exhibit signs of having been infected by the Epstein–Barr (EB) virus? The answer appears to be 'No' (see Chapter 7), although it might always be argued that such exceptions are not genuine examples of Burkitt's lymphoma. If they are, we have to discard the hypothesis that the EB virus is *the* essential infective agent, while retaining the idea that it might be essential under certain special circumstances.

Where malignancies of adult onset are concerned, host-to-host 'horizontal' transmission should reveal itself through a high concordance for cancer in spouses. Walach and Horn (1973) investigated 20 000 new cancer cases at the Department of Oncology, Hadassah–Hebrew University Medical Centre, Jerusalem, Israel over the period 1958–72. Only 15 couples were identified in which both husband and wife had malignant tumours; in seven of these, the wife had breast cancer and the husband lung cancer. Walach and Horn (1973) concluded that the observed concordances were coincidental, and not the result of a contagious phenomenon involving an oncogenic virus. It could be argued, however, that the effective age of infection with oncogenic viruses occurs before marriage.

To summarize, if oncogenic viruses in man behave as classical host-to-host transmitted agents such as the poliovirus, mumps or influenza viruses, we should have little difficulty in inferring their existence from studies of the patterns of seasonal and annual onset and, for adult-onset cancers, through concordance among spouses. Unfortunately, no malignancy in man has yet been discovered that exhibits epidemicity analogous to that of the classical non-malignant viral diseases. The hypothesis of a 'slow virus' infection is more difficult to disprove, because the slow and variable progress of disease would mask seasonal fluctuations of infectivity.

Gross's hypothesis of vertical transmission (see below, page 264) is even more difficult to refute outright because, given sufficient ingenuity, it could always be framed in a form that would render its 'segregation' properties indistinguishable from that of gene transmission. However, special ingenuity would be needed to give a convincing explanation of familial evidence that pointed to an explicit scheme of *polygenic* inheritance. If ingenuity prevailed, we would then have to rely entirely on laboratory tests and demonstrations of the invariable contribution of the virus—at some stage or other—to the pathogenesis of the cancer.

Although ideal situations can be envisaged that would be virtually definitive the inconclusive ones are our main concern. The unambiguous demonstration of a specific virus in association with every tumour examined, coupled with a much lower prevalence in unaffected controls, would provide strong corroboration but not, perhaps, 'proof'—if that is ever forthcoming in empirical science. But if the *only* role of the virus was to compete for defence antibodies, we might be reduced to showing that antiviral antibodies were invariably present in affected patients, at a titre in excess of some arbitrary level. The main difficulty in that situation would be with endemic viruses; antibodies to them might be present in virtually every immunologically normal person. Such a virus might or might not be essential to the development of the tumour. Hopefully, populations could be found in which the suspected virus was not endemic.

I conclude, in company with Bryan (1965) and Rowe (1965), that 'proof' or 'disproof' of a viral aetiology for a malignancy in man presents formidable problems. In Chapter 7, I was able to interpret a wide range of evidence without once having to invoke the concept of oncogenic viruses but, as argued above, the lack of definitive evidence for significant epidemics and connubial cancers does not conclusively dispose of the idea. We can be certain that oncogenic viruses make no contribution to initiating events for the great majority of natural malignant and non-malignant diseases—if not all of them. But until we have a thorough understanding of tumour development from the initiation of the (last) forbidden clone to the clinical detection of onset we shall not know whether a specific virus is essential to any one or more of the stages of malignant development. At present, I know of no evidence that *demands* the postulation of oncogenic viruses in the aetiology of cancers in man.

Vertical Transmission of Oncogenic Viruses: Oncogene and Protovirus Hypotheses

Gross (1974), who has developed his theory over two decades, believes that familial aggregations of cancer and leukaemia can be explained by the transmission of oncogenic viruses in a latent form, from one generation to the next. In certain instances, however, horizontal transmission, within the same generation, can occur. The virus is supposed to be activated by endogenous or exogenous factors to cause malignant development: the nature of the activation process is not defined. Huebner and Todaro (1969) have proposed that the cells of most or all vertebrates have C-type RNA virus genomes that are vertically transmitted from parent to offspring. The occurrence of a cancer is said to depend on the spontaneous and/or induced derepression of one or more viral oncogenes in a genetically susceptible host. Because horizontal transmission of the C-type virus is considered to be of rare occurrence, cancer can scarcely be regarded as an *infectious* disease either in Huebner's or Gross's theories. Accordingly, both theories predict that epidemic characteristics will be either of rare occurrence, or non-existent.

The initiating somatic mutations described in the last chapter would be interpreted, presumably, as activating events in Gross's theory and spontaneous derepression events in Huebner's oncogene theory. However, the observed kinetics of onset and death from cancer would appear to argue powerfully against such interpretations. Special and implausible *ad hoc* postulates would be necessary to explain why activating or derepressing events during embryogenesis and foetal life are ineffective. In other words, such theories need to explain why the time-scale for initiation begins at a period close to birth. Similarly, the constancy of k during the phase of postnatal growth, and the conformity of age-distributions to Yule, Weibull and combined statistics, also have to be accounted for. Neither do these theories offer any plausible interpretation of the distinction between unilateral and bilateral, or unicentric and multicentric cancers. The reproducibility of, for example, the ratio of unilateral to bilateral cancers in specific paired organs points to a biological, genetically determined, site-specificity. These several difficulties could be overcome if my theory of these essentially biological phenomena were adopted and if all the properties of MCP–TCF genes were attributed to oncogenic viruses.

Similar problems are implicit in Temin's (1971, 1972) protovirus hypothesis. Temin postulates that germ cells carry in their chromosomal DNA the 'potential' for the *de novo* production of the 'information for cancer'. He argues that, in normal development, a region of DNA in cell A is transcribed and the resulting RNA is then transferred to cell B. In cell B the transferred RNA directs the synthesis of new DNA through an RNA-dependent DNA polymerase, that is, *reverse transcriptase*. The new DNA becomes integrated into the DNA of cell B. This process might be repeated to involve further cells C, D . . . etc. Through this form of addition of genetic information to cells B, C, D . . . cellular differentiation is supposed to be accomplished. Temin suggests that the information transfer, DNA→ RNA→DNA is unstable: variants arise through interference at any stage of transfer. Certain variants may contain the 'information' necessary for cancer.

To reconcile these theories of oncogenic viruses with the evidence described and analysed in Chapter 7 many additional postulates are needed. Nevertheless, for the reasons stated above, it would be premature to assert that viruses play no part in the pathogenesis of cancers in man. On the basis of my theory, it is surprising that no clearcut evidence exists for the horizontal transmission and precipitating action of oncogenic viruses in man.

Conclusions

The analysis in this chapter of the biological basis of acute infectious diseases has some interesting implications for immunology. Many investigators believe that the primary role of the immune system is the protection of the host against invading and potentially pathogenic micro-organisms. Hitherto, the nature of 'susceptibles' has not been defined. Furthermore, it is widely supposed that infection alone often produces natural immunity. The age-dependence of acute, self-terminating infectious diseases forces us to adopt radically different perspectives.

Only persons with a particular genetic predisposition are able to become 'susceptible' and to develop a specific infectious disease. Although in the examples of whooping cough, chickenpox and measles, it is clear that a majority of the population is genetically predisposed to and, in the absence of artificial immunization, develops these diseases (Collins *et al.*, 1942), the same is not true of the rarer infectious diseases such as the several forms of poliomyelitis. Susceptibility results from the emergence of a forbidden clone' at the time of the infection. Infection in the absence of the forbidden clone fails to produce natural immunity. However, the emergence of a potentially pathogenic forbidden clone in the absence of the precipitating micro-organism does confer long-term natural immunity.

These considerations suggest that the *primary* role of the humoral immune system should be regarded as the protection of the host against his endogenous forbidden clones. If this suggestion is correct then we might expect to find a specific, complementary steric relation between the variable sections of immunoglobulin L and H chains and certain polypeptide components of pathogenic MCPs (Burch and Burwell, 1965).

In the non-infectious and non-allergic degenerative and malignant diseases, the humoral defence system evidently fails to protect completely, although it may well prolong the interval (latent period) between the end of initiation and first onset. Even in the acute, self-terminating infectious diseases themselves, the infective agent—in the absence of the pathogenic forbidden clone—fails to produce long-term immunity. This protection is brought about by the forbidden clone regardless of the presence or absence of the precipitating micro-organism. The history of epidemics shows that certain potentially pathogenic forbidden clones never manifest in given environments because they are effectively suppressed by the immune defence system and because no environmental infective or allergic agents are capable of competing effectively for the defence antibodies. This version of *immunological surveillance* differs from the one expounded by Burnet (1970).

CHAPTER 9

Carcinogenesis by Chemical and Physical Agents: Promotion Phase of Carcinogenesis

Although connections between natural and artificial carcinogenesis must be sought they will not necessarily be simple. Thus, physical and chemical carcinogens can induce tumours that do not normally arise under natural conditions, although not all tumours can be induced in all strains of animals. Any adequate theory needs to account for the similarities and the differences between natural and artificial carcinogenesis.

Studies of chemical carcinogenesis have delineated at least two distinctive phases: *initiation* and *promotion* (Berenblum, 1941). This separation accords with my theory of natural carcinogenesis. (I should interpolate that the term 'stage' is generally used in place of 'phase'. However, in some instances at least, initiation and promotion may well turn out to be complex processes themselves, involving multiple events and steps. Should this prove to be the case, the term 'stage' might be better employed to describe the separate steps within the broad 'phases' of initiation and promotion.) Generally, chemicals that act as initiators have little promoting action, and vice versa, although some substances, *complete* or *total carcinogens*, are efficient in both roles. Clayson (1962) has reviewed the earlier literature of chemical carcinogenesis.

Despite the recognized distinction between initiation and promotion, no consensus exists as to the biological and molecular bases of either phase. Most, if not all, initiators appear to bind either covalently, or by hydrogen bonds, to DNA, but binding to RNA and proteins is also observed—see Ryser's (1971) review. It is widely suspected, but not established, that initiators produce mutations or hereditable change—of one form or another —in cells whose descendants eventually acquire malignant properties.

Promoters, or co-carcinogens, of which croton oil is the best known, cause *proliferation* of the target tissue. This has prompted the suggestion that proliferation as such causes promotion. In keeping with this view, wound-healing and regenerative growth have been shown to be efficient promoters. However, anticarcinogens also provoke hyperplasia (Riley, 1968) and hence the simple suggestion that cell division causes promotion cannot be sustained without modification. The paradox could be resolved if the *type* of pro-liferation is important. Thus, *symmetric* mitosis stimulated by a mutant (initiated) MCP might be necessary for promotion while *asymmetric* mitosis—not involving MCPs, normal or mutant—might be ineffective. Alternatively, anticarcinogens, while provoking hyperplasia, might block some other step necessary to neoplastic transformation.

Dose-response relations for initiators indicate that they act through random 'hits'. In large-scale experiments in which benzopyrene was painted regularly on the backs of mice, age-specific onset-rates both of benign tumours and of infiltrating carcinomas were found to be proportional to the square of the dose of carcinogen (Lee and O'Neill, 1971). This quadratic relation suggests that benzopyrene, directly or indirectly, initiates both types of neoplasm through a two-hit stochastic process.

Possible Links between Natural and Chemical Carcinogenesis

From Chapter 7, I conclude that a specific natural tumour, at a given site, develops only in those individuals who have a particular genetic predisposition. It is therefore most important that, in certain instances, chemical carcinogens can induce a high incidence of tumours that never, or very seldom, arise under natural conditions; it is equally important that genetic factors can also determine susceptibility to chemical carcino-genesis.

I hold that natural tumours are initiated by the occurrence of r specific random somatic mutations in each of n distinctive growth-control stem cells. The fully mutant n stem cells propagate n forbidden clones of de-scendent cells. Products (mutant MCPs) of descendant cells in the forbidden clone interact with target cells to induce malignant change. Because the n mutant stem cells are probably located in the bone marrow this scheme is inapplicable to the local induction of tumours by locally applied carcinogens. When chemical carcinogens are applied to the skin, we cannot readily conceive that tumours arising within the painted area will have been initiated by mutations in *central* growth-control stem cells. Indeed, it is usually taken for granted that in the induction of, say, epithelial tumours, the initiator affects epithelial cells directly. Nevertheless, it is far from clear whether this assumption is valid: some ingenious transplantation experiments tend to undermine it.

Initiation: experimental evidence

Billingham, Orr and Woodhouse (1951) treated a small area of the skin on the thorax of mice with 20-methylcholanthrene, in weekly applications, for 12 weeks. When the treated epidermis, or thin Thiersch grafts of the treated area, were transplanted orthotopically to untreated body sites, no tumours appeared in the transplants. Occasional tumours developed in transplants when thick Thiersch grafts, or whole-thickness grafts, of treated skin were used. These observations suggest that initiated cells reside either in the dermis or in the proximal regions of hair follicles. But, when a denuded carcinogen-treated area was resurfaced with untreated epidermis taken from the tail, a considerable yield of tumours was obtained. Some of these tumours appeared at skin sites where no hair follicles could be seen.

Orr (1958) considered that some experiments with 0·5 per cent 9-10-dimethyl-1: 2-benzanthracene (DMB) virtually ruled out the idea that tumours at the denuded treated site arose from residual hair follicle cells. The DMB treatment totally destroyed the epidermis and hair follicles in a few days. Regenerative epidermis grew in from the periphery, and tumours eventually appeared near to the centre of the treated area and never at the periphery. Orr (1958) favours the hypothesis that the carcinogen affects all the elements in the treated area including the supporting and nutrient stroma; neoplastic transformation of epidermal cells depends on their interaction with the altered stroma.

In further experiments with three inbred strains of mice using 7, 12-dimethylbenz (α) anthracene (DMBA) in acetone as the initiator, and croton oil in acetone as the promoter, Bond and Orr (1969) observed that tumours arose from the superficial epidermis. The hair follicles played no part: none of the tumours showed tricho-epitheliomatous structure. Arundel, Karasek and Gates (1969) treated hairless, hairless-asebic and asebic groups of inbred mutant mice with 0·5 per cent DMBA in acetone. These mutants when adult have either no hair-growth (hairless, hairless-asebic) or greatly reduced hair-growth (asebic), but the skin shows remnants of hair follicles. Squamous cell carcinomas were obtained in each group of treated animals but none were found in untreated controls.

In an attempt to resolve the problem concerning the origin of epidermal tumours, Steinmuller (1971) treated the skin of F_1 hybrid mice with methylcholanthrene. He then used the inbred parent strains as the donors of untreated epidermal grafts. Of 14 carcinomas that arose at the graft sites in the primary hosts, none grew progressively when transplanted to the parent strain, whereas all grew in the F_1 hybrids. Steinmuller concluded that the tumours arose from epidermal cells of the F_1 host. However, this conclusion is by no means certain. Steinmuller demonstrated that progressive growth of the tumours is F_1-dependent but that does not establish their tissue of origin. To evaluate the tissue of origin, chromosome markers (such as the T6), would be preferable to histocompatibility markers. The latter may change as the result of graft *adaptation* (Barrett and Deringer, 1950); this phenomenon, which may well be important in carcinogenesis generally—see the section on promotion, page 273—has been reviewed recently by Jacobs and Uphoff (1974).

Cherry and Glucksmann (1971) found an optimal dose for the induction of skin tumours in rats by DMBA and in relating this phenomenon to their histological observations, they concluded that the epidermis should not be considered in isolation from its *interaction* with the dermis and supporting structures. From electron microscopic observations of skin treated with carcinogenic, or non-carcinogenic irritant chemicals (benzene, turpentine), Tarin (1968, 1969) deduced that changes seen at the dermo-epidermal junction in carcinogen-treated skin are directly related to the carcinogenic process. He argued that the disturbance in the interaction between epithelium and connective tissue is probably causally related to the carcinogenic process (Tarin, 1968, 1969, 1972(a)).

On balance, the experimental evidence—reviewed in a book edited by Tarin (1972(b))—favours the idea that interactions between stroma and epithelium are important, perhaps essential, to the induction of skin tumours *in vivo* by chemical carcinogens. However, the cells in connective tissue involved in these interactions have not been clearly identified.

Riley (1966, 1968) has emphasized the intimate involvement of the mast cell in the promotion phase of skin carcinogenesis. This view harmonizes well with our hypothesis that tissue mast cells might in some instances be the final effector cells in the humoral system of growth-control and the cells that undergo mutation during the initiation process. Promotion then involves the interaction between the products of these mutated (initiated) cells and the target epithelial cells. In the course of carcinogenesis, the initial epidermal hyperplasia is accompanied by a morphological change in mast cells within the dermis of the treated area; small, poorly granulated ortho-chromatic mast cells appear immediately under the hyperplastic epidermis (Riley, 1966, 1968). Papillomatous development is concomitant with an increase in the number, size and granularity of the adjacent mast cells (Riley, 1968). With the final progression to carcinoma, the number of mast cells in the upper part of the dermis declines.

In further experiments, Riley (1968) studied the effects of anticarcinogens such as ethyl phenyl propiolate, which also produce epidermal hyperplasia. As suggested above, this form of hyperplasia might involve asymmetrical mitosis. It is therefore interesting that the type of mast cell reaction that characterizes co-carcinogenesis fails to develop; slight reactivity takes place, but deep in the dermis, rather than proximal to the epidermis (Riley, 1968). Hence the findings from anticarcinogenesis further support the hypothesis of mast cells involvement during the promotion phase of chemical carcinogenesis.

The nature of initiation

Experiments investigating *in vivo* chemical carcinogenesis, coupled with the evidence from natural carcinogenesis (Chapter 7), suggest the following unifying scheme: Whereas in natural carcinogenesis initiating somatic mutations occur spontaneously in growth-control stem cells, the predominant site of induced mutation in local chemical carcinogenesis is in the *peripheral* cells (mast cells?) of the central system of growth-control. This contrast in the location of initiating mutations can explain why chemical carcinogens cause cancers in strains of animals in which the natural incidence of that type of cancer is very small or zero. We must presume that the mutations induced by chemical carcinogens in peripheral growth-control cells may also occur spontaneously in central growth-control stem cells. However, in the last chapter I deduced that many mutant growth-control stem cells stay suppressed: they produce active forbidden clones only when the body is invaded by extrinsic factors (microorganisms, allergens) bearing specific antigens. When such precipitating factors are absent from the environment and therefore never enter the host, the related mutant growth-control stem cells stay suppressed and never manifest their pathogenic potentiality. According to this interpretation the defence mechanism that often operates so effectively against mutant central growth-control stem cells fails to suppress similarly mutant peripheral growth-control cells when these are induced by extrinsic carcinogens.

This general scheme of initiation also explains certain forms of genetic susceptibility to chemical carcinogenesis. Only when locally mutant MCPs bear the appropriate *relation* to the TCFs of target cells will the latter be transformed. This relation is genetically determined.

We now have to ask: What is the connection between central and peripheral growth-control cells in the course of natural carcinogenesis? Suppose, for example, that five somatic mutations in a single growth-control stem cell ($n = 1$, $r = 5$) are needed to initiate a cancer. When the stem cell acquires 1, 2, 3 then 4 initiating somatic mutations, does it propagate descendent cells at each stage that replace the previous set of peripheral growth-control cells? An experiment of Ebbesen (1973) suggests this does occur. He transplanted skin grafts (evidently full-thickness) from (a) young mice and (b) old mice, to young host mice: after one year DMBA in acetone was applied to the graft. At seven weeks after this application, a maximum yield of papillomas was observed. Ebbesen (1973) found that the yield from grafts taken from old donors was more than double that from corresponding grafts from young donors. If peripheral growth-control cells (mast cells?) in the dermis of old grafts had contained a larger complement of mutant MCP genes than corresponding cells in young grafts, Ebbesen's findings are readily explained.

So far, I have considered only those mutations, spontaneous or induced, that occur in growth-control cells. We have, however, to account for the voluminous evidence relating to the immunogenicity of tumour cells. Evidently, the TCFs of tumour cells differ (sometimes or always) from the TCFs of their normal counterparts. This change constitutes part of the process of promotion.

Promotion

According to the arguments above, promotion in chemical carcinogenesis requires that mutant MCPs should be secreted from local (peripheral) growth-control cells and interact with complementary TCFs of target, for example epithelial cells, to induce malignant transformation. Factors such as cocarcinogens that promote symmetrical mitosis in target cells promote malignant transformation. Transformation is associated with the synthesis of 'not-self' mutant TCFs.

This theoretical scheme leaves open the nature of the transformation. Is this a purely deterministic process requiring only the interaction of an appropriately mutant MCP with a complementary TCF that undergoes inductive change? Or does the mutant MCP act by 'fixing' one or more spontaneous changes—such as DNA strand-switching mutations—of genes that code for TCFs in target cells? Or are both mechanisms effective? Experiments that determine the frequency of onset of tumours as a function of time after initiation should throw light on these questions.

Van Duuren et al. (1969) initiated skin tumours in female ICR/Ha Swiss strain mice with a single application of DMBA in acetone. Promotion was effected through the regular application (three times weekly) of a mixture of phorbol esters. The number of papillomas greater than 1 mm diameter was scored in relation to time after the commencement of promotion (see Figure 9.1). In one series of experiments actinomycin D in acetone, at doses of 5 or 20 μg, was applied to treated areas of skin 30 days after initiation.

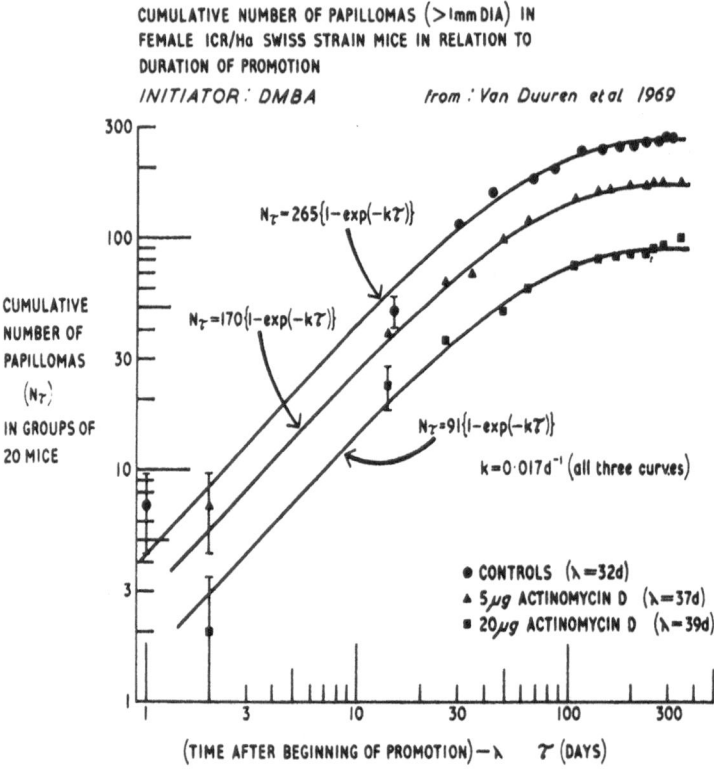

CUMULATIVE NUMBER OF PAPILLOMAS (>1mm DIA) IN
FEMALE ICR/Ha SWISS STRAIN MICE IN RELATION TO
DURATION OF PROMOTION

INITIATOR: DMBA   *from : Van Duuren et al 1969*

$N_T = 265\{1-\exp(-k\tau)\}$

$N_T = 170\{1-\exp(-k\tau)\}$

$N_T = 91\{1-\exp(-k\tau)\}$

$k = 0.017 d^{-1}$ (all three curves)

CUMULATIVE
NUMBER OF
PAPILLOMAS
(N_T)
IN GROUPS OF
20 MICE

● CONTROLS (λ=32d)
▲ 5 μg ACTINOMYCIN D (λ=37d)
■ 20 μg ACTINOMYCIN D (λ=39d)

(TIME AFTER BEGINNING OF PROMOTION) $-\lambda$ τ (DAYS)

Figure 9.1 Cumulative number (N_τ) of induced papillomas greater than 1 mm diameter, and persisting for at least 30 days in female ICR/Ha Swiss mice, in relation to (adjusted) time (τ) after beginning of promotion with a mixture of phorbol esters (Van Duuren et al., 1969). The failure of some animals to survive to the end of the experiment will lead to a slight underestimate of N_τ beyond $\tau = 130$ days. Top curve: controls (DMBA and promoter but no inhibitor); middle curve: 5 μg of actinomycin D applied 30 days after initiation; bottom curve: 20 μg of actinomycin D applied 30 days after initiation. Promotion was begun 14 days after the application of the inhibitor, actinomycin D

At 160 days, when animal survival was 90 per cent or more, the number of tumours per mouse was: 11.4 ± 1.6 in 'controls' (treated for initiation and promotion but without actinomycin D); 7.9 ± 1.0 in the group treated with 5 μg actinomycin D; and 4.0 ± 1.0 in the group treated with 20 μg actinomycin D. However, for each group, the time-dependence of the cumulative number of papillomas (N_τ) followed the simple stochastic relation: $N_\tau = N_A\{1 - \exp(-k_\tau)\}$, where N_A, the (hypothetical) number of papillomas per group at $\tau = \infty$, was a function of the dose A of actinomycin D; k, the average rate of 'random promoting events' (≈ 0.017 d^{-1}), was effectively independent of that dose; and $\tau =$ time after promotion, minus 32 days (controls), 37 days (group receiving 5 μg actinomycin), and 39 days (group receiving 20 μg actinomycin).

These data of Van Duuren *et al.*, together with the preceding arguments, suggest the following interpretation

(1) treatment with initiator converted N_O peripheral growth-control cells per group of mice into the carcinogenic form secreting mutant MCPs, and leading to the potential induction (at $\tau = \infty$) of N_O papillomas: N_O is the

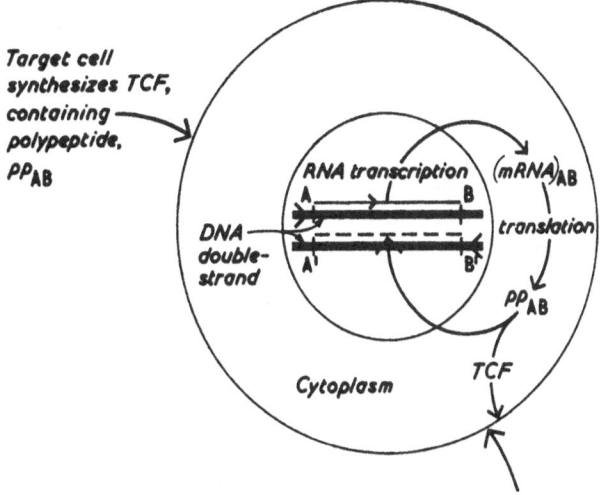

MCP molecules complementary to pp_{AB}, interact with target cell, promote mitosis and complex with pp_{AB} :

$$(MCP)_{B'A'} + pp_{AB} \rightarrow Complex$$

Concentration of free pp_{AB} in target cell reduced.

At next division of target cell, insufficient pp_{AB} polypeptides are available to complex with B'A' strand of DNA and to block transcription from it.

If RNA transcribed from B'A', then polypeptide $pp_{B'A'}$ is synthesized, enters nucleus, complexes with DNA strand AB and 'fixes' DNA strand-switching.

Figure 9.2 Possible mechanism whereby mitotic control proteins (MCPs), normal or mutant, can fix DNA strand-switching at certain tissue coding factor (TCF) genes in target cells

value of N_A in the above equation for zero dose of actinomycin D;

(2) treatment with actinomycin D at dose A reduced the number of initiated growth-control cells secreting mutant MCPs to N_A;

(3) the formation of a papilloma required the interaction of a mutant (tumorigenic) MCP with a *mutant* target epithelial cell;

(4) mutation of a target epithelial cell—the type of event that leads to the antigenicity of tumours—entailed a single random event, of average rate k per day ($\simeq 0.017$ d^{-1}), per distinctive mosaic of epithelial cells;

(5) the 'single random event' was the mutation—perhaps DNA strand-switching—of a TCF gene;

(6) promotion was necessary to 'fix' the mutated state of the TCF gene in the target epithelial cell—see below and Figure 9.2; and

(7) although actinomycin had a negligible effect on k, it retarded the growth-rate of papillomas so that λ, the average interval between the random promoting event and growth of the papilloma to 1 mm diameter increased with the dose of actinomycin.

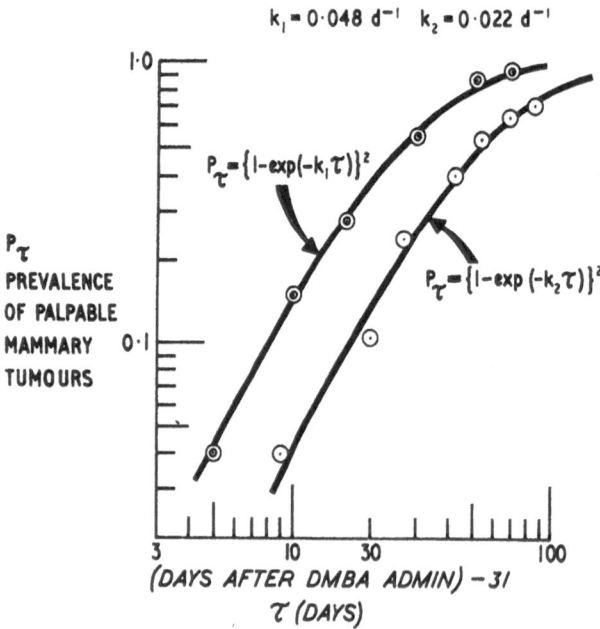

Figure 9.3 Prevalence (P_τ) of palpable mammary tumours initiated by DMBA in female Sprague–Dawley rats, in relation to time (τ) after initiation minus 31 days (Carroll and Khor, 1970). Left and upper curve relates to animals on a diet containing 20 per cent corn oil; right and lower curve relates to animals on a diet containing 0.5 per cent corn oil.

Similar experiments by Carroll and Khor (1970)—see Figure 9.3—and by Chan, Goldman and Wynder (1970)—see Fig. 9.4—are consistent with the general features of this interpretation. The promotion of palpable mammary tumours initiated by DMBA in female Sprague–Dawley rats appears to require two independent ($n = 2$, $r = 1$) random events (Figure 9.3), the

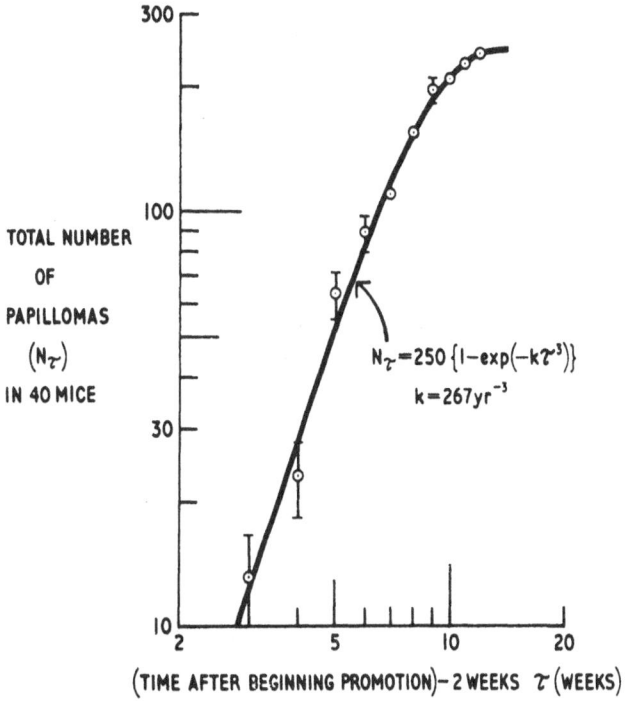

Figure 9.4 Total number (N_τ) of papillomas larger than 1 mm diameter, initiated in the control series of female Swiss mice by a single application to skin of 50 μg DMBA, and promoted by croton oil twice weekly, in relation to time (τ) after beginning of promotion minus 2 weeks (Chan, Goldman and Wynder, 1970)

average rate of which is affected by the percentage of corn oil in the diet (Carroll and Khor, 1970). For a 0·5 per cent content, the average rate of each random promoting event is 0·022 d^{-1}, but this increases to 0·048 d^{-1} for a 20 per cent corn oil diet.

From the experiments of Chan *et al.* (1970), it appears (Figure 9.4) that three random promoting events ($n = 1$, $r = 3$), perhaps in a single target cell, are needed to bring about the growth of a papilloma.

Similar conclusions regarding the biological nature of the promotion phase can be drawn from experimental radiation leukaemogenesis. Upton,

Jenkins and Conklin (1964) determined the time-specific onset-rate of myeloid leukaemia, in male RF mice, following a single, acute, whole-body irradiation. Bimodal or trimodal distributions were found, depending on the dose level: results obtained at the level of 450 rads are analysed in Figure 9.5. The distribution is well represented by the sum of two 'standard'

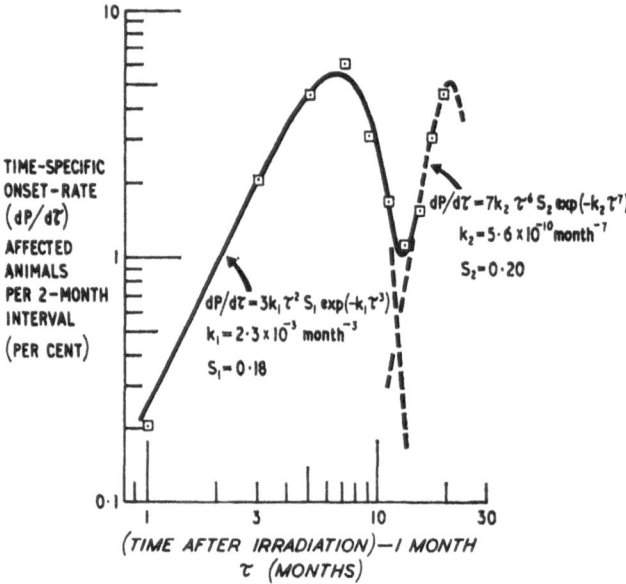

Figure 9.5 Time-specific onset-rate ($dP/d\tau$) of myeloid leukaemia in RF male mice, in relation to time (τ) after irradiation (Upton, Jenkins and Conklin, 1964). The lag, λ, between the last random promoting event and the detection of leukaemia is deduced to be approximately 1 month

stochastic functions, with $n=1$, $r=3$, $S_1=0\cdot18$ and $n=1$, $r=7$, $S_2=0\cdot20$ respectively. That is to say, two distinctive forms (at least) of myeloid leukaemia are induced at this level, in the almost equal proportions of $0\cdot18$ and $0\cdot20$ of the irradiated group of animals. This time–distribution of promotion has special interest because Gray (1965) showed that the overall incidence, I, of induced leukaemia in these experiments gives a good fit to the equation $I \propto D^2 f_c(D)$, where $f_c(D)$ defines cell survival at dose D. This relation will be discussed in detail below but here it is sufficient to note the conclusion that the D^2 term may signify a two-hit initiating mechanism (Gray, 1965). Hence, the number of random promoting events in each instance (three and seven respectively) probably exceeds the number (two) of radiation-induced initiating events. If this conclusion is correct, the steric relation between the mutant MCP and the target mutant TCF that results in neoplastic change can be complicated. It is not necessarily one of identity. However, radiation might induce mutations in cells that have already acquired a complement of spontaneous mutations. Quantitative considerations based on the estimated number of spontaneously mutant cells and the likely value of the radiation mutation coefficient tend to exclude this latter possibility. Nevertheless, it would be interesting to study the incidence of radiation-induced leukaemia in RF male mice as a function of animal age at irradiation.

It is important to observe that the time scale for the random promoting events commences with the time of initiation. This implies that any such events occurring prior to initiation are ineffective and/or reversed by a monitoring system. In conformity with general theory this monitoring will be carried out by MCPs from the central system of growth-control.

To summarize the argument, promotion requires the spontaneous mutation of one or more TCF genes (probably by DNA strand-switching) in one or more distinctive target cells and the 'fixation' of the mutant genes by appropriately mutant MCPs from cognate growth-control cells. In carcinogenesis, 'fixation' of the final mutant TCF gene in, say, an epithelial cell, is followed by symmetrical mitosis of that cell, stimulated by the cognate mutant MCP. If promoters such as croton oil and phorbol esters act primarily by increasing the frequency of symmetrical mitosis, this raises the possibility that DNA strand-switching of TCF genes in target cells is not entirely random but occurs (spontaneously) only during mitosis.

In the experiments of Van Duuren et al., the (deduced) average interval between the occurrence of the mutation in the target cell, and the first detection of the promoted papilloma, ranged from 32 to 39 days. The corresponding interval in the experiments of Carroll and Khor was about 31 days. In the experiments of Chan et al., the average interval between the last random promoting event and growth of the papilloma to 1 mm diameter was about 14 days: in those of Upton et al., the average interval between the final random promoting event and the detection of leukaemia was about one month. The average rate (k) of random promoting events is high— about 6·2 per year in the experiments of Van Duuren et al.—and from eight to 18 per year in those of Carroll and Khor.

The interpretation of the induction of papillomas and carcinomas by locally applied carcinogens and co-carcinogens also explains the familiar observations, emphasized by Prehn (1974), that spontaneous tumours generally show little or no capacity to induce an immune reaction that is sufficiently vigorous to inhibit tumour growth, whereas tumours induced by chemical carcinogens or laboratory-selected viruses are often markedly antigenic. According to the above theory, a markedly antigenic growth-control stem cell will be suppressed by the central defence mechanism: only weakly antigenic stem cells survive. On the other hand, those tumours that are induced *only* by carcinogens that mutate peripheral growth-control cells—not subject to the central defence mechanism—may be markedly antigenic. This agreement with observation further supports the theory of initiation and promotion for both natural and artificial carcinogenesis.

In his discussion of the nature of genes in the cancer cell, Temin (1974) points out that, in conventional mutation hypotheses, a normal cell does not contain the genes for cancer; during the process of carcinogenesis, such genes arise through mutation. In conventional differentiation hypotheses, normal cells contain the genes for cancer in an inactive form; during carcinogenesis these potential cancer genes become activated and their phenotypic expression leads to the formation of a cancer cell. My hypothesis of DNA strand-switching of TCF genes during the promotion phase of carcinogenesis combines features of both the mutation and the differentiation hypotheses. The DNA sequence remains invariant during carcinogenesis (as in differentiation hypotheses) but its phenotypic expression changes spontaneously (as in mutation hypotheses) through the switch in transcription from the normal, to the antiparallel strand, of DNA. It has to be borne in mind that, under certain circumstances, an oncogenic virus might effect DNA strand-switching.

Finally, the types of curves in Figures 9.1 and 9.3 to 9.5, considered in conjunction with the arguments of Chapter 4, show that promotion, as much as initiation, depends on *relational* phenomena. That is to say, in the initiation of any natural autoaggressive disease, the determining factor is the steric relation between the mutant (pathogenic) MCP and TCF of the target tissue. In promotion, whether of natural or artificially induced neoplasia, the factor that governs neoplastic growth is, similarly, the steric relation between the mutant MCP (whether of central or peripheral origin), and the mutant TCF of the target tissue. The relation between the number of induced random initiating events and the number of random promoting events may be complicated, as Figure 9.5 and the dose-response relation for the induction of myeloid leukaemia in RF mice suggest.

In Vitro Carcinogenesis

The above scheme distinguishes clearly between *initiation* which affects growth control cells, and *promotion* which involves the interaction of mutant MCPs with target cells that also become mutant. It also sheds light on *in vitro* carcinogenesis.

The phenomenon of the *in vitro* transformation of cells that can occur either spontaneously, or can be induced by chemical and physical agents (such as x-rays), implies that TCF genes undergo, and under certain conditions retain, the same type of mutational change *in vitro* as that which is fixed by mutant MCPs *in vivo*. Why then do TCF genes not undergo irreversible carcinogenic changes directly, under *in vivo* conditions? I have argued that, both during embryogenesis, and under normal conditions in the mature organism, MCPs (normal and mutant) generally exert a controlling influence over the induction of TCF genes in cognate target cells (Burch, 1968(a)). Thus, if a TCF becomes temporarily changed *in vivo* to a mutant form through spontaneous or induced DNA strand-switching of one or more TCF genes it will only become fixed by a similarly mutant MCP. If the cognate MCP is non-mutant, it will usually convert the mutant TCF back to the non-mutant form by reversing the switch of transcription (see Figure 9.2). Irreversible change of TCF genes, entailing the fixing of strand-switching, needs to be established *in vitro* before transformed cells will grow progressively *in vivo*. Even then, growth requires the presence in the host of a suitable MCP.

From experiments on x-ray-induced transformation using hamster embryo cells *in vitro*, Borek and Sachs (1968) concluded that two post-irradiation cell generations are needed to fix the transformed state. Klein (1974) found that cultured mouse spleen cells could not readily be made malignant by x-irradiation: close contact between viable and non-viable cells, and the presence of cell debris, was necessary to effect malignant transformation. This suggests that when a cell with early-stage mutant TCFs is surrounded *in vitro* by other non-mutant viable cells, these, and/or their secreted TCFs, can inhibit the fixing of spontaneous or induced DNA strand-switching. If the fixing of DNA strand-switching requires two cell divisions as suggested by Borek and Sachs, then the contact inhibition of mitosis arising from contact between viable cells would obviously inhibit the fixing of strand-switching.

Plastic Film Carcinogenesis

The preceding concepts lead to an interpretation of plastic film carcinogenesis (Burch, 1970(a)). Insertion of a plastic film between the cells of an organized tissue damages cells and also interferes with the contact inhibition of mitosis. This intervention elicits an inflammatory infiltration and localized hyperplasia. When plastic film is implanted in subcutaneous connective tissue the main hyperplastic cells are fibroblasts (Oppenheimer *et al.*, 1958; Vasiliev *et al.*, 1962). A tumour eventually develops from cells in close proximity to the implant.

I propose the following interpretation of the multiple steps in plastic film carcinogenesis:

(1) Initially, the plastic film causes localized hyperplasia of fibroblasts through interference with the contact inhibition of mitosis.

(2) The increase in the number of local fibroblasts results in an increased output of affector TCFs: this cuts off the flow of effector cognate MCPs and reduces or eliminates their monitoring function.

(3) When a fibroblast acquires a carcinogenic complement of mutant TCF genes the pre-malignant state becomes fixed through successive cell divisions and the failure of normal MCPs to monitor mutant TCFs. The experiments of Brand, Buoen and Brand (1967) and Johnson et al. (1970) show that daughter cells of a pre-malignant cell cover one side of a plastic film (15 × 22 mm) and generally remain in close contact with it.

(4) The synthesis and secretion of mutant TCFs by the clone of pre-malignant fibroblasts replaces that of normal TCFs. (Mutant TCFs might well interact with, and neutralize, normal complementary TCFs synthesized by non-mutant fibroblasts.) The displacement of normal TCFs by mutant ones permits normal MCPs to resume their normal monitoring role. Although the fixed mutant TCFs in pre-malignant fibroblasts persist, and cannot be restored to normal, the resumption of normal MCP secretion inhibits the formation of second and further foci of pre-malignant fibro-blasts. This failure of *multiple* neoplastic foci to emerge—when, statistically, they would be predicted—is one of the most important features of the experimental findings of Brand et al. (1967) and Johnson et al. (1970). These authors conclude that a specific inhibitory mechanism comes into play after the formation of the first pre-malignant clone and that it prevents the emergence of further pre-malignant clones.

(5) The development of a tumour depends on the emergence of an appropriately mutant MCP and/or further mutations of TCF genes in pre-malignant fibroblasts. As in other forms of carcinogenesis, the promotion of neoplastic growth requires a specific steric relation between the mutant MCP and the mutant TCF.

Lability of Normal and Mutant TCFs: Induced Adaptation

If the concept of limited lability of TCFs applies beyond the stage of embryo-genesis we might expect that transplanted malignant cells bearing mutant TCFs could in some instances be converted by complementary MCPs of the host back to the non-malignant state. In other words, mutant TCFs appropriate to the transformed state, in common with the TCFs of normal cells, might not always be irreversibly fixed.

Experiments relating to the lability of normal TCFs have been described by Billingham and Silvers (1967). We are all familiar, literally at first hand, with the great variety shown by epidermis. Embryologists and developmental biologists have established that the character of epithelium is determined during development, and maintained throughout normal life, by interactions between mesenchyme (mesoderm) and ectoderm (epithelium)—see the review by Billingham and Silvers (1963) and the proceedings of the 18th Hahnemann Symposium edited by Fleischmajer and Billingham (1968). Mesenchyme plays the initiating role during development and it is responsible for the site-to-site differences that are seen in epidermal differentiation. Billingham and Silvers (1967) were able to demonstrate that, at certain sites, dermis of the adult organism is able to govern the differentiation of overlying epidermal autografts. Recombinant grafts were studied in adult guinea-pigs and hamsters. The dermis determined the character of transplanted epidermis at the ear, the sole of the foot and the trunk, but not at the tongue, esophagus or cheek pouch. Billingham and Silvers concluded that the basal layer cells of the epidermis at some, but not all, sites behave as though they are equipotential and that, in the adult animal, the maintenance of their special characteristics depends on persistent specific stimuli from the underlying dermis. In our theory, the specific inductive stimuli for normal differentiation are MCPs secreted by peripheral growth-control cells; carcinomas develop when the normal stimuli are replaced by specifically mutant MCPs and when the TCFs of target epithelial cells have become suitably mutant. The neoplastic state is therefore associated with aberrant differentiation (as many authors have pointed out), but abnormal inductive and mitogenic stimuli (the mutant MCPs) are also needed to establish the state *in vivo*.

The lability of certain TCFs in the transformed, neoplastic state, is implied by some important but rather neglected experiments of Barrett and Deringer (1950). In accordance with the well-established rules of transplantation, a tumour that originated in a C3H mouse grew in all animals tested of that strain, and in (C3H × C)F$_1$ hybrids, but not in strain C mice. This tumour was inoculated into (C3H × C) backcross animals under the following conditions. In the first, the tumour was transplanted directly from a C3H donor to a backcross recipient. In the second, the tumour was first transplanted from a C3H donor to a (C3H × C)F$_1$ hybrid and then, after a three-week period of growth, tumour cells were inoculated into backcross recipients. Under these latter conditions of intermediate transfer to a hybrid host, three times as many recipient animals ($P < 0.001$) were killed by a progressively growing tumour as in the first case. Barrett and Deringer described the effect of tumour residence in the F$_1$ hybrid as *induced adaptation*.

Support for the concept of restricted lability of the mutant TCFs of malignant cells has also been obtained by Pierce and Wallace (1971). They used a carcinogen-induced rat squamous cell carcinoma that did not metastasize; a large inoculum grew slowly and caused death by cachexia with terminal infection. Tumour cells were found to be heterogeneous. Proliferative cells took up tritiated thymidine and were histologically undifferentiated. 'Pearls' of well-differentiated squamous cells formed within the tumours, and at 56 hours after a pulse of tritiated thymidine, radioautography revealed relatively few such cells with large numbers of grains per nucleus. In other words the cells in the 'pearls' seldom underwent division. On transplantation into Irish rats, 27 of 82 transplants of undifferentiated tumour cells had developed into tumours (presumed to be potentially fatal) by 7 months. None of the 78 transplanted 'pearls', with a cell number similar to that used in the transplants of undifferentiated cells, had grown into a squamous cell carcinoma by 7 months. Pierce and Williams (1971) concluded that some of the progeny of malignant cells developed into non-proliferating and well-differentiated squamous cells. Although the mechanism of change was not elucidated, their experiments clearly demonstrated the lability of factors (TCFs in our theory) that determine malignancy and cellular differentiation.

De Cosse et al. (1973) were able to induce differentiation of tumour cells into tubules. A mouse mammary adenocarcinoma was maintained in vitro for 14 days, separated by a $0.45~\mu$m pore-size Millipore filter from embryonic mammary mesenchyme. Not only did tubules develop, but DNA synthesis declined, and a presumptive acid mucopolysaccharide matrix appeared that was absent from control cultures. Embryonic inductive stimuli were able to change adenocarcinomatous cells into organized structures.

The phenomenon of tumour maturation—see the review by Smithers (1969)—can also be explained along similar lines. An initially malignant tumour will have been induced by one or more forbidden clones. Further mutation of appropriate MCP genes, forward or backward, in one or more of the stem cells giving rise to the forbidden clone(s), should change target cells from the malignant to the benign state. Spontaneous regression might be explained in the same way (see also Chapter 11). Such phenomena require that most or all of the cells in the original forbidden clones should be replaced by non-carcinogenic successors.

To summarize: in certain combinations, normal MCPs in an adult animal can convert and/or fix a normal TCF in an autograft into a different normal TCF, appropriate to the new anatomical site and the peripheral growth-control cells within it. A hybrid between two inbred strains of mice can, in certain instances, convert a tumour that originated in one of the inbred strains into a form that grows progressively in the other inbred strain. I interpret this to mean that MCPs of the hybrid can convert genes coding for histocompatibility antigens (TCFs) in tumour cells, so that the converted cells become histocompatible with the other inbred strain. Also, a normal MCP can in some instances probably convert malignant cells with a mutant TCF into normal or benign cells with a changed TCF.

My theory of promotion is based on the idea that a mutant MCP converts a normal TCF into a mutant TCF and/or fixes a mutant TCF that arises spontaneously. This general scheme of inductive change represents only a minor extension of the well-established phenomenon of ectodermal induction by mesenchyme during embryogenesis.

Radiation Carcinogenesis

Following the explosion of nuclear bombs at Hiroshima and Nagasaki at the end of the Second World War, ionizing radiation achieved notoriety as a mutagenic, leukaemogenic and carcinogenic hazard. If we should be compelled to resort increasingly to controlled nuclear fission as a source of energy (as seems likely) continued preoccupation with the biological hazards of ionizing radiation can be expected and would be justified. At present, the main contribution to the radiation dose received by the population from man-made sources comes, not from the use of fission for power production, but from the use of x-rays in medical diagnosis. In the United Kingdom, this contribution probably remains substantially less than that from natural background radiation, which averages a little over 100 mrem per year, but shows considerable variation with geological formation and, to a lesser extent in this country, with altitude.

The mutagenic and carcinogenic (including leukaemogenic) properties of ionizing radiation are well established, but quantitative dose-response relations for human populations are poorly defined, especially in the region of background levels of radiation. Ideally, policies for protection from radiation would be based on precise dose-response relations for each of the important biological effects of radiation on man. These depend on dose-rate, dose-fractionation, dose-distribution within the body, radiation quality (LET), and other modifying factors such as oxygen tension. The biological consequences of small doses and low dose-rates of radiation are of paramount interest to those whose occupation entails routine exposure to radiation. Inevitably, small effects are difficult to assess: epidemiological data become sparse and difficult to interpret as we approach background levels of radiation. The most reliable dose-response estimates come from investigations of effects at doses well in excess of those likely to be encountered occupationally.

We are therefore faced with the problem of extrapolating from large to small doses and, very often, from high to low dose-rates. Such extrapolations have generally to be based on theoretical assumptions, and to make reliable extrapolations, we need to understand the fundamental radiobiological mechanisms. My personal interest in carcinogenesis was largely stimulated by such needs. Together with others, I soon reached the conclusion that the understanding of radiation carcinogenesis requires a similar insight into natural carcinogenesis.

Possible mechanisms of radiation carcinogenesis

As in the case of chemical carcinogens, radiation might (at least in principle) initiate cancers in any one or more of several ways.

(1) By supplementing the spontaneous process through the induction of DNA strand-switching mutations in growth-control stem cells. For a life-time exposure to radiation at a constant (low) dose-rate, R, a supplementing mechanism would simply increase the value of the kinetic constant $k(=Lm^r)$. On the average, m would be increased by an amount αR. The constant of proportionality, α, represents the average radiation mutation coefficient at low or chronic dose-rate in terms of the number of mutations induced per gene at risk per cell at risk per unit dose (usually 1 rem); and R is the dose-rate, measured as rem per year. When the curve of dP/dt versus t for a specific cancer exhibits a mode under natural conditions (negligible dose-rate), we would expect that a sufficiently high dose-rate R would shift the mode to a lower age. Values of dP/dt on the low t side of the mode would be elevated but, beyond the mode, values of dP/dt would eventually fall below those in unirradiated populations. In this model, the average, modal and median ages at death from the cancer would all be reduced in the irradiated population. Whether or not the proportion of deaths attributable to a specific cancer would show an increase would depend on the effects of radiation on the incidence of other fatal diseases.

Obviously, this mechanism becomes important only when αR becomes comparable in magnitude with m. From experiments on the mutagenic effectiveness of ionizing radiation on mouse spermatogonial cells (Russell, 1965), we would expect the value of α at low dose-rate to be $\sim 10^{-7}$ muta-tions per gene per rem. With a value of $m \sim 10^{-3}$ mutations per gene per year (Burch, 1968(a)), R would need to be as high as ~ 1000 rem per year before $\alpha R = 0.1\ m$. Only for very low values of m would this mechanism be of any consequence in those practical situations where R is less than the maxi-mum permissible occupational level of 5 rems in any year.

(2) By inducing DNA strand-switching mutations, not only in growth-control stem cells, but in their clonal descendants as well. Although the

broad consequences of such a mechanism would be similar to those of (1), a much larger effect of radiation can be anticipated (Burch, 1970(a), 1971). The observed constancy of k with age in general populations suggests that if mutations occur spontaneously in the clonal descendants of growth-control stem cells then: (a) their average rate per gene per cell is constant with age; and (b) the average number of descendant cells per clone is also constant with age. In this latter situation, and the one in which spontaneous mutation is wholly, or almost wholly confined to the stem cells, the effect of radiation relative to that of mechanism (1) is multiplied by the average number of cells per clone. For reasonable values of the latter (~ 10 to 100 cells), I find that the generalized life-shortening effects of chronic irradiation on the heavily exposed (pre-1940) US radiologists (Seltser and Sartwell, 1966), can be plausibly explained (Burch, 1971).

(3) By inducing DNA strand-switching of TCF genes directly in target cells. Experimental dose-response relations suggest that this does not contribute to initiation although it might hasten promotion (Burch, 1971).

(4) By inducing malignant change of a type that does not occur naturally in the unirradiated genotype. It will be recalled that the evidence for the age-dependence of infectious diseases (Chapter 8) implies that many mutant growth-control cells are normally suppressed and fail to propagate forbidden clones. In general, we would expect that *some* centrally suppressed mutant MCPs are potentially carcinogenic. If the appropriate mutation(s) could be induced in a *peripheral* growth-control stem cell the defence that is directed against *central* growth-control cells would be ineffective. Hence, as in the case of chemical carcinogenesis, tumours that would otherwise fail to develop could be induced through local irradiation.

This latter mechanism has important consequences for dose-response relations (Burch, 1971). Mechanisms (1) and (2) imply that, for a uniform distribution of dose, D, the mathematical function describing *initiation* will generally have r terms, and be of the general polynomial form: $\alpha L_{r-1} D + \alpha^2 L_{r-2} D^2 + \ldots \alpha^r L_o D^r$; where L_{r-1} is the number of cells with $r-1$ specific mutations, etc. (Burch, 1965). At low D, this series tends to a linear dose-response relation, whereas at high enough D the D^r term will dominate.

Let us now consider mechanism (4) and the case where a once-, twice- etc., mutant growth-control stem cell fails to propagate a descendant clone. If, say, two mutations in a peripheral growth-control cell are required to initiate a cancer, and if neither mutation occurs spontaneously in such cells, then the mathematical function describing initiation will have a single term only, and, for a uniform dose distribution, will be of the form: $\alpha^2 LD^2$. We now need to consider the influence of cytotoxicity.

Cytotoxic action of ionizing radiation

In all the above mechanisms of initiation we have to bear in mind that radiation can also impair cellular function in ways that will modify dose-response relations. An outstanding property of ionizing radiation is its ability to eliminate the proliferative capacity of cells. If the induction of a neoplasm requires: (a) one or more specific gene mutations in a cell, and (b) the propagation of a tumour from that mutant cell, then by definition, the cell and at least some of its descendants must have the capacity to proliferate and form the tumour. Such a mechanism—for example (1) above—might be expected to operate in the induction of those types of leukaemia that involve the transformation either of growth-control T-lymphocytes, or of bone marrow granulocytes (?) of the humoral system of growth-control.

Dose-response relations (mentioned above) for the induction of myeloid leukaemia in RF mice by acute x- or γ-irradiation (Upton *et al.*, 1964) are remarkably consistent with this model. The induced leukaemia is clinically and pathologically indistinguishable from the form that arises, generally much later in life, in unirradiated animals. It closely resembles chronic granulocytic leukaemia in man (Upton *et al.*, 1964). The dose-response curve is bellshaped and the mode occurs between 200 and 300 rads. Gray (1965) showed that the curve can be interpreted in terms of a two-hit initiating mechanism combined with a cell survival (cytotoxicity) function represented by a D_o of 120 rads and an extrapolation number (E) of three. That is

$$I = AD^2 f_c(D) \tag{9.1}$$

Where I is the proportion of animals irradiated at dose D that develop leukaemia, A is a constant, and $f_c(D)$ is the cytotoxicity function described by Gray (1965). The parameters of this latter function are typical of those obtained when mammalian cells are subjected to acute x- or γ-irradiation *in vitro* or *in vivo*, and when cytotoxicity is defined in terms of the inhibition of the *proliferative capacity* of cells.

The dose-response curve for the induction of myeloid leukaemia in RF mice is unusual, however, in exhibiting a mode at such a low dose. More often, the mode lies at doses in the region of one to several thousand rads (see the literature review, United Nations, 1972).

For the induction of bone sarcomas in man by long-term radium burdens, the mode occurs at an average skeletal dose of nearly 10^4 rads (Rowland *et al.*, 1971). In instances such as these, the value of D_o for the cytotoxicity function greatly exceeds that associated with cell survival, when this is defined in terms of the retention of proliferative capacity. Theories that postulate the proliferation of a tumour from an initiated, directly mutated cell, are incompatible with such very high values of D_o.

Hulse, Mole and Papworth (1968) interpreted the dose-response relation for the induction of epithelial tumours in CBA/H mice, by a single external exposure to ^{204}Tl beta-particles, in terms of the equation

$$I = A D^2 f_c(D) \tag{9.2}$$

Where $f_c(D)$ has a D_o of 2440 rads. The equation suggests a two-hit initiating mechanism. An equation of the same form, but with $D_o = 2280$ rads, describes the dose-response relation for dermal tumours.

Rowland et al. (1971) also used a similar equation to describe the induction of bone sarcomas in radium patients

$$I = A D^2 \exp(-D/D_o) \tag{9.3}$$

Where $D_o = 4700$ rads. Most of the dose to these patients is delivered by α-particles which are much more effective than x-, γ-, or β-rays at preventing cellular proliferation; they are also more efficient at inducing several types of mutation. An important complication, however, that is likely to affect the interpretation of the observed dose-response relation, is provided by the marked heterogeneity of distribution of radium in the skeleton. The dose to cells at carcinogenic risk can be expected to show a wide distribution about the estimated average value D. This will have the effect of broadening the observed bellshaped dose-response curve, relative to that which would be observed for a uniform dose distribution. Consequently, the number of radiation hits needed to initiate bone sarcomas might well be greater than two and the true value of D_o is probably less than 4700 rads. However, the survival curve for the inactivation of the proliferative capacity of mammalian cells by natural α-particles is a negative exponential with a D_o of about 70 rads. It is exceedingly unlikely that the corrected value of D_o in the dose-response relation will even approach 70 rads. Hence, any model that postulates the proliferation of a radiation-induced osteogenic sarcoma from a directly mutated cell must be regarded as implausible.

Another important feature of this dose-response relation should be mentioned at this point. The incidence of bone sarcomas at the mode was found to be about 50 per cent. From Chapter 7 we see that the proportion of the England and Wales population genetically predisposed to bone sarcoma (excluding jaw) is less than 1 per cent. It follows that long-term radium burdens generally induce bone sarcomas by a mechanism that differs from the one responsible for natural tumours.

For relatively uniform β-irradiation, and the induction of skin tumours, values of D_0 in excess of 2000 rads are also incompatible with a direct initiating mechanism. I have proposed an indirect mechanism, analogous to that for chemical carcinogenesis, in which initiation requires a peripheral growth-control cell to be mutated by ionizing particles (Burch, 1968(a), 1971). The mutated growth-control cell does not have to divide to promote tumour growth: it needs only to synthesize and secrete a mutant MCP capable of interacting with one or more suitable target cells. Protein synthesis, for example of immunoglobulins by plasma cells, is known to be highly refractory to radiation. In accordance with the suggestions relating to chemical carcinogenesis, the peripheral growth-control cell for certain target tissues might be a mast cell.

Experiments designed to determine the depth beneath the epidermal surface of cells at radiation risk in skin carcinogenesis give results that agree with the mast cell hypothesis. Glucksmann (1963) reported that 0·3 MeV electrons failed to induce skin tumours in the mouse whereas 0·7 MeV electrons *were* carcinogenic. Albert, Burns and Heimbach (1967) found that protons penetrating only 0·17 mm into the skin of rats did not induce tumours. From experiments with beams of electrons, these workers estimated that the cells at risk lie about 0·3 mm below the surface. Mast cells reside specifically in this zone (Riley, 1959).

As in the case of chemical carcinogenesis, it is difficult from this evidence to eliminate the hypothesis that epithelial cells in hair follicles are the cells at risk. However, the dose-response relation greatly weakens this latter hypothesis. By implication, directly mutated epidermal cells do not divide to propagate a tumour, and hence such cells in hair follicles are most unlikely to be at risk with respect to the process of initiation.

In conclusion, the dose-response relations for radiation carcinogenesis offer strong support for my general theory. This theory predicts that certain types of leukaemia should be propagated from directly mutated growth-control stem cells. Dose-response relations for the induction of such leukaemias should show a 'conventional' value of D_0, relevant to the elimination of the proliferative capacity of stem cells. The experiments of Upton *et al.* (1964) described above, page 288, in which myeloid leukaemias were induced in mice, bear out this prediction. However, my theory requires an indirect mechanism for the induction by radiation, *in vivo*, of non-leukaemic neoplasms such as adenomas, carcinomas and sarcomas. The cell that is directly mutated by radiation does not itself divide to propagate the tumour: it has to synthesize and secrete a mutant (carcinogenic) MCP that interacts with and transforms spontaneously mutant target cells into the neoplastic state. Accordingly, the dose-response relations for malignancies of this type are expected to show much higher values of D_0 than those associated with the induction of myeloid leukaemias in mice. These expectations are realized: D_0 values of several thousand rads are observed.

Radiation Carcinogenesis in Man

Much of the evidence for radiation-induced tumours in man is too imprecise to shed light on mechanisms. However, if the claim is valid that very small doses (~ 1 rad) of radiation to the foetus increase the risk of all childhood malignancies by a factor of about 1·5 then a remarkably high sensitivity can be manifested. Obviously, the claim calls for careful investigation.

The age-dependence of autoaggressive disease during the early years indicates that MCPs and TCFs are not fully induced or 'committed' until around birth. Generally, the starting time, $t=0$, for the process of initiation occurs within about ± 0.1 year of birth (Burch, 1968(a)). Hence, if the mutation of an MCP gene should take place prior to $t=0$, it cannot contribute to the kinetics of initiation of early-onset autoaggressive disease. However, the somatic mutation of an MCP gene during early development might, in principle, have the same effect as the inheritance of the gene in its mutant form via the germ cell line. But whereas an inherited gene will be transmitted to all cells of the developing organism—though often not expressed in all—the influence of a somatic mutation will generally be limited to fewer descendant cells. Thus, during the third trimester, a somatic mutation in a single cell will generally affect many fewer descendant cells than if it should occur, say, during the first. In considering the claim that small doses of radiation to the foetus enhance the risk of childhood malignancies we need first to investigate the age-dependence of malignancies (a) in those children who were irradiated *in utero* and (b) in those who were not.

The findings of the Oxford Survey of Childhood Cancers conducted by Dr. Alice Stewart enable us to examine these age-patterns (Stewart and Kneale, 1968, 1970(a), (b)).

Childhood malignancies and prenatal irradiation

The age-distributions of the onset of childhood malignancies in those who were irradiated *in utero*, and in those who were not, are shown in Figures 9.6 to 9.13. For simplicity, numbers of cases for each series, rather than age-specific onset-rates are plotted on the ordinate. These numbers will be approximately proportional to age-specific onset-rates (dP/dt). To obtain the true value of dP/dt we would need to know (as always) the survival, during childhood, of individuals genetically predisposed to each of the malignancies considered: this may well differ from the average survival for the general population. This information is unattainable, but because we are

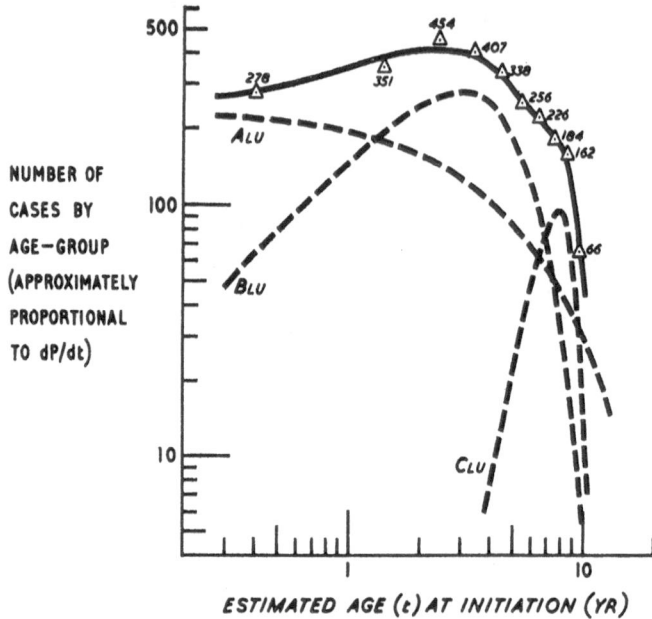

NUMBER OF
CASES BY
AGE–GROUP
(APPROXIMATELY
PROPORTIONAL
TO dP/dt)

ESTIMATED AGE (t) AT INITIATION (YR)

Figure 9.6 Numbers of cases of leukaemia (all types) in children of unirradiated mothers, in relation to estimated age (*t*) at initiation. Latent period correction $=0.1$ year. Data from the Oxford Childhood Cancer Survey (Stewart and Kneale, 1970(b)). The parameters describing the three theoretical curves are given in Tables 9.1 and 9.2. Curves A_{LU} and A_{LI} (Figure 9.7) correspond largely or wholly to acute myeloid and monocytic leukaemias. Curves B_{LU} and C_{LU} and, in Figure 9.7, B_{LI} and C_{LI} correspond to acute lymphocytic leukaemia. Sen and Borella (1975) examined blast cells from 48 children with acute lymphocytic leukaemia for the presence of receptors for sheep erythrocytes. For patients under 10 years of age, the positive cases evidently belong mainly or wholly to group C and the negative cases, most of whom were under 6 years of age, belong mainly or wholly to group B. The presence or absence of sheep erythrocyte receptors correlated not only with age at onset, but also with characteristic clinical features

comparing irradiated with unirradiated populations the deficiency is only of minor concern. Estimated values of latent period and *k* should be only slightly affected by the approximation.

Table 9.1 gives the parameters *n*, *r* and *k* that describe the theoretical curves in Figures 9.2 to 9.9. The same values are used, for corresponding curves, in the irradiated and unirradiated series. Although numbers are small in some age-groups of the irradiated series, the graphical analysis suffices to show that corresponding parameters (*n*, *r* and *k*) are essentially similar, and perhaps the same, in the two series. However, the proportions (S_I) of the irradiated series that developed childhood malignancies differed,

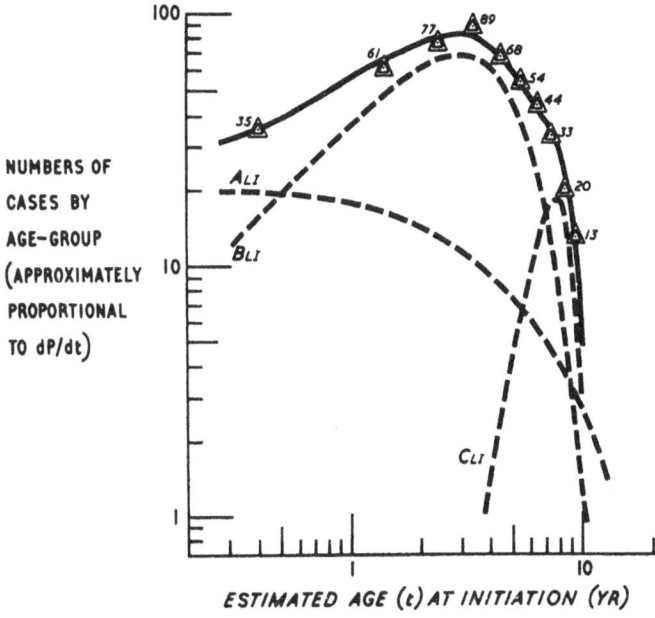

NUMBERS OF
CASES BY
AGE-GROUP
(APPROXIMATELY
PROPORTIONAL
TO dP/dt)

ESTIMATED AGE (t) AT INITIATION (YR)

Figure 9.7 As for Figure 9.6. Data for cases of leukaemia in children irradiated *in utero*

often quite markedly, from those (S_U) in the unirradiated series (Table 9.2). Although problems of latent period, heterogeneity of tumour type, size of population at risk, among other factors, preclude a rigorous statistical analysis of the exact significance of these differences, most are obviously real. In the ten categories into which cases are analysed, S_I is probably genuinely greater than S_U in the following six instances: leukaemia B and C, Wilms's B, neuroblastoma A, and cerebral A and C. However, S_I is

Table 9.1 Parameters n, r and k of Theoretical Curves in Figures 9.6 to 9.13

Malignancy	Curve	n	r	k
Leukaemia	A_{LU}, A_{LI}	1	1	0.22 yr^{-1}
	B_{LU}, B_{LI}	1	2	$5.6 \times 10^{-2} \text{ yr}^{-2}$
	C_{LU}, C_{LI}	1	6	$3.7 \times 10^{-6} \text{ yr}^{-6}$
Wilms's tumour	A_{WU}, A_{WI}	1	1	1.6 yr^{-1}
	B_{WU}, B_{WI}	1	2	$5.9 \times 10^{-2} \text{ yr}^{-2}$
Neuroblastomas	A_{NU}, A_{NI}	2	1	1.1 yr^{-1}
	B_{NU}, B_{NI}	1	2	$3.9 \times 10^{-2} \text{ yr}^{-2}$
Cerebral tumours	A_{CU}, A_{CI}	1	1	2.8 yr^{-1}
	B_{CU}, B_{CI}	1	2	$2.3 \times 10^{-1} \text{ yr}^{-2}$
	C_{CU}, C_{CI}	1	3	$3.8 \times 10^{-3} \text{yr}^{-3}$

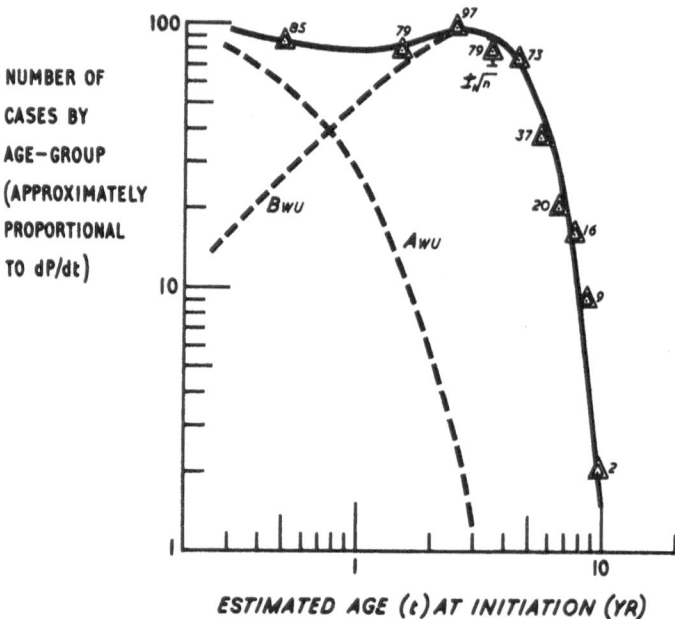

NUMBER OF CASES BY AGE-GROUP (APPROXIMATELY PROPORTIONAL TO dP/dt)

ESTIMATED AGE (t) AT INITIATION (YR)

Figure 9.8 As for Figure 9.12. Data for cases of Wilms's tumour in children of un-irradiated mothers. No correction for latent period. Clinical studies indicate the existence of at least two types of Wilms's tumour. Thus, 11 of 19 patients with bilateral nephroblastoma were under the age of one year (Jereb, 1971) and hence such cases belong largely, or wholly, to the early-onset group A_W

approximately equal to S_U in three instances: Wilms's A, neuroblastoma B, and cerebral B. For leukaemia A, S_I appears to be appreciably less than S_U. If the association between childhood malignancy and foetal irradiation is causal (or preventive, for negative associations), then relative inducibility (or prevention) clearly differs from tumour to tumour. It is equally clear that no appreciable differences in the statistical character (n, r) and kinetics (k) of postnatal initiating events emerge between the two series. Hence, if radiation to the foetus causes the increases in S_I, then the induction of a single mutation in a growth-control stem cell, or a precursor growth-control stem cell, is 'transmitted' in some way to all L stem cells that are at risk at birth and during postnatal life with respect to tumour initiation.

Mole (1974) used the data for twins from the Oxford Childhood Cancer Survey to support the causal hypothesis. Whereas only 10 per cent of singleton foetuses culminating in live births were x-rayed, the corresponding figure for twins was 55 per cent. Consistent with the causal hypothesis, the ratio of the x-rayed to the non-x-rayed for cases of leukaemia among twins was 2·2 (not markedly different from 1·5 for singletons); and the cor-

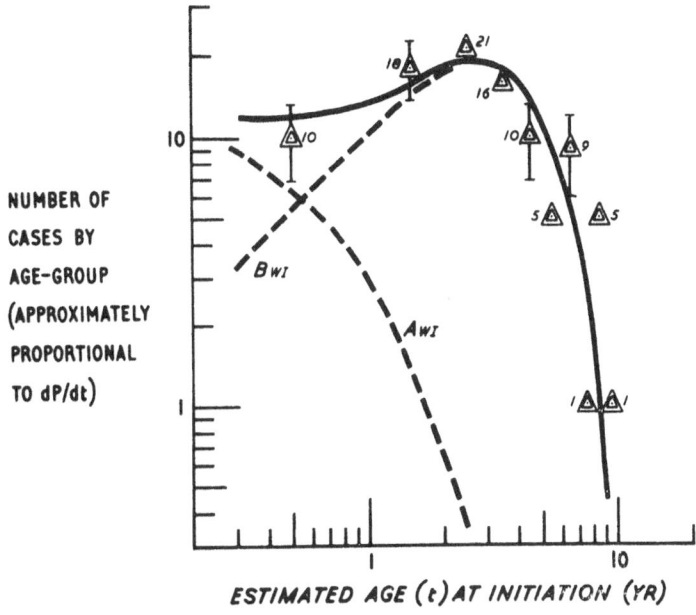

NUMBER OF

CASES BY

AGE-GROUP

(APPROXIMATELY

PROPORTIONAL

TO dP/dt)

ESTIMATED AGE (t) AT INITIATION (YR)

Figure 9.9 As for Figure 9.8. Data for cases of Wilms's tumour in children irradiated *in utero*

responding ratios for solid cancers were 1·6 (twins) and 1·5 (singletons). However, Mole failed to point out that, despite the high proportion of x-rayed twins, the absolute frequency of leukaemia in the whole twins series was only $1·98 \times 10^{-4}$—in contrast to $2·35 \times 10^{-4}$ for singletons—and the absolute frequency of solid cancers was only $2·58 \times 10^{-4}$ in twins, as opposed to $2·75 \times 10^{-4}$ in singletons. Although these comparisons raise interesting questions about the genetic comparability of twins and singletons, they do not resolve the problem as to whether foetal x-rays cause an increase in the incidence of childhood malignancies.

Many authors have questioned whether the association is causal in nature (Miller, 1969; Jablon and Kato, 1970; Burch, 1970(d); Russell, 1970; MacMahon, 1972; UN Scientific Committee, 1972; Jablon, 1973; Shore, Robertson and Bateman, 1973; Oppenheim, Griem and Meier, 1974, 1975).

The findings from Hiroshima and Nagasaki (Jablon and Kato, 1970) suggest a different interpretation. Jablon and Kato discovered only one case of juvenile cancer among the 1292 children who suffered nuclear bomb irradiation *in utero*. The number expected on the basis of the 1960 Japanese national death-rates (assuming no carcinogenic action of radiation) was 0·75. On a straightforward application of Stewart and Kneale's (1970(a)) dose-response relation (572 ± 133 deaths per million person-rad in ten years), the

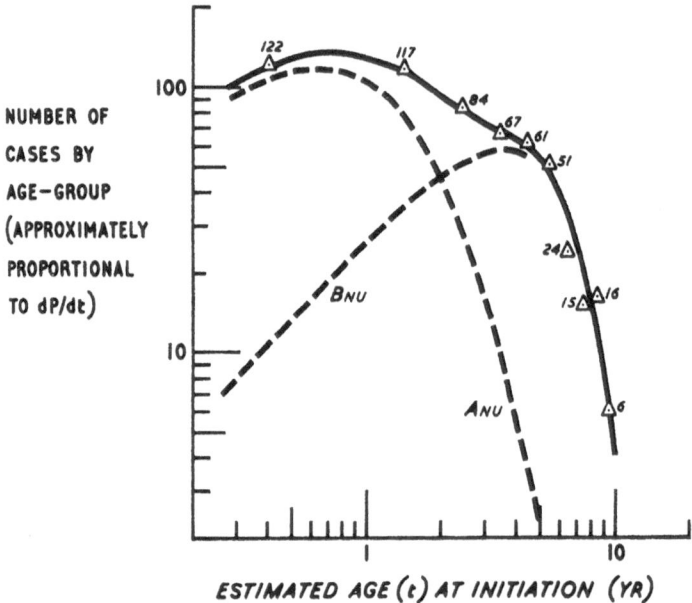

Figure 9.10 As for Figure 9.6. Data for cases of neuroblastoma in children of un-irradiated mothers. Latent period correction = 0·1 year. Clinical studies point to the existence of at least two types of neuroblastoma. Most of the children enjoying spontaneous regression of disseminated neuroblastoma are under one year of age (Schwartz *et al.*, 1974) and therefore belong, perhaps exclusively, to the early-onset group

number of induced cases was expected to be 36·9 (Jablon and Kato, 1970). Although there are various reasons for supposing that Stewart and Kneale's (1970(a)) estimate of the radio-inducibility of childhood cancers might not be directly applicable to the circumstances at Hiroshima and Nagasaki (they include population and environmental differences, and widely different dose-levels) the discrepancy is so large it cannot readily be explained by the causal hypothesis (Jablon, 1973).

Graham *et al.* (1966) have found that exposure of mothers or fathers to diagnostic x-rays, up to a decade *before* conception, associates with an excess risk (1·3 to 1·6) of childhood leukaemia in the offspring; this risk is numerically similar to that connected with foetal irradiation. It is very difficult to account for the association between childhood leukaemia and preconception diagnostic x-rays in causal terms. The radiomutability of genes as determined in mouse experiments is some three orders of magnitude lower than that implied by the findings of Graham *et al.* (1966).

Interpretation in causal terms of the association between medically requested x-irradiation of the pregnant mother and foetus, and subsequent

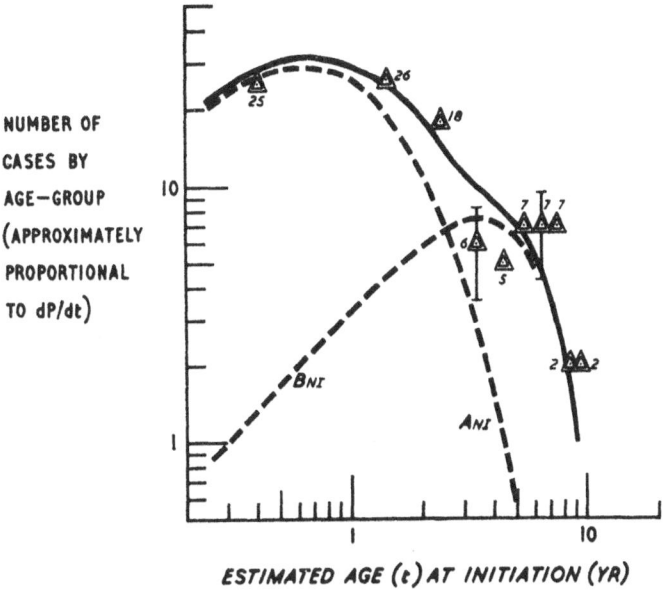

Figure 9.11 As for Figure 9.10. Data for cases of neuroblastoma in children irradiated *in utero*. Latent period correction = 0·1 year.

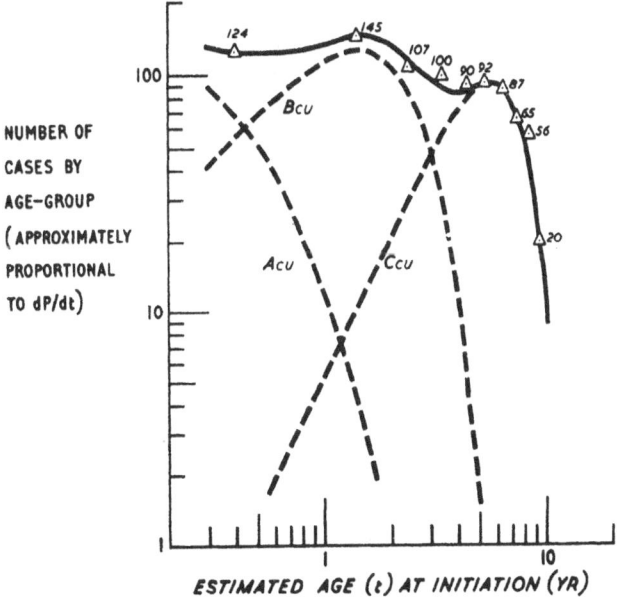

Figure 9.12 As for Figure 9.6. Data for cases of cerebral tumour in children of un-irradiated mothers. Latent period correction = 0·1 year

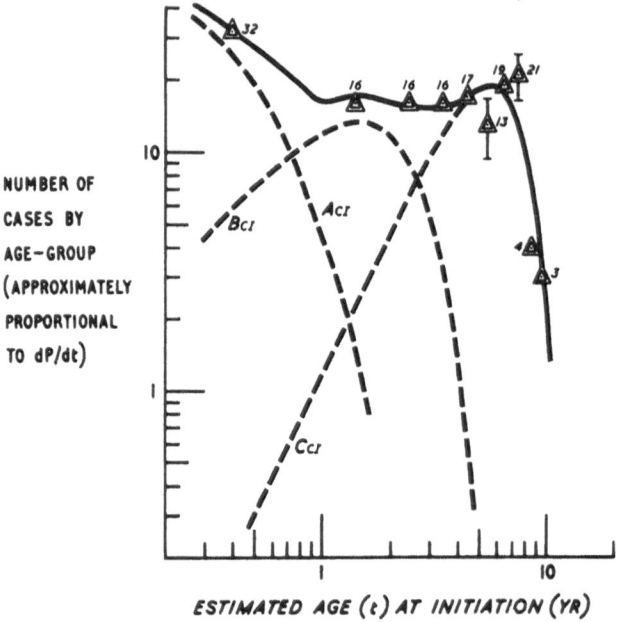

NUMBER OF
CASES BY
AGE-GROUP
(APPROXIMATELY
PROPORTIONAL
TO dP/dt)

ESTIMATED AGE (t) AT INITIATION (YR)

Figure 9.13 As for Figure 9.6. Data for cases of cerebral tumour in children irradiated *in utero*

childhood malignancy, requires independent corroboration; women chosen for investigation do not constitute a random sample from the general population of pregnant women. Russell and Richards (1971) found that the obstetrician is very efficient at referring for pelvimetry the patient who will experience trouble in labour. Oppenheim *et al.* (1975) show that women x-rayed during pregnancy suffer markedly higher rates of complications of pregnancy, and of operative deliveries, than women not x-rayed. Accordingly, the potential complications that attend selection bias cannot be disregarded. Thus the medical reasons for selecting a woman for obstetric x-ray examination might well associate, positively or negatively, with the risk of bearing a child predisposed to a given disorder. In particular, genetic factors that predispose to obstetric x-rays might associate, positively or negatively, with those that predispose offspring to particular childhood malignancies.

An objection to this constitutional hypothesis is that it does not automatically account for the roughly linear dose–response relation found by Stewart and Kneale (1970(a)). Constitutionalists need to postulate, for example, that the foetus predisposed to a childhood malignancy is more likely to suffer an examination involving a large number of films than the non-predisposed foetus. (A supplementary hypothesis linking maternal and foetal genetically determined characteristics is, of course, implicit in constitutional theories.) On the other hand, the constitutional hypothesis has no difficulty in accounting for the association between *preconception* x-ray examinations and the risk of leukaemia in the offspring, the negative association between leukaemia A and perhaps cerebral B tumours and foetal irradiation, and for the negative findings at Hiroshima and Nagasaki. It also receives some support from a critique of the conclusions of Stewart and Kneale given by Shore *et al.* (1973).

These latter authors demonstrated a marked change in the supposed dose-response relation for irradiations carried out over the period 1943–65 and for deaths reported over the period 1953–65. The ratio (cancer frequency per rad in irradiated series)/(cancer frequency in control series), as derived from the Stewart–Kneale study, changed with time for the successive cohorts as follows: $1·53 \pm 0·03$ for irradiation in 1943–49; $0·40 \pm 0·17$ for 1950–54; $1·17 \pm 0·19$ for 1955–59; and $-0·05 \pm 0·25$ for the 1960–65 cohort. Moreover, the dose-response relation depended on the reasons for ordering the obstetric x-ray examination (Shore *et al.*, 1973). This finding, and the secular shifts in the 'dose-response' relation, are both incompatible with a simple causal hypothesis. The secular shifts reflect the analysis given in Table 9.2 as the following argument shows. Truncated cohorts were studied. For those irradiated during 1943–49, the lowest age at death was 3 years. Hence for the early period irradiations the average age at death of children in the study group was greater than that of children who were irradiated in the later periods. Table 9.2 and Figures 9.6 to 9.13 show that the apparent. carcinogenic effectiveness of radiation decreases with decreasing age of onset. The ratio S_I/S_U tends to be low for the majority of early-onset cases: thus, for the relatively large subgroup leukaemia A of predominantly early onset, $S_I/S_U = 0·79$.

No support for the causal hypothesis is forthcoming from experimental studies of the effect of radiation on animal embryos and foetuses: only developmental abnormalities, but not malignancies, are readily induced.

The random allocation of a sufficiently large number of pregnant women to: (a) irradiation and (b) non-irradiation, could decide between causal and constitutional hypotheses but would be justifiable only in special circumstances. Routine pelvimetry for 1006 primaparas, without medical selection, was in fact practiced in 1948 at the Chicago Lying-In Hospital in the belief that delivery, and outcome of labour, would be made more predictable (Griem, Meier and Dobben, 1967; Oppenheim *et al.*, 1974). Before and after 1948 routine pelvimetry was not practiced, and first-born children born before 1948 (some 829 children) and after 1948 (some 981 children) were chosen as two sets of controls. The median age of the study population at the time of the second (and last) survey of results was 19 years. On a

Table 9.2 Relative Frequencies of Leukaemias, Wilms's Tumour, Neuroblastomas and Cerebral Tumours in the Irradiated and Unirradiated Populations

| Malignancy | | *Normalized values of S | | Ratio $\dfrac{S_I}{S_U}$ |
		Population unirradiated in utero S_U	Population irradiated in utero S_I	
Leukaemia	A	22·67	17·88	0·79
	B	29·01	60·89	2·10
	C	7·14	11·41	1·60
Wilms's	A	1·72	1·67	0·97
	B	9·32	15·71	1·69
Neuroblastoma	A	4·60	9·42	2·05
	B	7·25	7·72	1·06
Cerebral	A	1·43	4·58	3·20
	B	6·48	5·79	0·89
	C	10·39	17·72	1·71
Normalized totals		100·0	152·8	

* Values are proportional to the fractions of the unirradiated population (column 2) summed and normalized to 100·0 and the irradiated population (column 3) summed and normalized to 152·8 that appear to be predisposed at birth and develop the childhood malignancy in question. The overall incidence of childhood malignancies in the irradiated series was $1·5_{28}$ times that in the unirradiated series (Stewart and Kneale, 1970(a)). More significant figures are quoted than is warranted by their accuracy to facilitate the normalization procedure.

chi-square test, the only neoplasms showing a significantly raised incidence ($P < 0·05$) in the pelvimetry group were benign skin neoplasms (in one subgroup of the pelvimetry group attending one of the clinics) and haemangiomas in the total pelvimetry group. However, only a small percentage of the frequently occurring benign skin neoplasms and haemangiomas was actually recorded and hence the scope for bias was large; Oppenheim et al. (1974) concluded that the apparently raised incidence was probably an artefact of observation and recording associated with the routine pelvimetry programme. (About 70 per cent of these children had five films of the entire body and head shortly after birth and were subjected to more detailed examination.) Unfortunately, the study was far too small to detect an association between pelvimetry and rare diseases such as leukaemia. Only one death from leukaemia was found in the pelvimetry group and two in the control groups.

Where all deaths before the age of ten are concerned, Oppenheim et al. (1975) recorded nine deaths (1·05 per cent) in the routine pelvimetry group and 16 deaths (1·42 per cent) among controls. This nominally *lower* death-rate in the routine pelvimetry group conflicts ($P = 0.01$) with the finding by Diamond, Schmerler and Lilienfeld (1973), of a raised death-rate ($\times 1.87$) in a medically selected x-rayed group over non-irradiated controls. Oppenheim et al. (1975) believe that the process of selection is the most likely source of the discrepancy.

Conclusions

In view of: (a) the overwhelming methodological objections to inferences drawn from studies of non-random, medically selected groups; (b) the demonstration of complications of pregnancy and total deaths before the age of ten associated with selection; (c) the existence of negative as well as positive associations between malignancies and foetal irradiation in the data of Stewart and Kneale; (d) the absence of support for a causal mechanism from animal studies; and (e) the conflict between Stewart and Kneale's 'dose-response' relation and the findings at Hiroshima and Nagasaki, we have to regard the alleged carcinogenic hazards of foetal x-ray examinations as non-proven.

Postnatal irradiation

The follow-up of adult patients irradiated for ankylosing spondylitis (Court-Brown and Doll, 1957, 1965) and the findings at Hiroshima and Nagasaki (Ishimaru et al., 1971) demonstrate clearly the leukaemogenic effect of ionizing radiation, but they fail to define a clearcut dose-response relation. This should not surprise us. Heterogeneity of several factors, including irradiation conditions and distribution, population, leukaemia type, sex, etc., precludes the selection of simple homogeneous categories containing adequate numbers.

The data both from Hiroshima and from Nagasaki approximate to a linear regression of overall incidence on dose, but formal statistical tests reject an exact linear relation ($P < 0.01$) for both series (Ishimaru et al., 1971). In the ankylosing spondylitis series, the relation between mean dose to the spinal marrow and the total incidence of leukaemia was found to be approximately linear from 250 rem to 2000 rem, but markedly supralinear beyond 2000 rem (Court Brown and Doll, 1957; Burch, 1965). At the highest dose-range, just over 10 per cent of the irradiated group developed leukaemia of one kind or another. This high response suggests that some leukaemias, at least, were induced in patients who were not genetically predisposed to a natural leukaemia. It is of interest that chronic lymphocytic leukaemia has not been associated with radiation exposure.

Survivors of the nuclear bombs, and patients irradiated for ankylosing spondylitis, were all subjected to acute irradiations, which were fractionated in the latter series. The early US radiologists, however, accumulated large total doses prior to 1930—perhaps in the region of 3000 rads (Braestrup, 1957)—but from numerous small assaults approximating to chronic exposure. Seltser and Sartwell (1966) found a 'mortality ratio'—death-rates in radiologists, versus those in low risk medical consultants serving as controls—of around 1·4 for each of the selected main categories of causes of death: cancers other than leukaemia, cardiovascular and renal disease, and all other causes. The ratio remained effectively constant for death-rates in the age-groups 35 to 49 years; 50 to 64 years; and 65 to 79 years. However, the mortality-ratio for death-rates from leukaemia in the age-group 50 to 64 years, was just over seven. During the period 1945 to 1958, no indication of excessive mortality was discovered among the younger radiologists in the age-group 35 to 49 years. This latter finding suggests that: (a) improved radiological practice had largely or wholly eliminated the occupational hazards of diagnostic x-rays; and (b) the positive findings for older and heavily exposed radiologists should probably be attributed to radiation exposure, rather than selection bias.

Findings for the heavily irradiated radiologists (except, perhaps, for the substantial increase in leukaemia) agree with the hypothesis that chronic irradiation increased the rate of natural processes, and raised the value of the kinetic constant k for many fatal diseases. Nevertheless, very large occupational dose-rates (probably as high as ~ 100 rads per year (Braestrup, 1957)) produced a surprisingly small effect—an increase in death-rates from all causes, over the age-range 35 to 79 years, of a factor of 1·4.

General Conclusions

The evidence from chemical and radiation carcinogenesis usefully corroborates my general theory and sheds important light on the nature of the promotion phase of carcinogenesis. Promotion in chemical and radiation carcinogenesis appears to involve a random, as well as a deterministic process. Similarly, the interval between the end of initiation in *natural* carcinogenesis and the beginning of malignant growth *might*, like the kinetics of initiation, be governed by one or more random changes. However, whereas initiation involves the mutation of genes in central growth-control cells, promotion involves the mutation of TCF genes in target cells. In principle, this hypothesis of random events in promotion could be tested in the context of natural carcinogenesis by measuring the distribution of time intervals in a large enough series of patients, between the emergence of successive foci belonging to visible multicentric malignancies such as bilateral retinoblastomas, certain skin tumours, and, possibly, bilateral breast cancer.

CHAPTER 10

Smoking and Cancer

The idea that cigarette smoke causes lung cancer makes a strong intuitive appeal. We can readily envisage airborne carcinogens passing through the mouth, past the larynx and pharynx, down the trachea to the bronchi and lodging in the lungs. Animal experiments reveal chemical carcinogens in the condensate of cigarette smoke and no great imaginative feat is needed to connect such carcinogens with the initiation of cancers of the respiratory and gastrointestinal tracts. Positive associations between smoking and various types of tumour, but conspicuously cancers of the pharynx, larynx, bronchus and lung, have been observed in many surveys. It is less immediately obvious how 'cigarette-associated' cancers of the kidney, bladder and prostate might arise, although in principle, a general systemic effect due to circulating carcinogens can be invoked.

That smoking causes lung cancer is widely regarded as unequivocal: objections to the causal thesis '. . . are found to be without substance' (Royal College of Physicians, 1971). Indeed, I was once so persuaded of this thesis (not then having studied the evidence for myself) that I thought it would be a waste of time and effort to examine the age-dependence of lung cancer. A powerful cohort effect—such as the increase during the first half of this century in the habit of cigarette smoking—would be expected to distort the equilibrium form of curves of dP/dt versus t, both for horizontal (cohort) and vertical (longitudinal) analyses, thus rendering them totally unsuited to studies of the kind presented in Chapter 7. Eventually, I decided to examine the statistics for lung cancer because they promised to be able to settle the unresolved question as to whether cigarette smoke acts as an initiator and/or promoter.

Before turning to such details it will be helpful to discuss first the evidence for associations between smoking and other diseases. Although statisticians and logicians have told us *ad nauseam* that association is no proof of cause, conspicuous associations have, historically, been the first pointers to causal connections.

Associations between Cigarette Smoking and Diseases other than Lung Cancer

If cigarette smoking causes various cancers then, other things being equal, we would expect to find a rise in the death-rates from such cancers during

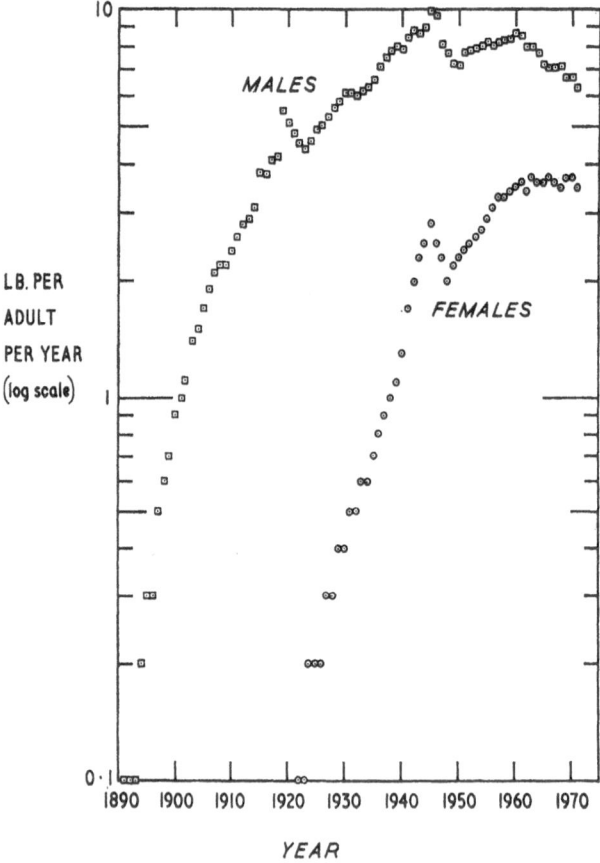

Figure 10.1 Consumption of manufactured cigarettes in the United Kingdom (lb per adult male or female per year) on log scale, against calendar year for the period 1891 to 1971 (Todd, 1972)

the first half of this century resulting from the increase in that habit. We are greatly aided in testing secular correlations in the England and Wales population by a fortunate difference in the smoking habits between the two sexes. Figure 10.1 shows that the sharp post-1920 increase in cigarette smoking among women lagged some 30 years behind the correspondingly sharp post-1890 increase among men. Assuming approximately equal induction periods in the two sexes, we would expect to find that cigarette-associated increases in disease incidence would occur about 30 years later in women than in men.

Associations between smoking and disease are often described in terms of a mortality ratio, which is usually the death-rate in a selected population, characterized by a given smoking habit, divided by the corresponding death-rate in non-smokers of the same sex and age-group. From the Dorn study of US male war veterans, Kahn (1966) obtained mortality ratios for many diseases—malignant and non-malignant—by smoking category.

Figures 10.2 to 10.4 summarize secular trends in age-standardized mortality-rates (SMR) as calculated by the Registrar General (General Register Office, 1957) for cancer sites that, in Kahn's (1966) report, show mortality ratios: (all current cigarette smokers)/(non and occasional smokers) of 1·5 or more. These ratios relate to the age-range 35 to 84 years. (It would be preferable to use mortality ratios for the England and Wales population, but in Doll and Hill's (1964) study of British doctors (the largest available) no deaths were recorded in non-smokers for cancers of the mouth, pharynx, or larynx.)

From Figure 10.2 we see that the SMR for cancer of the prostate rose

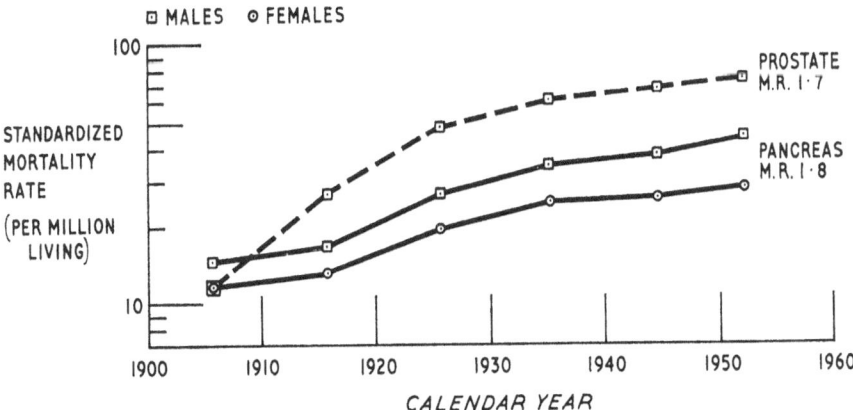

Figure 10.2 Standardized recorded death-rates, England and Wales (log scale) for cancers of the pancreas and prostate, against calendar year for the period 1901–54 (General Register Office, 1957)

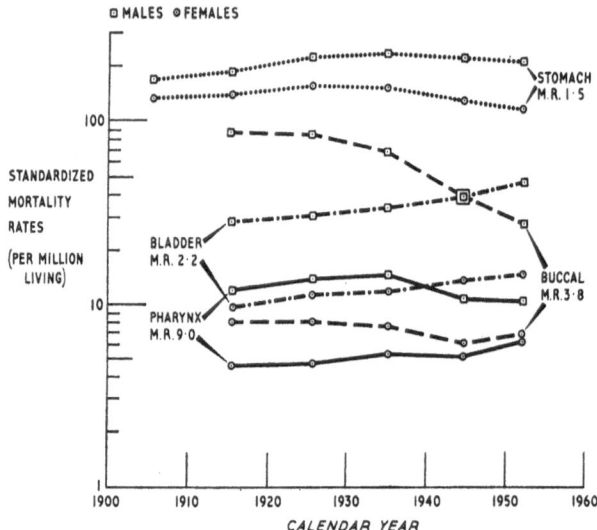

Figure 10.3 Standardized recorded death-rates, England and Wales (log scale), for cancers of the stomach, bladder, buccal sites and pharynx, against calendar year for the period 1901–54 (General Register Office, 1957)

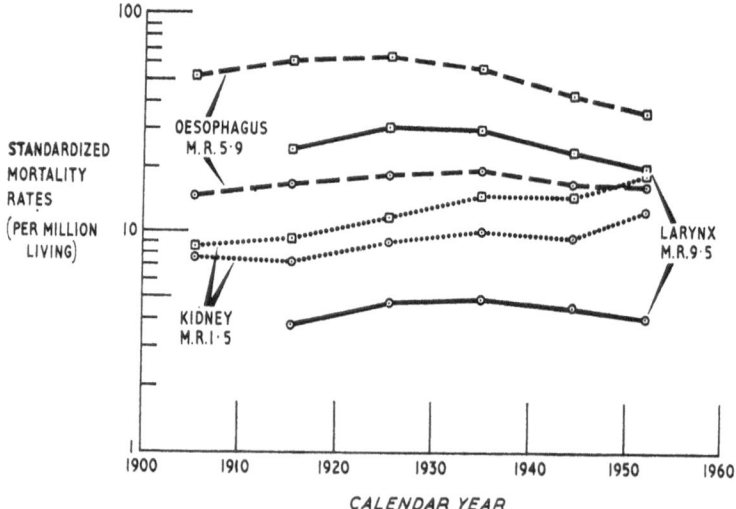

Figure 10.4 Standardized recorded death-rates, England and Wales (log scale) for cancers of the oesophagus, larynx and kidney, against calendar year for the period 1901–51 (General Register Office, 1957)

from 11·8 per million per year, 1901–10, to 74·2 per million per year, 1950–54. The increase, a factor of 6·2, is far too large to be accounted for solely in terms of cigarette smoking: the mortality ratio in Kahn's study was only 1·7 for cancers at this site. (In Doll and Hill's (1964) study, the mortality ratio: (cigarette smokers)/(non-smokers) was 0·5—suggesting a *negative* association between cigarette smoking and cancer of the prostate.) Factors other than smoking must have been responsible for the bulk of the secular change although we cannot rule out the possibility that smoking made some contribution.

For cancer of the pancreas, we are able to compare the secular trends in the two sexes. These run almost parallel and we see no suggestion of an initial rise in death-rates among men preceding a rise among women by about 30 years. (In the prospective study by Hirayama (1967, 1972) of large populations in Japan, from which volunteer bias was virtually eliminated, the mortality ratio—cigarette smokers/non-smokers—for cancer of the pancreas was 2·05 for men and 1·94 for women.)

In Figure 10.3 none of the secular trends in death-rates bear the expected relation to the secular trends in cigarette consumption. The data for cancer of the pharynx, with a mortality ratio of 9·0 (which approaches that (10·9) for lung and bronchus) are most surprising. They show a slight increase in both sexes from 1911–20 to 1931–40, followed by a slight decrease over the next decade, which continued for males but reversed for females over the final period. Again, and despite the large mortality ratio, factors other than smoking obviously dominated the secular trends.

Also intriguing are the decreases in death-rates from buccal cancer, which has the moderately large mortality ratio of 3·8. (In Hirayama's (1972) study, the mortality ratio for cancers of the mouth was 10·0.) We might feel tempted to attribute the fall in the death-rates among men to the decline in the consumption of pipe tobacco. From 1890 to 1939 consumption fell, at the most, by about a factor of 2 (Todd, 1972). However, the fall in SMR, 1911–20 to 1950–54, was a factor of 3·2 for men. When we bear in mind that non-smokers also develop buccal cancer this discrepancy is serious enough, but the explanation in terms of pipe-smoking is still further embarrassed by the magnitude of the mortality ratio for men who smoked pipes only. This was a mere 3·1 in Kahn's study (based, however, on only four deaths among pipe smokers) as compared with 3·8 for current cigarette smokers and 4·1 for smokers of cigars only.

Where stomach and bladder cancers are concerned, it is perhaps sufficient to note that the secular trends in SMR for the two sexes diverge at the end of the studied period when they might be expected to converge.

The data plotted in Figure 10.4 also fail to show the secular trends that

would be expected if mortality ratios greater than unity signify a carcinogenic action of cigarette smoke. In particular, cancer of the larynx, with the
high mortality ratio of 9·5, presents the same kind of problem as cancer of
the pharynx. Stell (1972) has drawn attention to this contradiction between
the secular trends in SMR and the mortality ratio. The overall decline in
SMR for men actually exceeded that for women; the causal hypothesis
predicts a fairly substantial secular rise in both sexes, but larger in men than
in women.

Overall, Figures 10.2 to 10.4 show that, when both sexes are at risk, the
secular trends of SMRs for men roughly parallel those for women. No sign
of the expected 30-year lag of increase in women can be discerned in any of
the data. If we wish to retain the causal hypothesis, we have to invoke a
different set of *ad hoc* arguments to explain the trends for each site. Factors
that were responsible for the changes in SMR at a given site with time had,
in the main, a rather similar and *simultaneous* impact on the two sexes.
Generally, the timing of the impact of these factors differed from site to site.
Clearly, no corroboration of the causal interpretation of mortality ratios
can be extracted from this study of secular trends. Stell (1972) excepted, it
is curious that so little attention should have been directed to these paradoxes;
we might have expected cigarette manufacturers to have been encouraged
by them.

Negative associations

In connection with the possibility that cigarette smoking produces a general
systemic carcinogen we must note that in Kahn's (1966) study, cancer of the
rectum shows a tendency towards a negative association with cigarette
smoking (mortality ratio = 0·90). Hammond (1966) found a mortality ratio
for colorectal cancer (history of cigarette smoking)/(never smoked regularly)
of 1·01 for men aged 45 to 64 years; 1·17 for men 65 to 79 years; but 0·78
for women 45 to 64 years with a history of cigarette smoking, and 0·66
for women 45 to 64 years classed as 'heavier' smokers. In Hirayama's (1972)
Japanese study, the mortality ratio for rectal cancer in men was 0·86, but
1·06 for women. In Doll and Hill's study of British male doctors the mortality
ratio for bowel cancer (cigarette smokers)/(non-smokers), was 0·84, but for
rectal cancer the association was positive, with a corresponding mortality
ratio of 2·4.

Choi, Schuman and Gullen (1970), in a case-control study of subjects aged
20 years and over, found that primary central nervous system neoplasms
(glioma, astrocytoma, glioblastoma and meningioma) are negatively
associated ($P = 0·017$) with cigarette smoking. No disparity between cases
and controls was found in the frequency of cigar or pipe smokers. A negative

association was also found between CNS neoplasms and alcohol consumption $(P = 0.007)$.

These several findings conflict with the idea that positive associations between cigarette smoking and cancers should be attributed to a general, non-specific carcinogen, with a systemic distribution.

Another very intriguing finding concerns the connections between smoking, oral leukoplakia, the histological character (dysplasic, non-dysplasic) of the epithelium in oral leukoplakia, and the development of oral carcinoma. Oral leukoplakia is much more common among tobacco users than non-users. In a Swedish series of 782 patients (522 M and 260 F), only 17 per cent did not use tobacco (Einhorn and Wersäll, 1967). Roed-Petersen, Bánóczy and Pindborg (1973) studied 345 Danish and 184 Hungarian patients with oral leukoplakia. They found that epithelial dysplasia was as common among non-smokers (21 per cent) as among smokers (20 per cent). However, the development of oral carcinoma is much *more* frequent among *non*-smoking than smoking patients (Einhorn and Wersäll, 1967; Roed-Petersen, 1971; and Bánóczy and Sugár, 1973). In the large Swedish series studied by Einhorn and Wersäll (1967), the frequency of oral carcinoma in non-smoking leukoplakia patients was eight times that in smokers. In the smaller series followed up by Roed-Petersen (1971) the corresponding ratio was five to one. It is difficult to believe that cigarette smoke is anti-carcinogenic with respect to the induction of oral carcinoma in patients with oral leukoplakia.

Negative associations have been found consistently between smoking and the non-malignant neurologic disorder, Parkinson's disease. In Kahn's (1966) study, the mortality ratio: (current smokers)/(never smoked or occasional only), was 0·26. In Hammond's (1966) study, the mortality ratio for men 45 to 64 years, (cigarette smoking only)/(never smoked regularly) was 0·76, and for the age group 65 to 79 years, was 0·81. Nefzger, Quadfasel and Karl (1968) found that among 138 patients with Parkinson's disease only 70 per cent had ever smoked compared with 84 per cent of 166 controls. The differences in smoking habits are seen prior to the onset of Parkinson's disease and hence the negative association is not brought about by the disease itself. Nefzger *et al.* (1968) also found that those diseases that are positively associated with smoking are infrequently reported in patients with Parkinson's disease. Kessler (1972) reported similar findings and in a community-based survey confirmed results previously obtained from a study of hospital patients; only 45·9 per cent of male patients with Parkinson's disease had ever smoked compared with 68·9 per cent of male controls; the corresponding values for women were 24·5 per cent and 36·8 per cent respectively.

Westlund (1970) used data from Norwegian counties to test the hypothesis of a negative correlation between lung cancer and Parkinson's disease. For deaths at all ages, he found a rank correlation coefficient of -0.17 and for disability from Parkinson's disease in relation to the incidence of lung cancer the coefficient was -0.44.

If smoking has a prophylactic effect Westlund pointed out that we would expect to find: (a) a secular *decrease* in morbidity and mortality from Parkinson's disease, as the result of the secular *increase* in smoking; and (b) a higher mortality in rural than in urban areas. He was unable to confirm either expectation; secular trends in mortality, 1951 to 1968, were upward in both sexes and age- and sex-adjusted death-rates were higher in urban than in rural municipalities.

If cigarette smoking does not protect against Parkinson's disease, how then do we account for the negative association? As we have seen, the problem is a more general one. In addition to the instances quoted above, Rothman and Manson (1973) found a negative association between smoking and another neurological disorder, trigeminal neuralgia. In his prospective Japanese study involving a total of 11858 deaths, Hirayama (1972) found, among other negative associations with cigarette smoking, mortality ratios for diabetes of 0.71 in men and 0.81 in women.

Dose-response relations

We saw in Chapter 9 that no universal relation exists between the dose of carcinogen and incidence of induced tumours. However, at fairly low levels, incidence often increases approximately linearly, or with the square of dose. For most cancers positively associated with smoking, a more or less linear relation with the rate of smoking is observed, but cancer of the stomach provides an interesting exception. Thus, in Kahn's (1966) study, the mortality ratio for males smoking one to nine cigarettes a day is 1.7; at ten to 30 cigarettes a day it is 1.4; at 31 to 39 cigarettes a day it is 1.6; and for more than 39 cigarettes a day the ratio is 1.8. Doll and Hill (1964) found that standardized death-rates for stomach cancer in non-smokers closely resembled those in smokers of cigarettes: however, corresponding death-rates in 'mixed' smokers were approximately halved. In a survey of stomach cancer among the Japanese in Hawaii, Haenszel *et al.* (1972) found that males smoking more than 20 cigarettes a day had a lower incidence than those smoking fewer than 20 cigarettes a day.

A similar 'dose-response' relation has been proposed in connection with poorly differentiated squamous cell carcinoma of the lung (Weiss *et al*, 1972). At one to ten cigarettes per day, the age- and race-adjusted rate was 0.7 per 1000 per year (based on only two cases); at ten to 19 per day, the equivalent rate was 0.4 per 1000 per year (based on six cases); and at 20+

per day the rate was 1·0 per 1000 per year (based on five cases). Numbers are small, but the indications are intriguing. For other histological types of lung cancer—well-differentiated squamous cell carcinoma, small cell carcinoma, adenocarcinoma, but excepting large cell carcinoma of which only four cases were recorded—adjusted mortality rates increased with the daily rate of smoking (Weiss *et al.*, (1972).

Flat dose-response relations (which will be discussed later), in common with negative associations between smoking and disease, pose difficulties for causal theories.

Alternative Interpretations

In principle, the simplest way to assess rigorously the disease-inducing effects of an agent A, is to study two populations, one not treated with A to serve as a control group, and the other, experimental group, which we treat with A: in all other pertinent respects, the two groups should be alike. These desiderata can be closely approached in experiments with animals. Genetic differences can be minimized (but not always completely eliminated) by the use of highly inbred strains; age and sex can be accurately controlled; and environmental factors such as diet, housing, exposure/non-exposure to pathogenic micro-organisms can often be satisfactorily manipulated and standardized by the experimenter. When all such precautions have been taken and we then find that disease D_i appears consistently in the treated group but not in the control group—or, say, at a repeatable and significantly higher level in the treated than in the control group—then we are entitled to conclude that some form of causal relation exists between A and D_i. Of course, such an experiment tells us nothing about the existence of other causal factors. The agent A might effect or facilitate only one step in a complex causal chain. Also, we might carry out a closely similar experiment using a different strain of animal, to find that A fails to induce D_i in this second strain.

Obviously, the requirement of the strictly controlled experiment cannot be met or even approached in epidemiological studies of disease in man. Many potential complications can be recognized. In studies of the effects of smoking in an outbred population such as man we could, in principle, hope to allow for the genetic factor, at least approximately, by suitable randomization. Unfortunately, this principle cannot be realized in practice. Under no circumstances short of absolute compulsion could I be persuaded to smoke 20 or even two cigarettes a day. In a free society, smokers remain self-selected although they may be subjected to various and conflicting pressures, including those from cigarette advertisers on the one hand, and those from the Royal College of Physicians on the other. Because of this factor of self-selection, the usual studies of simple associations between smoking and disease fail to satisfy the minimum requirements for valid scientific inference. There is always the possibility that a common cause might influence the decision to smoke and affect the risk of contracting a certain disease. Also, in logic, we need to consider the possibility that the disease, or, say, a pre-disease associated condition, might influence the smoking habit of the subject (Fisher, 1959).

This is not to say that studies of simple associations are useless, or that we can never draw valid conclusions from epidemiological surveys. But we have to recognize, and with appropriate ingenuity to try to circumvent, the effects of self-selection and other biases.

Yerushalmy (1972) went a long way towards achieveing these objectives in connection with the well-known association between the low birth-weight of babies and maternal smoking. He first discovered that although the mean birth-weight of babies born to smoking mothers was indeed lower than that of babies born to non-smokers, the low birth-weight babies of smokers had a *lower* neonatal death-rate than the low birth-weight babies of non-smokers (Yerushalmy, 1971). Various other paradoxical findings alerted Yerushalmy to the possibility that the association between maternal smoking and low birth-weight might not be causal. These included the discovery that the age at menarche was lower for smoking than for non-smoking mothers. Doubts about the validity of the causal interpretation were carried an important stage further when Yerushalmy (1972) found that women who subsequently became smokers had a high incidence of low birth-weight infants during the period *before they started to smoke*. This evidence, if confirmed in other studies, supports the hypothesis that the higher incidence of low birth-weight infants is due to the *smoker* rather than the *smoking*.

Constitutional theories

Yerushalmy's (1971, 1972) findings lead us to one of the two main alternatives to causal interpretations of positive associations. If the constitution of the mother is largely responsible both for her small babies and her decision to smoke, then we may reasonably seek an explanation in terms of genetics. We would need to postulate a net positive association between the genes that predispose to smoking, and those that predispose to low birth-weight babies. In view of the anthropometric differences found between smoking and non-smoking males (Seltzer, 1963, 1967), and even between cigar and pipe-smoking males (Seltzer, 1972), such a theory is not implausible. (Further evidence for the role of genetic factors in smoking will be considered later.)

Fisher (1958(a), (b), 1959) and Berkson (1959) put forward a constitutional hypothesis of the association between smoking and lung cancer and this will also be considered later in this chapter.

At this stage, it is sufficient to point out that constitutional hypotheses are not embarrassed by the lack of consistency between mortality ratios and secular change illustrated in Figures 10.2 to 10.4 and discussed above. Neither do they have any difficulty in accounting for negative associations: on the contrary, such relations are predicted by them. Similarly, the observed differences in mortality ratios from one genetically distinctive population to another are to be expected.

Approximately linear dose-response relations can be explained if social as well as complex genetic factors contribute to certain smoking habits. As Seltzer's (1972) survey shows, different genetic factors are likely to be associated with different forms of smoking; in certain persons, the genetic influence might be minimal and social factors might dominate. If these 'social' smokers tend not to be predisposed to, say, lung cancer, and if their proportion in any smoking category is roughly inversely proportional to the daily rate of smoking, then an approximately linear (pseudo) dose-response relation would be observed. More complicated models, involving different genotypes for different rates of cigarette smoking, are not excluded.

In the case of stomach cancer, and the absence of a dose-response gradient, we would need to postulate a net positive association between a gene or genes that help to predispose to any form of cigarette smoking—so called 'social' and 'compulsive'—and a gene or genes that predispose to stomach cancer.

Disease causes habit—Another possibility should be remembered in connection with positive associations: the disease D_i, or an associated pre-disease condition, might cause the habit H (Fisher, 1959). Although Fisher believed the 'common cause' or 'constitutional' explanation to be the more likely where lung cancer is concerned, he was not prepared to exclude entirely the idea that the pre-cancerous condition causes smoking.

Lung Cancer

Antismoking propaganda has relied heavily on the strength of the association between cigarette smoking and lung cancer in men. Most of the large retrospective and prospective epidemiological studies have involved Caucasian populations and these have generally given a mortality ratio: (male cigarette smokers)/(male non-smokers) in the region of nine to 14 (Surgeon General's Report, 1971). So far as I am aware, only one large-scale prospective survey has been made of a non-Caucasian population—that of

Hirayama (1972) in Japan. For men aged 40 years and over he found a mortality ratio of only 3·85, in contrast to 10·0 for cancer of the mouth and 11·0 for cancer of the larynx; for women aged 40 years and over he obtained the following ratios: 2·44 (lung), 1·22 mouth and 9·0 larynx.

This lack of reproducibility in mortality ratios between genetically dissimilar populations, and between Japanese males and females shows, quite apart from the secular trends discussed above and below, that no *simple* causal interpretation of positive associations can be sustained. The findings highlight the need for a deeper study of the factors that complicate the relation between smoking and disease and, in particular, an understanding of the role of the 'host'.

The importance of secular trends has been acknowledged, but mainly (for obvious reasons) in the context of lung cancer. Thus, the 1971 Report of the Royal College of Physicians states (p. 63): 'The chief reason for rejecting the genetic hypothesis is its inability to account for the enormous rise in death rates from lung cancer in the past half century'. I shall consider this objection in detail below, but the reader will scarcely be surprised to learn that I also wish to emphasize the importance of the sex- and age-dependence of the disease.

Secular trends in lung cancer according to sex-dependence and age-dependence

The sex- and age-dependence of recorded death-rates from lung cancer in England and Wales are shown in Figures 10.5 to 10.11. These data cover the entire period from 1901 to 1970 in five-year steps. Throughout, data for men above the age of about 40 years are fitted to the same basic equation with $n = 2$, $r = 5$; the values of k and S are adjusted to give a good fit by eye. Data for women above about the age of 40 years are fitted to the equation with $n = 1$, $r = 6$; appropriate adjustments to k and S are made to give a good fit. (As we shall see, this is a slight oversimplification.) For both sexes, a latent period correction of 2·5 years has been applied throughout. (The curve with $n = 3$, $r = 4$ has a very similar shape to the one with $n = 2$, $r = 5$, over a restricted range of t on both sides of the mode, and it gives a generally satisfactory fit to these and other data for males in other countries.)

This curve-fitting procedure should be regarded as a convenient device for obtaining a form of age-standardized death-rate—in terms of the parameters S_M and S_F. As we shall see, it would be unwise to place heavy biological emphasis on the detailed form of these particular age-patterns.

Sex-differences in the apparent number and type of initiating events which, despite the many uncertainties described below are probably real, imply that the genetic predisposition to the major forms of lung cancer differs between the two sexes. The possibility of a Y-linked predisposing

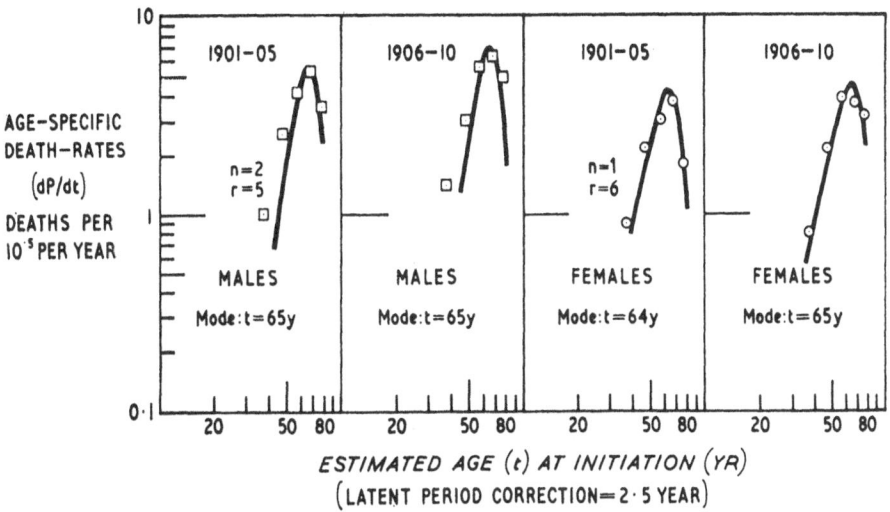

Figure 10.5 Sex-specific and age-specific death-rates (log scale) from malignant neo-plasms of the lung and pleura, England and Wales, 1901–10, against estimated age at initiation (log scale) (General Register Office, 1950)

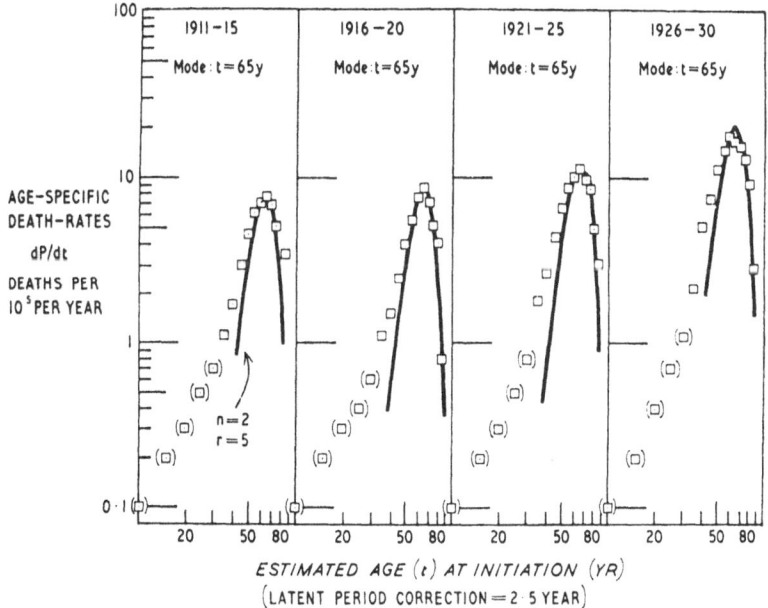

Figure 10.6 Age-specific death-rates, males (log scale) from malignant neoplasms of the lung and pleura, England and Wales, 1911–30, against estimated age at initiation (log scale) (General Register Office, 1957)

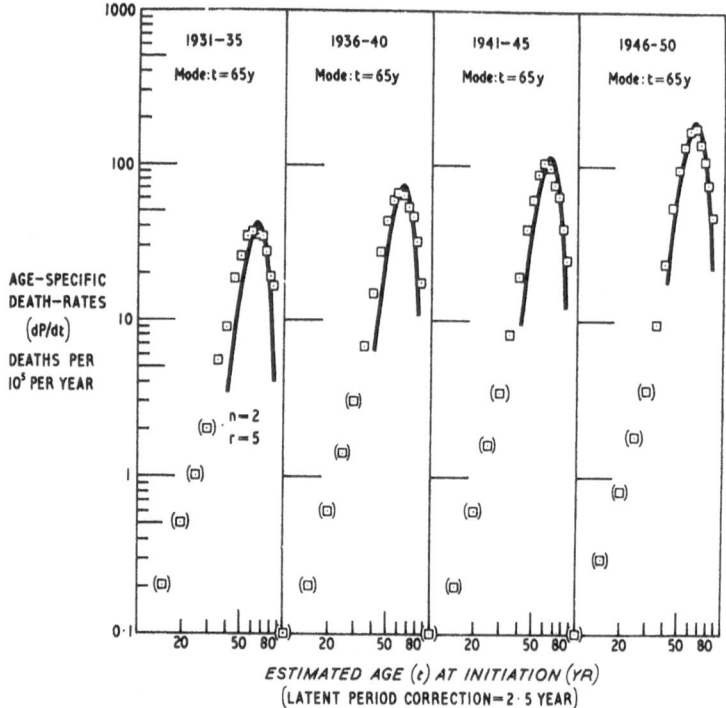

Figure 10.7 As for Figure 10.6. Period 1931–50

factor (and/or Y-linked somatic mutation) in males has to be considered as well as autosomal and X-linked factors. (It will be interesting to discover whether predisposition to certain forms of smoking also entails sex-linkage (X and/or Y).) Sex-differences are seen in the survival time between the diagnosis of lung cancer and death: on average, women survive longer than men (Ederer and Mersheimer, 1962; California Tumour Registry, 1963). This is unlikely to be due to the fact that the smoking rates of women are generally lower than in men because, among men, heavy smokers have the best survival and non-smokers the worst (Linden et al., 1972).

Following Case (1956(a), (b)), I had expected that vertical analysis of mortality statistics for lung cancer would fail to show any simple form of reproducibility because of the enormous cohort changes. However, as pointed out in Chapter 6, the choice between vertical, horizontal and other analyses, depends on the *cause* of secular change and the objectives of the analysis. Such regularities as are shown in Figures 10.5 to 10.11 were unexpected because I had assumed, in common with others, that cigarette smoking was a major cause of the secular increase.

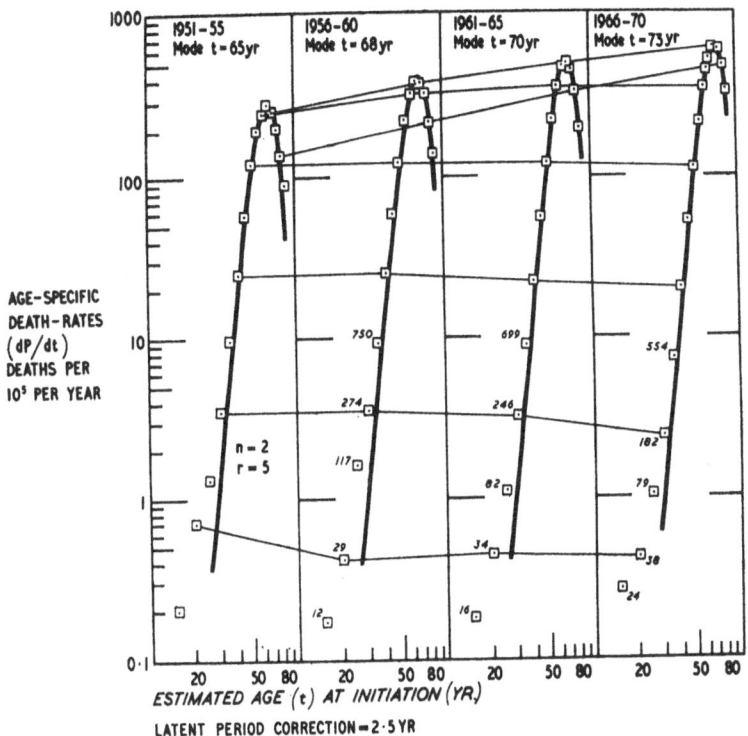

Figure 10.8 As for Figure 10.6. Period 1951–70. Data from General Register Office (1957) and annual reports (Medical) of the Registrar General

Above $t = 30$ to 50 years, depending on the period, we find unexpectedly that the curves of age-specific death-rates (dP/dt), versus initiation age (t), stay fairly constant in *shape*. Throughout, but especially during the past 20 years, all the data above $t = 40$ years give a reasonable fit to unmodified theoretical curves, despite the very large increase in absolute death-rates. The age for the modal dP/dt remained almost constant at about 65 years in the data for men from 1901 to 1955 and then increased to about 73 in 1966–70. For women, the modal age was about 64 to 66 years from 1901 to 1930 and it then shifted upwards to 75 years in 1951–55, followed by a slight decline to 73 years in 1966–70.

Possible Causal Mechanisms

Consider the effects to be expected if cigarette smoke acts as (a) an initiator; (b) a promoter; or (c) a precipitator—directly or indirectly—after the manner of a micro-organism or allergen (see Figure 10.12). An initiator might act by increasing the average rate of those somatic mutations that would otherwise

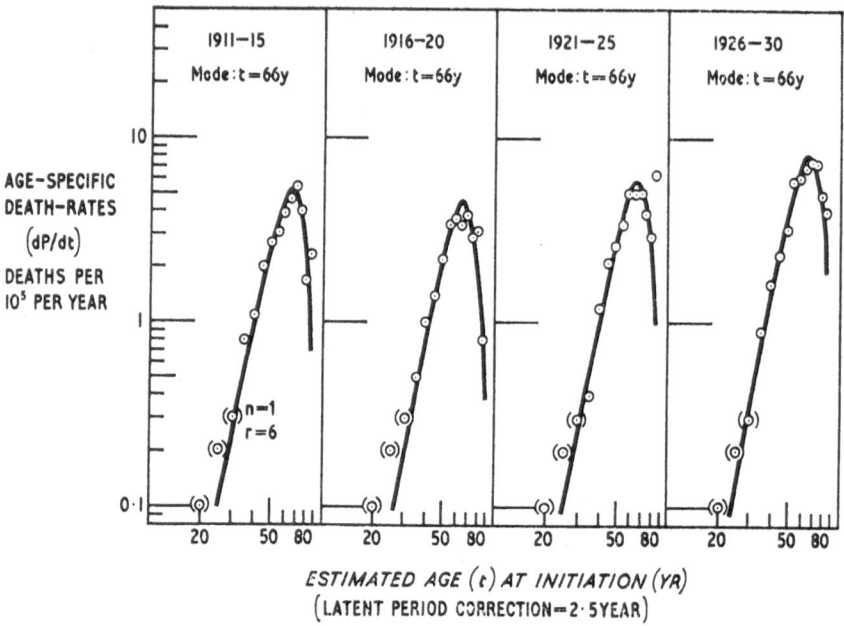

Figure 10.9 Age-specific death-rates, females (log scale), from malignant neoplasms of the lung and pleura, England and Wales, 1911–30, against estimated age at initiation (log scale) (General Register Office, 1957)

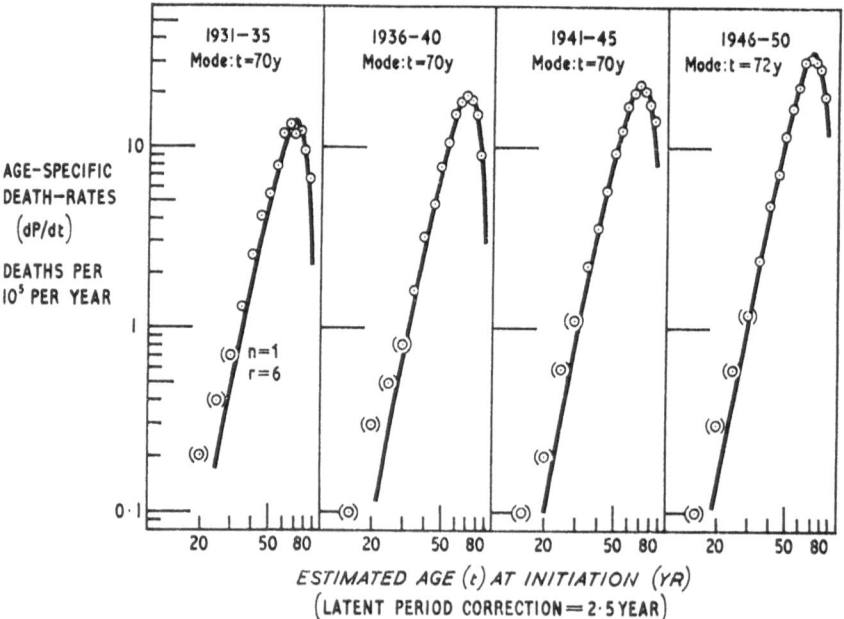

Figure 10.10 As for Figure 10.9. Period 1931–50

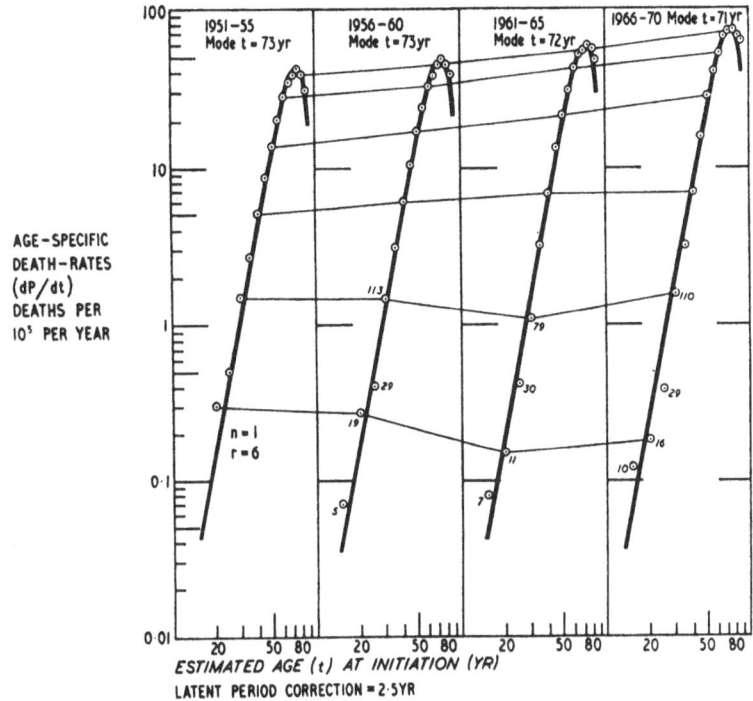

Figure 10.11 As for Figure 10.9. Period 1951–70. Data from General Register Office (1957) and the Registrar General's Annual Medical Reports

occur spontaneously (thus producing an increase in k) and/or by initiating changes in peripheral growth-control cells of a kind that would not occur under natural conditions (see Chapter 9). In either event, the shape of the age-pattern and/or the position of the mode would be expected to differ between smokers and non-smokers. Figures 10.5 to 10.11 support neither of these initiator mechanisms. The calculated value of k remained constant for the earlier part of the century, but in recent years it *decreased*, especially in males.

Mortality ratios in relation to age (Hammond, 1966; Kahn, 1966), show no consistent trends, suggesting that k has a similar or identical value in male smokers and non-smokers. In Kahn's (1966) report, the mortality ratio for males: (total current cigarette smokers)/(never smoked or occasional only) is 13·8 at 35 to 64 years; 9·4 at 65 to 74 years and 8·8 at 75 to 84 years—showing a decline with age; but in Hammond's (1966) study, the mortality ratio: (cigarettes only)/(never smoked regularly) increases with age from 7·2 at 35 to 54 years; to 9·8 at 55 to 59 years; and 10·7 at 70 to 84 years. Clearly, no marked or consistent differences in the form of the age-dependence of

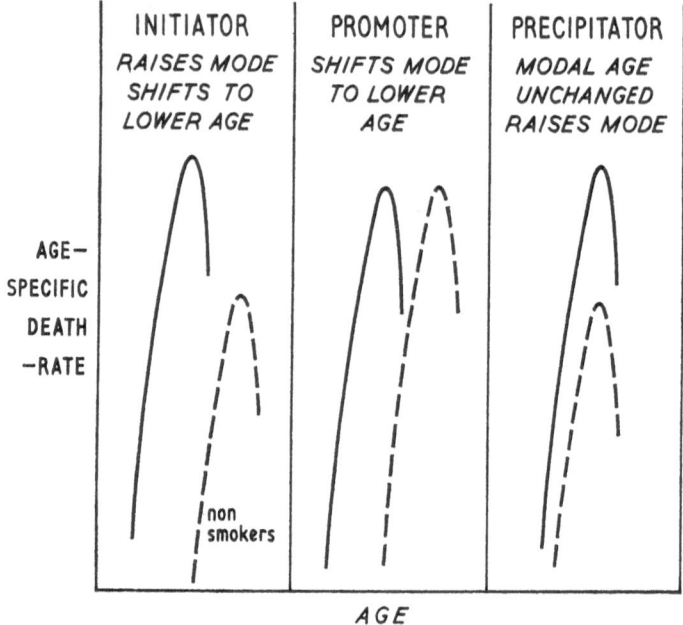

Figure 10.12 Predicted effects of hypothetical initiating, promoting and precipitating carcinogens in cigarette smoke on the age-distribution of death-rates from an induced cancer. Broken curves represent age-specific death-rates in non-smokers. Continuous curves show predicted effects of carcinogens in tobacco smoke, according to type of carcinogen. The initiator is assumed to increase the value of the kinetic constant, k: it might, however, produce a drastic change in the shape of the age-pattern (see Chapter 9)

lung cancer exists between smokers and non-smokers above 35 years, and hence the statistical character and rate of initiating events appear to be similar, or identical, in both types of person.

That the rate of smoking does not appreciably affect the mean age of onset in men was shown vividly by Passey (1962). He examined the records of 499 men with lung cancer who attended the Joint Consultation Clinic of the Royal Marsden Hospital and the Brompton Hospital during the period 1948–56. The mean age at onset of lung cancer in 90 men smoking one to ten cigarettes a day was 58·6 years; for 178 men smoking 11 to 20 it was 57·0 years; for 132 men smoking 21 to 30 it was 57·1 years; for 52 smoking 31 to 40 it was 55·9 years and for 43 smoking 41 to 50 it was 56·6 years. The overall average was 57·3 years. (A criticism of Passey's paper by Pike and Doll (1965) was based in part on the false assumption that age-specific death-rates from lung cancer are simply proportional to a power of (adjusted) age, throughout the lifespan.) Passey also showed that rates of smoking for early age of onset were not higher than those for late age of onset: for cases with age of onset at 20 to 34 years, the average rate was 20 a day; at 35 to 39 years, 22 a day; at 40 to 44 years, 23 a day; at 45 to 49 years, 25 a day; at 50 to 54 years, 24 a day; at 55 to 59 years, 24 a day; at 60 to 64 years, 22 a day; at 65 to 69 years, 20 a day; at 70 to 74 years, 21 a day; and at 75 to 79 years, 25 a day. Passey's findings have been confirmed recently by Herrold (1972) in her study of 2241 US war veterans (from Dorn's series) for whom lung cancer was listed on the death certificates either as the underlying or contributory cause of death.

The scope of promoting action—given an average latent period of perhaps one or a few years between the completion of initiation and onset—is small and hence (b) can be discounted as an important influence.

That leaves us with (c). Neglecting the recent apparent decreases in k_M and k_F, we see that the data in Figures 10.5 to 10.11; those for mortality ratios as a function of age (Hammond, 1966; Kahn, 1966); and Passey's (1962) and Herrold's (1972) findings for the independence of age at onset on rate of smoking; are all reasonably consistent with the view that smoking acts directly or indirectly as a precipitator of the forbidden clones that induce lung cancer.

Secular trends in death-rates and tobacco consumption

It will be seen that the secular increases in dP/dt have been largely confined to the higher age-groups. In 1911–15, the value of dP/dt for men at $t=20$ years was 0·3 deaths per 10^5 per year, and in 1966–70 it was only 0·4 deaths per 10^5 per year; for women, the corresponding values of dP/dt were 0·1 and 0·2 respectively. Even the most recent statistics for men show a 'surplus mortality' above the theoretical curve below $t=30$ years. This surplus might be attributable to oat cell carcinoma, which has a relatively early age of onset. Among 40 persons who developed lung cancer before the age of 40, Kennedy (1972) found that 26 (19 male, 7 female) or 65 per cent, had oat cell carcinoma.

Increases in dP/dt at higher ages are best reflected in the calculated values of S, the apparent proportions of the population at risk with respect to recorded death from late-onset lung cancer. For men, S rose from $1·47 \times 10^{-3}$ in 1901–05, to 187×10^{-3} in 1966–70, a factor of 127; for women, a much smaller rise was recorded over the same period: $1·19 \times 10^{-3}$ to $25·1 \times 10^{-3}$, a factor of only 21. These secular changes in S_M and S_F, and in cigarette consumption by 5-yearly averages, are illustrated in Figure 10.13.

A serious complication strikes us immediately. The sharp upturn in S_M and S_F around 1920 was simultaneous in both sexes although the upsurge

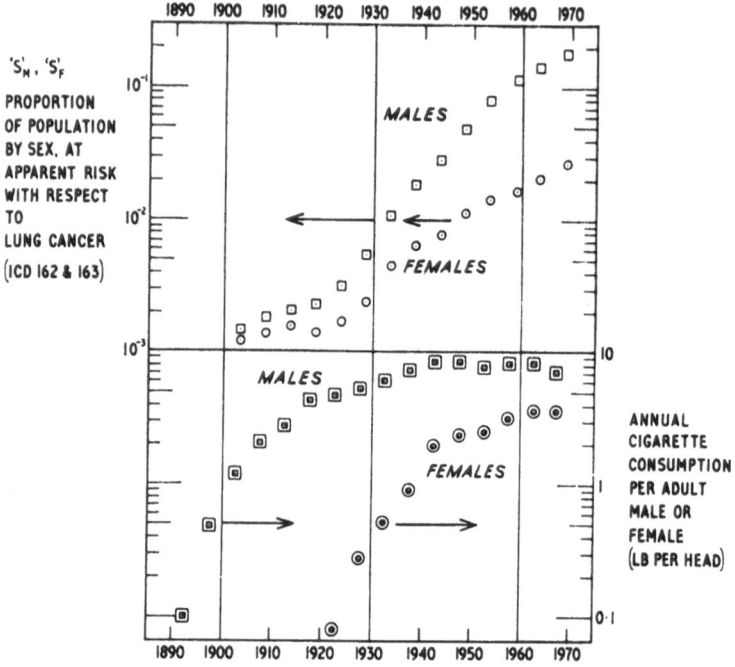

Figure 10.13 Upper panel: Results of analysis of data shown in Figures 10.5 to 10.11 in terms of the proportions of the male (S_M) and female (S_F) populations at apparent risk with respect to recorded death from lung cancer (log scale), in relation to calendar year. Lower panel: Average annual cigarette consumption per adult male, or female, by quinquennia (log scale), in relation to calendar year. The sharp post-1920 increases in S_M and S_F are synchronous

in the consumption of cigarettes by women lagged some 30 years behind that for men. This feature, coupled with the similarity of the time-dependence of S_M and S_F (apart from the magnitudes), at once raises the doubt as to whether any of the secular increases in death-rates were due to tobacco.

A more revealing way of examining the relation between S_M and S_F, and time, is to plot the proportionate increase from period to period as a function of time (Figure 10.14). Increments in S_M and S_F due to certain common causes unrelated to tobacco consumption (such as diagnosis, atmospheric pollution from motor car exhausts and other factors) are likely to be approximately in phase in the two sexes, whereas increments in S_M due to cigarette consumption should precede those in S_F by about 30 years. Figure 10.14 shows that proportionate increments in the two sexes (ΔS_M, ΔS_F) have been overwhelmingly in phase. Thus, minima occurred in both sexes between 1911–15 and 1916–20; 1936–40 and 1941–45; and 1956–60 and 1961–65.

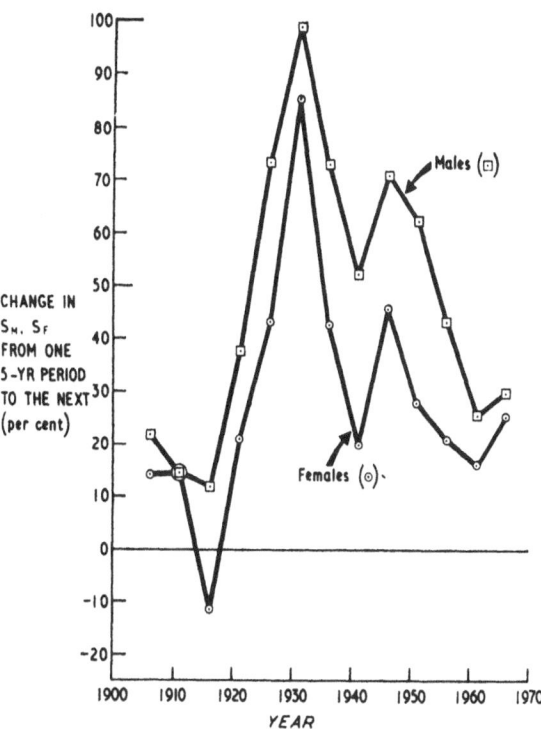

Figure 10.14 Data in Figure 10.13 analysed to show the fine structure of secular change in S_M and S_F. The ordinate gives the increments in S_M and S_F from one five-year period to the next. With one exception, these increments are larger for men than women, but in step. The cause(s) of secular change in S_M and S_F are largely or wholly synchronous and unrelated to the secular increases (see Figures 10.1 and 10.13) in cigarette consumption

Maxima in both sexes were also coincident in time: between 1926–30 and 1931–35; and 1941–45 and 1946–50.

Because the sharp rise in cigarette smoking by women lagged some 30 years behind that in men, cigarette-associated increases in S_F should have lagged some 30 years behind those in men, provided the induction period is similar in the two sexes. In Figure 10.15, the increments (ΔS_M) in S_M, from one five-year period to the next, 1906 to 1936, are compared with the increments, ΔS_F, in S_F that occurred 30 years later, 1936 to 1966. Apart from the initial fall in increments for both sexes, the directions of all the other changes in ΔS_M and S_F are opposite in the two sexes. Thus, the 'in phase' changes in the two sexes expected on the basis of the causal hypothesis, are conspicuously absent. Figures 10.14 and 10.15 show, therefore, that the changes in recorded death-rates from lung cancer in both

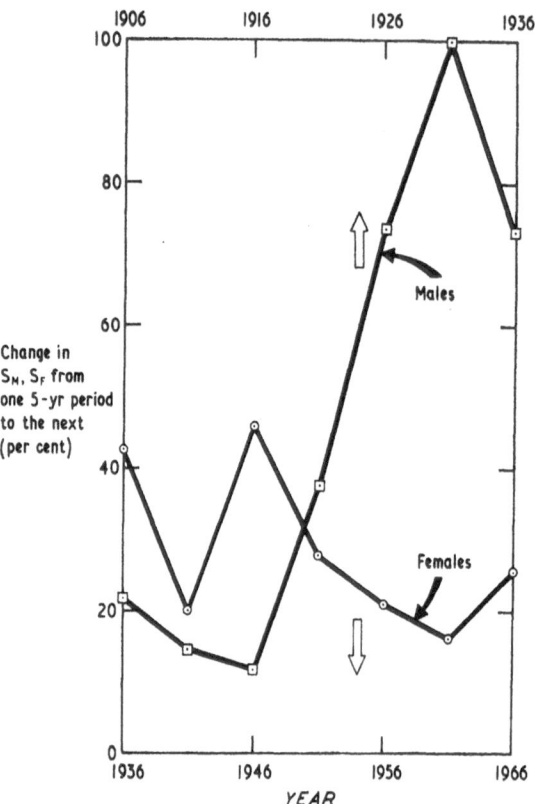

Figure 10.15 Data in Figure 10.14 replotted to allow for the 30-year lag in the rise of cigarette consumption by women behind that of men. The curve for males shows the increments in S_M from 1906 to 1936 and the curve for females shows increments in S_F from 1936 to 1966. If the increases in cigarette consumption by the two sexes had been responsible for the increases in S_M and S_F the two curves would have been approximately in step, with the curve for women lying consistently below that for men—roughly as in Figure 10.14.

sexes, between 1901 and 1970, were largely and perhaps wholly unconnected with the increase in tobacco consumption. Thus, we cannot conclude from these data that the major part of the increments in S_M and S_F was caused by smoking, acting as an initiator, promoter or precipitator. However, the overall increases in the higher age-groups are so large they might conceal a small causal effect.

Expected secular increase in lung cancer

From: (a) the supposed dose-response relation between the rate of cigarette smoking and the death-rate from lung cancer (Doll and Hill, 1964); (b) death-rates from lung cancer in pipe and/or cigar smokers (Doll and Hill, 1964); and (c) data for the total consumption of cigarette and tobacco goods per adult male (Todd, 1972), we can estimate the expected approximate increase in death-rates from lung cancer in males during this century that should be attributed to smoking.

In 1956, the earliest year for which detailed statistics of smoking in the United Kingdom are available (Todd, 1972), 1·7 million men smoked pipes only, and 2·1 million were 'mixed' smokers. From the point of view of pipe smoking, we can regard these two categories as being roughly equivalent to a population of 2·7 millions smoking a total of 19·5 million pounds of pipe tobacco. Some 3740 manufactured cigarettes per adult man were consumed in 1956 (Todd, 1972). Because of the approximate linearity of the presumed dose-response relation (Doll and Hill, 1964), we can estimate the total carcinogenic hazard of tobacco by 'spreading' the total consumption of cigarettes and pipe tobacco over the whole male population. From Figure 1 of Doll and Hill (1964), the annual standardized death-rate from lung cancer per 10^3 men from 3740 cigarettes per man would be expected to be about 0·77, as compared to 0·07 in non-smokers. Pipe and/or cigar smokers had a standardized death-rate of 0·47 per 10^3 per year (that is 0·40 above non-smokers). This rate, spread through the entire adult male population of 18·3 millions, would produce an increase of about 0·4 × (2·7/18·3) or 0·06 above that of non-smokers. Consumption of all forms of tobacco by males was fairly steady for about 20 years before 1956 and has tended to fall in recent years (Todd, 1972). Hence, we would expect recent standardized death-rates in men due to smoking alone to be about 0·76 per 10^3 per year above that of non-smokers, or 0·83 per 10^3 per year, overall.

For death-rates at the beginning of the century, we can neglect the small consumption of cigarettes (which had only just begun) and consider tobacco, cigars and snuff, the sale of which increased from 63·5 million pounds in 1880 to 80·4 million pounds in 1900. Thus the average consumption of such tobacco over this period was about 3·7 times that in 1956. Consequently, the expected standardized death-rate in males around the turn of the century attributable to pipe smoking would have been about 0·06 × 3·7 or 0·22, giving 0·29 per 10^3 per year in all, allowing for the rate in non-smokers.

Thus the expected increase in standardized death-rates for males between about 1901–05 and recent years is about 0·83/0·29, or a factor of around 2·9. (Although the consumption of cigarettes has greatly increased, that of pipe tobacco has fallen by about one-third.)

When we contrast this expected factor of about 2·9 with the observed change in S_M between 1901–05 and 1966–70 (a factor of 127) we can appreciate that increases resulting from causes unrelated to tobacco must have swamped any increase due to smoking, as Figure 10.14 implies quite clearly.

The data for women also show a big discrepancy between expected and observed increases. In 1956, some 1430 cigarettes were consumed per adult woman, in contrast to 3740 by men, From Hammond's (1966) survey, lung cancer mortality ratios for women, at comparable levels of smoking, appear to be about one-third of those in men, although the data do not allow an accurate cross-comparison. In men, smoking 3740 cigarettes per year, the mortality ratio: (cigarette smokers)/(non-smokers) was about ten. Hence, for women, the increase in lung cancer death-rates in recent years compared to those at the beginning of the century (when women did not smoke to any extent) should, on the causal hypothesis, be about a factor of $\{1 + (10 \times 0.33 \times 1430/3470)\}$, or 2·3—in contrast to the observed factor of 21.

The Royal College of Physicians (1971) use a somewhat different argument. As mentioned above, they state that the chief reason for rejecting the genetic hypothesis is its inability to explain the 'enormous rise in death-rates from lung cancer in the past half-century'. With a superb *non sequitur*, they dismiss the idea that the increase is 'fictitious, and due to doctors having mistaken lung cancer for other diseases in the earlier part of this century', because the 'rise has been far greater in men than in women'—as, indeed, it has been. That the recorded increases in the higher age-groups have been many times higher than the causal theory predicts (by a factor of around 44 in men and nine in women) are among the quantitative details the Royal College overlooked. We might be tempted to argue that because recorded increases in S_M and S_F have been so large, some small part at least must be genuine and caused by tobacco; such temptations to spurious logic should again be resisted. If a causal relation between cigarette smoking and lung cancer should eventually be established (against all the odds) cynics will observe that the right suspicions were aroused for the wrong reasons.

It might be claimed that increases in recorded rates of lung cancer due to causes unrelated to tobacco, including diagnosis, should have the same ratios in the two sexes and that the greater increments of S_M compared with S_F shown in Figure 10.14 reflect true increases in males over females due to heavier smoking by males. Such an argument can be readily refuted. The expected increases due to smoking have similar ratios in the two sexes— a factor of about 2·9 in men and of 2·3 in women—whereas the observed ratios of increases in S_M and S_F (1906 to 1966) show a large sex difference— a factor of 127 for men and only 21 for women. Furthermore, the *per capita* consumption of manufactured cigarettes and all tobacco goods by men has fallen (in both categories by about 36 per cent over the period 1945 to 1971, whereas for women, the corresponding consumption of cigarettes has risen fairly steadily, by an overall factor of 2·4, between 1948 and 1971 (Todd, 1972). Consequently, we would expect increments in S_F during recent years to be conspicuously greater than those in S_M. In fact, the opposite relation is seen in Figure 10.14.

We have to conclude, therefore, in conflict with the Royal College of Physicians (1971), that a quantitative study of secular trends offers no support for the causal hypothesis. Neither, however, does it fully reject that hypothesis. In any case, we are obliged to explain the enormous secular increase in recorded death-rates from lung cancer.

Problems of diagnosis

Many authors realize that great advances in the diagnosis of lung cancer have been achieved during this century. A fascinating review of the nineteenth-century literature, showing an appreciation by the 'old masters' of their under-diagnosis of lung cancer, has been given by Onuigbo (1971). Sehrt (1904) described 178 cases of lung cancer discovered at necropsy, only six of which had been recognized during life. When we consider that the increase in recorded deaths in early-onset cases has been very small from 1901 to 1971 (Figures 10.5 to 10.11), Sehrt's (1904) observations suggest that a large part, if not all, of the increase in the higher age-groups may well have been due to diagnosis.

Smithers (1953) wrote a most entertaining review of the earlier literature and described the difficulties of arriving at a reliable diagnosis of lung cancer. He tells us that in 1912, Adler repudiated the then current view that lung cancer was rare and maintained, on the contrary, that it was a common disease. Smithers (1953) presented death-rates, for men and women separately for (a) respiratory cancer and (b) all other respiratory diseases, for the period 1921 to 1949. He pointed out: 'Without taking any account of patients dying from cardiac disease with similar symptoms there would still have been little difficulty in losing our entire present lung cancer death-rate in the general death-rate from respiratory diseases in the past if these cases were really there to lose'. The greater increase of S_M over S_F could well be related to the higher frequency of 'all other respiratory diseases' in men.

Doll (1955) reported that most members attending a conference at Louvain in 1952 agreed that 'a significant part of the increase in mortality' from lung cancer represented a genuine increase due to cigarette smoking. It would be interesting to know how this conclusion was reached. Figure 10.14 and the above calculations of the increase expected on the causal theory both imply that any genuine increase due to tobacco must have constituted an *insignificant* part of the total. Rigdon and Kirchoff (1952) believed—in line with my deductions—that claims of a genuine increase in the frequency of lung cancer were '. . . open to question'. Willis (1967) emphasized the difficulties of clinical and pathological diagnoses of lung cancer and the high frequency of error. From his extensive review of the literature and his own experience he concluded: '. . . it is not possible either to affirm or to deny that there has been a real increase'.

Feinstein (1968) gives a fascinating description of the many problems involved in diagnosing and recording the cause of death. He describes how, about 50 years ago in the USA, most clinical conditions affecting the lungs were called 'pneumonia' or 'pleurisy' if acute, and 'tuberculosis' if chronic. The use of the chest x-ray did not become common until after 1919. Cancer of the lung first appeared as a separate entity in the mortality data for 1923 and thereafter its recorded annual rates rose steadily. In discussing secular changes in disease-rates generally, Feinstein (1968) concludes that diagnostic changes have played the most important role.

The reliability of the diagnosis given on more recent death certificates has been investigated by various authors. Frequent disagreement between clinicians and pathologists over the diagnosis of lung cancer has been demonstrated. In a survey conducted in 1959 in 75 hospitals of the National Health Service in England and Wales, post-mortem examinations were made routinely on every deceased person, provided relatives did not object (Heasman and Lipworth, 1966). Overall, some 65 per cent of deaths were followed by necropsy. Clinicians diagnosed 338 cases of primary cancer of the lung (7th ICD 162); 417 were diagnosed at necropsy, but only 227 of these agreed with the clinicians' assessment. Assuming the pathologists' diagnosis to be correct, 111, or 33 per cent of the clinicians' diagnoses were false-positive, while 190 genuine cases (46 per cent) of lung cancer were missed, giving rise to a net deficit. Heasman and Lipworth (1966) concluded that a large part of the increase in recorded mortality from cancer of the lung resulted from advances in diagnosis. In 1959 there was '. . . still considerable room for further improvement'.

The accuracy of clinical diagnoses at the Boston City Hospital, US, was investigated by reviewing all necropsies performed from 1955 to 1965 (Beuer and Robbins, 1972). Necropsies disclosed 446 cases of cancer of the lung. The overall clinical diagnostic error for these cases was 49·1 per cent: some 98 cases (22 per cent) were unsuspected. By contrast, the clinical diagnostic error for breast cancer was only 10·7 per cent.

The history of the diagnosis of lung cancer has been reviewed by Rosenblatt (1969). He described the great advances in diagnosis brought about, mainly or wholly in this century, by radiology, bronchoscopy, sputum examination and surgery. His literature survey also shows that in the post-

1930 period, false-positive clinical diagnoses of lung cancer have often been reported due to metastases in the lung from primaries at many different sites. This demonstration agrees with the findings of Heasman and Lipworth (1966). Rosenblatt (1969) believes that the 'prodigious' increase in recorded lung cancer over the past three decades was not due to an extrinsic carcinogen but has resulted from the use of new diagnostic techniques. He also argues that the more recent intense interest in lung cancer has produced a tendency towards overdiagnosis based on radiologic, biopsy and cytologic evidence, in the absence of necropsy. (Smithers (1953) found that even specialists in thoracic diseases made an appreciable proportion of false-positive diagnoses from 1944 to 1950.) Overdiagnosis could explain the shift in the mode in the data for men, from $t \simeq 65$ years in 1951–55, up to $t \simeq 73$ years in 1966–70, and a similar shift in the data for women. Many cancers (see Chapter 7) have a rising age-dependence beyond $t = 65$ years; their occasional false diagnosis as lung cancer will tend to produce a larger increase in dP/dt at a very high t than at medium or low t.

Rosenblatt's (1969) arguments regarding the recent tendency to over-diagnose lung cancer were confirmed by a study of 1000 consecutive necropsies at the Doctor's Hospital, New York, over the period 1st January 1960 to 6th February 1971 (Rosenblatt et al., 1971(a), (b)). Some 493 malig-nant conditions were discovered in 1000 consecutive necropsies, only 27 of which (5·5 per cent of all malignancies) proved to be lung cancer. Among the total of 2779 deaths at the Hospital over this period, some 139 cases, or 11·4 per cent of all malignancies, were diagnosed clinically as lung cancer. Carcinoma of the lung was the only neoplasm to be greatly overdiagnosed clinically and in which no unsuspected cases were found at necropsy. At the other main sites, clinical diagnosis was confirmed by necropsy in some 85 to 100 per cent of instances. Primary lung cancer had been simulated by pulmonary metastases from carcinomas of the pancreas, kidney, stomach, breast and thyroid; and by malignant melanoma (Rosenblatt et al., 1971(a)). It is of great interest that the 5·5 per cent of lung cancers found in this recent New York necropsy series of malignancies is *lower* than the proportions found among several necropsy series from Austria, Germany and the US published at the end of the nineteenth and the beginning of the twentieth centuries (Rosenblatt et al., 1971(b)). In five such series in which necropsy findings were the main basis of diagnosis, lung cancer diagnoses ranged from 8·3 to 11·5 per cent of all cancers. A strict comparison between these early and the recent studies would call for the control of histological criteria, country, age, sex, etc., and the evaluation of possible bias in selecting cases for necropsy. The detailed statistics from the Swedish Cancer Registry (1971) for incidence during the years 1959–65 are largely free from the bias of selection because they cover the whole country. They show that registered cancers of the trachea, bronchus and lung constituted only 5·3 per cent of all cancers.

That the chance of clinical overdiagnosis of lung cancer is now substantial can be appreciated from Berge's (1974) large-scale post-mortem study of the anatomical distribution of metastases in Swedish cancer cases. A total of 747 primary lung cancers was recorded, but some 2097 metastases to the lung were found from primaries at sites outside the lung.

When we consider that in many countries only a minority of certified lung cancer deaths are confirmed by necropsy, the risk of incorrect diagnosis must be regarded as high. Bonser and Thomas (1959) found that in Leeds only 28 per cent of lung cancer deaths had been confirmed by necropsy, while 48 per cent of diagnoses were made without histological examination of any kind. In a study of mortality in US war veterans, Herrold (1972) found that 2241 had been diagnosed as lung cancer patients. Of these, 183 were excluded because of incorrect diagnosis or becauses no diagnostic information was available. Some 1107 cases were diagnosed without necropsy and of these 342 were diagnosed by unreliable methods. No histological slides were available, or were ever made, in about one-third of the whole series. Of the 1477 cases for which histologic material was available for review, lung cancer was definitely confirmed in only 1047, or 70·9 per cent. Thus, of the original series of 2241 cases of lung cancer, only 1047 (46 per cent) were definitely established. Although some of the unconfirmed cases of lung cancer were probably genuine, in the absence of histological evidence the diagnosis was unjustified.

There can be no doubt, therefore, that diagnostic artefacts have contributed massively to the secular increases in recorded death-rates from lung cancer illustrated in Figures 10.5 to 10.11. The beginning of the century was characterized by severe underdiagnosis, especially above the age of 40 years. However, in 1959, Heasman and Lipworth's (1966) study showed that although false-negative diagnoses were still common (46 per cent), false-positive diagnoses were already making an appreciable contribution (33 per cent). The upward shift in the modal age during recent years is doubtless largely, if not wholly, due to false-positive diagnoses of the kind described by Rosenblatt et al. (1971(a), (b)) and Herrold (1972). This view is strongly supported by Haenszel and Taeuber's (1964) direct study of age-specific death-rates in the United States (1958 men; 1958–59 women), for: (a) all diagnoses and (b) well established histological diagnoses of lung cancer. Above the age of 60 years (men) and 50 years (women) the ratio: {rates for (b)}/{rates for (a)} declined progressively with increasing age. In the lower age-ranges this ratio is almost unity. Although Figure 10.14 implies that most (but not necessarily all) of the secular increase has been due to factors other than tobacco, it does not in isolation automatically implicate diagnostic error. A role for extrinsic carcinogens with a precipitating action is not excluded by this evidence. Nevertheless, the very sharp rise in rates between 1921 and 1935 (Figures 10.13 and 10.14) coincided with improvements in radiological apparatus and techniques, and the widespread use of bronchoscopy (Rosenblatt, 1969).

Before leaving the subject of diagnostic accuracy an intriguing set of coincidences should be mentioned. Figure 4.1 of the report of the Royal College of Physicians (1971) shows a striking inverse relationship between death-rates in men aged 45 to 64 years (England and Wales) from pulmonary tuberculosis, and corresponding death-rates from lung cancer, over the period 1916 to 1965. The rise in death-rates from lung cancer is accompanied by an almost equivalent fall in death-rates from pulmonary tuberculosis. This relationship suggests the hypothesis that during the earlier part of the century when tuberculosis was a common disease, the actual cause of death in many cases of pulmonary tuberculosis was, in fact, a supervening lung cancer. The sex- and age-specific death-rates from pulmonary tuberculosis in England and Wales, 1956–59 (Figure 10.16) support this hypothesis. Late mortality cases (males) are fitted to the same equation ($n=2$, $r=5$), with the same mode ($t=68$ years), as lung cancer cases for 1956 to 1960 (Figure 10.8). Similarly, late mortality cases (females) are fitted to the same equation ($n=1$, $r=6$) with almost the same mode ($t=74$ years against $t=73$ years), as lung cancer cases, 1956–60 (Figure 10.11). Furthermore, active tuberculosis, even during 1950 to 1971 at the Memorial Hospital, New York, was a fairly common complication of neoplastic disease, especially lung cancer (Kaplan, Armstrong and Rosen, 1974). The prevalence of tuberculosis was highest in Hodgkin's disease (96 per 10^4), but was next highest in cancer of the lung (92 per 10^4)—in contrast, for example, to a prevalence of only four cases of tuberculosis per 10^4 cases of bladder cancer. More than half the cases of tuberculosis in lung cancer were of the pulmonary type.

Either we are dealing with a set of remarkable coincidences, or many instances of death from lung cancer in tuberculous patients, especially prior to 1950, were recorded (not unreasonably) as pulmonary tuberculosis.

We have now reached the following position: (a) a positive association between a habit such as smoking, and a disease such as a specific cancer, is an unreliable indicator of a causal connection—to *assume* that a positive association implies a causal connection is, of course, a methodological outrage; and (b) the bulk of the enormous secular increase in death-rates from lung cancer recorded during this century was the consequence of

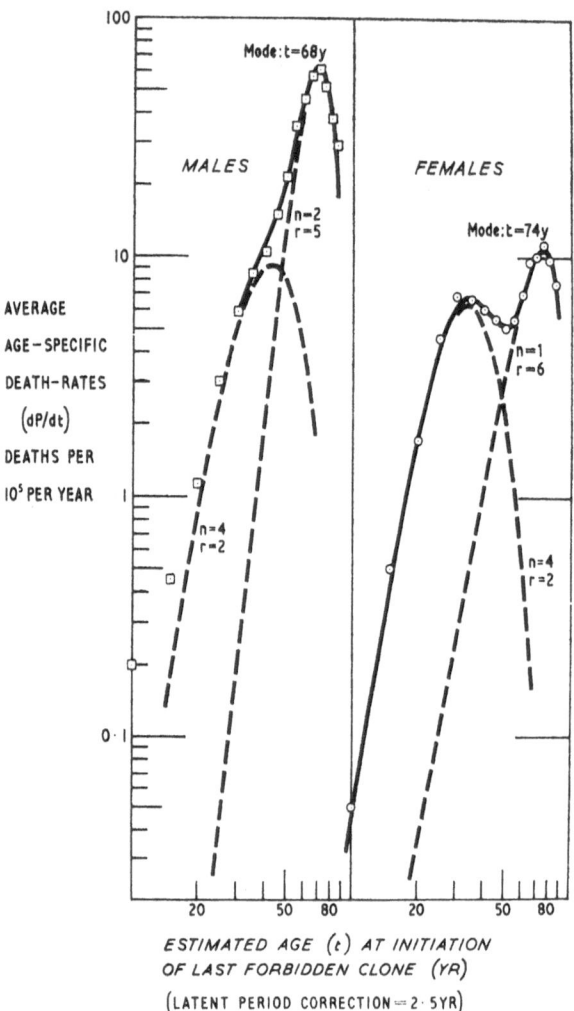

ESTIMATED AGE (*t*) AT INITIATION
OF LAST FORBIDDEN CLONE (YR)

(LATENT PERIOD CORRECTION = 2·5YR)

Figure 10.16 Sex-specific and age-specific death-rates from tuberculosis of the respiratory system, England and Wales, 1956–59, in relation to the estimated age at initiation of fatal forbidden clones. (Data from Registrar General's Annual Medical Reports.) Data points below $t=20$ years (males) are insufficient to define the age-pattern for deaths among young males. The form of the curve for late deaths (males), with $n=2$, $r=5$ and mode at $t=68$ years, is the same as that for lung cancer deaths, 1956–60—see Figure 10.8. Similarly, the curve for late deaths from tuberculosis (females), with $n=1$, $r=6$ and mode at $t=74$ years, closely resembles the curve for lung cancer deaths, 1956–60—see Figure 10.11

diagnostic error and cannot be attributed to tobacco. Nevertheless, the type of evidence considered so far does not allow us to reject decisively the hypothesis that smoke in the lung can cause cancer. Before considering whether discriminatory evidence can be obtained the sex- and age-dependence of lung cancer as recorded in other countries will be examined.

Sex- and Age-dependence of Lung Cancer in other Countries

Mortality statistics

In Figs. 10.17 to 10.20, age-specific death-rates for men, 1960–61, in countries of relatively high incidence—shown in the left panel—are contrasted with those for countries of relatively low incidence, shown in the right panel (Finland versus Portugal; German Federal Republic versus Norway; US White versus Japan; and Scotland versus Sweden). Statistics are taken from Segi and Kurihara (1966). Figures 10.21 to 10.24 illustrate the corresponding data for women. Table 10.1 lists the parameters used to fit these statistics and others taken from a WHO publication (WHO, 1970).

My conclusion that secular influences have had little effect on the *shape* of curves of log (dP/dt) versus log (t) above $t \simeq 50$ years has been based, so far, on mortality statistics for England and Wales, 1901 to 1970; the mortality ratios for US cigarette smokers versus non-smokers obtained by Hammond (1966) and Kahn (1966); and studies by Passey (1962) and Herrold (1972) of age at onset or death from lung cancer in relation to smoking habits. False-positive diagnoses have latterly caused an increase in the modal age without any marked change of the shape of the curve. It is therefore most interesting to see that the shapes of the curves in countries of low and of high incidence in males are remarkably similar. This may be a consequence, in part, of the period chosen for study—1960–61. To judge from Heasman and Lipworth's (1966) England and Wales study, the impact of false-negative and false-positive diagnoses was probably close to a minimum in 1960–61.

The pattern of secular change in death-rates throughout this century in relation to sex-specific tobacco consumption in these various countries would be most interesting, but sex-specific data for tobacco consumption are not available. However, mortality statistics, mainly for the period 1950 to 1963, show similar upward trends in the 25 populations covered by Segi and Kurihara's (1966) compilation. The similarity of these trends would seem to favour a common cause, and the diagnosis–artefact hypothesis, rather than the hypothesis of a tobacco-independent precipitator. It is unlikely that an antigenically specific precipitator, such as a virus or allergen, would exhibit a similar time-dependent increase in widely separated and disparate populations, in different countries.

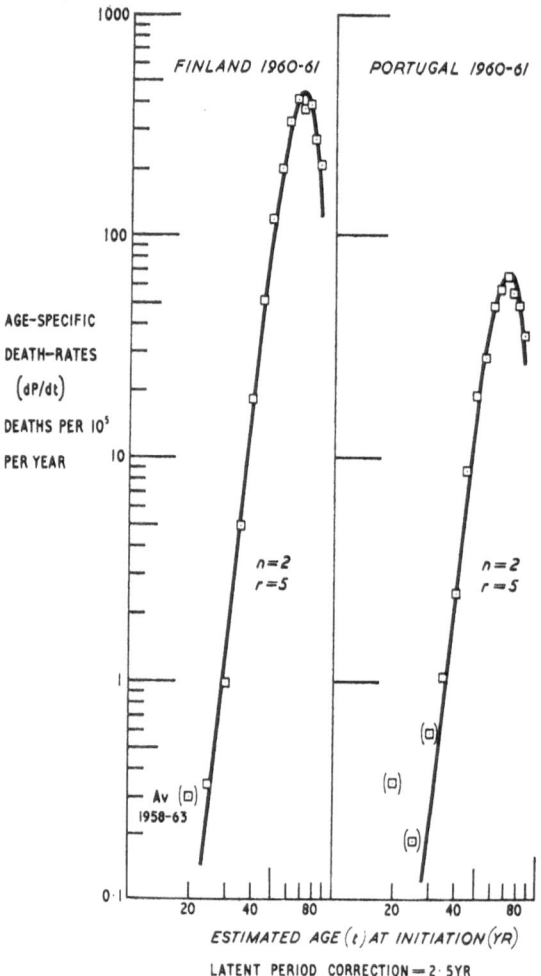

Figure 10.17 Age-specific death-rates (males), 1960–61, Finland (left panel) and Portugal (right panel), in relation to estimated age at initiation (Segi and Kurihara, 1966). Despite the very different levels of recorded rates (see Table 10.1), the form of the age-patterns ($n = 2$, $r = 5$) and the modal ages ($t = 70$ years) are the same in the two populations (see Table 10.1)

Statistics of onset of lung cancer

The analysis of Registry statistics for onset requires a slightly smaller latent period correction than mortality statistics, but only a few countries have comprehensive registries, covering the whole population. (The statistics from the California Tumour Registry (1963) indicate that the average interval between onset and death in males, 1942 to 1956, was about 0·73

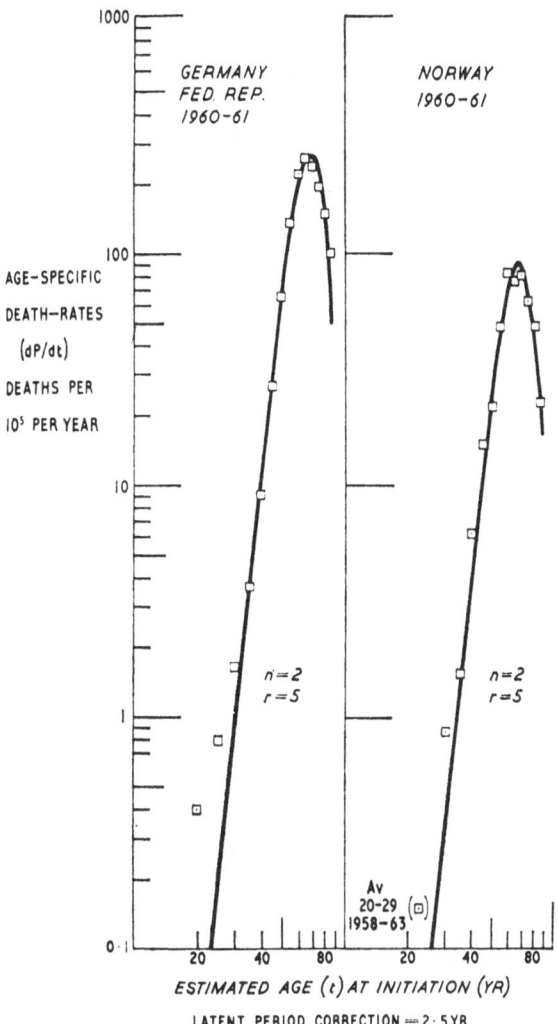

Figure 10.18 As for Figure 10.17. Data for German Federal Republic (left panel) with a modal age of 69 years and Norway (right panel) with a modal age of 68 years.

years.) Registry statistics for onset suffer from the risk of under-registration and, in some instances, the absence of necropsy evidence.

Statistics from the Swedish Cancer Registry, 1959 to 1965, are available by tumour type: adenocarcinoma (Figure 10.25), squamous carcinoma (Figure 10.26) and undifferentiated carcinoma (Figure 10.27). Cases of adeno-carcinoma in males up to $t = 40$ years, exceed those expected on the basis of the theoretical curve, $n = 2$, $r = 5$: they might result from a single forbidden

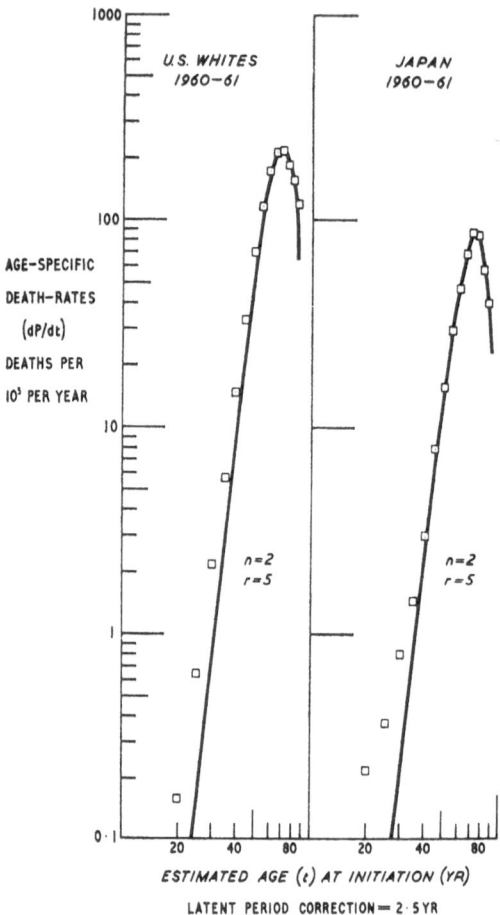

Figure 10.19 As for Figure 10.17. Data for US Whites (left panel) with a modal age of 69 years and for Japan (right panel) with a modal age of 72 years

clone ($n=1$, $r=5$). The two highest age-groups also show an excess above the theoretical curve. Data for squamous carcinoma (both sexes) and un-differential carcinoma (males) give a good fit to the theoretical curves used to fit other data. However, the data for undifferentiated carcinoma in women (Figure 10.27) fit the curve $n=1$, $r=7$, in contrast to $n=1$, $r=6$ used to fit the other data. Hence the broad category, 'cancer of the trachea, bronchus and lung' appears to be a complex of genetically distinctive as well as histologically distinctive diseases.

Other registry statistics (not available by histological type) are illustrated in Figures 10.28 to 10.32. In many instances, surprisingly good fits to the

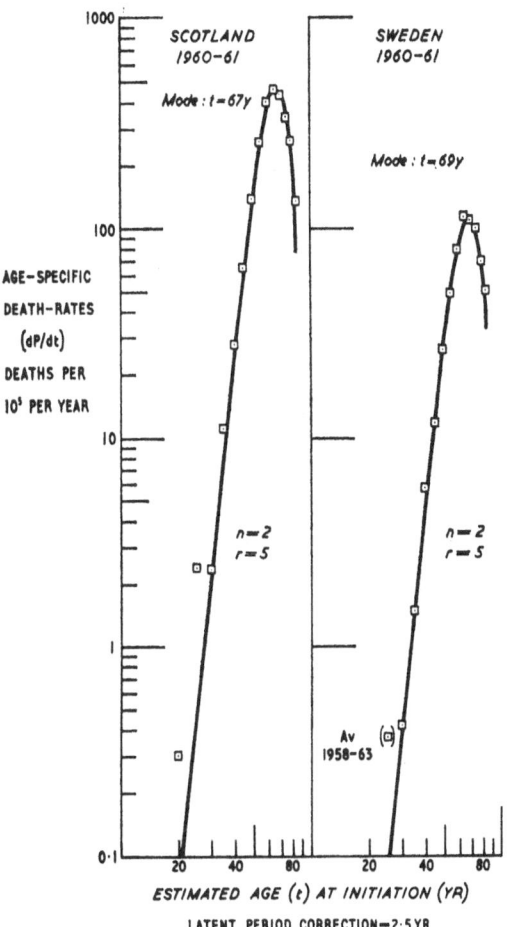

Figure 10.20 As for Figure 10.17. Data for Scotland (left panel) with a modal age of 68 years and for Sweden (right panel) with a modal age of 69 years

'standard' theoretical curves are obtained. The overall measure of reproducibility of the shapes and modes of curves of onset-rates (as well as of death-rates) for populations with low and high incidences of lung cancer, restrict the possible theories of tobacco-carcinogenesis (see Figure 10.12). If lung cancer is indeed 'almost entirely due to cigarette smoking' then any appreciable contribution from initiating or promoting action is ruled out by these statistics: only the precipitator hypothesis survives this test.

Another interesting approach to the problem of age-dependence was made by Passey (1962) and repeated by Herrold (1972) who confirmed Passey's findings. Passey (1962) listed the age at onset of lung cancer in the

Table 10.1 Values of k and S Calculated from Mortality Statistics for Cancer of the Lung, Bronchus and Trachea, 1960–61, for Various Populations

Population	k_M $\times 10^{10}$ yr^{-5} $(n=2, r=5)$	k_F $\times 10^{12}$ yr^{-6} $(n=1, r=6)$	S_M	S_F	S_M/S_F
Australia	7·4	4·4	$6·2 \times 10^{-2}$	$8·9 \times 10^{-3}$	7·0
Austria	7·4	2·8	$1·09 \times 10^{-1}$	$2·02 \times 10^{-2}$	5·4
Belgium	9·3	3·8	$7·3 \times 10^{-2}$	$1·16 \times 10^{-2}$	6·3
Canada	7·4	3·5	$5·8 \times 10^{-2}$	$1·09 \times 10^{-2}$	5·3
Chile	6·9	3·8	$2·9 \times 10^{-2}$	$1·46 \times 10^{-2}$	1·98
Denmark	8·6	2·8	$6·2 \times 10^{-2}$	$2·3 \times 10^{-2}$	2·7
Eire	10·9	8·5	$4·7 \times 10^{-2}$	$1·12 \times 10^{-2}$	4·2
Finland	7·4	3·3	$1·24 \times 10^{-1}$	$1·04 \times 10^{-2}$	11·9
France	9·3	3·3	$4·1 \times 10^{-2}$	$1·09 \times 10^{-2}$	3·8
German Federal Republic	8·6	4·1	$7·0 \times 10^{-2}$	$1·23 \times 10^{-2}$	5·7
Greece	6·4	3·8	$5·9 \times 10^{-2}$	$1·26 \times 10^{-2}$	4·7
Israel	5·9	2·8	$4·9 \times 10^{-2}$	$2·36 \times 10^{-2}$	2·1
Italy	12·9	5·2	$3·38 \times 10^{-2}$	$9·6 \times 10^{-3}$	3·5
Japan	6·9	5·6	$2·46 \times 10^{-2}$	$8·5 \times 10^{-3}$	2·9
Netherlands	8·6	2·8	$8·1 \times 10^{-2}$	$1·26 \times 10^{-2}$	6·4
New Zealand	6·9	4·4	$7·0 \times 10^{-2}$	$1·26 \times 10^{-2}$	5·6
Norway	8·6	3·8	$2·52 \times 10^{-2}$	$7·2 \times 10^{-3}$	3·5
Portugal	7·4	4·8	$1·94 \times 10^{-2}$	$5·5 \times 10^{-3}$	3·5
Scotland	9·3	5·6	$1·27 \times 10^{-1}$	$1·92 \times 10^{-2}$	6·6
South Africa	6·9	4·4	$7·9 \times 10^{-2}$	$1·69 \times 10^{-2}$	4·7
Sweden	8·0	3·8	$3·18 \times 10^{-2}$	$1·12 \times 10^{-2}$	2·8
Switzerland	9·3	3·1	$5·8 \times 10^{-2}$	$1·01 \times 10^{-2}$	5·7
UK (England, Wales, Scotland, N. Ireland)	8·6	5·2	$1·23 \times 10^{-1}$	$1·89 \times 10^{-2}$	6·5
US White	8·0	4·4	$6·24 \times 10^{-2}$	$1·18 \times 10^{-2}$	5·3
US Non-white	10·9	8·5	$5·2 \times 10^{-2}$	$8·5 \times 10^{-3}$	6·1
US All races	8·6	4·8	$6·1 \times 10^{-2}$	$1·14 \times 10^{-2}$	5·4

Sources: Segi and Kurihara, 1966; WHO, 1970

13 men who were the youngest to commence smoking (at 6 to 10 years of age, average 9 years), and in the 14 men who were the oldest to take up smoking (at 26 to 41 years, average 30 years). The average age of onset of lung cancer in the early smokers was $61·4 \pm 2·0$ years (the standard error of $\pm 2·0$ years is based on a normal distribution); and in the late smokers it was astonishingly similar: $61·3 \pm 2·4$ years. The earliest age of onset, in either group, was 42 years.

Figueroa, Raszkowski and Weiss (1973) found that the incidence of lung cancer in men exposed to chloromethyl methyl ether was eight times the

Table 10.2 Values of S_M from Mortality Statistics, 1960–61, Cigarette and Tobacco Consumption, 1950, by Country

Country	S_M (1960–61)	Cigarette consumption* Number per adult 1950	Tobacco consumption* lb per adult 1950
Australia	$6 \cdot 2 \times 10^{-2}$	1280	6·3
Austria	$1 \cdot 09 \times 10^{-1}$	1100	3·2
Belgium	$7 \cdot 3 \times 10^{-2}$	1240	6·1
Canada	$5 \cdot 8 \times 10^{-2}$	1790	7·6
Denmark	$6 \cdot 2 \times 10^{-2}$	1290	8·1
Finland	$1 \cdot 24 \times 10^{-1}$	1640	3·6
France	$4 \cdot 1 \times 10^{-2}$	930	4·1
German Federal Republic	$7 \cdot 0 \times 10^{-2}$	630	4·1
Greece	$5 \cdot 9 \times 10^{-2}$	1600	4·0
Ireland (Republic)	$4 \cdot 7 \times 10^{-2}$	2510	6·9
Italy	$3 \cdot 4 \times 10^{-2}$	815	2·3
Japan	$2 \cdot 46 \times 10^{-2}$	1220	3·1
Netherlands	$8 \cdot 1 \times 10^{-2}$	1120	7·5
New Zealand	$7 \cdot 0 \times 10^{-2}$	1420	7·2
Norway	$2 \cdot 5 \times 10^{-2}$	510	4·3
Portugal	$1 \cdot 94 \times 10^{-2}$	610	1·9
South Africa	$7 \cdot 9 \times 10^{-2}$	1170	4·9
Sweden	$3 \cdot 2 \times 10^{-2}$	810	4·1
Switzerland	$5 \cdot 8 \times 10^{-2}$	1500	6·0
UK	$1 \cdot 23 \times 10^{-1}$	2180	5·7
USA	$6 \cdot 1 \times 10^{-2}$	3250	10·2

* From Beese (1968)

Table 10.3 Values of k and S Derived from Cancer Registry Statistics for Cancer of the Lung, Bronchus and Trachea (ICD 162–163)

Population and period	k_M $\times 10^{10}$ yr^{-5} $(n=2, r=5)$	k_F $\times 10^{12}$ yr^{-6} $(n=1, r=6)$	S_M	S_F	S_M/S_F
England and Wales, four regions 1960–62	8·0	6·1	$1 \cdot 32 \times 10^{-1}$	$1 \cdot 78 \times 10^{-2}$	7·4
Finland 1959–65	7·4	2·8	$1 \cdot 50 \times 10^{-1}$	$1 \cdot 51 \times 10^{-2}$	9·9
German Democratic Republic 1964–66	8·0	5·2	$1 \cdot 04 \times 10^{-1}$	$9 \cdot 6 \times 10^{-3}$	10·8
Norway 1959–66	8·0	4·4	$2 \cdot 98 \times 10^{-2}$	$7 \cdot 5 \times 10^{-3}$	4·0
Scotland 1962–65	9·3	7·2	$1 \cdot 24 \times 10^{-1}$	$1 \cdot 70 \times 10^{-2}$	7·3
Sweden 1959–61	8·0	3·8	$3 \cdot 18 \times 10^{-2}$	$1 \cdot 05 \times 10^{-2}$	3·0
Sweden 1962–65	6·9	2·2	$4 \cdot 39 \times 10^{-2}$	$1 \cdot 89 \times 10^{-2}$	2·3
Sweden 1966–68	6·4	2·2	$5 \cdot 43 \times 10^{-2}$	$2 \cdot 02 \times 10^{-2}$	2·7

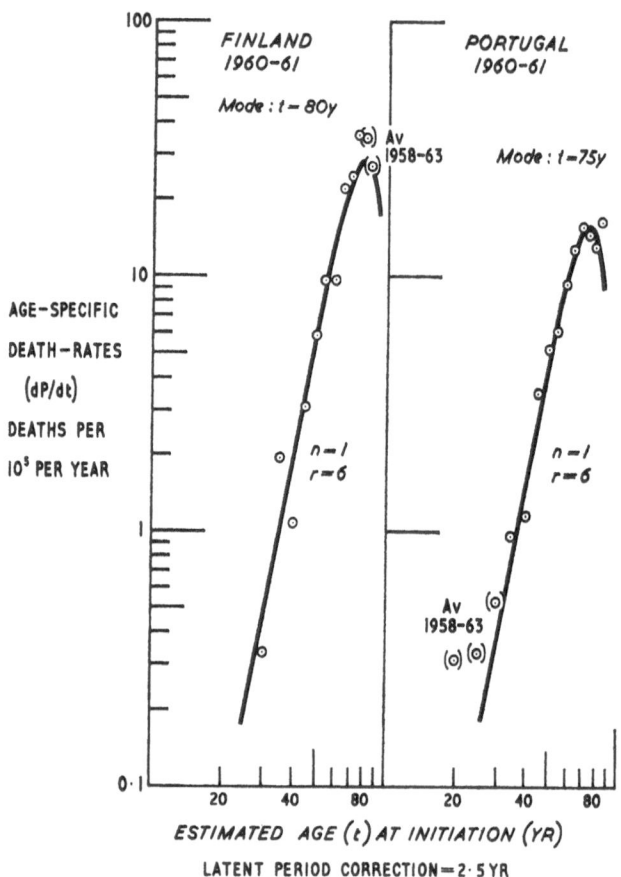

Figure 10.21 Age-specific death-rates (females), 1960–61, Finland (left panel), and Portugal (right panel), in relation to estimated age at initiation (Segi and Kurihara, 1966)

expected value: in this series the average age of onset was only 44·9 years. Langård and Norseth (1975) carried out a cohort study in Norway of workers producing chromate pigments. Three cases of bronchial carcinoma were found (as against 0·079 expected) and the average age at diagnosis was 50 years. As in experimental carcinogenesis, it appears that carcinogens at an effective concentration not only increase the incidence of associated tumours, but they also induce an unusually early onset.

Once again, quantitative data cast grave doubt on the validity of the hypothesis that cigarette smoking causes nearly all cases of lung cancer, but they do not reject it decisively. However, agreement with the constitutional hypothesis could scarcely be better.

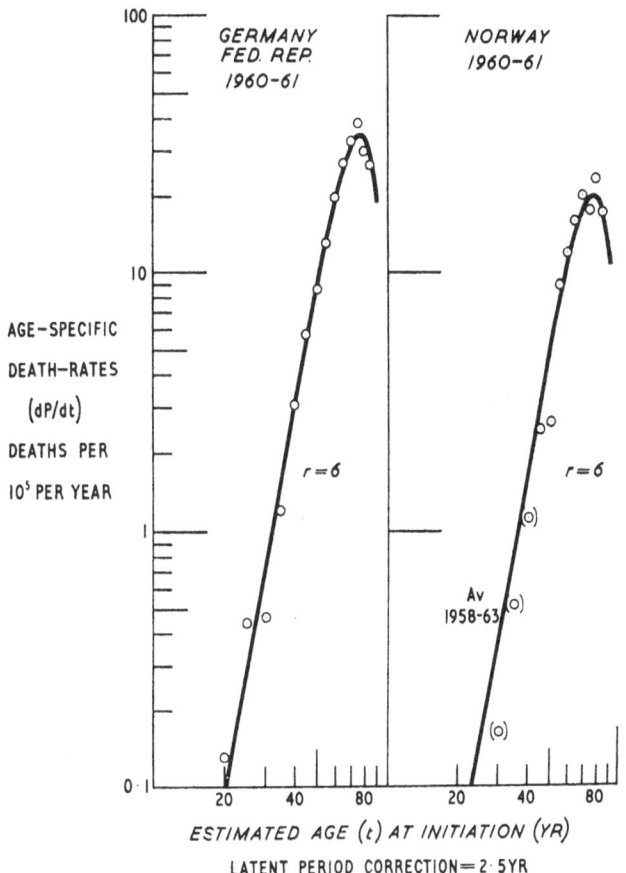

Figure 10.22 As for Figure 10.21. Data for German Federal Republic (left panel) and Norway (right panel)

Death-rates and tobacco consumption by country

On a simple causal hypothesis, and with no concessions to genetic factors, we would expect national death-rates from lung cancer to correlate with the effective tobacco consumption in that country. Because of differences in the type of tobacco smoked, manner and history of smoking, use or non-use of filters, levels of diagnosis and many other factors, we would not expect to find a perfect correlation. The scattergrams shown in Figures 10.33 (for cigarette consumption) and 10.34 (for total tobacco consumption) depart so drastically from a simple linear regression, they seem somewhat at variance with a straightforward causal hypothesis. Table 10.2 lists the values plotted in Figures 10.33 to 10.34.

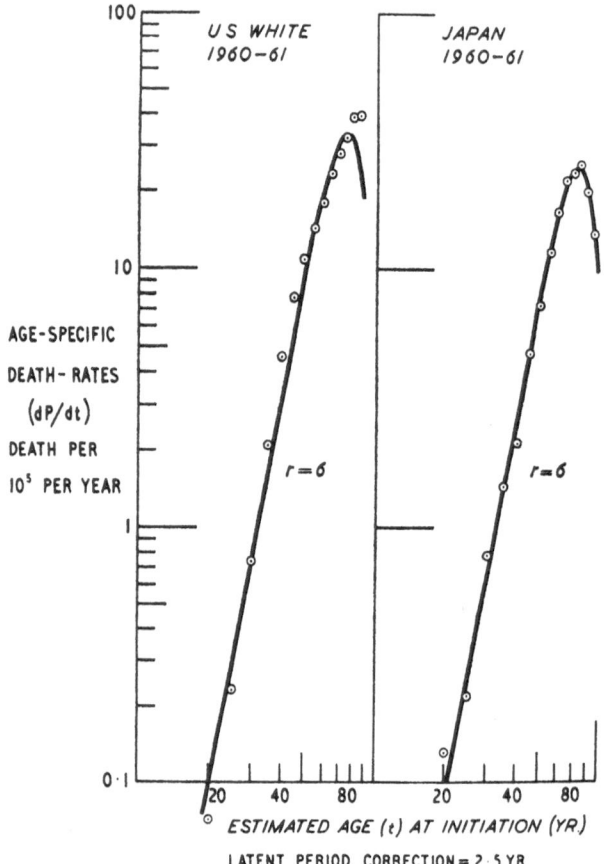

Figure 10.23 As for Figure 10.21. Data for US Whites (left panel) and Japan (right panel

Stocks (1970) tested for correlations between the mean annual consumption of cigarettes, 1951–54, and the mean age-adjusted death-rates from cancer at various sites, 1964–65, in 20 countries. For cancer of the lung and bronchus, the association was just significantly positive ($P=0\cdot05$) for males, but it failed to reach conventional significance for females ($P=0\cdot085$). Out of a total of 26 statistical tests (males and/or females), applying to 15 sites, some 15 of the tests gave nominally negative associations, with four of them giving $P<0\cdot05$, while the remaining 11 gave positive associations, only one of which (lung and bronchus, male) attained a P value of $0\cdot05$. The negative associations with national cigarette consumption were found for cancers at the following sites: buccal cavity and pharynx in males only; stomach in

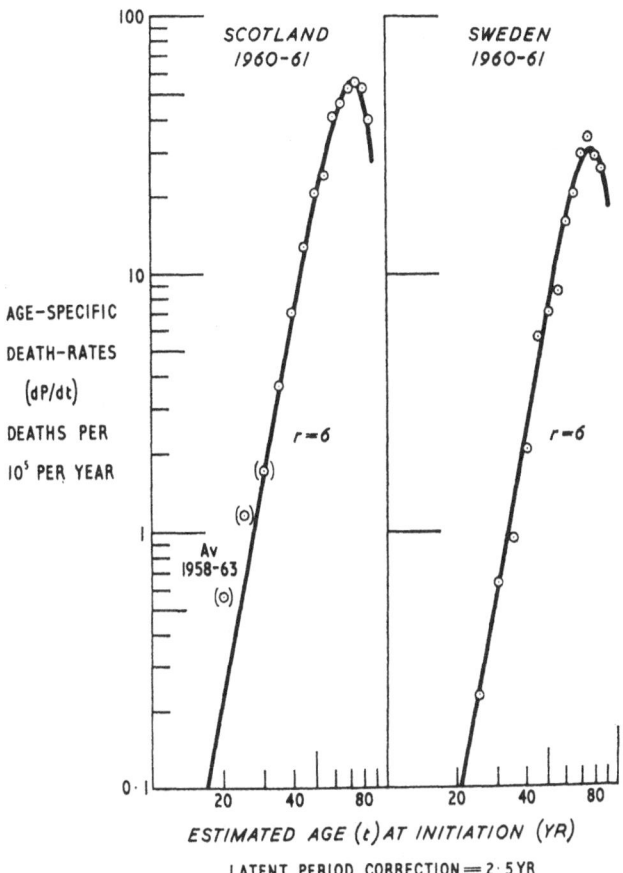

Figure 10.24 As for Figure 10.21. Data for Scotland (left panel) and Sweden (right panel)

males and females; rectum in males and females; liver and bile passages in males ($P=0.05$) and in females ($P=0.08$); larynx in males only; bladder in males ($P=0.009$) and in females; prostate ($P=0.05$); ovary; uterus ($P=0.0008$); and leukaemia in males and females (Stocks, 1970).

The meaning to be attached to correlations and P values in this context is somewhat obscure, but I find it difficult to believe that the negative associations, even the highly significant ones, signify a prophylactic action of cigarette smoking. But what should we conclude from negative associations between national cigarette consumption and cancers of the buccal cavity, pharynx and larynx in men, for which sites Kahn (1966) obtained mortality ratios of 3·8, 9·6 and 9·5 respectively? Perhaps the chief merit of

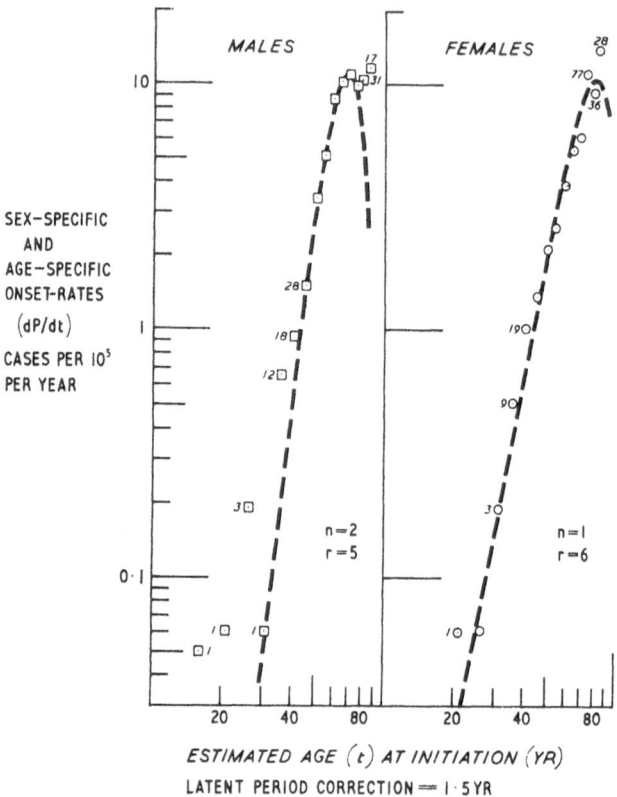

Figure 10.25 Data from Swedish Cancer Registry (1971) for sex-specific and age-specific onset-rates for adenocarcinoma of the trachea, bronchus and lung in relation to estimated age at initiation. The excess of male cases above the theoretical curve at low t suggests the possibility of an early-onset group (perhaps $n=1$, $r=5$). At very high t we see a suggestion of a third, late-onset group

such studies is to demonstrate the utter absurdity of relying upon mortality ratios, and/or correlations between national death-rates and cigarette consumption, as evidence for causal relations. If *recorded* national death-rates from specific cancers depend primarily on the frequency of genetically predisposed persons and the accuracy of diagnosis, the apparent contradictions disappear. But it then becomes very difficult to test the hypothesis that, say, a small number of cases in any country might be due to smoking. Whatever else they might do, these data, and Stocks's (1970) studies cast doubt on the advisability of using words such as 'unequivocal' in connection with the idea that smoking causes cancers of the lung, buccal cavity, pharynx and larynx.

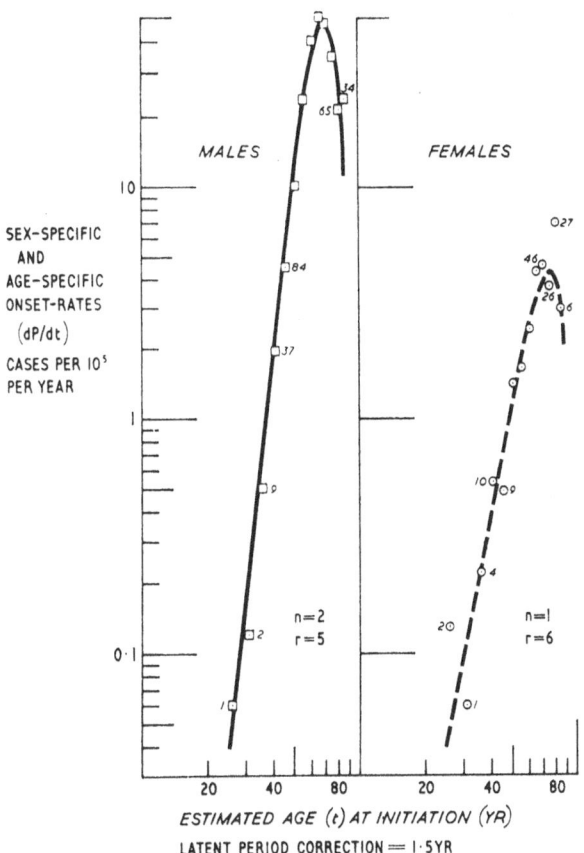

Figure 10.26 As for Figure 10.25. Onset data for squamous carcinoma of the trachea, bronchus and lung. The fit to the 'standard' theoretical curves is satisfactory

Genetics of lung cancer and smoking

Despite the international concern with lung cancer the possible role of genetic factors has attracted little attention. Doll (1974) has remarked that 'few scientists have been sufficiently attracted by the hypothesis to mount the effort required [to study] large numbers of twins'. The report of the Royal College of Physicians (1971) states: 'There is, however, little evidence of any inherited tendency to lung cancer'. To be more precise, few studies have been made of the genetics of lung cancer. Indeed, only one large-scale familial study has been carried out but, fortunately for the genetic hypothesis, it gave unambiguous results (Tokuhata, 1964; Tokuhata and Lilienfeld, 1963(a), (b); Tokuhata, 1973). First-degree relatives of 270 lung cancer probands were compared with first-degree relatives of 270 controls, matched

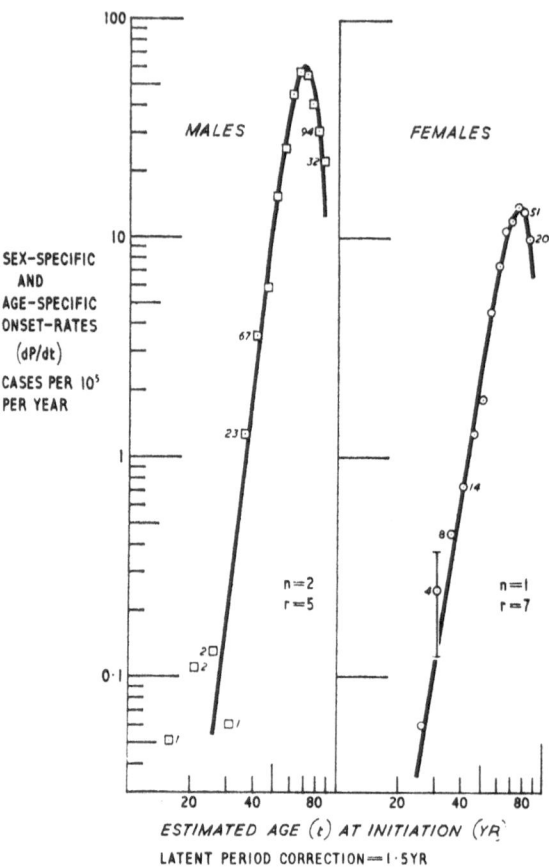

Figure 10.27 As for Figure 10.25. Onset data for undifferentiated carcinoma of the trachea, bronchus and lung. Data for women are more steeply age-dependent than in Figures 10.25 and 10.26. They give a good fit to the curve with parameters $n=1$, $r=7$

with cases for race, sex, age and residence. Deaths from lung cancer among non-smoking first degree relatives of cases were found to be 3·8 times greater than expected on the basis of those observed in non-smoking first-degree relatives of controls; among smokers, the corresponding ratio was reduced to 2·3. For both sexes, and smokers and non-smokers combined, Tokuhata and Lilienfeld (1963(b)) calculated that the probability that these differences between case and control relatives would arise by chance was 0·0006.

Some ancillary findings of this study are equally important for our understanding of genetic associations and the connections between smoking and disease. For all causes of death, rates in case relatives were 1·09 times

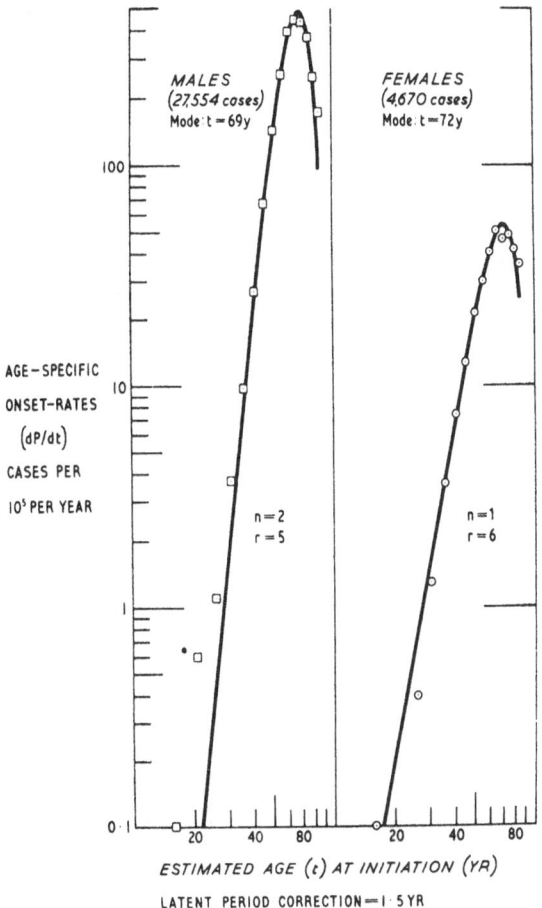

Figure 10.28 Registry data for onset of cancer of the lung, bronchus and trachea from four regions of England and Wales, 1960–62, in relation to estimated age at initiation (Doll *et al.*, 1966)

higher than expected from the rates in control relatives ($P=0.01$). For all cancers, the corresponding ratio was somewhat higher, at 1·62, and the level of significance was very high, at $P=0.000\,06$ (Tokuhata and Lilienfeld, 1963(b)). They found that 32 per cent of cancer diagnoses in the relatives of cases were of the respiratory system, in contrast to 20 per cent in the control relatives. Deaths from non-malignant diseases of the respiratory system (tuberculosis, asthma, influenza, pneumonia, bronchitis) were also more common in case relatives than in control relatives, by a factor of 1·66 ($P=0.000\,06$). To check the possible influence of the home and local environment, deaths in case spouses were compared with those in control spouses;

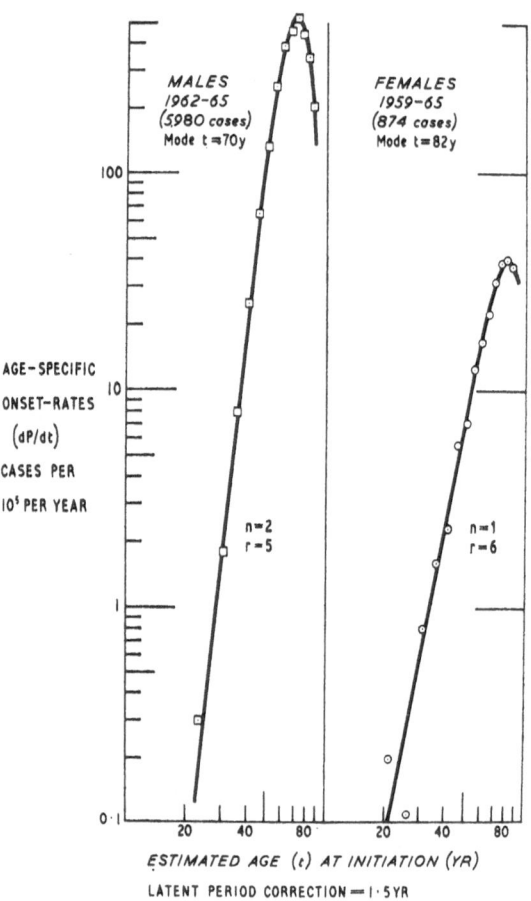

Figure 10.29 As for Figure 10.28. Data from the Finnish Cancer Register, males 1962–1965, and females 1959–65 (Doll *et al.*, 1966, 1970)

no significant differences were found (Tokuhata and Lilienfeld, 1963(b)).

Among the 270 lung cancer cases, 250 were smokers, but among the 270 controls only 160 were smokers, illustrating the well-established association between lung cancer and smoking. Among the relatives of cases, 41·0 per cent were smokers in contrast to 37·2 per cent among control relatives (*P* = 0·01). This is consistent with independent evidence (see below) that points to genetic factors in smoking, but it might also reflect intrafamilial social pressures. Another interesting statistic can be extracted from Tokuhata and Lilienfeld's (1963(b)) findings. The total number of deaths observed among case relatives was 796, as against 727·9 expected on the basis of mortality among control relatives. When we subtract the contribution to

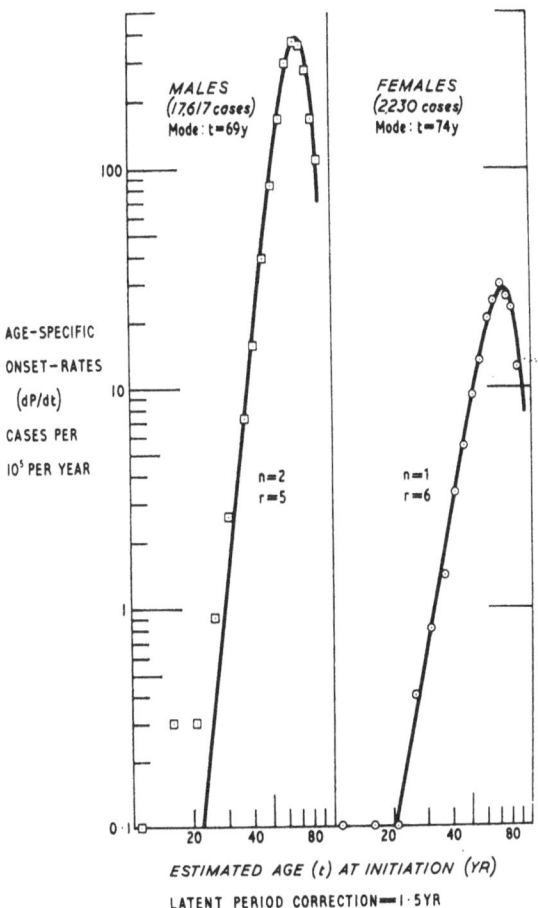

MALES
(17,617 cases)
Mode: t = 69y

FEMALES
(2230 cases)
Mode: t = 74y

AGE-SPECIFIC

ONSET-RATES

(dP/dt)

CASES PER

10⁵ PER YEAR

n=2
r=5

n=1
r=6

ESTIMATED AGE (t) AT INITIATION (YR)

LATENT PERIOD CORRECTION = 1·5YR

Figure 10.30 As for Figure 10.28. Data from the German Democratic Republic, 1964–66 (Doll *et al.*, 1970)

total deaths from all cancers and non-malignant respiratory diseases, we obtain for the remaining deaths, 463 observed among case relatives as against 523·1 expected. Remembering that these deaths include the large category of total cardiovascular disease, which is positively associated with smoking, it follows that many of the other causes of death must be appreciably negatively associated both with smoking and with lung cancer.

These findings of Tokuhata and Lilienfeld corroborate the following hypotheses: (a) smoking and lung cancer are positively associated; (b) certain genes predispose to lung cancer; (c) certain genes predispose to smoking; (d) the net positive familial association between lung cancer and all causes of death is genetically based; (e) the net positive familial association

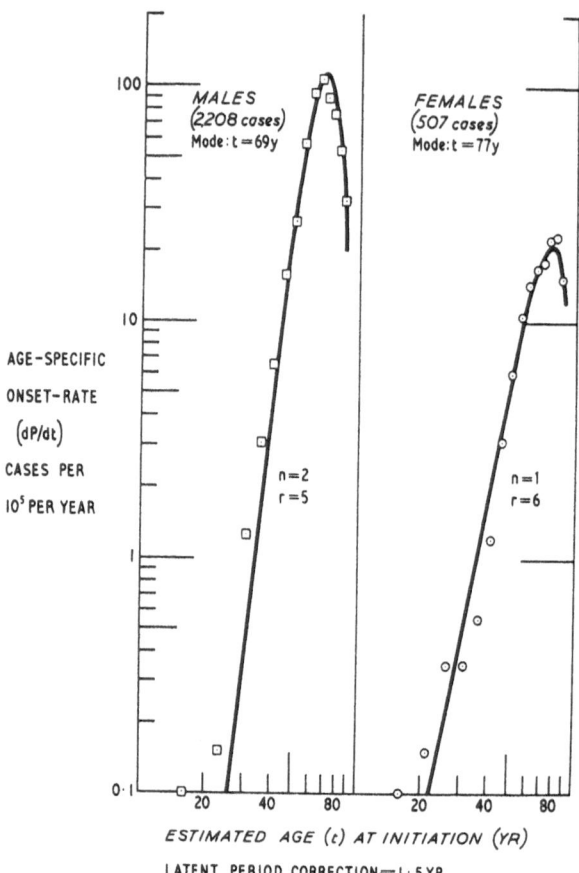

Figure 10.31 As for Figure 10.28. Data from Norway, 1959–66 (Doll *et al.*, 1970)

between lung cancer and all cancers has a genetic basis; (f) the net positive familial association between lung cancer and fatal, non-malignant respiratory diseases has a genetic basis; and (g) the net negative familial association between lung cancer and fatal diseases other than those under (e) and (f) has a genetic basis.

It must be added that (e) does not exclude negative associations between lung cancer and *some* other cancers, and similarly, (f) does not exclude negative associations between lung cancer and *some* non-malignant respiratory diseases. Although these data support genetic hypotheses of positive and negative associations between smoking and disease, they do not exclude additional causal factors.

In a further and most important analysis of the findings from this study, Tokuhata (1973) determined the frequency of cigarette smokers among the

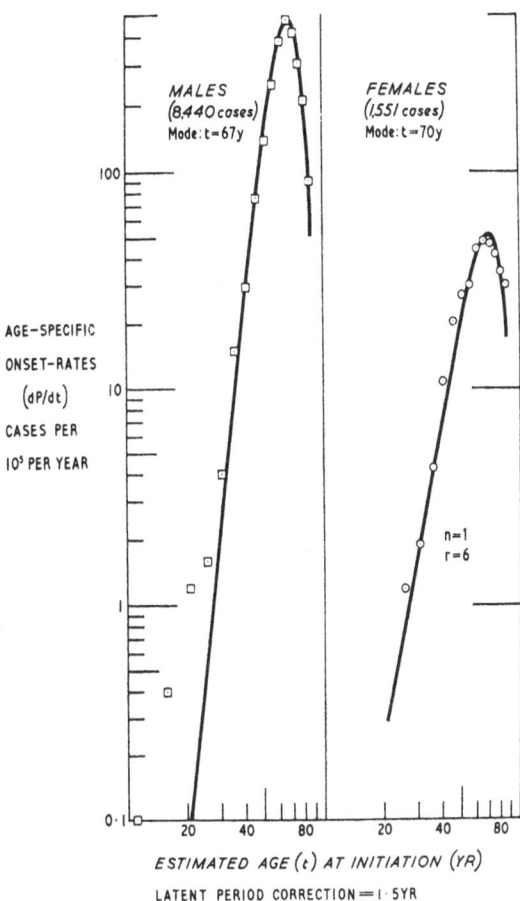

MALES
(8,440 cases)
Mode: t = 67y

FEMALES
(1,551 cases)
Mode: t = 70y

100

AGE–SPECIFIC

ONSET–RATES

($\partial P/\partial t$)   10

CASES PER

10^5 PER YEAR

n = 1
r = 6

1

0·1

20   40   80   20   40   80

ESTIMATED AGE (t) AT INITIATION (YR)

LATENT PERIOD CORRECTION = 1·5YR

Figure 10.32 As for Figure 10.28. Data from Scotland, 1963–66 (Doll *et al.*, 1970)

first-degree relatives of: (a) smoking and (b) non-smoking probands and controls. In the proband group, when the lung cancer index subject was a smoker, 41·1 per cent of relatives smoked; when the index subject was a non-smoker, 40 per cent of relatives smoked. In the control group, 41·8 per cent of the relatives of smoking index subjects were smokers, in contrast to only 30·7 per cent of the relatives of non-smoking index subjects (Tokuhata, 1973). These, and particularly other more complicated familial connections described by Tokuhata (1973) indicate: (a) some non-smoking cancer cases nevertheless had a genetic predisposition to smoking and/or (b) marked positive associations exist between the genotypes for lung cancer and cigarette smoking.

Further large-scale familial studies of this kind would be valuable. Careful attention would need to be given to the inference from age-patterns that

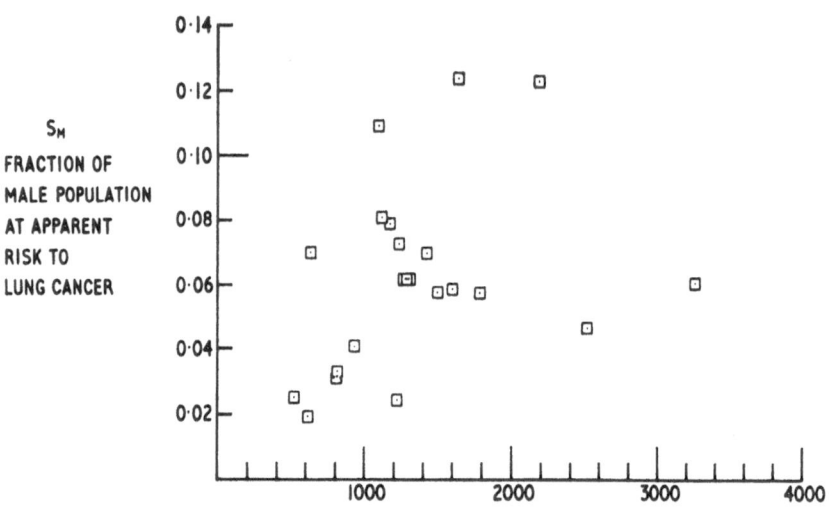

Figure 10.33 Death-rates from lung cancer in males (in terms of S_M) for 21 different populations, 1960–61, in relation to national consumption of manufactured cigarette tobacco in 1950

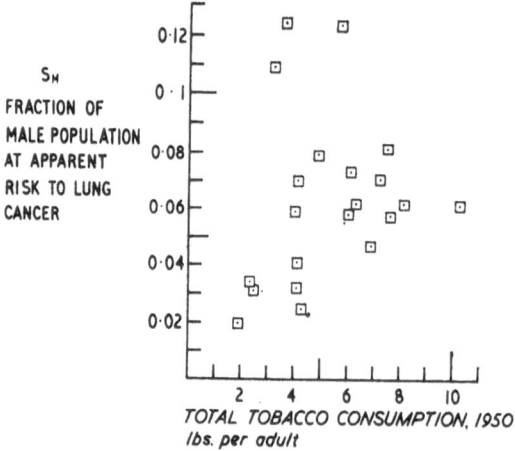

Figure 10.34 Death-rates from lung cancer in males (in terms of S_M) for 21 different populations, 1960–61, in relation to national consumption of all forms of tobacco in 1950

for most, if not all, cases of lung cancer, genetic predisposition in males should differ, in at least one factor, from that in females. Swedish Registry statistics (Figures 10.25 to 10.27) indicate at least two major predisposing genotypes among women. Sex-differences between the genotypes that predispose to the various forms of smoking should also be anticipated.

Mortality from lung cancer in Jews has been compared with that in other ethnic and religious groups in Montreal (Horowitz and Enterline, 1970), and Pittsburgh (Herman and Enterline, 1970). In both cities, Jewish males had low rates compared with non-Jews, while the opposite relation was found among women. It was estimated that differences in smoking might account for the lower mortality among Jewish males but not for the higher mortality among Jewish females (Horowitz and Enterline, 1970; Herman and Enterline, 1970). The extent of medical care and diagnostic procedures might have accounted in part for the differences between Jewish and non-Jewish women (Herman and Rao, 1971), but genetic differences (which were not mentioned) are probably implicated, as they surely are among males. The value of S_F in Israel, 1960–61 ($2 \cdot 4 \times 10^{-2}$), is the highest of those countries listed in Table 10.1. Belcher (1971), from detailed studies of the sex-ratio of bronchial carcinoma in 49 different countries, invoked a genetic explanation of the wide spread in values (more than one order of magnitude) that arose mainly from differences in the frequencies of affected males.

Even more valuable than studies of first-degree relatives would be extensive surveys of twins on an international scale along the lines followed by Friberg et al. (1970). The importance of this type of investigation will be discussed later.

Kellerman, Shaw and Luyten-Kellerman (1973) studied the frequency of people with low, intermediate and high inducible aryl hydrocarbon hydroxylase activities, and found a highly significant ($P < 0 \cdot 001$) difference in distribution between 50 patients with bronchogenic carcinoma and 85 healthy controls. They pointed out that their findings support Tokuhata's hypothesis that susceptibility to lung cancer is inherited.

Urban–Rural Differences

Many authors have described a high ratio of urban-to-rural mortality from lung cancer among men (see, for example, Haenszel, Loveland and Sirken, 1962; and Stocks, 1966). These high ratios persist when 'corrections' are applied to allow for differences in smoking habits. Among women, the urban–rural gradient of mortality is less consistent; in certain regions of the United States, lung cancer mortality, adjusted for age and smoking history is higher in rural than in urban environments (Haenszel and Taeuber, 1964).

I need hardly add that urban–rural differences are nearly always attributed to environmental factors, especially atmospheric pollution. However, from their detailed studies and analysis, Haenszel et al. (1962) recognized the difficulties of a simple causal interpretation and referred to '. . . a need to introduce modifications into models concerned with environmental background effects'. Thus, they found that men with a lifetime residence in urban areas had a substantially *lower* mortality from lung cancer than those whose period of urban residence was under 1 year, 1–9 years, 10–39 years, and 40 years and over, but less than a lifetime residence. Allowances were made for age and smoking history and for each group a standardized lung cancer mortality ratio was calculated. Substantially similar findings were obtained for women (Haenszel and Taeuber, 1964). Haenszel *et al.* (1962) also found that the 'standardized lung cancer mortality ratio' (SLCMR based on an average index of 100) for men born on farms who migrated to metropolitan areas was much higher than for those who were born in, and continued to reside in, metropolitan areas.

These data and the 'anomalous' findings for women (Haenszel and Taeuber 1964), suggest that the *type of person*, rather than residence as such, determines the risk of lung cancer. In general, the city dweller has a higher risk than his rural counterpart, but in the United States the man who migrates from his farm to the city has a particularly high risk. Migrancy and restlessness appear to be correlated with the risk of lung cancer. This generalization extends to immigrants to the United States (Haenszel *et al.*, 1962; Haenszel and Taeuber, 1964). For men who did not smoke regularly, the SLCMR for the foreign-born was 61 in contrast to 26 for the native-born (Haenszel *et al.*, 1962). For women, the corresponding SLCMR were 119 (foreign-born) and 69 (native-born). For regular male smokers, the SLCMR for the foreign-born was 277, and for the native-born 180; for women smokers, the corresponding SLCMRs were 320 and 249 respectively (Haenszel *et al.*, 1962; Haenszel and Taeuber, 1964).

The hypothesis that atmospheric pollution causes lung cancer appears at least as suspect as the assertion: 'lung cancer is almost entirely due to cigarette smoking'.

Inhaling

Those who must smoke are exhorted to inhale less (Royal College of Physicians, 1971). This advice may surprise those familiar with the evidence. The only numerically adequate survey in this country of the effect of inhaling was based on 399 inhalers and 249 non-inhalers. It showed that, after standardizing for the number of cigarettes smoked per day (1–4; 5–14; 15–24; 25–49; >49) inhalers suffered, on the average, a 10 per cent *lower* incidence of lung cancer than non-inhalers (Fisher, 1959). From the data supplied to him by Doll and Hill, Fisher (1959) was able to disprove ($P \simeq 0.01$) the hypothesis that inhalers and non-inhalers have the same incidence of lung cancer. He commented: 'Even equality would be a fair knockout for the theory that smoke in the lung causes cancer'. Doll and Hill's (1964) study of British doctors with lung cancer involved only 33 inhalers and 11 non-inhalers, but even that suggested that inhalers who were heavy smokers had a lower incidence than corresponding non-inhalers.

It must be said that the findings concerning inhaling are inconsistent. Thus, in the United States, Lombard and Snegireff (1959) found that the incidence of lung cancer in non-inhaling 'light' smokers was only 55 per cent of that in inhaling 'light' smokers, but that the incidence in non-inhaling 'heavy' smokers was 88 per cent of that in inhaling 'heavy' smokers. 'Light' smokers had smoked a total of 0 to 9124 equivalent packs, and 'heavy' smokers more than 20000 equivalent packs. Curiously, the findings for inhaling/non-inhaling 'medium' smokers were not given. Because inhaling correlates both with total amount smoked and the daily rate of smoking (Schwartz et al., 1961), the divisions into 'light' and 'heavy' by integral lifetime consumption seem to be too crude to test properly the hypothesis that inhaling is more hazardous than non-inhaling. The small difference found in the broad 'heavy' category casts further doubt on that hypothesis. Unfortunately, the statistical significance of differences was not given and no details of the numbers involved were stated.

Schwartz et al. (1961) carried out an elaborate study in France in which they compared the smoking habits of male lung cancer cases (and other cancer cases) with suitably matched controls. 'Pure' cigarette smokers who inhaled and smoked 1–9; 10–19; or 20–29 cigarettes a day suffered a significantly higher risk of lung cancer ($\times 2\cdot5$; $\times 1\cdot7$; $\times 1\cdot8$ respectively), than corresponding non-inhalers, but for those smoking 30+ cigarettes a day, the risk among inhalers was only 60 per cent of that in non-inhalers (significance not stated). Another peculiarity of these findings should be mentioned; if two men smoked the same number of cigarettes a day, the one who, in addition, smoked a pipe, incurred only half the risk of lung cancer (Schwartz et al., 1961). A similar paradox persisted when the factor of inhalation was controlled (Schwartz et al., 1961). Indeed, the 'prophylactic effect' of the additional pipe smoking was even more marked among those who smoked cigarettes at the rate of 30+ a day, and inhaled. Schwartz et al. (1961) came to the inescapable conclusion that the explanation of their paradoxical findings must be sought in the smoker himself.

Other investigators have failed to standardize either for the rate of smoking, or total consumption, and hence the overall evidence for the effects of inhaling is not only inconsistent, but unsatisfactory. Of course, the inconsistencies may well reflect genuine differences. On the constitutional hypothesis, inhalers and non-inhalers will tend to be genetically dissimilar. It is improbable that inhaling/non-inhaling genotypes will have the same quantitative associations with lung cancer genotypes in all populations.

Combining commonsense with the causal hypothesis, we would expect the risk of lung cancer in inhalers (other things being equal) to be overwhelmingly greater than in non-inhalers for all rates of smoking, and in all populations. The failure to confirm this expectation might appear to demolish the causal hypothesis. Alas, 'commonsense' is not always the best guide in biology and medicine. Strictly, the recorded age-dependence of lung cancer favours no form of (smoking) causal hypothesis, but it is least inconsistent with the idea that smoking precipitates the growth of forbidden clones. Precipitating action is more likely to take place centrally (perhaps in the bone marrow), than peripherally in the lungs and bronchi (see Chapter 9). Hence, even when the incidence of lung cancer in inhalers of certain types of tobacco smoke is indeed lower than in non-inhalers—as was shown in Fisher's (1959) analysis of extensive British data—this does not disprove the causal hypothesis as such. In this connection, we may note Fisher's choice of words: 'Even equality would be a fair knockout for the theory that *smoke in the lung causes cancer*' (my italics). Fisher was as renowned for his careful and precise use of words as for his development of the science of statistics and scientific logic.

We are forced to conclude that the evidence for the effects of inhaling cannot provide definitive tests of all causal hypotheses, although it might help to define some of those anatomical sites where cigarette smoke does *not* exert a direct carcinogenic action.

Cigar and Pipe Smoking

In view of the lack of consistent evidence for the effects of inhalation of cigarette smoke, we can conclude that the actual route of entry of carcinogens has rather little relevance. Accordingly, we might expect to find a simple correlation between the incidence of lung cancer and the concentration of chemical carcinogens in tobacco smoke. The yield of various polycyclic hydrocarbons, and notably 3,4-benzpyrene, is generally much higher from cigars and pipes than from cigarettes (Cardon et al., 1956; Campbell and Lindsay, 1957). These indications from chemical analysis were confirmed in a carefully controlled study of the carcinogenicity of tobacco smoke condensate applied to mouse skin (Davis and Day, 1969). The condensate from small cigars (C1) was compared with that from cigarettes made from a composite blend of flue-cured tobacco (T4) and from cigarettes made from the cigar tobacco (C2), which, instead of being granulated, was shredded and wrapped in normal cigarette paper. At 116 weeks, 16 animals (11·1 per cent) treated with cigar condensate (C1) had developed carcinoma, in contrast to 1 (0·7 per cent) treated with T4, and none treated with C2. Non-malignant tumours were also more readily induced by C1. Davies and Day (1969) concluded that the difference in the carcinogenicity of the condensates is due to the physical differences between cigars and cigarettes rather than the nature of the tobacco. Pursuing the implications of this type of experimental evidence, we would anticipate a much higher incidence of lung cancer in 'pure' cigar and pipe smokers than in smokers of equivalent masses of cigarette tobacco.

In most studies, the reverse relation is found; pipe and 'classical' cigar smokers suffer lower rates of lung cancer than cigarette smokers (Doll and Hill, 1964; Hammond, 1966; Kahn, 1966; Gsell and Abelin, 1972). In France, Schwartz et al. (1961) found that pure pipe smoking was far more common, and heavier, among controls than among lung cancer cases. However, cheroot smokers in Switzerland hàve rates comparable with cigarette smokers, and European smokers of cigars/pipes appear generally to be at higher risk than their US counterparts (Gsell and Abelin, 1972). Again, the important factor would appear to be the person who smokes (and his constitution) rather than the type of tobacco he smokes, and how he smokes it.

Overall, the incidence of lung cancer in pipe and cigar smokers supplies further evidence (if that were needed) against the 'initiating' version of the causal hypothesis. Those animal experiments that demonstrate the carcinogenic action of tobacco smoke condensate—such as the one carried out by Davies and Day (1969)—appear to have little or no relevance to lung cancer in man. The idea that trials on animals can test for 'safer' or 'less harmful' cigarettes should be treated with suspicion. It must also be doubted whether the 'tar league' published by the United Kingdom Government has any relevance to carcinogenic risks.

Fisher's Constitutional Hypothesis: Genetic Factors

It is not sufficient to question the 'unequivocal' causal theory and to demonstrate the weakness of its foundations: critics have an obligation to put forward an alternative theory. So far as I am aware, the only rival formulation that is at present superior to the causal theory is the constitutional hypothesis considered above (see also Fisher, 1958(a), (b); 1959; Berkson, 1959; Brownlee, 1965). However, the two theories are not mutually exclusive and both may contain some truth. For example, twins studies indicate that the higher prevalence in smokers of persistent cough and morbidity from chronic bronchitis results from genetic factors as well as a genuine causal action of smoking (Cederlöf, Friberg and Hrubec, 1969).

Many surveys testify to the involvement of genetic factors in certain forms of smoking, from classical twins studies (Fisher, 1958(a), (b); Friberg et al., 1959; Todd and Mason, 1959), to studies of morphology (Seltzer, 1962, 1967, 1972) and psychology (Eysenck, 1965; Thomas, Fargo and Enslein, 1970). Monozygotic (MZ) twins tend to be strikingly concordant for smoking habits; in one series of male pairs, only 24 per cent showed distinct differences such as a cigarette smoker and a non-smoker, or a cigar smoker and a cigarette smoker (Fisher, 1958). By contrast, distinct differences were seen in 52 per cent of dizygotic twin pairs (Fisher, 1958a). The finding of pairs of MZ twins discordant for smoking habits is important because it shows that inheritance is not the sole factor that determines the habit.

Among the many studies of personality differences between smokers and non-smokers, one reveals the influence of social pressures. Thomas et al. (1970) found that medical students who were heavy smokers in their early 20s were a heterogeneous population. In the ensuing years, which was a period of intensive pressure to give up smoking, less than a third did so. However, the 14 persons who gave up smoking resembled the original non-smoking group in vocational interest, even though they smoked cigarettes heavily in their early 20s (Thomas et al., 1970). This evidence suggests the obvious hypothesis that people who relinquish the habit tend to be those who are genetically predisposed only to 'social' smoking rather than 'compulsive' smoking. Evidence for lung cancer in ex-smokers has, therefore, to be analysed with circumspection.

The distribution of blood groups and the ability to taste phenylthio-carbamide (PTC) differ between smokers and non-smokers (Thomas and Cohen, 1960; Cohen and Thomas, 1962). Freire-Maia (1960) concluded that smoking in itself is not the cause of the heightened ability to test PTC.

That the various forms of smoking tend to involve different genetic factors is illustrated in Seltzer's (1972) study of anthropometric, somatotype, occupational and educational differences between 'pure cigar' and 'pure pipe' smokers in the US. Significant differences between these types of smoker, often at the level of $P < 0.01$, were found among the measured characteristics.

In certain respects, cigar and pipe smokers as a group differ from non-smokers and cigarette smokers. An interesting study of medical absenteeism among men aged 55 to 59 years by Holcomb and Meigs (1972) revealed an average of 4·2 days lost per man year by non-smokers, 5·80 for smokers of less than one pack per day, 5·94 for smokers of one pack per day, 8·16 for smokers of more than one pack per day, but only 3·22 for smokers of cigars and/or pipes. Holcomb and Meigs (1972) suggested that constitutional rather than (tobacco) causal factors might underlie these differences.

From these many lines of evidence there can be no serious doubt, therefore, that genetic factors predispose to certain types of smoking and that different types of smoking tend to involve genotypic differences. Tokuhata's (1973) analysis (see above) of evidence for the frequency of smokers among the first-degree relatives of (a) non-smoking lung cancer probands and (b) non-smoking controls, agrees with Fisher's suggestion of a positive association between smoking genotypes and lung cancer genotypes.

Mortality in Ex-smokers

Superficially, findings for the incidence of lung cancer in ex-smokers might appear to corroborate the causal hypothesis and dispose of the constitutional hypothesis. In their Figure 2, Doll and Hill (1964) illustrate the annual death-rate from lung cancer in those doctors who had given up smoking, versus 'years stopped smoking'. Death-rates fell abruptly at first, then more slowly, and at around 20 years they had flattened out. Unfortunately, these characteristics are predicted by both the causal and the constitutional hypotheses. Most people who give up smoking are self-selected even though many may be yielding to social pressures. The constitutional hypothesis predicts that ex-smokers will tend to be the social smokers, few of whom will be genetically predisposed to lung cancer, and hence the initial fall in death-rates will be steep. The longer an ex-smoker can relinquish the habit the more likely it is that he is a social, rather than a compulsive smoker. Hence, although the fall in death-rates will continue and eventually approach that in non-smokers, the rate of fall will diminish with increasing time after ceasing to smoke. These predictions of the constitutional hypothesis fit the observations.

The nature of supposed causal mechanisms has, unfortunately, not been propounded in a way that enables them to be tested quantitatively, or even semiquantitatively, against this evidence. As we have seen, a long induction period of around 30 years is usually claimed for the carcinogenic action of smoking and the problem is to reconcile this slow process with the immediate drop in death-rates that follows the cessation of smoking. If we regard precipitating action as the only remotely plausible causal mechanism, then the long induction period implies that smoking produces some form of cumulative damage that eventually permits the entry into the body of specific antigenic material. On this view, the cessation of smoking would need to be followed by an initially rapid repair of the damaged barriers. We are then left with the problem of explaining the incidence of lung cancer in non-smokers and how it is that the kinetics are the same in smokers and non-smokers.

A good test of causal/constitutional hypotheses would be forthcoming if the (genuine) mortality from lung cancer could be followed in a total population in which tobacco consumption falls, and a proportion of the members give up smoking. The causal theory predicts that a genuine fall in mortality would follow immediately upon the decline in the smoking habit: the constitutional theory predicts no consequent change.

One total population approaching these requirements has been described by Doll and Pike (1972). This comprised all those doctors who had responded to the questionnaire sent out originally by Doll and Hill on 31st October, 1951. Unfortunately, only 69 per cent of men and 60 per cent of women responded to the initial request for information (Doll and Hill, 1964). The risk of self-selection bias was therefore severe; analysis of standardized overall death-rates, using a one in ten random sample of all doctors, confirmed the suspected bias. In those doctors who replied, death-rates were found to be only 63 per cent of those in all doctors in the second year of the inquiry and 85 per cent in the third year (Doll and Hill, 1964). In the fourth to tenth years the corresponding proportion fluctuated about an average of 93 per cent (Doll and Pike, 1972). Hence, with regard to all deaths, selection effects persisted, though at a fairly low level. But with respect to specific causes of death, and in particular lung cancer, we have no information. In comparing the mortality experience in male doctors with that in the general male population, Doll and Pike (1972) omitted the experience of the first and second years of the inquiry to avoid the worst effects of self-selection bias. The percentage of ex-smokers in the age-group 35 to 64 years increased from 18·1 in 1951 to 29·5 in 1966: the corresponding increase for the age-group 35 to 84 was from 19·5 to 32·0. Those doctors who continued to smoke cigarettes only, smoked on the average, fewer per day, although the percentage of pipe or cigar smokers increased over the study period.

For the age-range 35 to 84 years, the standardized annual death-rates from lung cancer per 1000 male doctors in the sample, were as follows: 1953–57, 1·10; 1957–61, 0·85; and 1961–65, 0·83. Because 1953–57 included a period during which selection bias was still marked with respect to all causes of death (but what of lung cancer?), it is of doubtful value to the estimate of trends. For the remaining two periods, no significant trend emerges. However, in doctors aged 35 to 64 years, standardized annual death-rates per 1000 were as follows: 1953–57, 0·60; 1957–61, 0·56; and 1961–65, 0·37. Neglecting the first unreliable period, we see a large fall (34 per cent) from 1957–61 to 1961–65, to which much attention has been directed. Numbers of deaths were not given (I estimate there were about 30 in the last period), and hence we cannot assess reliably the significance of the trend. Nevertheless, this fall, in this age-group—coupled with the near constant rates for the age-group 35 to 84 years—implies that a substantial *increase* must have occurred over this period in the recorded death-rate from lung cancer in the age-group 65 to 84 years. Doll's (1974) table, published in response to criticism (Burch, 1974b), shows this to have been 37 per cent, which is larger than the fall recorded for the age-group 35 to 64 years! Furthermore, we can infer from Table 4 of Doll and Pike (1972) that the age-group 65 to 84 years is the one in which the percentage of ex-smokers was highest and increasing, and in which the rate of cigarette smoking was lowest and declining.

These paradoxical trends, by age-group, are not unlike those observed in the general population—see Figure 10.8 in particular. From 1951 onwards, a tendency to declining death-rates is seen for men under 55 years of age; increases have been confined to *older* men. In the general male population of the United Kingdom, manufactured cigarette consumption per smoker above the age of 50 remained almost constant from 1958 to 1971, although the percentage of ex-smokers over 60 years of age increased steadily from 27 per cent in 1961 to 37 per cent in 1969 (Todd, 1972). At 50 to 59 years of age, the percentage of ex-smokers was fairly steady, but in lower age-groups the percentage actually tended to fall over this period, while the rate of consumption of manufactured cigarettes per smoker steadily increased from 1958 to 1971 (Todd, 1972). These secular trends in recorded age-specific smoking habits among men show, therefore, a negative association with the corresponding secular trends in age-specific death-rates. They do not favour a causal hypothesis, but the reality of the apparent trends in death-rates must, of course, be doubted in view of the unreliability of diagnosis.

Strict comparability of the statistics for doctors and those for the general population should not be expected. Thus, in Doll and Hill's (1964) report of mortality in British doctors we read that Dr. J. R. Bignall 'advised on the diagnosis in particularly difficult cases'. The standards of diagnosis for doctors differed, therefore, from those for non-doctors. Wynder (1955) reported that '. . . physicians use the smoking history of patients as an aid in differential diagnosis of lung conditions'. This acknowledged bias of US physicians cannot be assumed to be entirely absent from this country and it threatens the validity of any distinctions that depend on rather small differences, especially between groups in which the accuracy of diagnosis and the degree of bias might not be comparable—as between male doctors and the general male population.

The overall evidence for death-rates from lung cancer in ex-smokers fails, therefore, to distinguish clearly between causal and constitutional hypotheses and it throws up the usual crop of apparent inconsistencies. Diagnostic error may well be responsible for the divergent and paradoxical secular trends below and above the age of 55 years. Even in Doll and Hill's (1964) study of British doctors, histological, cytological, or necropsy evidence, was available for only 56 per cent of presumed deaths from lung cancer. The survey of Rosenblatt *et al.* (1971(a), (b)) in New York, if broadly applicable to this country, indicates that part of the recent increase in the higher age groups should be attributed to false-positive diagnoses. The upward shift between 1951 and 1970 in the modal age for age-specific death-rates from lung cancer (Figure 10.8), points to the impact of false-positive diagnoses in England and Wales.

Other Evidence

We might hope to obtain definitive tests from what can best be termed bizarre evidence. One example is provided by a study of Seventh-Day Adventists, a religious group in which the consumption of tobacco and alcohol is rare (Wynder, Lemon and Bross, 1959). In men, they found only two hospital cases of lung cancer against 16·7 expected, based on controls. For every other category of cancer considered, fewer than expected numbers of male cases were found in the Seventh-Day Adventists, although for colorectal cancer (25 against 31·7 expected) and cancer of the prostate (31 against 33·8 expected) differences were small and not significant. However, for women, a surprising result was obtained that attracted no comment. The observed number of lung cancer cases was 6 against 3·8 expected from the study of controls. Perhaps the numbers were too small to excite comment. For cancers of the mouth, larynx, and esophagus only one female case was found against 6·4 expected. At most other sites the observed number was slightly smaller than expected, although for uterine cancer (22 versus 18·6 expected) and for all metastatic cancers where the primary was not determined (21 versus 16·7) a slight but not significant excess was found in the Seventh-Day Adventists.

If male members of this religious group were randomly selected from the general population, these findings would corroborate a causal hypothesis of the connection between cancer, especially lung cancer, and tobacco and/or alcohol. We must, however, withhold judgement. Seventh-Day Adventists do not represent a random selection from the general population and the problem of self-selection enters again. We have to bear in mind the strong possibility that genetically determined psychological factors could play a part in determining voluntary membership of a particular religious group, and that the predisposing genes might be negatively associated with those that predispose to smoking and to lung cancer. (The puritan in me finds it difficult to associate religious fervour with chain-smoking.) It would be interesting to discover whether the excess incidence of lung cancer in female Seventh-Day Adventists represents a mere statistical excursion, non-committed membership of the group, or some other feature.

Another example of bizarre evidence has been presented by Davies (1973). He described a remarkable Roman Catholic community, of Spanish origin, living in the large valley of Vilcabamba in the province of Loja in Ecuador and achieving remarkable longevity. Out of a total population of 819, some 46 (5·6 per cent) were alleged to be over 80 years of age, 16 (2 per cent) over 90, and 9 (1 per cent) over 100. According to Davies (1973), who is evidently well aware of the problems of substitution and confusion between generations, it is difficult to doubt the evidence of age, which is drawn from baptismal certificates. Anyway, Vilcabamba boasts some 6 per cent of its rural population as octogenarians, in contrast to the 0·7 per cent for rural Ecuador. All this is remarkable enough, but to cap it all, the inhabitants of Vilcabamba drink two to three cups of rum a day and smoke anything from 40 to 60 cigarettes each day! Happily, the rum is unrefined and the cigarettes are homemade, mainly from tobacco grown in their own gardens and wrapped in maize leaves, although toilet paper is preferred when available. I leave the interpretation to the reader.

Pathology: Carcinoma *in situ*

If we can place any reliance on the age-patterns for lung cancer in males —and despite errors of diagnosis a consistent *shape* is seen in different countries and at different times—then they suggest that n, the number of initiating forbidden clones, is greater than unity. It might be two or three. (A consistent level of underdiagnosis would not, of course, distort the shape of the age-pattern. It is a surprising and fortuitous result, however, that the main effect of recent overdiagnosis has been to raise the modal age—as well as levels—without appreciably altering the shape of the age-pattern.) Where women are concerned, it seems likely that adenocarcinoma, squamous carcinoma and undifferentiated carcinoma (Figure 10.24 to 10.26), are all initiated by a single forbidden clone. However, with the smaller numbers and the ill-defined mode, this conclusion is less reliable than that relating to males. Be that as it may, lung cancer in women bears a much better prognosis than in men (Ederer and Mersheimer, 1962).

According to my general theory, we would expect well-defined premalignant conditions of the lungs and bronchi, such as carcinoma *in situ*, to be common in males with overt carcinoma and rare, or absent, in similarly affected women.

Auerbach *et al.* (1957) studied the histologic changes in the tracheobronchial tree, by serial section of the lungs of 54 white men who, at necropsy, had bronchogenic carcinoma. Some 48 cases showed at least some signs of carcinoma *in situ*. In the 7993 usable slides, definite carcinoma *in situ* was seen in 735 (9 per cent) and borderline carcinoma *in situ* in 622 (8 per cent). In one (extreme) case, some 60 per cent of the slides revealed carcinoma *in situ*. Of special interest is the laterality of change. Gross carcinoma was found in the right lung in 29 cases and in the left 22 cases. In three cases, the major site of involvement was indeterminate. Of the 51 cases with well-defined unilateral carcinoma, 43 showed evidence of carcinoma *in situ* in the contralateral lung. We are thus presented with a fascinating situation in which bilateral carcinoma *in situ* is present in about 80 to 90 per cent of cases (at least), although bilateral carcinoma is rather rare, occurring with a frequency of about 2 per cent in large series (Willis, 1960).

If carcinogens in cigarette smoke are mainly responsible for both conditions (as many would have us believe) it is not easy to understand this striking disparity in the frequency of bilateral involvement. On a biological interpretation no difficulty arises. Assume (for males) that $n=1$ for carcinoma *in situ* and $n=2$ for carcinoma. Then the target cells for the single forbidden clone that induces carcinoma *in situ* are, in most genetically predisposed persons, distributed in the bronchial epithelium of both lungs. Following the deductions and arguments of Chapter 7, carcinomatous development requires the transformation in genetically predisposed persons of a minimum of two distinctive mosaic epithelial elements, probably contiguous. By inference, the genetically determined anatomical distribution of such contiguous elements is predominantly, but not exclusively, unilateral.

This line of reasoning receives remarkable support from the observations of Auerbach *et al.* (1957). Their slides strongly suggested to them that when carcinoma of the bronchus arose from carcinoma *in situ*, it did so from multiple, contiguous foci. Previously, McGrath, Gall and Kessler (1952) had arrived at a similar conclusion. In their necropsy study of 87 indisputable cases of bronchogenic carcinoma (sex not specified) they found 25 specimens in which pre-invasive or early-invasive plaques were either in close contiguity with the main tumour or at independent sites.

The studies of McGrath *et al.* (1952) and of Auerbach *et al.* (1957) both emphasize the multifocal origins of bronchial carcinoma. Corresponding studies for female cases would be most interesting.

Importance of Twins Studies

Finally we need to inquire how the distinction between causal and constitutional theories could best be drawn. Obviously, we should reap a huge reward if we could control the genetic variable. Probably the best way to do this in human populations is through the study of twins. Monozygotic (MZ) twins begin their embryonic life with the same complement of genes although somatic mutation must introduce some measure of postzygotic variation in somatic cells. To a first approximation, dizygotic (DZ) twins are no more alike, genetically, than ordinary siblings. If, therefore, we can find sufficient numbers of twin pairs in which one member smokes and the other does not, or in which one smokes heavily and the other lightly, then we can hope to answer some of our outstanding problems.

A 'pure' causal theory that ignores or denies the role of inheritance—that is, the one usually propounded—predicts for a specific disease, other things being equal, that the ratio: (incidence in smokers)/(incidence in non-smokers) should be greater than unity and have the same value in: (a) a series of MZ twins, discordant for smoking habits; and (b) a series of DZ twins, similarly discordant for smoking habits.

A 'pure' constitutional theory that denies causal effects of smoking predicts an equal incidence of a specific disease among the smoking and non-smoking members of a series of smoking-discordant MZ twins, assuming, of course, that other extrinsic causal agents have the same impact. For a disease that is positively associated with smoking, a 'pure' constitutional theory predicts a higher incidence in the smoking than in the non-smoking members of a series of smoking-discordant DZ twins, and the reverse relation for negatively associated diseases.

(A reservation needs to be mentioned in connection with constitutional hypotheses. It is conceivable that differences in smoking between the discordant members of a pair of MZ twins might, in some instances, be due to one or more postzygotic mutations: such mutations might also affect predisposition to disease. This is a subtle possibility, but that is no reason for overlooking it completely.)

Combined causal and constitutional theories make intermediate predictions. A situation in which a combined theory needs to be applied arises in connection with the prevalence of 'prolonged cough' (Cederlöf, Friberg and Hrubec, 1969). The prevalence in the non-smoking members of a series of discordant pairs of MZ twins was found to be 2·4 per cent and in the smoking members of the series, 5·4 per cent. In the non-smoking members of a series of DZ twins discordant for smoking habits, the prevalence in the non-smokers was 2·0 per cent (effectively the same as in the MZ non-smokers), but in the smokers it was 9·8 per cent (Cederlöf *et al.*, 1969). The higher prevalence of 'prolonged cough' in smoking, over non-smoking members of the MZ series, points to the causal action of smoking, but the higher ratio: (prevalence in smokers)/(prevalence in non-smokers) in the DZ series ($\simeq 5$) as compared with the MZ series ($\simeq 2\cdot2$), points to a genetic contribution in addition. The genetic influence was confirmed in a study of Swedish twins which revealed a substantially higher 'coincidence rate' of respiratory symptoms in MZ than in DZ twins of similar smoking habits (Cederlöf et al., 1969). ('Coincidence rate' is defined as the percentage of twin pairs in which both members have the same symptoms.)

The largest published study of mortality in series of twins discordant for smoking habits still yields rather small numbers. Table 10.4 condenses some of the information from this study (Friberg et al., 1973). Mortality over an 11-year period (1961–72) was followed in 1487 pairs of DZ-, and 572 pairs of MZ twins, born between 1901 and 1925. Hence, 'early' deaths predominated and in only 19 pairs had both members died within the survey period. The bottom row of Table 10.4 gives the distribution of 'first' deaths. (Eventually, all twins will die, but in this survey we are interested in the smoking habits of the first member of a pair to die. On the causal hypothesis, the smoking-twin will tend to die before the non-smoking co-twin. Thus, when both members of a pair had died, only the 'first' death is included in the bottom row Table 10.4.)

For all causes of death among MZ twins (both sexes), no significant difference is seen between the low smoking group (31 first deaths) and the high smoking groups (32 first deaths). A similar result was obtained for all cancers, with seven deaths among low MZ smokers and eight among high MZ smokers. However, among DZ twins, sexes combined, the number of first deaths from all causes in the high smoking group (97), is significantly higher ($P = 0.006$) than among the low smoking group (62). The difference for women alone, 31 first deaths in the low group versus 42 first deaths in the high group is not significant ($P = 0.24$). For men, with 31 first deaths low, versus 55 first deaths high, the difference is significant ($P = 0.011$).

These findings of Friberg et al. (1973) for all causes of death are strikingly consistent with a 'pure' constitutional hypothesis. They show that the fatal (causal) effects of smoking are not pronounced and might well be non-existent.

For cancer of the lung, the findings are nominally in line with the constitutional hypothesis (one male MZ low, versus one male MZ high, no female MZ cases; one male DZ low, versus seven male DZ high; no female DZ low, versus one female DZ high), but numbers are far too small as yet for an adequate test.

Clearly, a very large survey along the lines being pursued by Professor Friberg and his colleagues, preferably on a coordinated and world-wide basis, will be necessary to provide better discrimination between causal and constitutional hypotheses. If we allow a complex (causal-plus-constitutional)

Table 10.4 Cause of Death, by Sex and Zygosity, in Twin Pairs Discordant for Smoking Habits

Cause of death	Men 706 DZ pairs Low group	Men 706 DZ pairs High group	Men 246 MZ pairs Low group	Men 246 MZ pairs High group	Women 781 DZ pairs Low group	Women 781 DZ pairs High group	Women 326 MZ pairs Low group	Women 326 MZ pairs High group	Sexes combined 1487 DZ pairs Low group	Sexes combined 1487 DZ pairs High group	Sexes combined 572 MZ pairs Low group	Sexes combined 572 MZ pairs High group
Cancer of lung	1	7	1	1	0	1	0	0	1	8	1	1
Other cancer	9	10	0	1	18	18	6	6	27	28	6	7
All cancer	10	17	1	2	18	19	6	6	28	36	7	8
All causes	35	58	20	23	34	44	13	14	69	102	33	37
All causes 'first' deaths in a pair	31	55	18	18	31	42	13	14	62	97	31	32

Source: adapted from Friberg et al. (1973)

hypothesis, findings from twins studies will never be able to exclude some small causal contribution. Nevertheless, world-wide studies of twins discordant for smoking habits could establish helpful upper limits for possible morbid and fatal actions of smoking.

Conclusions

The report of the Royal College of Physicians (1971) states (page 48) that many countries have set up 'authoritative committees and commissions' to study the cause of lung cancer ('this modern scourge'), and that all have concluded 'that it is almost entirely due to cigarette smoking'. They concede that the 'experts' have been challenged by 'a small number of individuals'. I regret I have no option but to join that small band, although in 1975, I am unable to go beyond Fisher (1959) who argued '. . . that the data so far do not warrant the conclusions based upon them'.

Although unable to disprove the restricted hypothesis: '*some* cases of lung cancer are caused by cigarette smoking', I have shown that the bulk of the enormous increase in death-rates recorded during this century in England and Wales has been due to factors unconnected with tobacco. The seemingly paradoxical findings for: (a) inhaling; (b) mixed (cigarette and pipe) smoking; and (c) ex-smokers, are more elegantly and economically interpreted by the constitutional hypothesis: unconvincing *ad hoc* assumptions are needed to rescue the causal hypothesis. The age of onset of lung cancer in early and late smokers (Passey, 1962; Herrold, 1972), argues strongly (but not conclusively) against the restricted causal hypothesis. When we compare: (a) mortality ratios (smokers)/(non-smokers) for various cancers with secular trends; and (b) death-rates from various cancers with national cigarette consumption, we encounter so many paradoxes that the value of both forms of evidence for interpreting causal relations becomes completely undermined.

Negative associations between smoking and various diseases, that cannot be attributed to genuine prophylaxis or artefacts, lie beyond the scope of traditional causal theories. They are, however, predicted by constitutional hypotheses. It would be very strange if no positive associations could be traced to constitutional factors. Indeed, the studies of Tokuhata and Lilienfeld (1963(b)) show a positive association between the predisposition to smoking and the predisposition to lung cancer.

To judge from the studies of twins discordant for smoking habits, we are on firm ground in concluding with Cederlöf *et al.* (1969) that smoking and inheritance both contribute to the development of 'prolonged cough', and morbidity from chronic bronchitis. The same source of information (Friberg *et al.*, 1973) indicates that smoking does not play a major causal role—

according to present statistics it appears to have no role—in the pathogenesis of various fatal diseases including lung cancer, cancer at other sites and cardiovascular diseases. However, numbers are too small, as yet, to yield definitive answers.

Most of the misconceptions concerning positive associations between smoking and disease appear to arise from rather elementary lapses in scientific logic and a widespread failure to appreciate that genetic inheritance cannot be disregarded when we analyse the 'causes' of habits and diseases. This reluctance to take inheritance into account—or even to mention it in supposedly scientific papers—is commonplace within and outside medicine and it is characteristic of our epoch. The eagerness to identify causes of disease that (unlike inheritance) might be readily controlled, must be applauded as wholly admirable. Unfortunately, it seems that excessive zeal leads only too often to methodological shortcuts, spurious argument, premature conclusions and the sacrifice of truth.

CHAPTER 11

Survival from Malignant Disease

The question: Why does a patient die from cancer? is seldom asked. It is usually taken for granted that a malignant tumour proliferates, infiltrates, and perhaps metastasizes, until it kills. Progressive and remorseless growth tends to be regarded as the hallmark of cancer and a sufficient cause of death.

The need for reliable prognostic indicators and guides to the efficacy of different therapeutic techniques has stimulated many studies of the duration of survival of cancer patients. Extensive records of the survival of cancer patients in California, from diagnosis to death, have been compiled by the California Tumor Registry (1963). More recently, less detailed survival statistics from the Birmingham Regional Cancer Registry have been published by Waterhouse (1974). At the theoretical level, various attempts have been made to define and interpret survival curves (Boag, 1948; Berkson and Gage, 1952; Tivey, 1954; Berg, 1965; Myers, Axtell and Zelen, 1966; Berg and Robbins, 1967; Zelen, 1968; Blumenson and Bross, 1969), but the interpretation given here differs from previous ones. It entails a simple extension of my theory of carcinogenesis.

Survival: Descriptions and Definitions

The simplest description of survival in relation to time is known as *observed survival*. It defines the proportion of patients with a cancer that survive, after time τ from diagnosis, regardless of the cause of death. Hence, *observed survival* includes a contribution from deaths due to causes other than the cancer of interest. *Relative survival* attempts to correct for intercurrent mortality from other diseases and to estimate survival as though the diagnosed cancer were the only cause of death (Ederer, Axtell and Cutler, 1961; Axtell, 1963; Cutler, Axtell and Heise, 1967; Shedd, van Essen and Connelly, 1968). To obtain relative survival, the observed proportion of the patients in a cancer series surviving at time τ after diagnosis, is expressed as a fraction or percentage of the proportion of the general population that would be expected to survive under similar circumstances. In other words, the post-diagnostic mortality experience in the selected cancer subpopulation is compared with that in the corresponding group of the general population.

When interpreting relative survival, two potential complications arise. First, a group with a specific cancer constitutes a selected subgroup of the general population. Hence, members of this subgroup might be either more or less susceptible to other fatal diseases than members of the general population. Second, the presence of the cancer in the patient might of itself affect mortality from other diseases either directly or indirectly—for example, as the result of cancer therapy. These uncertainties can be reduced if deaths from other diseases in the cancer series can be recorded explicitly, and the appropriate correction applied—see Haybittle (1959) and Cutler, Axtell and Schottenfeld (1969). However, the primary cause of death cannot always be reliably assessed. Of course, if the patients in a given series are young, and if survival seldom extends beyond a few years, little error will be introduced by neglecting intercurrent mortality from other diseases.

It should be emphasized, however, that in most instances, the method of correction has little effect on the general mathematical character of curves of survival versus time, although, as shown below, it can alter appreciably the numerical values of the defining constants.

Analysis of Survival Data

Throughout this section, representative data are analysed graphically in terms of one, or the sum of two, negative exponential functions of the form: $S_\tau = \exp(-\lambda\tau)$. Where S_τ represents the corrected or uncorrected fraction of patients surviving at time τ after diagnosis, or admission to clinical trial. In general, the rate-constant λ depends not only on the method used to correct S_τ, but also on the specific cancer and the therapeutic regimen. The rate-constant λ is equal to $(1/\tau_{\frac{1}{2}})\ln 2$, where $\tau_{\frac{1}{2}}$ represents the time after diagnosis at which S_τ for a defined group become 0·5.

Breast cancer

Fig. 11.1 is calculated from the data of Haybittle (1959) for the survival of 705 women with breast cancer treated at the Radiotherapeutic Centre, Addenbrooke's Hospital, Cambridge, in the years 1947 to 1950 inclusive. I

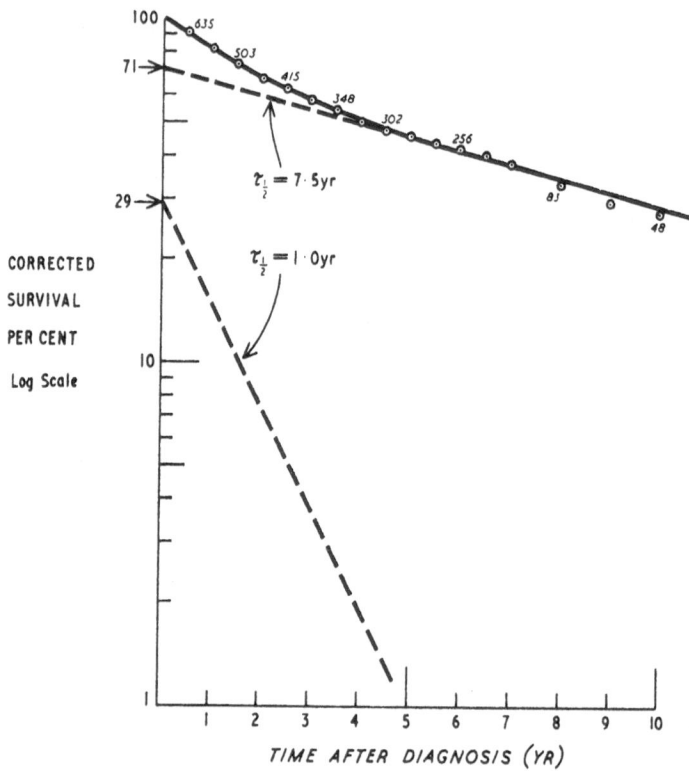

Figure 11.1 Survival of 705 women with breast cancer, treated at the Radiotherapeutic Centre, Addenbrooke's Hospital, Cambridge, 1947–50, in relation to time after diagnosis (Haybittle, 1959). The data are corrected for mortality from diseases other than breast cancer

have corrected the original data for intercurrent mortality from diseases other than breast cancer using the information given in Haybittle's (1959) paper. The survival curve ·can be analysed graphically in terms of two exponential functions. Using this probably oversimplified interpretation, it appears that approximately 29 per cent of the patients in the group had a poor prognosis, with $\tau_{\frac{1}{2}} \simeq 1$ year. The remaining 71 per cent had a much better survival, with $\tau_{\frac{1}{2}} \simeq 7.5$ years.

Figure 11.2 shows data from the California Tumor Registry (1963) for the observed survival of women with breast cancer, 1942–56. It will be recalled that observed survival represents survival from all causes of death. Women in all age groups are included (as in Figure 11.1), and again, the overall survival has been interpreted graphically in terms of two exponential functions. For 30 per cent of the patients, the value of $\tau_{\frac{1}{2}}$ is 1·2 years, and for 70 per cent, $\tau_{\frac{1}{2}}$ is about 9·1 years.

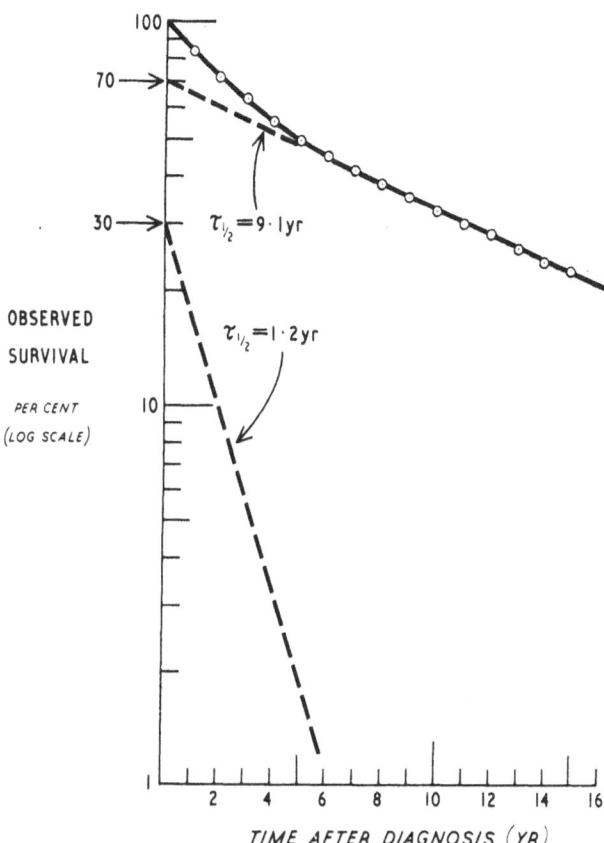

Figure 11.2 'Observed survival' (which records survival from all causes of death), for 13392 women in California with breast cancer, in relation to time after diagnosis (California Tumor Registry, 1963)

Figure 11.3 refers to the same patients as in Figure 11.2, but shows *relative* survival, which attempts to correct for deaths from causes other than breast cancer. Again, the overall survival curve can be quite well represented by the sum of two exponential functions, but with $\tau \simeq 1\cdot 7$ year and $16\cdot 6$ years respectively.

Figures 11.1 to 11.3 agree with the hypothesis that two *main* groups of women patients with breast cancer are involved, each exhibiting negative exponential survival of the form: $S_\tau = \exp(-\lambda\tau)$, one with a relatively good, and the other with a relatively poor prognosis. Nevertheless, because data for *observed survival*—which records all causes of death—can be fitted satisfactorily to the sum of only two exponential functions, we see that the method of analysis is insensitive to the total number of distinctive causes of death, when the relative contributions of some of these causes are small.

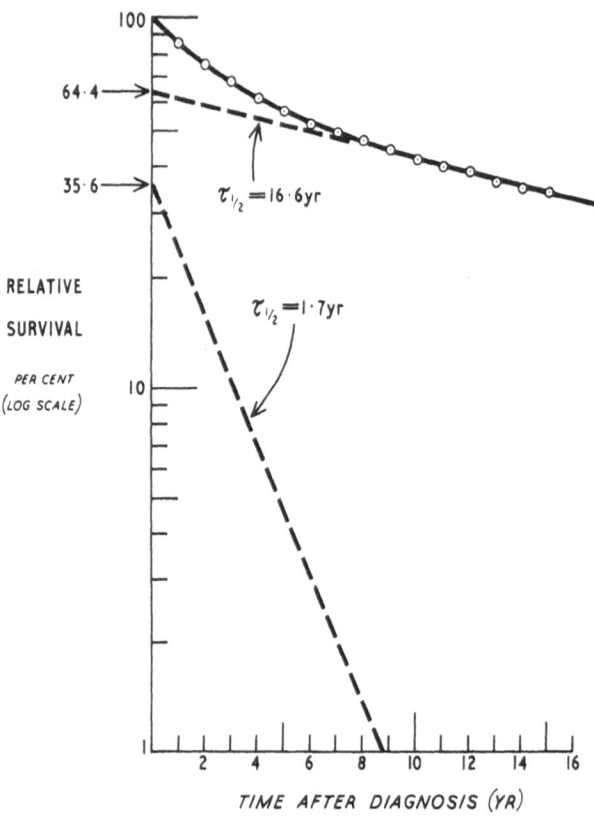

Figure 11.3 'Relative survival' (which attempts to correct for death from causes other than breast cancer), for the same 13 392 women to whom Figure 11.2 applies, in relation to time after diagnosis (California Tumor Registry, 1963)

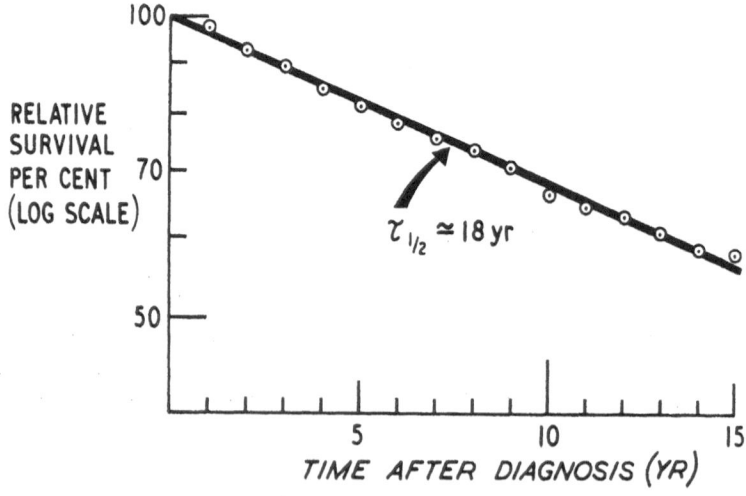

Figure 11.4 'Relative survival' from localized breast cancer, for 5159 women of all ages in California, in relation to time after diagnosis (California Tumor Registry, 1963)

Figure 11.4 shows relative survival, taken from the California Tumor Registry (1963), for women in all age groups with localized breast cancer. From Figure 11.3, illustrating data from the same Registry, we see that the total series of breast cancer patients contains about $0 \cdot 644 \times 13\,392$, that is 8624 patients with a relatively good prognosis ($\tau_{\frac{1}{2}} \simeq 16 \cdot 6$ years). Figure 11.4 refers to 5159 patients from the same total series who had localized breast cancer, and for whom $\tau_{\frac{1}{2}} \simeq 18$ years. It appears, therefore, that in the total series of breast cancer patients, a majority of the patients with good prognosis had the localized form of the disease at diagnosis.

Cutler, Asire and Taylor (1969) analysed the survival of women patients with disseminated breast cancer. They considered survival in relation to the interval between the first diagnosis of primary breast cancer and the subsequent diagnosis of disseminated disease. Prognosis was found to be related to this interval; the longer the interval, the better the prognosis. For each group, however, survival in relation to time after diagnosis of disseminated disease approximately followed a negative exponential curve. Values of $\tau_{\frac{1}{2}}$ ranged from about $0 \cdot 6$ to $2 \cdot 2$ years. Cutler *et al.* (1969) also assessed survival from disseminated breast cancer in relation to the number of metastatic sites. Again, most curves approximated to a negative exponential, and values of $\tau_{\frac{1}{2}}$ ranged from about $0 \cdot 5$ years for four or more metastatic sites, up to about $1 \cdot 6$ years for a single metastasis. It appears, therefore, that patients with a poor prognosis constitute several subgroups, each showing approximately negative exponential survival.

In Chapter 7, we found that the age-dependence of breast cancer pointed to a minimum of two genetically distinctive groups, one with onset predominantly before, and the other with onset predominantly after, 60 years of age. We might expect, therefore, that for a specific form of breast cancer, for example localized, survival will be related to age at onset. Figure 11.5 shows that for women with localized breast cancer and onset prior to 45 years of age, relative survival is described by a simple negative exponential with $\tau_{\frac{1}{2}} \simeq 21$ years; for onset between 65 and 74 years, $\tau_{\frac{1}{2}}$ (relative survival) $\simeq 14$ years. These data in isolation do not, of course, tell us whether age *per se*, or genetic differences, are responsible for the differences in relative survival.

Other cancers

Data for the relative survival of men, with onset of bladder cancer between 55 and 64 years (Figure 11.6), can be represented approximately by two exponential components with $\tau_{\frac{1}{2}} \simeq 0 \cdot 95$ year and $13 \cdot 4$ years, respectively. A better fit could be obtained if an additional group with poor survival was assumed. Similar data for rectal cancer (Figure 11.7) can be described, rather

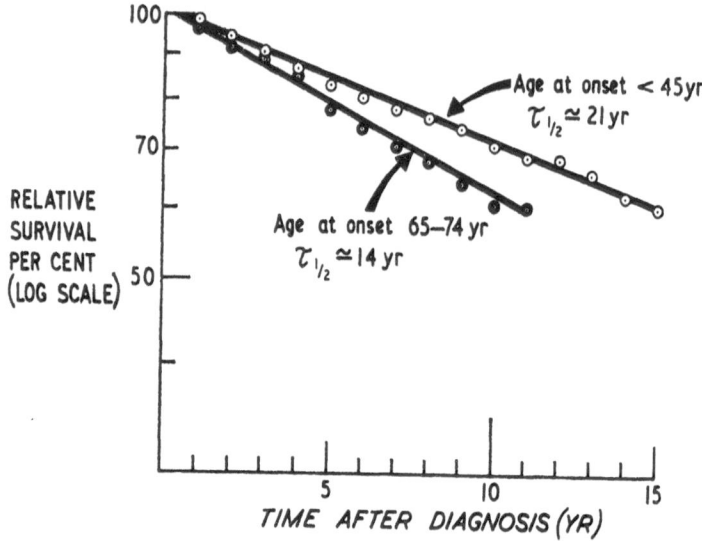

Figure 11.5 'Relative survival' from localized breast cancer for women (a) with onset prior to 45 years of age (upper curve), and (b) for onset between 65 and 74 years (lower curve), in relation to time after diagnosis (California Tumor Registry, 1963)

more accurately, by two components with $\tau_{\frac{1}{2}} \simeq 0 \cdot 8_2$ years and $16 \cdot 0$ years, respectively.

Effects of Therapy

The most dramatic effects of therapy have been obtained in connection with acute lymphocytic leukaemia occurring in children and adolescents. Cutler, Axtell and Heise (1967) describe survival trends by leukaemia type, and age group, for clinical series from 98 hospitals in the United States, 1940 to 1962. In many instances, relative survival followed an approximately negative exponential course during 1940–49. For acute lymphocytic leukaemia in the age-range 0 to 9 years, the relative survival at 6 months after diagnosis was 16 per cent, and at one year it was only about 1 per cent. For the period 1960–62, the *shape* of the relative survival curve had changed from a simple negative exponential curve, to a 'type C' curve with a conspicuous initial shoulder, followed by a negative exponential region. Moreover, the slope of the final negative exponential portion of the curve had changed, becoming markedly less steep. At six months after diagnosis, relative survival in 1960–62 was 73 per cent; at 1 year it was 43 per cent; and at 3 years, 6 per cent (Cutler *et al.*, 1967). The period 1940 to 1962 was marked by an increasing resort to chemotherapy. During 1940–49, only about 10 per cent

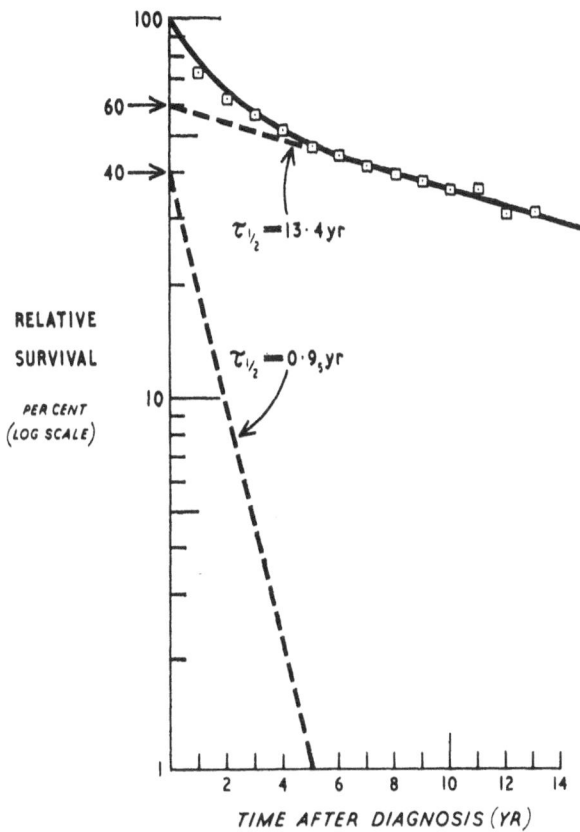

Figure 11.6 'Relative survival' from bladder cancer in 800 males, with onset 55 to 64 years, in relation to time after diagnosis (California Tumor Registry, 1963)

of patients with leukaemia received chemotherapy; in 1960–62, this proportion had increased to about 82 per cent (Cutler *et al.*, 1967).

A randomized trial provides the most reliable test of therapeutic measures. This procedure was used by Roswit, Patno and Rapp (1968) to assess the effects of radiation treatment for localized, but inoperable bronchogenic carcinoma in male patients. One group consisting of 308 men was given 4000 to 5000 rads when possible in four to six weeks: 246 similar patients, serving as concurrent controls, were given the inert compound lactose as a placebo. Observed survival for both groups is illustrated in Figure 11.8. For the placebo group, survival approximates to a negative exponential $(\tau_{\frac{1}{2}} \simeq 4 \cdot 2$ months) up to 12 months. Up to 6 months, survival in the radiation therapy group follows a curve parallel to that for the placebo group, but displaced by about 0·7 month to the right. (Beyond 6 months, statistical errors become large.) In other words, for the first 6 months after admission

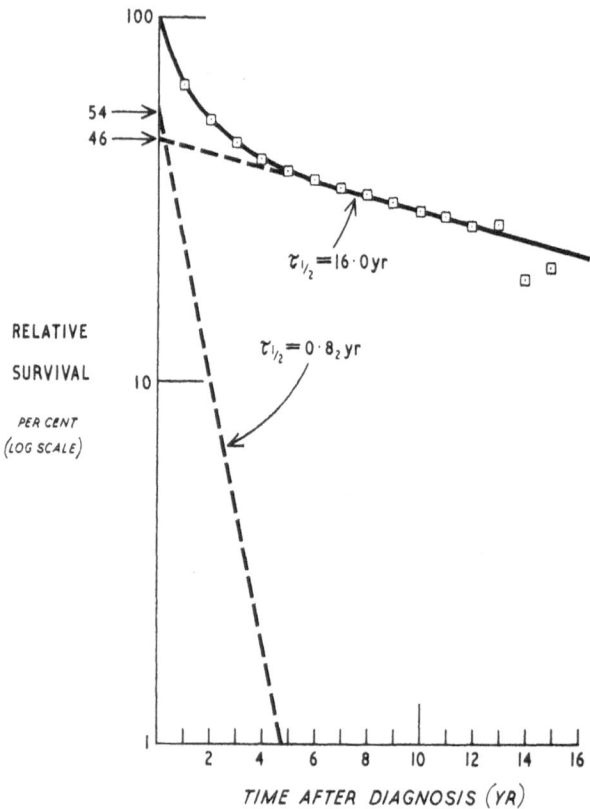

Figure 11.7 'Relative survival' from rectal cancer in 844 males, with onset 55 to 64 years, in relation to time after diagnosis (California Tumor Registry, 1963)

to the trial, death in the treated group was delayed by about 0·7 month. After the first month, and up to 6 months, the death-rate (percentage deaths per month) remained the same in treated and placebo groups.

Interpretation of Survival Statistics

Figures 11.4, 11.5, 11.8 and 11.9 show survival curves that approximate closely to simple negative exponentials. Curves of this kind are described in radiobiology as 'type A' survival curves. Other figures show 'type B' survival curves that can be represented as the sum of two type A curves, although in most instances this is probably a grossly oversimplified inter-pretation. Curves with a shoulder at low τ are known as 'type C' survival curves: the region at high τ may or may not approximate to a negative exponential.

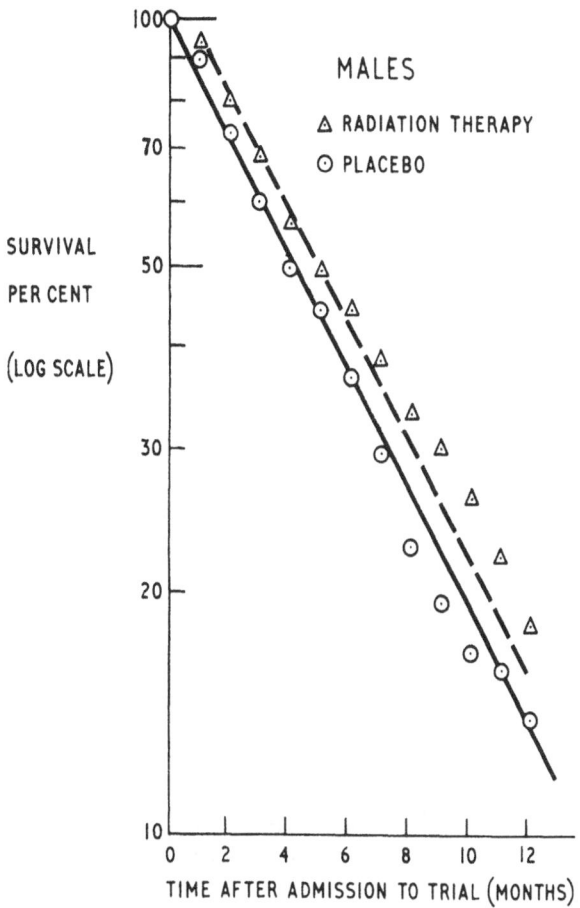

Figure 11.8 Survival of males from localized but inoperable lung cancer: ⊙ placebo group; △ radiation therapy group; in relation to time after admission to trial (Roswit *et al.*, 1968)

Type C curves with a negative exponential region at high τ are seen in connection with the survival of young patients (0 to 19 years), treated mainly by chemotherapy for acute lymphocytic leukaemia (Cutler *et al.*, 1967) (see also the curve for the treated group of lung cancer patients in Figure 11.8). Similar type C curves have been reported in connection with the *observed* survival of treated and untreated patients suffering from chronic myelogenous leukaemia—reviewed by Bergsagel (1967)—although type B curves were obtained for this type of leukaemia in the analysis of *relative* survival given by Cutler *et al.* (1967). This discrepancy might be explained, in part, by the choice of the parameter plotted on the abscissa. In the review by

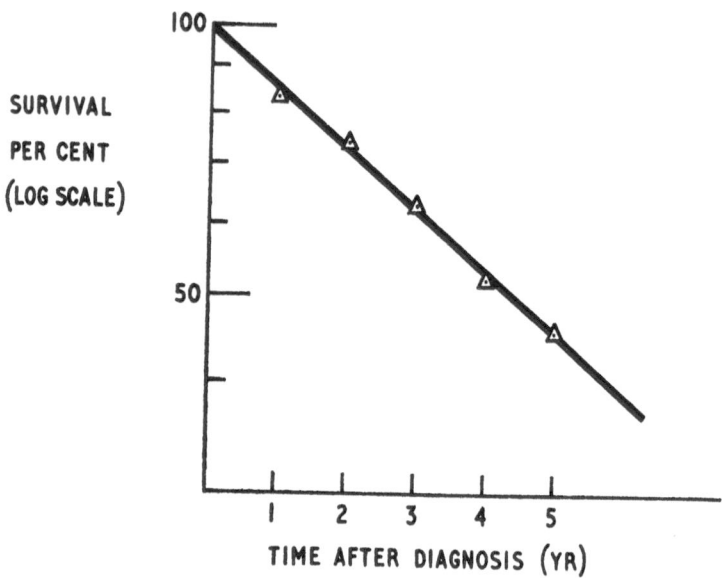

Figure 11.9 Survival from malignant melanoma of patients (both sexes) with age at onset under 25 years, in relation to time after diagnosis (Nathanson *et al.*, 1967)

Bergsagel (1967), survival was referred to the time from the onset of symptoms; in the survey of Cutler *et al.* (1967), survival was referred to the time from diagnosis. However, there seems little doubt that survival from polycythaemia vera is represented by a type C survival curve. Osgood (1965) showed that observed mortality in a group of patients with polycythaemia vera (unlike that in cancer patients) approximate to a normal distribution in time. Because the pattern of survival from polycythaemia vera differs so markedly from that found for most types of cancer, Osgood argued that polycythaemia vera is not a malignant process. From Chapter 7 we can infer that survival of multiple polyposis patients, from diagnosis of colorectal cancer to death, will also be described by a type C curve. Similarly, the survival of women from the first diagnosis of either cervical dysplasia, or carcinoma *in situ* of the uterine cervix, to death, will also be represented by a type C curve.

We see therefore that type A curves, or type B curves compounded of two or more negative exponential (type A) curves, often arise in connection with survival from malignant disease. Although this feature has long been recognized, many investigators have assumed that negative exponential distributions of survival must greatly oversimplify what is intrinsically a highly complex relation. There is a sense in which this assumption is true, but not, I believe, the sense intended.

The simplest interpretation of any type-A survival curve postulates that death results from a single random event that is rate-determining: the average rate of occurrence of this event remains constant, from the time of diagnosis to death.

At first sight, such an interpretation of death from cancer seems so unpromising that we might be tempted to dismiss it out of hand. It fails to correspond with the commonsense view mentioned above in the introduction which can be broadly outlined thus: The duration of survival after diagnosis depends on: (a) the stage of the cancer at the time of diagnosis; (b) the rate of growth of the cancer including not only the primary but any metastases; (c) the degree of invasiveness; and (d) the sites invaded.

This picture of progressive growth and/or invasion leading remorselessly to death can be characterized as being essentially deterministic, rather than stochastic, in character. We would, therefore, expect that death-rates from a specific cancer (per affected person, per unit time after diagnosis) would tend to be low initially, and to increase with time after diagnosis, because of progressive growth, invasiveness and the formation of metastases. An increasing death-rate with time after diagnosis—that is, an increase of λ with τ—would give rise to a type C survival curve, with a continuously increasing (negative) slope. However, this expected type of curve is only occasionally seen. For most narrowly defined malignancies, and in the absence of effective therapy, we see an approximate type A survival curve which implies that the average death-rate from cancer itself (λ) remains approximately constant from the time of diagnosis onwards. It is very difficult to conceive how the combined factors (a) to (d) should so frequently and fortuitously result in a type A survival curve, or a type B curve, compounded of two or more such contributions.

The biological and biochemical causes of fatal crises in cancer are obscure. Sylvén (1969) points out that many cancer patients die without advanced malnutrition, uraemia, infection or haemorrhage; death seldom coincides with the rapid growth of the tumour, but rather with tumour deterioration and arrest of further growth. Before pursuing the problem of the fatal crisis it will be helpful to consider the time-dependence of tumour growth.

Growth of Tumours

According to my basic theory, the growth of a natural tumour, benign or malignant, follows from interactions between specific mutant MCPs and their cognate promoted target tissues. Hence, tumour size should depend on: (a) the output of mutant MCPs, which might be affected by the endogenous defence system and/or by the functioning of a residual homeostatic control mechanism; (b) the access of mutant MCPs and the supply of nutrients to target cells; and (c) the loss of cells from the tumour resulting from necrosis and/or the host's immune mechanism. If the host survives long enough and if homeostatic control is preserved the tumour will eventually attain a limiting size.

Laird (1964, 1965), McCredie et al. (1965), Sullivan and Salmon (1972) and subsequently others have found that many spontaneous, induced and transplanted tumours in experimental animals, and spontaneous tumours in man, exhibit a similar growth pattern, culminating in a limiting size. This pattern can often be described accurately by the following Gompertz function:

$$N = N_o \exp\left[(A/\alpha)\{1 - \exp(-\alpha\tau)\}\right] \qquad (11.1)$$

Where N = number of cells in the tumour at time τ; N_o = number of cells in the tumour at $\tau = 0$; A and α are constants. (In place of cell number, N and N_o sometimes refer to tumour volume or mass.)

Equation (11.1) is the solution of the following differential equations

$$dN/d\tau = \gamma N \qquad (11.2)$$

and

$$d\gamma/d\tau = -\alpha\gamma \qquad (11.3)$$

whence

$$\gamma = A \exp(-\alpha\tau) \qquad (11.4)$$

When $\tau = \infty$, N attains a finite limiting size

$$N_\infty = N_o \exp(A/\alpha) \qquad (11.5)$$

These equations indicate that the growth of many tumours, primary or transplanted, is initially exponential, but that the effective growth stimulus, γ, falls off approximately exponentially with time (equation 11.4). From the mathematical form of the growth curve, Laird (1965) argued that a tumour does not grow as a population of individual cells, but as though it were a single organism. Indeed, the growth of whole organisms, through the embryonic and postnatal stages, can be fairly well represented by the Gompertz equation (11.1) above (Laird, Tyler and Barton, 1965; McCredie et al., 1965).

When we consider that different organs in the body grow at different rates, it is somewhat surprising that the growth curves of: (a) the whole body; and (b) of many different tumours, should have similar characteristics. Just as surprising, perhaps, is the similarity of the growth patterns of primary and transplanted tumours. A transplanted tumour will generally be introduced into a host with an intact growth-control system and hence, when the Gompertz relation is followed, it would appear that the growth of the tumour might well depend on the interaction between normal MCPs of the host and the (in part) complementary TCFs of the target cells in the tumour. In all these instances we are probably concerned with the growth of heterogeneous structures (recall the vasculature of solid tumours) and the operation of complex feedback systems.

That the growth of Lewis lung carcinoma transplanted to C57BL/6 male mice is under the control of the host, and that the ultimate size of the tumour is also host-controlled, is strongly indicated by some ingenious experiments of De Wys (1972). An implant of 2×10^5 tumour cells was made into the right hind leg muscles. For about the first 7 days, tumour growth was exponential, but the rate then declined to approach zero at 25–30 days. Metastatic growth in the lungs was first detected (about 10^2 cells) at 9 days after transplantation. Again, growth was approximately exponential for about 7 days, after which the rate declined rapidly to approach zero at 25–30 days after the original transplant (De Wys, 1972). An important finding was that of exponential growth in the small metastasis (10^2–10^5 cells) during a period when the growth of the large primary transplant (at 10^8–10^9 cells) was markedly subexponential. Metastatic growth was first observed in the kidney 17 days after transplantation, but the small size of the metastasis and errors of measurement prevented an accurate characterization of the mathematical form of growth (De Wys, 1972). Nevertheless, it was clear that the initial rate of growth in these late metastases was much lower than in the early lung metastases.

These important data suggest that a substantial part of the *initial departure* from exponential growth in the large primary transplant relates to the number of cells in that transplant. Thus, the growth of a small metastasis in the lung proved to be exponential during the period when the growth of the primary implant began to deviate substantially from the exponential characteristic. Lala (1972) found that within a solid tumour, zones of high growth-rate were associated with proximity to capillaries. (For discussions of this aspect of growth-limitation in tumours, see Burton (1966) and Burns (1969).) However, De Wys (1972) found that the *late* approach to zero growth occurred simultaneously in the large primary transplant and the smaller metastases to the lung and kidney. Other observations, both in man and experimental animals, have shown that when the volume of a tumour is reduced by radiation, a period of accelerated growth follows (Van Peperzeel, 1972). Barendsen and Broerse (1970) observed the effect of various radiation treatment schedules on the growth of a rhabdomyosarcoma, transplantable in an inbred strain of rats. After three weeks of fractionated irradiation, surviving cells proliferated initially with a doubling time of

2 days, as compared with 4 to 5 days in the large tumour mass before irradiation.

Hence, the good approximation of the growth curve for many tumours to the Gompertz function appears to be somewhat coincidental. The initial departure from exponential growth in a large mass of tumour tissue probably results mainly from a failure of mitotic stimuli and/or nutrients to reach the more inaccessible tumour cells. However, the limiting size reached by the entire tumour mass (primary plus metastases) is probably governed by feedback control. Thus, in another set of experiments, De Wys (1972) showed that in animals that received a second transplant 8 or 15 days after the first, not only did the large first tumour influence the growth of the second, but the smaller second tumour also influenced the growth of the first. Indeed, the total mass of tumour in animals with: (a) one transplant; and (b) with two transplants, the second being given 8 days after the first, was almost the same (within 3 per cent) throughout the observation period of 15 to 25 days after the first transplant. From his experiments, De Wys concluded that retardation of tumour growth increases with *total* tumour mass and that the retardation effect manifests systemically. However, he did not consider the possibility that the final size of the tumour might be determined by a central—if physiologically inappropriate—homeostatic system.

Bichel (1971) suggested that the growth of the experimental ascites tumour depends on the amount of tumour tissue present in the mouse and is analogous to the regulation of the growth of normal tissue. The number of tumour cells usually reaches a plateau before the host dies. Bichel found that for pairs of mice in parabiotic union, a fully developed ascites tumour (a transplantable plasmacytoma) in one animal retarded the growth of an aspirated tumour in the partner. He proposed that an inhibiting principle diffuses through the peritoneum from one animal to its partner. However, essentially *dissimilar* results were obtained by Rockwell and Kallman (1972) who observed the growth curves for: (a) single KHT sarcomas implanted in syngeneic C3H/Km mice; and (b) for nine or ten similarly implanted tumours per mouse. Each tumour, whether implanted singly or as one of multiple tumours, showed the same growth curve. However, the experiment was terminated well before the plateau region was reached, but after departure from exponential growth had occurred. There was no indication that the departure from exponential growth resulted from a negative feedback mechanism. Either no such mechanism operates in this tumour–host system or the extent of tumour growth was inadequate to reveal it.

Tumour Growth and Body Weight

Many cancer patients develop asthenia and severe wasting. De Wys (1972) found that total body weight in mature C57BL/6 mice receiving an implant of Lewis lung carcinoma had increased by about 20 per cent at 30 days post-implantation. However, when the weight of tumour tissue was subtracted, he found that 'carcass' weight had fallen by about 15 per cent.

These phenomena suggest that a high rate of flow of affector 'not-self' or mutant TCFs from a tumour might interfere with non-cognate central growth-control elements. The complementarity of components of 'not-self' or mutant TCFs for components of non-homologous MCPs, might cause them to be intercepted by receptors in the central growth-control elements and to be 'mistaken' for normal affector TCFs. Such errors would reduce or eliminate the output of normal MCPs from disturbed elements and interfere with homeostasis.

Conclusions

Studies of the growth of tumours *in vivo* suggest that, in many instances, the eventual size is regulated, at a physiologically *inappropriate* level, by a central homeostatic system that exports mitogenic effectors and responds to tumour-derived affectors.

Observations of the growth of tumours of human origin *in vitro* point to the presence of mitogenic factors in the serum. If in the culture medium, heterologous foetal calf or horse serum, or pooled human serum, is replaced by autologous serum, growth of tumour cells then takes place more rapidly (Cobb and Walker, 1961; Kahn and Donaldson, 1970). Similarly, Röller, Owen and Heidelberger (1966) found that when human tumours were cultivated in Eagle's MEM medium supplemented with various sources of protein, the supplement that yielded the highest tumour viability was the patient's own serum. Various authors have reported that, under certain circumstances, immunoglobulin antibodies can stimulate tumour growth. Shearer *et al.* (1975) found that immunostimulation *in vitro* is greatly augmented by complement, with utilization of both the classical and alternate pathways via C3. This raises the possibility that the humoral system of normal growth-control might be connected, in some way, with the complement system. Some ingenious experiments on tumour-bearing mice by Vaillier (1974) demonstrate the presence of tumour mitogenic factors *in vivo*. Using cells from RV2 tumours chemically induced in the C3H/He strain of mouse, he compared their growth in diffusion chambers implanted in (a) normal and (b) RV2 tumour-bearing C3H/He mice. The diffusion chambers incorporated Millipore filters of 0·1 μm pore size. Such chambers are impermeable to cells, but diffusible substances can be exchanged between the host and the enclosed tumour cells. In five separate experiments, each involving five diffusion chambers per mouse, the growth of tumour cells in the chambers was always significantly higher in the tumour-bearing mice than in the normal mice.

I have argued that, in the control of the growth (symmetrical mitosis) of epidermal cells, the peripheral representatives of the control system (possibly mast cells) reside in the local stroma. The induction of dermal and epidermal tumours by the local application of chemical carcinogens, or by local irradiation, probably requires specific mutation of controlling mast cells (see Chapter 9). Van Scott and Reinertson (1961) confirmed the importance of the local stroma to tumour growth in man. Tumours unaccompanied by their associated connective tissue failed to grow when autotransplanted to distant sites. Metastasis as a general phenomenon undoubtedly involves site specificity. Probably complementarity between tumour TCFs and site TCFs is needed for metastasis, together with a sufficiently high concentration of mitogenic MCPs.

Support for the existence of central controlling factors comes from a study of 423 women with breast cancer (clinical stages I or II) who had undergone simple mastectomy and radiotherapy (Bruce, Carter and Fraser, 1970). In 112 patients, recurrences were observed to occur synchronously, or nearly so, at both local and distant metastatic sites (Bruce et al., 1970). These findings, in common with those quoted above, imply that recurrences were caused by systemic factors of central origin that affected target cells at multiple sites, more or less simultaneously. The distribution of time intervals between mastectomy and the first detectable recurrence was similar in each of three distinctive groups: (a) patients developing distant metastases only; (b) patients developing distant metastases and local recurrence; (c) patients developing local recurrence only (Bruce et al., 1970). This common distribution (Figure 11.10) can be represented by the following simple stochastic function

$$P = 1 - \exp(-k\tau)$$

where P is the probability of recurrence at time τ after mastectomy, and $k \simeq 0·26$ year^{-1} for each group. The fit of the distributions to this equation suggests that the development of a local and/or distant recurrence is triggered by a single random event. Hence, the pathogenesis of this form of recurrence resembles, kinetically, that commonly found for lethality. The rate of the random event that triggers recurrence is comparable to the rates found for lethal random events. Clearly, the biological nature of such events could be of considerable importance to therapists.

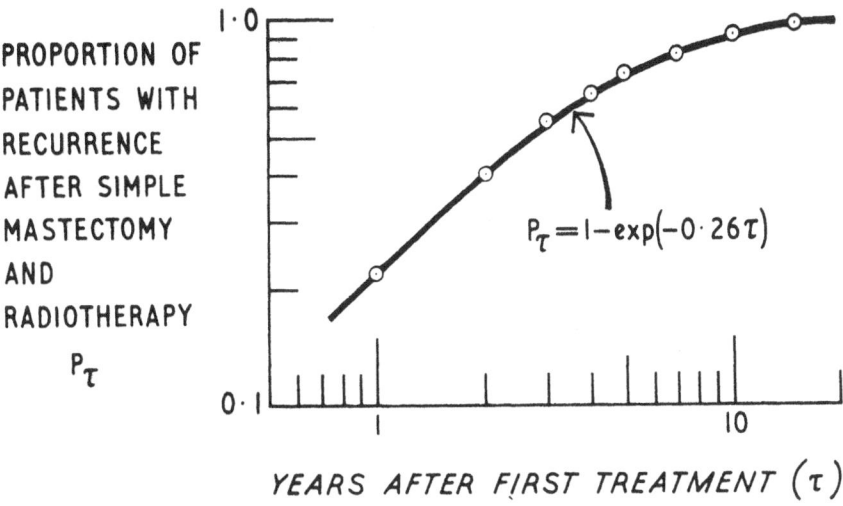

Figure 11.10 Prevalence of patients with recurrence after simple mastectomy and radiotherapy in relation to time after first treatment (Bruce *et al.*, 1970)

The nature of the lethal event

We need to be able to explain the following evidence relating to the hypothetical lethal event.

(1) For many cancers, the average rate of the random event is constant, or nearly so, from diagnosis to death.

(2) Radiotherapy for inoperable lung cancer, which reduces tumour volume, does not alter the average rate of the lethal event although it delays its impact by about 30 days (Roswit *et al.*, 1968).

(3) Chemotherapy for acute lymphocytic leukaemia slows the rate of the lethal event and delays its impact.

(4) The survival of male or female patients with thymic tumours in association with myasthenia gravis follows a negative exponential (Hale, 1968). However, the slope of the survival curve for men is approximately twice as steep as that for women. For men, the value of $\tau_{\frac{1}{2}}$ (diagnosis to death) is 4·5 years, but for women it is approximately 9·5 years, effectively double the value for men (Hale, 1968).

This latter evidence could well have special significance for the understanding of the nature of the lethal event in cancer and also for sex-differences in the distribution of the latent period between initiation and onset, and initiation and death, in various diseases. For those spontaneous autoaggressive diseases that involve forbidden clones of T-lymphocytes (these include myasthenia gravis) the average latent period in *XX* women is generally (perhaps always) double that in *XY* men, with a similar predisposing genotype (Burch, 1968(a); Burch and Rowell, 1968, 1970). The most plausible interpretation of this sex-difference, bearing in mind (1) to (4) above, is that the average number of pathogenetic T-lymphocytes in a forbidden clone in affected women is half that in similarly affected men. Apparently, the size of the clone is determined in some way by the total number of *X*-chromosomes in cells of the clone, rather than the number of cells. If death from thymic tumour depends on a single random event—as suggested by the negative exponential survival curves (Hale, 1968)—and if this event is the spontaneous somatic mutation of an autosomal gene in a 'cell at risk' in the forbidden clone, then the sex-difference in survival can be explained. The two-to-one difference in clone size will also explain the two-to-one ratio in the duration of the latent period in diseases such as myasthenia gravis.

Carcinomas are not induced by forbidden clones of T-lymphocytes but, in theory at least, by forbidden clones of cells that synthesize and secrete mutant *humoral* MCPs. Very often, carcinomas at comparable anatomical sites entail sex-differences in genetic predisposition. Also, the proportion of, say, early- and late-onset cases may differ between the sexes (see Chapter 7). Consequently, relative survival from cancer at defined sites in men and women often shows a sex-differential. Nevertheless, the basic principles that apply to survival from thymic tumours probably apply also to carcinomas and other types of malignancy. When survival—from the diagnosis of a malignancy to death—follows a simple negative exponential, I suggest the single random lethal event is a spontaneous somatic mutation in a cell of a forbidden clone. This forbidden clone will have promoted, or have assisted in promoting, the malignant transformation of target cells. If a typical average rate of initiating somatic mutation is $\sim 10^{-3}$ per growth-control stem cell at risk, per year; and if a typical average rate of lethal somatic mutational events is ~ 1 per year, then the number of cells at risk in the forbidden clone, with respect to the lethal event, should be ~ 1000. (This assumes that the average rates of somatic gene mutation in growth-control stem cells and daughter forbidden clone cells, are similar.)

Spontaneous regression

A brief reference was made in Chapter 9 to the phenomenon of spontaneous regression. Various reviews and case reports leave little doubt as to its authenticity (Nelson, 1962; Smithers, 1962, 1964; Boyd, 1966; Everson and Cole, 1966; Cole, 1974), although its rarity has precluded the collection of adequate data concerning the frequencies of regression and recurrence at a particular site in relation to time after onset. It would be valuable to establish whether the relation between regression frequency and time can be described by a simple stochastic equation.

Among the possible hypotheses of spontaneous regression the following, which are not mutually exclusive, are perhaps among the more plausible.

(1) The host's immune system eliminates most, or all, of the cells of the tumour by virtue of the antigenicity of their mutant TCFs.

(2) The host's immune system eliminates most, or all, of the cells in the promoting carcinogenic forbidden clone(s).

(3) Somatic mutation (especially a back mutation) of an MCP gene in the growth control stem cell propagating a carcinogenic forbidden clone, leads to the replacement of cells in the forbidden clone by non-carcinogenic cells from the altered stem cell.

(4) A change in hormonal status modulates the growth of those tumours subject to homeostatic regulation.

In view of the astronomical number of cells in a typical tumour we cannot easily accept that the host's immune system—hypothesis (1)—passes from a state of non-suppression of tumour cells to one of complete or near-complete suppression. However, a somatic mutation in, for example, a stem cell of the T-lymphocyte series, might just conceivably give rise to a new clone of lymphocytes cytotoxic for tumour cells. Because the source of immunogenicity of cells in a natural tumour (mutant TCFs) is analogous to that of initiating mutant MCPs—and hence also of mutant T-lymphocytes—I regard this as a rather improbable mechanism. But a change in the hormonal status of the host might lead to greatly enhanced immune activity.

If the above estimate of the number of cells (~ 1000) in a promoting forbidden clone is correct, then the host's immune system would be much more likely to diminish substantially the size of the forbidden clone than that of the tumour. Against this hypothesis (2) is the extreme rarity of spontaneous regression. We could argue, however, that spontaneous regression is confined to a small genetically specific subpopulation with a very effective immune system. If that were the case, it would be difficult to understand how the tumour flourished in the first place. But again, we could always invoke, either the concept of hormonal change and stimulation of the immune system, or spontaneous somatic mutation in the immune system.

Hypothesis (3) has the advantage that the postulated back mutation must occur occasionally. Its most serious apparent drawback concerns the requirement that cells of a carcinogenic forbidden clone should be largely or wholly eliminated. Experimental chemical and radiation carcinogenesis indicates that carcinogenic peripheral growth-control cells are not usually eliminated by the host's immune system. However, this apparent objection might, in fact, constitute support, because spontaneous regression is seen relatively frequently in connection with only a few types of tumour—notably hyper-nephroma and neuroblastoma—and very rarely with the common carcinomas (Everson and Cole, 1966). If this mechanism does operate, then the relation between regression frequency and time should reveal the random nature of the somatic mutation of the MCP gene.

A further hypothesis needs to be considered in connection with the regression of metastases that sometimes follows the excision of a bulky primary lesion (Cole, 1974). For those tumours whose ultimate size is governed by a homeostatic control, a rate of flow of affector tumour TCFs in excess of some minimum will be needed to maintain the output of effector carcinogenic MCPs (see Chapter 3 and Figure 3.3). If through the removal of a large primary tumour the rate of flow of affector (mutant) TCFs from remaining metastases falls below the critical minimum, the output of effector carcinogenic MCPs will be cut off and metastases will regress. The initial growth of a carcinogenic forbidden clone occurs because normal target cells 'feed back' non-mutant affector TCFs.

Cyclic non-malignant disorders are not uncommon and these can be attributed to an oscillation set up through the tendency of forbidden clones both to proliferate and to elicit a defence mechanism (Burch, 1968(a)). Cyclic leucocytosis has been observed in untreated (Morley, Baikie and Galton, 1967) and treated (Kennedy, 1970) patients with chronic myeloid leukaemia. Defence, or other feedback controls, might be implicated in such instances. Because oscillation of the peripheral-blood leucocyte count can also be observed in healthy individuals, the oscillation seen in patients with chronic myeloid leukaemia might reflect the residual operation of a normal homeostatic control (Morley et al., 1967).

The growth of certain tumours—for example, of the prostate and breast—appears to be subject to hormonal regulation. Presumably, the functioning of the central system of growth-control, both in normal and neoplastic growth, is to some extent hormone-dependent. A change in hormonal status brought about by, for example, ovariectomy in pre-menopausal women, often effects a temporary (three to nine months) regression of breast cancer (Cole, 1974). The short-lived nature of such regressions suggests that hormones modulate the activity of homeostatic growth-control without changing permanently the level of control.

Therapeutic issues

My interpretation of the cause of death from malignant disease raises some new issues and possibilities for cancer therapists. Hitherto, therapy has been directed to the elimination of cancerous tissue by physical, chemical and/or immunological means. In principle, the total elimination of target tissue should always result in cure although this might be only temporary if the formation of a new forbidden clone gives rise to a new tumour. Such a tumour would usually be classed as a recurrence. So far as I am aware, the idea that the growth and fate of a cancer is determined by a central control mechanism has not been considered in the therapeutic context. From the study of Roswit et al. (1968)—see Fig. 11.8—we see that the radiation-induced partial regression of a malignant lung cancer delayed death by about one month only; the average rate of the lethal event appeared to be unaffected by the irradiation. Chemotherapy, at least of leukaemia, slows the average rate of the lethal event. This suggests that the number of cells in forbidden clones can be reduced by chemotherapeutic agents. These cells are likely to be located, at least in part, in the bone marrow.

Because of the lack of specificity of available chemotherapeutic agents, it seems unlikely that pathogenetic forbidden clones could in general be completely eliminated without destroying much of the bone marrow. We need, therefore, to discover whether forbidden clones can be localized by using, say, tagged antibodies.

This would entail the preparation of specific anti-forbidden-clone anti-bodies: antitumour antibodies should suffice in certain instances. The anti-bodies would then need to be labelled with a suitable γ-ray-emitting radioisotope. If localization could be achieved in this way, then massive local irradiation of the appropriate zone(s) might be used to eliminate the for-bidden clone(s) while leaving the bulk of bone marrow unirradiated and intact. Elimination of the cancer-promoting forbidden clone(s) should be followed by regression of the cancer, without further treatment.

Another line of attack might consist in blocking the action of the products (mutant MCPs) of the lethal forbidden clone by immunological methods. However, it is difficult to envisage how blocking action could be maintained effectively over a period of years.

Although death from a cancer appears generally to follow the occurrence of a single random event in a cell of a forbidden clone, this event in itself does not represent the ultimate cause of death. The additionally mutant cell in the forbidden clone presumably gives rise to a lethal forbidden clone, the products of which interact with complementary malignant cells. Sylvén (1969) has proposed that a fatal toxic factor is released from tumour cells. Such an effect, or, say, increased invasiveness, might constitute the terminal phase. But in any case, it is difficult to conceive effective therapeutic inter-vention at this late and essentially unpredictable stage.

Outside conventional approaches, the main therapeutic promise would appear to lie in the identification and elimination of forbidden clones. Although elimination by immunological methods should not be overlooked, the prospects for consistent success seem slender. The host's endogenous defence is generally ineffective, although, as suggested above, the occurrence of rare, spontaneous regressions might signify occasional success.

Summary

The following brief summary of the main conclusions drawn in this chapter may be helpful.

Tumour growth, in common with that of non-neoplastic tissues, is often under homeostatic control. Of course, the extent of growth is inappropriate to the physiological needs of the organism. Control is exercised by the forbidden clone or clones that promote tumour growth. These clones arise as the result of spontaneous somatic mutations in cells of the central system of normal growth-control.

Generally, death from a cancer does not result merely from its growth, which may attain a plateau. The distribution of the time intervals between diagnosis and death, together with other evidence, indicates that death from many cancers follows the occurrence of a single somatic gene mutation in a cell of a promoting forbidden clone. This additionally mutant clonal cell probably gives rise to the formation of the lethal forbidden clone. The interaction of the products of the lethal clone with the target cells in the cancer gives rise to the terminal phase.

Conventional therapeutic methods aim at the elimination of cancer cells. Certain forms of chemotherapy and radiotherapy succeed, however, in reducing the number of cells in the forbidden clones that promote malignant transformation. They thereby slow the rate of occurrence of the lethal event. Theoretically, selective elimination of forbidden clones appears to be a therapeutic alternative to the removal of cancer cells. The main barrier to the attainment of this objective is likely to be the difficulty of localizing the cells of the forbidden clone. In principle, this barrier could be overcome if anti-forbidden-clone antibodies could be prepared and labelled with a suitable γ-emitting radioisotope. 'Visualization' of the zone occupied by the forbidden clone—using a gamma camera or a scanning technique— would enable large doses of radiation to be delivered locally. In this way, it might be possible to destroy the forbidden clone without inflicting excessive damage on healthy tissues.

CHAPTER 12

Summary and Concluding Remarks

In this treatise I have deployed what must be regarded in biomedical science as unconventional methods, in an attempt to elucidate those enigmas that still surround the tantalizing subject of cancer. Instead of pursuing the customary intensive line of experimental research, I have: (a) surveyed a wide range of biological and medical evidence, both experimental and observational; (b) modified and elaborated the insights and seminal concepts of Burnet (1959) (forbidden clones), and Burwell (1963) (lymphoid control of morphostasis); and (c) resorted extensively to mathematical and logical analysis of quantitative observations. The resulting mixture of analysis with synthesis, and reductionism with holism, has generated a fairly comprehensive but basically simple description of cancer and carcinogenesis. This account derives from a unified theory of normal growth, cytodifferentiation and age-dependent disease. The theory of age-dependent disease was formulated originally to explain the aetiology and pathogenesis of the so-called autoimmune diseases; only after some five years or so did I appreciate that it applies, with equal validity, to natural neoplastic and malignant diseases. The interrelations described between the phenomena of embryonic induction, cytodifferentiation, tissue organization, postnatal growth-control, age-dependent disease and neoplastic change are, perhaps, among the most interesting features of our unified theory.

All disorders with a reproducible age-dependence—malignant and non-malignant, infectious and non-infectious, acute and chronic, lethal and non-lethal—are seen to be *initiated* by specific somatic mutations (probably DNA strand-switching events) in stem cells of the central system of growth-control. We describe such disorders as *autoaggressive*.

Normally, the cells propagated by growth-control stem cells form part of the efferent limb of a negative feedback (homeostatic) system of growth-control (see Chapters 3 and 4). The peripheral descendant cells of specific growth-control stem cells, or their humoral products (the effectors), control symmetrical mitosis of cells in specific mosaic elements of a classical 'tissue', at one or more anatomical sites. In order to do this, a particular effector needs to locate and interact with a cognate target cell, in a specific mosaic element. The process of identification, which is extremely demanding in a complex organism such as man, necessitates a highly specific interaction between mutual recognition elements associated with the effector and the target cell. The recognition elements comprise major and minor histocompatibility antigens, conventional tissue-specific antigens and subtler determinants that distinguish one mosaic element of a classical 'tissue' from other similar, but not identical, elements.

We call effector molecules (humoral and cellular) mitotic control proteins or MCPs; and affector molecules from target cells and the corresponding recognition molecules carried on the cytoplasmic membrane of target cells, tissue coding factors or TCFs. The TCFs synthesized by target cells also determine their cytodifferentiation. Mutual recognition between cognate MCPs and TCFs, at both ends of the feedback loop, depends on the identity of the recognition protein components of the interacting molecules. The London–van der Waal's 'self-recognition' forces of interaction are weak and short-range, but highly specific. This scheme of MCP–TCF recognition in growth-control constitutes the core of my unified theory. Two independent arguments (see Chapter 4), both entailing logical deductions from simple and well-founded empirical premises, establish this theory of recognition in normal growth-control with a fair degree of confidence. Experimental testing will require the isolation, purification and amino acid sequencing of cognate MCPs and TCFs.

The random events that initiate natural autoaggressive disorders obey unexpectedly simple stochastic laws (see Chapter 6): the events entail the spontaneous mutation of MCP genes in growth-control stem cells. Mutation converts the relation of identity between the recognition components of normal MCPs and TCFs, into one of complementarity between the mutant MCP and the normal TCF. In various forms of carcinogenesis (experimental, certainly; natural, by implication), the *promotion* phase entails spontaneous mutation of one or more specific TCF genes in one or more target cells and the fixing of these mutations by the interacting mutant MCP. Neoplastic growth of specifically mutant target cells is then stimulated by the mutant MCPs.

Those neoplastic diseases that exhibit qualitatively distinctive stages of *progression* involve multiple initiating forbidden clones (see Chapter 7).

Progression towards clinical invasiveness corresponds to an increase in the number of forbidden clones. Invasiveness depends on molecular complementarity between the mutant TCFs of cancer cells and the normal TCFs of invaded tissues. The anatomical specificity of metastasis has a similar interpretation. When the stage of clinical invasiveness has been reached, death from the malignancy follows, in many instances, from the occurrence of a single random event (see Chapter 11). This event is probably a DNA strand-switching somatic mutation in a mitotically competent cell of an initiating forbidden clone.

Contrast with Orthodox Views of Cancer

The informed reader will appreciate that the interpretation of cancer given in this book and summarized above departs radically from orthodox views. On certain basic issues, I find myself in sympathy with Smithers (1962), Willis (1967) and Foulds (1969) and hence in conflict with the prevailing philosophy. Preoccupation with the cancer cell has obscured the key issue of inter-cellular *relations*: neoplastic growth should be regarded as a breakdown, or aberration, in *biological organization*. Cancer is primarily a biological problem.

More specifically, the great majority of cancers in man result, not from the action of extrinsic carcinogenic agents, but from spontaneous changes of genes in stem cells of the central system of growth-control, and, during promotion, from similar changes in cells of the target tissue. The contribution from occupational and extrinsic carcinogens is too small to be detected in national onset and death statistics against the overwhelming background of natural cancers. Those epidemiological studies that purport to show a causal connection between cigarette smoking and various cancers, but particularly lung cancer, fail when examined critically to establish the causal claim. In this context I have no option but to reject the conclusions of 'authoritative committees and commissions' and to concur with Fisher (1959), Berkson (1959) and others in proposing that the positive (and negative) associations between smoking and various malignant diseases have a genetic origin (see Chapter 10).

The question as to whether oncogenic viruses are implicated in the pathogenesis of cancers in man is not resolved by the available evidence; it is discussed at length in Chapter 8. Although epidemiological studies have generally failed to show that the horizontal transmission of oncogenic viruses is an important phenomenon in man, theories of vertical transmission can be devised that are very difficult or almost impossible to refute. Because my general theory holds that acute infectious disease is that form of autoaggressive disease in which an invading micro-organism precipitates the growth of forbidden clones, I find it difficult to understand why oncogenic viruses have not been clearly identified in the pathogenesis of at least some malignancies in man. Of course, the identification may yet be made.

Despite this failure to demonstrate infectious malignant disease in man, the following features of natural carcinogenesis are probably shared by all diseases that have a reproducible age-dependence.

(1) A specific autoaggressive disorder, including any specific natural cancer, is restricted to a genetically specific subpopulation. (It would be possible so to narrow the definition of 'specific' as to make every cancer virtually unique. Seldom will the same mosaic element(s) of a given target tissue be involved in different persons at the same age. However, the overall kinetics of initiation of many conventionally homogeneous cancers, involving different sets of mosaic elements, are often indistinguishable in genetically similar populations—see Chapter 7.)

(2) The disease process is *initiated* through the spontaneous (random) occurrence of mutations of MCP genes in stem cells of the central system of growth-control. Some r specific mutations, in one or n distinctive stem cells, are needed for initiation. The value of r may range from one to perhaps twelve; the value of n may range from one to at least seven, depending on the particular cancer (see Chapter 7).

(3) In ordinary environments, the average rate of any specific initiating somatic mutation, probably depends only on the DNA base sequence. The average rate remains effectively constant from around birth, to the onset of disease, even when this occurs at the end of the normal lifespan.

For accurately diagnosed and well-defined age-dependent diseases I have failed so far to find any clearcut violations of features (1) to (3). They may well prove to be wide-ranging biological laws applicable to all warm-blooded (homeothermic) animals.

My analysis of neoplastic and malignant growth in terms of a breakdown in biological organization and growth-control offers no easy panacea for the elimination of cancer although Chapter 11 examines some new therapeutic possibilities. Because most malignant diseases have their predominant onset beyond the reproductive years, natural selection has failed to eliminate those genes that predispose to cancer. Those malignancies with predominantly early onset are of relatively low frequency (see Chapters 7 and 9).

The need for theory

To describe cancer as a breakdown in normal growth-control verges on the tautologous, but few previous theories have tried to make explicit the nature of the normal control of growth and its breakdown in cancer. Accordingly, no other reasonably comprehensive theory exists with which the present one can be compared and contrasted. Even in such restricted (but important) areas as the age-dependence and anatomical distribution of malignant and pre-malignant disease, no other quantitative theory of carcinogenesis is capable of interpreting most of the observations discussed in Chapter 7.

Although the methods used in this book are commonplace throughout physics, they have so far failed to find much application, or even to achieve respectability, in medicine and oncology. The contemporary climate of opinion with respect to the status of ideas and observations in biomedical research has been perceptively described by Horrobin (1975). Although we have a *Journal of Theoretical Biology*, we have no journals of *Theoretical Medicine* or *Theoretical Oncology*. However, *Medical Hypotheses*, of which Horrobin is the Editor and in which his article appeared, has just been launched and it may help to inaugurate an epoch during which systematic argument and analysis will eventually displace the intuitive hunches that often masquerade as theory in medicine.

In physics, the most highly developed discipline in the natural sciences, it has long been obvious that only the rare and exceptionally versatile genius, such as the late Enrico Fermi, has the capacity to excel in both theory and experiment. In the less developed field of medicine, we tend to assume that every competent clinician and experimentalist should be able to generate his or her own theories. Consequently, much of what passes for hypothesis— even in the 'Hypothesis' section of the *Lancet*—lacks profundity.

The frequency with which association is identified with cause—despite numerous warnings from the most distinguished statisticians and logicians— stands out as one of the most serious defects in the medical literature. Problems raised by the genetic heterogeneity of human populations and the associated phenomenon of self-selection tend to be overlooked or ignored. This or that habit or dietary factor is said to *cause* this or that cancer, on the evidence of mere association. Furthermore, incautious claims of this kind are usually rewarded with scare headlines in the national press and even in medical journals. Neither can we rely on the 'peer review' system to stamp out the methodological abuses: many of the 'peers' perpetrate the same malpractices.

At the deeper levels of inquiry, the time needed for contemplation and the thorough exploration of ideas is a luxury in which the busy clinician and the highly specialized experimentalist can seldom indulge. The very harvesting of countless data in their perplexing variety—coupled with the neglect of mathematical and logical analysis—leads inevitably to mental indigestion, paralysis of the imagination and an impoverishment of the scientific under-

standing of disease. Those trained in medicine or biology tend to be mathematically incompetent, while those trained in mathematics or the physical
sciences usually have little awareness of the subtleties and complexities of
biology and medicine.

The depth and quality of the emotions engulfing the subject of cancer
constitute further hindrances to rational and detached inquiry. When
medical scientists announce that 'the cure for cancer is imminent' (or words
to that effect) many of us shudder with apprehension. (Shall we not be
expected to fulfill our promises?) Apart from the absurdity of such generali-
zations, the raising of unjustified expectations constitutes gross irresponsi-
bility. But in an era when much research is supposed to satisfy the needs and
demands of the consumer we must expect that a few unscrupulous scientists
will bolster their applications for research funds with extravagant promises.

My concept of cancer as a large group of genetically determined and
usually fatal diseases, whose onset obeys the laws of chance, is as unlikely to
appeal to grant givers as to laymen. Truth, however, is not necessarily
palatable and the analysis and conclusions of this book highlight a conflict
that permeates much of medicine. Where he cannot cure his patient the
clinician would welcome measures that would prevent the fatal disease; he
cannot be expected to feel enthusiastic about a theory that offers neither
simple cure nor prophylaxis.

The basic medical scientist on the other hand must be primarily concerned
with the pursuit of truth, and the elucidation of the causes and mechanisms
of disease, however unwelcome they may appear to his clinical colleagues.
In what we might like to regard as an 'ideal' world, understanding of cause
would lead automatically to cure and prevention. Alas, I see no reason to
believe that we inhabit an 'ideal' world.

References

Abbondandolo, A. and Bonatti, S. (1970). The production, by nitrous acid, of complete and mosaic mutations during nuclear stages in cells of *Schizosaccharomyces pombe*. *Mutation Res.*, **9**, 59–69

Abercrombie, M. and Ambrose, E. J. (1962). The surface properties of cancer cells: a review. *Cancer Res.*, **22**, 525–48

Achord, H. L. and Procter, H. D. (1963). Malignant degeneration and metastasis in Peutz–Jeghers syndrome. *Arch. Internal Med.*, **111**, 498–502

Adatia, A. K. (1966). Burkitt's tumour in the jaws. *Brit. Dent. J.*, **120**, 315–26

Adler, I. (1912). *Primary Malignant Growths of the Lungs and Bronchi: A Pathological and Clinical Study*. New York and London: Longmans, Green and Co.

Aita, J. A. (1967). Genetic aspects of tumours of the nervous system. Chapter 6 in: *Hereditary Factors in Carcinoma*. Editor: H. T. Lynch. Berlin and New York: Springer-Verlag

Albers, J. J. and Dray, S. (1969). Allelic exclusion and phenogroup expression in individual molecules of rabbit low-density lipoprotein allotypes. *J. Immunol.*, **103**, 163–69

Albert, R. E., Burns, F. J. and Heimbach, R. D. (1967). The effect of penetration depth of electron radiation on skin tumor formation in the rat. *Radiation Res.*, **30**, 515–24

Aloni, Y. and Attardi, G. (1971). Symmetrical *in vivo* transcription of mitochondrial DNA in HeLa cells. *Proc. Nat. Acad. Sci. USA*, **68**, 1757–61

Amiel, J. L. (1967). A study of the leukocyte phenotypes in Hodgkin's disease. In: *Histocompatibility Testing*, pp. 79–81. Editors: E. S. Curtoni, P. L. Matting, and M. R. Tosi. Copenhagen: Munksgaard

Anderson, D. E. (1971(a)). Clinical characteristics of the genetic variety of cutaneous melanoma in man. *Cancer*, **28**, 721–25

Anderson, D. E. (1971(b)). Some characteristics of familial breast cancer. *Cancer*, **28**, 1500–04

Anderson, D. E. (1972). A genetic study of human breast cancer. *J. Nat. Cancer Inst.*, **48**, 1029–34

Anderson, D. E., Smith, J. L. Jr. and McBride, C. M. (1967). Hereditary aspects of malignant melanoma. *J. Amer. Med. Ass.*, **200**, 741–46

Anderson, D. E., Taylor, W. B., Falls, H. F. and Davidson, R. T. (1967). The nevoid basal cell carcinoma syndrome. *Amer. J. Human Genet.*, **19**, 12–22

Andrews, J. C. (1968). Malignant melanoma in siblings. *Arch. Dermatol.*, **98**, 282–83

Antley, R. M. and Fox, A. S. (1970). The relationship between RNA and protein synthesis and the aggregation of *Drosophila* embryonic cells. *Develop. Biol.*, **22**, 282–87

Armitage, P. and Doll, R. (1954). The age distribution of cancer and a multistage theory of carcinogenesis. *Brit. J. Cancer*, **8**, 1–12

Armitage, P. and Doll, R. (1957). A two-stage theory of carcinogenesis in relation to the age distribution of human cancer. *Brit. J. Cancer*, **11**, 161–69

Armitage, P. and Doll, R. (1961). Stochastic models for carcinogenesis. *Proc. Fourth Berkeley Symposium on Mathematical Statistics and Probability*, **4**, 19–38. Berkeley and Los Angeles: University of California Press

Arundell, F. D., Karasek, M. A. and Gates, A. H. (1969). 7, 12-dimethylbenzanthracene tumor induction in mutant (hairless, asebic, and hairless–asebic) mice. *J. Investigative Dermatol.*, **52**, 119–25

Asboe-Hanson, G. (1964). Dermatologic aspects of mast cell activity. *Dermatologica*, **128**, 51–67

Ashley, D. J. B. (1969(a)). Oesophageal cancer in Wales. *J. Med. Genet.*, **6**, 70–75

Ashley, D. J. B. (1969(b)). Gastric cancer in Wales. *J. Med. Genet.*, **6**, 76–9

Ashley, D. J. B. (1969(c)). Colonic cancer arising in polyposis coli. *J. Med. Genet.*, **6**, 376–78

Ashley, D. J. B. (1969(d)). The two-'hit' and multiple-'hit' theories of carcinogenesis. *Brit. J. Cancer*, **23**, 313–28

Ashley, D. J. B. (1970(a)). Incidence and mortality of intestinal cancer. *Cancer*, **25**, 959–965

Ashley, D. J. B. (1970(b)). A systematic sex difference in intestinal carcinoma. *Cancer*, **25**, 966–71

Ashley, D. J. B. and Davies, H. D. (1966). Gastric cancer in Wales. *Gut*, **7**, 542–48

Asman, H. B. and Pierce, E. R. (1970). Familial multiple polyposis. A statistical study of a large Kentucky kindred. *Cancer*, **25**, 972–81

Aster, R. H., Miskovich, B. H. and Rodey, G. E. (1973). Histocompatibility antigens of human plasma. Localization to the HDL-3 lipoprotein fraction. *Transplantation*, **16**, 205–10

Auerbach, O., Gere, J. B., Pawlowski, J. M., Muehsam, G. E., Smolin, H. J. and Stout, A. P. (1957). Carcinoma *in situ* and early invasive carcinoma occurring in the trachobronchial trees in cases of bronchial carcinoma. *J. Thorac. Surg.*, **34**, 298–307

Axelsson, U. and Hällén, J. (1968). Review of fifty-four subjects with monoclonal gammopathy. *Brit. J. Haematol.*, **15**, 417–20

Axtell, L. M. (1963). Computing survival rates for chronic disease patients. A simple procedure. *J. Amer. Med. Ass.*, **186**, 1125–28

Aylett, S. (1971). Cancer and ulcerative colitis. *Brit. Med. J.*, **ii**, 203–5

Baccarani, M., Zaccaria, A. and Tura, S. (1973). Philadelphia–chromosome–positive preleukaemic state. *Lancet*, **ii**, 1094

Bailey, D. W. and Kohn, H. I. (1965). Inherited histocompatibility changes in progeny of irradiated and unirradiated inbred mice. *Genet. Res.*, **6**, 330–40

Baker, J. B. and Humphreys, T. (1971). Serum-stimulated release of cell contacts and the initiation of growth in contact-inhibited chick fibroblasts. *Proc. Nat. Acad. Sci. USA*, **68**, 2161–64

Bakker, P. M. and Tjon A Joe, S. S. (1971). Multiple sebaceous gland tumours, with multiple tumours of internal organs. A new syndrome? *Dermatologica*, **142**, 50–7

Bánóczy, J. and Sugár, L. (1973). Longitudinal studies in oral leukoplakias. *J. Oral Pathol.*, **1**, 265–72

Barendsen, G. W. (1969). Tumour induction in rat skin by 300-kV x-rays and 15-MeV neutrons. In: *Radiation-induced Cancer*, pp. 413–21. Vienna: International Atomic Energy Agency, ST1/PUB/228

Barendsen, G. W. and Broerse, J. J. (1970). Experimental radiotherapy of a rat rhabdomyosarcoma with 15 MeV neutrons and 300 kV x-rays. II. Effects of fractionated treatments, applied five times a week for several weeks. *Eur. J. Cancer*, **6**, 89–109

Barrett, M. K. and Deringer, M. K. (1950). An induced adaptation in a transplantable tumour of mice. *J. Nat. Cancer Inst.*, **11**, 51–9

Barron, B. A. and Richart, R. M. (1971). An epidemiologic study of cervical neoplastic disease. Based on a self-selected sample of 7000 women in Barbados, West Indies. *Cancer*, **27**, 978–86

Barron, S. L., Roddick, J. W. Jr., Greenlaw, R. H., Rush, B. and Tweeddale, D. N.

(1968). Multiple primary cancers of the ororespiratory tract and the cervix. *Cancer*, **21**, 672–81

Bart, R. S. and Schnall, S. (1973). Eye color in darkly pigmented basal-cell carcinomas and malignant melanomas. *Arch. Dermatol.*, **107**, 206–07

Bauer, F. W. and Robbins, S. L. (1972). An autopsy study of cancer patients. I. Accuracy of the clinical diagnoses (1955 to 1965) Boston City Hospital. *J. Amer. Med. Ass.*, **221**, 1471–74

Beese, D. H. (1968) (Editor). *Tobacco Consumption in Various Countries*. Research Paper 6, 2nd edition. London: Tobacco Research Council

Belcher, J. R. (1971). World-wide differences in the sex ratio of bronchial carcinoma. *Brit. J. Dis. Chest*, **65**, 205–21

Berenblum, I. (1941). The cocarcinogenic action of croton resin. *Cancer Res.*, **1**, 44–8

Berendes, U. (1974). Multiple tumors of the skin: clinical, histopathological, and genetic features. *Humangenetik*, **22**, 181–210

Berg, J. W. (1965). The distribution of cancer deaths in time. A survey test of the lognormal model. *Brit. J. Cancer*, **19**, 695–711

Berg, J. W., Hajdu, S. I. and Foote, F. W. Jr. (1971). The prevalence of latent cancers in cancer patients. *Arch. Pathol.*, **91**, 183–86

Berg, J. W., Hutter, R. V. P. and Foote, F. W. Jr. (1968). The unique association between salivary gland cancer and breast cancer. *J. Amer. Med. Ass.*, **204**, 771–74

Berg, J. W. and Robbins, G. F. (1967). The failure of a model to predict cancer survival. *J. Chronic Dis.*, **20**, 809–14

Berg, K. and Bearn, A. G. (1966). An inherited X-linked serum system in man. The Xm system. *J. Exp. Med.*, **123**, 379–97

Berge, T. (1974). Splenic metastases. Frequencies and patterns. *Acta Patholog. Microbiolog. Scand.*, **82A**, 499–506

Bergsagel, D. E. (1967). The chronic leukemias: a review of disease manifestations and the aims of therapy. *Canad. Med. Ass. J.*, **96**, 1615–20

Berkson, J. (1959). The statistical investigation of smoking and cancer of the lung. *Proc. Staff Meetings Mayo Clinic*, **34**, 206–24(a)

Berkson, J., and Gage, R. P. (1952). Survival curve for cancer patients following treatment. *J. Amer. Statistical Ass.*, **47**, 501–15

Bernard, C. (1865). *Introduction à l'étude de la médecine expérimentale*. Paris: J. B. Baillière et Fils

Bernardis, L. L. and Goldman, J. K. (1972). Renal compensatory hypertrophy in weanling rats with ventromedial hypothalamic lesions. *Growth*, **36**, 209–15

Berne, B. H., Dray, S. and Knight, K. L. (1970). Identification and genetic control of the Mt-3 and Mt-4 allotypes of rabbit serum α_2-macroglobulin. *J. Immunol.*, **105**, 856–64

Berne, B. H., Dray, S. and Knight, K. L. (1972). Contribution of the allelic *Mtz*[3] and *Mtz*[4] allotype genes to the formation of individual rabbit serum α_2-macroglobulin molecules. *Biochem. Genet.*, **7**, 95–110

Beutler, E., Collins, Z. and Irwin, L. E. (1967). Value of genetic variants of glucose-6-phosphate dehydrogenase in tracing the origin of malignant tumours. *New Eng. J. Med.*, **276**, 389–91

Bhargava, P. M., Pallaiah, T. and Premkumar, E. (1970). Aminoacyl-transfer RNA synthetase recognition codewords in yeast transfer RNAs: a proposal. *J. Theoret. Biol.*, **29**, 447–69

Bichel, P. (1971). Feedback regulation of growth of ascites tumours in parabiotic mice. *Nature, London*, **231**, 449–50

Billingham, R. E., Orr, J. W. and Woodhouse, D. L. (1951). Transplantation of skin components during chemical carcinogenesis with 20-methylcholanthrene. *Brit. J. Cancer*, **5**, 417–32

Billingham, R. E. and Silvers, W. K. (1963). The origin and conservation of epidermal specificities. *New Eng. J. Med.*, **268**, 477–80; 539–45

Billingham, R. E. and Silvers, W. K. (1967). Studies on the conservation of epidermal specificities of skin and certain mucosas in adult mammals. *J. Exp. Med.*, **125**, 429–46

Bisno, A. L., Barratt, N. P., Swanston, W. H. and Spence, L. P. (1970). An outbreak of acute respiratory disease in Trinidad associated with para-influenza viruses. *Amer. J. Epidemiol.*, **91**, 68–77

Black, M. M., Barclay, T. H. C., Cutler, S. J., Hankey, B. F. and Asire, A. J. (1972). Association of atypical characteristics of benign breast lesions with subsequent risk of breast cancer. *Cancer*, **29**, 338–43

Bloodgood, J. C. (1914). Carcinoma of the lower lip; its diagnosis and operative treatment. *Surg. Gynecol. and Obstet.*, **18**, 404–22

Bloth, B., Chesebro, B. and Svehag, S.-E. (1968). Ultrastructural studies of human and rabbit αM-globulins. *J. Exp. Med.*, **127**, 749–56

Blumenson, L. E. and Bross, I. D. J. (1969). A mathematical analysis of the growth and spread of breast cancer. *Biometrics*, **22**, 95–109

Boag, J. W. (1948). The presentation and analysis of the results of radiotherapy. *Brit. J. Radiol.*, **21**, 128–38

Boll, I. T. M. and Fuchs, S. (1970). A kinetic model of granulocytopoiesis. *Exp. Cell Res.*, **61**, 147–52

Bond, B. and Orr, J. W. (1969). The effects of a single dose of 7, 12-dimethylbenz(α)-anthracene on the epidermis and hair follicles of mice, with notes on concurrent changes in the ovaries and adrenals. *Brit. J. Cancer*, **23**, 188–96

Bonnevie, O., Binder, V., Anthonisen, P. and Riis, P. (1974). The prognosis of ulcerative colitis. *Scand. J. Gastroenterol.*, **9**, 81–91

Bonser, G. M. and Thomas, G. M. (1959). An investigation of the validity of death certificates of cancer of the lung in Leeds. *Brit. J. Cancer*, **13**, 1–12

Borek, C., and Sachs, L. (1968). The number of cell generations required to fix the transformed state in x-ray-induced transformation. *Proc. Nat. Acad. Sci. USA*, **59**, 83–5

Boyd, J. T., Doll, R., Hill, G. B. and Sissons, H. A. (1969). Mortality from primary tumours of bone in England and Wales, 1961–63. *Brit. J. Prevent. and Social Med.*, **23**, 12–22

Boyd, W. L. (1966). *The Spontaneous Regression of Cancer*. Springfield, Illinois: C. C. Thomas

Boyse, E. A., Old, L. J. and Luell, S. (1963). Antigenic properties of experimental leukemias. II. Immunological studies *in vivo* with C57BL/6 radiation-induced leukemias. *J. Nat. Cancer Inst.*, **31**, 987–95

Boyse, E. A., Old, L. J. and Stockert, E. (1966). The TL (thymus leukemia) antigen. A review. In: *Immunopathology. Fourth International Symposium*, pp. 23–40. Editors: P. Grabar and P. A. Miescher. Basel, Switzerland: Benno Schwabe and Co.

Boyse, E. A., Stockert, E. and Old, L. J. (1967). Modification of the antigenic structure of the cell membrane of thymus-leukaemia (TL) antibody. *Proc. Nat. Acad. Sci. USA*, **58**, 954–57

Braestrup, C. B. (1957). Past and present radiation exposure to radiologists from the point of view of life expectancy. *Amer. J. Roentgenol.*, **78**, 988–92

Brand, K. G., Buoen, L. C. and Brand, I. (1967). Carcinogenesis from polymer implants:

new aspects from chromosomal and transplantation studies during premalignancy. *J. Nat. Cancer Inst.*, **39**, 663–79

Britten, R. J. and Kohn, D. F. (1968). Repeated sequences in DNA. *Science*, **161**, 529–540

Broca, P. (1866). *Traité des Tumeurs*. Paris: Asselin

Brownlee, K. A. (1965). A review of 'Smoking and Health'. *J. Amer. Stat. Ass.*, **60**, 722–39

Brubaker, G., Geser, A. and Pike, M. C. (1973). Burkitt's lymphoma in the North Mara district of Tanzania 1964–70: failure to find evidence of time–space clustering in a high-risk isolated rural area. *Brit. J. Cancer*, **28**, 469–72

Bruce, J., Carter, D. C. and Fraser, J. (1970). Patterns of recurrent disease in breast cancer. *Lancet*, **i**, 433–35

Brues, A. M., Drury, D. R. and Brues, M. C. (1936). A quantitative study of cell growth in regenerating liver. *Arch. Pathol.*, **22**, 658–73

Bruni, H., Lilly, J., Newman, W., McHardy, G. (1971). Small bowel carcinoma as a complication of regional enteritis. *Southern Med. J.*, **64**, 577–80

Bryan, W. R. (1962). The search for causative viruses in human cancer: a discussion of the problem. *J. Nat. Cancer Inst.*, **29**, 1027–34

Bryan, W. R. (1965). Formal discussion of: a survey of the tumor virus problem from an epidemiologic standpoint. *Cancer Res.*, **25**, 1283–85

Bucher, N. L. R. (1963). Regeneration of mammalian liver. *Int. Rev. Cytol.*, **15**, 245–300

Bucher, N. L. R. (1967). Experimental aspects of hepatic regeneration. *New Eng. J. Med.*, **277**, 686–96; 738–46

Bucher, N. L. R., Swaffield, M. M. and Di Troia, J. F. (1964). Influence of age upon incorporation of thymidine-2-C^{14} into DNA of regenerating rat liver. *Cancer Res.*, **24**, 509–12

Buehler, S. K., Firme, F., Fodor, G., Fraser, G. R., Marshall, W. H. and Vaze, P. (1975). Common variable immunodeficiency, Hodgkin's disease, and other malignancies in a Newfoundland family. *Lancet*, **i**, 195–97

Bullough, W. S. (1962). The control of mitotic activity in adult mammalian tissues. *Biolog. Rev.*, **37**, 307–42

Bullough, W. S. (1965). Mitotic and functional homoeostasis: a speculative review. *Cancer Res.*, **25**, 1683–1727

Bullough, W. S. (1972). The control of epidermal thickness. *Brit. J. Dermatol.*, **87**, 187–199 and 347–54

Bullough, W. S., Lawrence, E. B., Iversen, O. H. and Elgjo, K. (1967). The vertebrate epidermal chalone. *Nature, London*, **214**, 578–80

Bullough, W. S. and Rytomaa, T. (1965). Mitotic homoeostasis. *Nature, London*, **205**, 573–78

Burachik, M., Craig, L. C. and Chang, J. (1970). Studies of self-association and conformation of peptides by thin-film dialysis. *Biochemistry*, **9**, 3239–3300

Burbank, F. (1972). US lung cancer death rates begin to rise proportionately more rapidly for females than for males: a dose-response effect? *J. Chronic Dis.*, **25**, 473–79

Burch, P. R. J. (1963(a)). Auto-immunity: some aetiological aspects. *Lancet*, **i**, 1253–57

Burch, P. R. J. (1963(b)). Mutation, auto-immunity and ageing. *Lancet*, **ii**, 299–300

Burch, P. R. J. (1964(a)). Cardiovascular diseases: new aetiological considerations. *Amer. Heart J.*, **67**, 139–40

Burch, P. R. J. (1964(b)). Schizophrenia: some new aetiological considerations. *Brit. J. Psychiatry*, **110**, 818–24

Burch, P. R. J. (1965). Natural and radiation carcinogenesis in man, I, II and III. *Proc. Roy. Soc. Lond.*, **B162**, 223–87

Burch, P. R. J. (1966). Spontaneous auto-immunity: equations for age-specific prevalence and initiation-rates. *J. Theoret. Biol.*, **12**, 397–409

Burch, P. R. J. (1967). Radiation Biophysics. Chapter 11 in: *Principles of Radiation Protection*, pp. 366–97. Editors: K. Z. Morgan and J. E. Turner. New York, London and Sydney: John Wiley and Sons, Inc.

Burch, P. R. J. (1968(a)). *An Inquiry Concerning Growth, Disease and Ageing.* Edinburgh: Oliver and Boyd; also Buffalo, N.Y.: University of Toronto Press (1969)

Burch, P. R. J. (1968(b)). Huntington's chorea. Age at onset in relation to aetiology and pathogenesis. Chapter 14 in: *Handbook of Clinical Neurology*, **6**, 379–98. Editors: P. J. Vinken and G. W. Bruyn. Amsterdam: North-Holland Publishing Co.

Burch, P. R. J. (1969(a)). Ionizing radiation and life shortening. *Nuclear Safety*, **10**, 161–70

Burch, P. R. J. (1969(b)). Radiation and 'natural' carcinogenesis. Does somatic mutation provide a common link? In: *Radiation-induced Cancer*, pp. 29–44. Vienna: International Atomic Energy Agency, ST1/PUB/228

Burch, P. R. J. (1970(a)). New approach to cancer. *Nature, London*, **225**, 512–16

Burch, P. R. J. (1970(b)). The Hodgkin maze. *Lancet*, **i**, 469–70

Burch, P. R. J. (1970(c)). Leucocyte phenotypes in Hodgkin's disease. *Lancet*, **ii**, 771–772

Burch, P. R. J. (1970(d)). Prenatal radiation exposure and childhood cancer. *Lancet*, **ii**, 1189

Burch, P. R. J. (1971). Radiation-induced disease. Problems of response in relation to dose, dose-rate and radiation quality. In: *International Congress on Protection Against Accelerator and Space Radiation.* CERN, Geneva. *Proceedings*, Vol. 1, pp. 13–37

Burch, P. R. J. (1974(a)). What limits the life span? In: *Population and the New Biology*, pp. 31–56. *Proceedings of the Tenth Annual Symposium of the Eugenics Society, London 1973.* Editors: B. Benjamin, P. R. Cox and J. Peel. London and New York: Academic Press

Burch, P. R. J. (1974(b)). Does smoking cause lung cancer? *New Scient.*, **61**, 458–63

Burch, P. R. J. and Burwell, R. G. (1965). Self and not-self: a clonal induction approach to immunology. *Quart. Rev. Biol.*, **40**, 252–79

Burch, P. R. J. and Dawson, J. B. (1969). Aetiological implications of the sex- and age-distribution of renal lithiasis. In: *Renal Stone Research Symposium.* Editors: A. Hodgkinson and B. E. C. Nordin, pp. 71–84. London: J. and A. Churchill Ltd.

Burch, P. R. J., de Dombal, F. T. and Watkinson, G. (1969) Aetiology of ulcerative colitis. II. A new hypothesis. *Gut*, **10**, 277–84

Burch, P. R. J., Jackson, D. and Rowell, N. R. (1972). Growth, disease and ageing: a unified approach. *Zeit. für Alternsforschung*, **26**, 1–18

Burch, P. R. J., Jackson, D., Fairpo, C. G. and Murray, J. J. (1973). Gingival recession ('getting long in the tooth'). Colorectal cancer. Degenerative and malignant changes as errors of growth control. *Mechanisms Ageing and Develop.*, **2**, 251–73

Burch, P. R. J. and Milunsky, A. (1969). Early-onset diabetes mellitus in the general and Down's syndrome populations. Genetics, aetiology and pathogenesis. *Lancet*, **i**, 554–58

Burch, P. R. J., Murray, J. J. and Jackson, D. (1971). The age-prevalence of arcus senilis, greying of hair, and baldness. Etiological considerations. *J. Gerontol.*, **26**, 364–72

Burch, P. R. J. and Rowell, N. R. (1965). Psoriasis: aetiological aspects. *Acta Derm.–Venereolog., Stockholm*, **45**, 366–80

Burch, P. R. J. and Rowell, N. R. (1968). The sex- and age-distributions of chronic discoid lupus erythematosus in four countries. *Acta Derm.–Venereolog., Stockholm*, **48**, 33–46

Burch, P. R. J. and Rowell, N. R. (1970). Lupus erythematosus. Analysis of the sex- and age-distributions of the discoid and systemic forms of the disease in different countries. *Acta Derm.–Venereolog., Stockholm*, **50**, 293–301

Burkitt, D. (1962). A children's cancer dependent on climatic factors. *Nature, London*, **194**, 232–34

Burkitt, D. and Wright, D. (1966). Geographical and tribal distribution of the African lymphoma in Uganda. *Brit. Med. J.*, **i**, 569–73

Burkitt, D. P. (1969). Etiology of Burkitt's lymphoma—an alternative hypothesis to a vectored virus. *J. Nat. Cancer Inst.*, **42**, 19–28

Burnet, F. M. (1959(a)). *The Clonal Selection Theory of Acquired Immunity*. London: Cambridge University Press

Burnet, F. M. (1959(b)). In: *Significant Trends in Medical Research*, p. 60, Ciba Foundation Symposium, London: J. and A. Churchill Ltd.

Burnet, F. M. (1965). Somatic mutation and chronic disease. *Brit. Med. J.*, **i**, 338–342

Burnet, F. M. (1969(a)). *Cellular Immunology*. Victoria: Melbourne University Press; London: Cambridge University Press

Burnet, F. M. (1969(b)). The evolution of adaptive immunity in vertebrates. *Acta Patholog. Microbiolog. Scand.*, **76**, 1–11

Burnet, F. M. (1970). *Immunological Surveillance*. Oxford: Pergamon Press

Burnet, F. M. (1972). *Auto-immunity and Auto-immune Disease*. Lancaster: Medical and Technical Publishing Co. Ltd.

Burnet, F. M. and Fenner, F. (1949). *Production of Antibodies*. 2nd Edition. Melbourne: Macmillan

Burns, E. R. (1969). On the failure of self-inhibition of growth in tumors. *Growth*, **33**, 25–45

Burns, F. J., Albert, R. E. and Heimbach, R. D. (1968). The RBE for skin tumors and hair follicle damage in the rat following irradiation with alpha particles and electrons. *Radiation Res.*, **36**, 225–41

Burton, A. C. (1966). Rate of growth of solid tumours as a problem of diffusion. *Growth*, **30**, 157–76

Burwell, R. G. (1962). Studies of the primary and secondary immune responses of lymph nodes draining homografts of fresh cancellous bone with particular reference to mechanisms of lymph node reactivity. *Ann. N.Y. Acad. Sci.*, **99**, 821–60

Burwell, R. G. (1963). The role of lymphoid tissue in morphostasis. *Lancet*, **ii**, 69–74

Byar, D. P. and Mostofi, F. K. (1972). Carcinoma of the prostate: prognostic evaluation of certain pathologic features in 208 radical prostatectomies. *Cancer*, **30**, 5–13

Cajano, A. (1960). Immunomorphological findings following the use of hetero-immune sera. Proceedings Seventh Congress European Society of Haematology, London, 1959. *Acta Haematolog.*, **24**, 71–80

Cajano, A. (1963). Immunomorphological implications in the mechanism of carcinogenesis. *Acta Unionis internationalis contra cancrum*, **19**, 213–15

Cajano, A. and Faiella, A. (1960). Acquisizioni e problemi nella immunologia cellulare e serica delle empotaie maligne. *Estratto*, **7**, 317–34

California Tumor Registry (1963). *Cancer Registration and Survival in California*. State of California Department of Public Health

Campbell, J. M. and Lindsey, A. J. (1957). Polycyclic hydrocarbons in cigar smoke. *Brit. J. Cancer*, **11**, 192–95

Canellos, G. P. and Whang-Peng, J. (1972). Philadelphia–chromosome–positive pre-leukaemic state. *Lancet*, **ii**, 1227–29

Cannon, M. M. and Leavell, B. S. (1966). Multiple cancer types in one family. *Cancer*, **19**, 538–40

Cardon, S. Z., Alvord, E. T., Rand, H. J. and Hitchcock, R. (1956). 3, 4–benzpyrene in the smoke of cigarette paper, tobacco, and cigarettes. *Brit. J. Cancer*, **10**, 485–97

Carrel, A. (1922). Growth-promoting function of leucocytes. *J. Exp. Med.*, **36**, 385–391

Carrel, A. (1924). Leucocytic trephones. *J. Amer. Med. Ass.*, **82**, 255–58

Carroll, K. K. and Khor, H. T. (1970). Effect of dietary fat and dose level of 7, 12-dimethylbenz(α)-anthracene on mammary tumor incidence in rats. *Cancer Res.*, **30**, 2260–64

Case, R. A. M. (1956(a)). Cohort analysis of mortality-rates as an historical or narrative technique. *Brit. J. Prev. and Soc. Med.*, **10**, 159–71

Case, R. A. M. (1956(b)). Cohort analysis of cancer mortality in England and Wales 1911 to 1954 by site and sex. *Brit. J. Prev. and Soc. Med.*, **10**, 172–99

Castor, L. N. (1968). Contact regulation of cell division in an epithelial-like cell line. *J. Cell. Physiol.*, **72**, 161–72

Castor, L. N. (1971). Control of division by cell contact and serum concentration in cultures of 3T3 cells. *Exp. Cell Res.*, **68**, 17–24

Catalona, W. J., Engelman, K., Ketcham, A. S. and Hammond, W. G. (1971). Familial medullary thyroid carcinoma, pheochromocytoma, and parathyroid adenoma (Sipple's syndrome). Study of a kindred. *Cancer*, **28**, 1245–54

Cebra, J. J., Colberg, J. E. and Dray, S. (1966). Rabbit lymphoid cells differentiated with respect to α-, γ-, and μ-heavy polypeptide chains and to allotypic markers Aa1 and Aa2. *J. Exp. Med.*, **123**, 547–58

Cederlöf, R., Friberg, L. and Hrubec, Z. (1969). Cardiovascular and respiratory symptoms in relation to tobacco smoking: A study on American twins. *Arch. Environ. Health*, **18**, 934–40

Chan, P. C., Goldman, A. and Wynder, E. L. (1970). Hydroxyurea: suppression of two-stage carcinogenesis in mouse skin. *Science*, **168**, 130–32

Chen, L. (1971). Studies on the relationship between thymus regeneration and lymphoma prevention in C57/Bl/6 mice irradiated and injected with syngeneic spleen cells. *Int. J. Cancer*, **7**, 491–98

Cherry, C. P. and Glucksmann, A. (1971). The influence of carcinogenic dosage and of sex on induction of epitheliomas and sarcomas in the dorsal skin of rats. *Brit. J. Cancer*, **25**, 544–64

Chevassu, M. (1906). *Tumeurs du Testicule*. Paris: G. Steinheil

Choi, N. W., Schuman, L. M. and Gullen, W. H. (1970). Epidemiology of primary central nervous system neoplasms. II: Case-control study. *Amer. J. Epidemiol.*, **91**, 467–85

Chorlton, S. H., Hughes, N. R. and Larkin, M. F. (1969). *Human Mammary Cancer*, Publication No. 16, New South Wales State Cancer Council. Sydney: Australasian Medical Publishing Co. Ltd.

Clayson, D. B. (1962). *Chemical Carcinogenesis*. London: J. and A. Churchill Ltd.

Clemmesen, J. (1948). Carcinoma of the breast. Symposium. Results from statistical research. *Brit. J. Radiol.*, **21**, 583–90

Clerici, E., Mocarelli, P. and Provini, L. (1964). Rat liver regeneration after partial hepatectomy and sympathetic denervation. *Exp. and Mol. Pathol.*, **3**, 569–82

Clinical Pharmacology Unit (1971). Relation between breast cancer and s blood antigen system. *Lancet*, **i**, 301–05

Cobb, J. R. and Walker, D. G. (1961). Effect of heterologous, homologous, and autologous serums on human normal and malignant cells *in vitro*. *J. Nat. Cancer Inst.*, **27**, 1–15

Cohen, B. H. and Thomas, C. B. (1962). Comparison of smokers and non-smokers. II. The distribution of ABO and Rh(D) blood groups. *Bull. Johns Hopkins Hosp.*, **110**, 1–7

Cohen, S. and Milstein, C. (1967). Structure and biological properties of immunoglobulins. *Adv. in Immunol.*, **7**, 1–89

Cole, P., MacMahon, B. and Aisenberg, A. (1968). Mortality from Hodgkin's disease in the United States. Evidence for the multiple-aetiology hypothesis. *Lancet*, **ii**, 1371–1376

Cole, W. H. (1974). Spontaneous regression of cancer: the metabolic triumph of the host? *Ann. N.Y. Acad. Sci.*, **230**, 111–41

Colley, D. G., Wu, A. Y. S. and Waksman, B. H. (1970). Cellular differentiation in the thymus. III. Surface properties of rat thymus and lymph node cells separated on density gradients. *J. Exp. Med.*, **132**, 1107–21

Collins, S. D., Wheeler, R. E. and Shannon, R. D. (1942). The occurrence of whooping cough, chickenpox, mumps, measles and German measles in 200 000 surveyed families in 28 large cities. Special Study Series No. 1, US Public Health Service, Washington

Comings, D. E. (1967). The duration of replication of the inactive X chromosome in humans based on the persistence of the heterochromatic sex chromatin body during DNA synthesis. *Cytogenetics*, **6**, 20–37

Conard, R. S. (1964). Indirect effect of X-irradiation on bone growth in rats. *Ann. N.Y. Acad. Sci., Art.*, **1**, 335–38

Condamine, H., Custer, R. P. and Mintz, B. (1971). Pure-strain and genetically mosaic liver tumors histochemically identified with the β-glucoronidase marker in allophenic mice. *Proc. Nat. Acad. Sci., USA*, **68**, 2032–36

Cook, G. B. (1966). A comparison of single and multiple primary cancers. *Cancer*, **19**, 959–66

Cook, P. J., Doll, R. and Fellingham, S. A. (1969). A mathematical model for the age distribution of cancer in man. *Int. J. Cancer*, **4**, 93–112

Cooper, E. L. (1969). Chronic allograft rejection in *Lumbricus terrestris*. *J. Exp. Zool.*, **171**, 69–73

Cooper, E. L. and Rubilotta, M. (1969). Allograft rejection in *Eisenia foetida*. *Transplantation*, **8**, 220–23

Court Brown, W. M. and Doll, R. (1957). Leukaemia and aplastic anaemia in patients irradiated for ankylosing spondylitis. Medical Research Council Special Report 295. London: HMSO

Court Brown, W. M. and Doll, R. (1965). Mortality from cancer and other causes after radiotherapy for ankylosing spondylitis. *Brit. Med. J.*, **ii**, 1327–32

Courville, C. B. (1950). *Pathology of the Central Nervous System*. 3rd Edition. Mountain View, California: Pacific Press Publishing Association

Cramer, F. (1971). Three-dimensional structure of tRNA. *Prog. in Nucleic Acid Res. and Mol. Biol.*, **11**, 391–421

Crawley, E. P. (1952). Genetic aspects of malignant melanoma. *Arch. Dermatol. and Syphilol.*, **65**, 440–50

Creagan, E. T. and Fraumeni, J. F. (1973). Familial gastric cancer and immunologic abnormalities. *Cancer*, **32**, 1325–31

Crichlow, R. W. (1972). Carcinoma of the male breast. *Surg., Gynecol. and Obstet.*, **134**, 1011–19

Crick, F. H. C. (1963). The recent excitement in the coding problem. *Prog. in Nucleic Acid Res.*, **1**, 163–217

Crick, F. H. C. (1968). The origin of the genetic code. *J. Molec. Biol.*, **38**, 367–79

Croizat, H., Frindel, E. and Tubiana, M. (1970). Proliferative capacity of the stem cells in the bone-marrow of mice after single and multiple irradiations (total- or partial-body exposure). *Int. J. Rad. Biol.*, **18**, 347–58

Crosby, W. H. (1970). Experience with injured and implanted bone marrow: relation of function to structure. In: *Hemopoietic Cellular Proliferation*, pp. 87–95. Editor: F. Stohlman, Jr. New York: Grune and Stratton

Curtis, H. J. (1967). Radiation and ageing. In: *Aspects of the Biology of Ageing*, pp. 51–63. Symposia of the Society for Experimental Biology. Editor: H. W. Woolhouse. London: Cambridge University Press

Curtis, H. J. (1969). Somatic mutations in radiation carcinogenesis. In: *Radiation-induced Cancer*, pp. 45–55. Vienna: International Atomic Energy Agency, ST1/PUB/228

Cutler, S. J., Asire, A. J. and Taylor, III, S. G. (1969). Classification of patients with disseminated cancer of the breast. *Cancer*, **24**, 861–69

Cutler, S. J., Axtell, L. M. and Heise, H. (1967). Ten thousand cases of leukemia: 1940 to 1962. *J. Nat. Cancer Inst.*, **39**, 993–1026

Cutler, S. J., Axtell, L. M. and Schottenfeld, D. (1969). Adjustment of long-term survival rates for deaths due to intercurrent disease. *J. Chronic Dis.*, **22**, 485–91

Czeizel, E., Vaczo, G. and Kertai, P. (1962). Effect of bone-marrow on regeneration of liver of X-irradiated rats. *Nature, London*, **196**, 240–41

Dahmus, M. E. and Bonner, J. (1970). Nucleoproteins in regulation of gene function. *Federation Proc.*, **29**, 1255–60

Dammacco, F., Trizio, D. and Bonomo, L. (1969). A case of IgA κ-myelomatosis with two urinary Bence-Jones proteins (BJK and BJL) and multiple chromosomal abnormalities. *Acta Haematolog.*, **41**, 309–20

Dameshek, W. and Gunz, F. (1964). *Leukaemia*, 2nd Edition. New York, London: Grune and Stratton

Davidson, J. W. and Clarke, E. A. (1970). The Hodgkin maze. *Lancet*, **i**, 1051–52

Davies, A. J. S., Leuchars, E., Doak, S. M. A. and Cross, A. M. (1964). Regeneration in relation to the lymphoid system. *Nature, London*, **201**, 1097–1101

Davies, D. (1973). A Shangri-la in Ecuador. *New Scient.*, **57**, 236–38

Davies, R. F. and Day, T. D. (1969). A study of the comparative carcinogenicity of cigarette and cigar smoke condensate on mouse skin. *Brit. J. Cancer*, **23**, 363–368

Dawkins, R. L., Aw, E. J. and Simons, P. J. (1972). The persistence of tissue specific antigen in muscle cells growing *in vitro*. *Immunology*, **23**, 961–66

Dawson, A. and Kember, N. F. (1974). Compensatory growth in the rat tibia. *Cell Tissue Kinet.*, **7**, 285–91

Dawson, W. B. (1968). Growth impairment following radiotherapy in childhood. *Clin. Radiol.*, **19**, 241–56

De Cosse, J. J., Gossens, C. L., Kuzma, J. F. and Unsworth, B. R. (1973). Breast cancer: induction of differentiation by embryonic tissue. *Science*, **181**, 1057–58

De Dombal, F. T., Watts, J. McK., Watkinson, G. and Goligher, J. C. (1966). Local complications of ulcerative colitis: stricture, pseudopolyposis and carcinoma of colon and rectum. *Brit. Med. J.*, **i**, 1442–47

Denison, E. K., Peters, R. L. and Reynolds, T. B. (1971). Familial hepatoma with hepatitis-associated antigen. *Ann. Internal Med.*, **74**, 391–94

Deonier, R. C. and Williams, J. W. (1970). Self-association of muramidase (lysozyme) in solution at 25°, pH 7·0, and $I = 0·20$. *Biochemistry*, **9**, 4260–67

De Waard, R., De Laive, J. W. J. and Baanders-Van Halewijn, E. A. (1960). On the bimodal age distribution of mammary carcinoma. *Brit. J. Cancer*, **14**, 437–48

De Wys, W. D. (1972). Studies correlating the growth rate of a tumor and its metastases and providing evidence for tumor-related systemic growth-retarding factors. *Cancer Res.*, **32**, 374–79

Diamond, E. L., Schmerler, H. and Lilienfeld, A. M. (1973). The relationship of intra-uterine radiation to subsequent mortality and development of leukemia in children. A prospective study. *Amer. J. Epidemiol.*, **97**, 283–313

Dicker, S. E. (1972). Inhibition of compensatory renal growth in rats. *J. Physiol.*, **225**, 577–88

Dicker, S. E. and Morris, C. A. (1972). Absence of compensatory renal hypertrophy in baboons. *J. Physiol.*, **223**, 365–73

Dicker, S. E. and Shirley, D. G. (1972). Compensatory hypertrophy of the contralateral kidney after unilateral ureteral ligation. *J. Physiol.*, **220**, 199–210

Dittmar, K., Kochwa, S., Zucker-Franklin, D. and Wasserman, L. R. (1968). Co-existence of polycythemia vera and biclonal gammopathy (γGK and γAL) with two Bence-Jones proteins (BJK and BJL). *Blood*, **31**, 81–92

Dmytryk, E. T. (1971). Familial breast carcinoma. *J. Amer. Med. Ass.*, **216**, 1350

Doll, R. (1955). Etiology of lung cancer. *Adv. Cancer Res.*, **3**, 1–50

Doll, R. (1968). The age distribution of cancer in man. In: *Thule International Symposia. Cancer and Ageing*, pp. 15–36. Stockholm: Nordiska Bokhandelus Forlag

Doll, R. (1971). The age distribution of cancer: implications for models of carcinogenesis. *J. Roy. Stat. Soc.*, Series A (General), **134**, 133–66

Doll, R. (1974). Smoking, lung cancer and Occam's razor. *New Scient.*, **61**, 463–67

Doll, R. and Hill, A. B. (1964). Mortality in relation to smoking: ten years' observations of British doctors. *Brit. Med. J.*, **i**, 1399–1410 and 1460–67

Doll, R., Muir, C. and Waterhouse, J. (Editors) (1970). *Cancer Incidence in Five Continents*, Vol. II. Berlin, Heidelberg and New York: Springer-Verlag

Doll, R., Payne, P. and Waterhouse, J. (Editors) (1966.) *Cancer Incidence in Five Continents*. International Union Against Cancer. Berlin, Heidelberg, New York: Springer-Verlag

Doll, R. and Pike, M. C. (1972). Trends in mortality among British doctors in relation to their smoking habits. *J. Roy. Coll. Physicians London*, **6**, 216–22

Druckrey, H. (1959). Pharmacological approach to carcinogenesis. In: Ciba Foundation Symposium on Carcinogenesis. *Mechanisms of Action*, pp. 110–127. Editors: G. E. W. Wolstenhome and M. O'Connor. London: J. and A. Churchill Ltd.

Duke-Elder, W. S. (1940). *Textbook of Ophthalmology*, Vol. III. London: Henry Kimpton

Duke-Elder, W. S. and Perkins, E. S. (1966). *System of Ophthalmology*, **Vol. 9**, *Diseases of the Uveal Tract*. London: Henry Kimpton

Dukes, C. (1952). Familial intestinal polyposis. *Ann. Eugen.*, **17**, 1–29

Dukes, C. E. (1958). Cancer control in familial polyposis of the colon. *Dis. Colon and Rectum*, **1**, 413–23

Dunn, J. E., Bragg, K. U., Sautter, C. and Gardipee, C. (1972). Breast cancer risk following a major salivary gland carcinoma. *Cancer*, **29**, 1343–46

Dunstone, G. H. and Knaggs, T. W. L. (1972). Familial cancer of the colon and rectum. *J. Med. Genet.*, **9**, 451–56

Duprat, P. (1964). Immunologie—mise en évidence de réaction immunitaire dans les homogreffes de paroi du corps chez le lombricieu *Eisenia foetida* typica. *Compte Rendu de l'Acad. Sci., Paris*, **259**, 4177–82

Dyson, J. L., Beilby, J. O. W. and Steele, S. J. (1971). Factors influencing survival in carcinoma of the ovary. *Brit. J. Cancer*, **25**, 237–49

Ebbesen, P. (1973). Papilloma induction in different aged skin grafts to young recipients. *Nature, London*, **241**, 280–81

Ederer, F., Axtell, L. M. and Cutler, S. J. (1961). The relative survival rate: a statistical methodology. *Nat. Cancer Inst. Monograph*, **6**, 101–21

Ederer, F. and Mersheimer, W. L. (1962). Sex differences in the survival of lung cancer patients. *Cancer*, **15**, 425–32

Edinin, M. (1964). Transplantation antigen levels in the early mouse embryo. *Transplantation*, **2**, 627–37

Edwards, F. C. and Truelove, S. C. (1964). The course and prognosis of ulcerative colitis. Part IV. Carcinoma of the colon. *Gut*, **5**, 15–22

Egorov, I. K. and Blandova, Z. K. (1972). Histocompatibility mutations in mice: chemical induction and linkage with the H-2 locus. *Genet. Res.*, **19**, 133–43

Einhorn, J. and Wersäll, J. (1967). Incidence of oral carcinoma in patients with leukoplakia of the oral mucosa. *Cancer*, **20**, 2189–93

Einstein, A. (1949). Autobiographical Notes. In: *Albert Einstein: Philosopher Scientist*. Editor: P. A. Schilpp. Evanston, Illinois: Library of Living Philosophers

Ekelund, G. R. and Pihl, B. (1974). Multiple carcinomas of the colon and rectum. *Cancer*, **33**, 1630–34

El-Hefnawi, H., Maynard Smith, S. and Penrose, L. S. (1965). Xeroderma pigmentosum —its inheritance and relationship to the ABO blood-group system. *Ann. Human Genet., London*, **28**, 273–90

Elwood, J. M. and Lee, J. A. H. (1974). Trends in mortality from primary tumours of skin in Canada. *Canad. Med. Ass. J.*, **110**, 913–15

Ertl, N. and Wieser, O. (1971). Changes in the thymus during the regenerative growth of the liver after partial hepatectomy in rats. *Oncology*, **25**, 505–11

Everson, T. C. and Cole, W. H. (1966). *Spontaneous Regression of Cancer*. Philadelphia, Pa: W. B. Saunders Co.

Eyring, H., Stover, B. J. and Brown, R. A. (1971). The dynamics of life. V. Applying the steady-state theory of mutations to human cancer. *Proc. Nat. Acad. Sci., USA*, **68**, 1670–72

Eysenck, H. J. (1965). *Smoking, Health and Personality*. London: Weidenfeld and Nicolson

Ezdinli, E. Z., Sokal, J. E., Crosswhite, L. and Sandberg, A. A. (1970). Philadelphia-chromosome–positive and –negative chronic myelocytic leukaemia. *Ann. Internal Med.*, **72**, 175–82

Fabrikant, J. I. (1967). The spatial distribution of parenchymal cell proliferation during regeneration of the liver. *Johns Hopkins Med. J.*, **120**, 137–47

Fairpo, C. G. (1968). Comparison of dental caries experience in identical and like-sexed fraternal twins. *J. Dent. Res.*, **47**, 971

Falk, J. and Osoba, D. (1971). HL-A antigens and survival in Hodgkin's disease. *Lancet*, **ii**, 1118–21

Farmer, R. G., Hawk, W. A. and Turnbull, R. B. Jr. (1971). Carcinoma associated with mucosal ulcerative colitis, and with transmural colitis and enteritis (Crohn's disease). *Cancer*, **28**, 289–92

Fechner, R. E. (1971). Ductal carcinoma involving the lobule of the breast. *Cancer*, **28**, 274–81

Feinstein, A. R. (1968). Clinical epidemiology. II. The identification rates of disease. *Ann. Internal Med.*, **69**, 1037–61

Fialkow, P. J., Klein, G., Gartler, S. M. and Clifford, P. (1970). Clonal origin for individual Burkitt tumours. *Lancet*, **i**, 384–86

Fialkow, P. J., Sagebiel, R. W., Gartler, S. M. and Rimoin, D. L. (1971). Multiple cell origin of hereditary neurofibromas. *New Eng. J. Med.*, **284**, 298–300

Figueroa, W. G., Raszkowski, R. and Weiss, W. (1973). Lung cancer in chloromethyl methyl ether workers. *New Eng. J. Med.*, **288**, 1096–97

Fine, R. N., Korsch, B. M., Stiles, Q., Riddell, H., Edelbrock, H. H., Brennan, L. P., Grushkin, C. M. and Lieberman, E. (1970). Renal homotransplantation in children. *J. Pediat.*, **76**, 347–57

Fisher, B., Szuch, P. and Fisher, E. R. (1971(a)). Evaluation of a humoral factor in liver regeneration utilizing liver transplants. *Cancer Res.*, **31**, 322–31

Fisher, B., Szuch, P., Levine, M. and Fisher, E. R. (1971(b)). A portal blood factor as the humoral agent in liver regeneration. *Science*, **171**, 575–77

Fisher, J. C. (1958). Multiple mutation theory of carcinogenesis. *Nature, London*, **181**, 651–52

Fisher, J. C. and Holloman, J. H. (1951). A hypothesis of the origin of cancer foci. *Cancer*, **4**, 916–18

Fisher, R. A. (1958(a)). Lung cancer and cigarettes? *Nature, London*, **182**, 108

Fisher, R. A. (1958(b)). Cancer and smoking. *Nature, London*, **182**, 596

Fisher, R. A. (1959). *Smoking. The Cancer Controversy. Some Attempts to Assess the Evidence*. Edinburgh: Oliver and Boyd

Fitzgerald, M. G. (1967). Clinical aspects of diabetes mellitus. *Abst. World Med.*, **41**, 825–41

Fitzgerald, P. H. and Hamer, J. W. (1969). Third case of chronic lymphocytic leukaemia in a carrier of the inherited Ch¹ chromosome. *Brit. Med. J.*, **iii**, 752–54

Flaks, A. (1967). Observations of the action of the thymus on the induction of lung tumours by 9,10-dimethyl-1,-2 benzanthracene (DMBA) in newborn A mice. *Brit. J. Cancer*, **21**, 390–92

Flamm, W. G. (1972). Highly repetitive sequences of DNA chromosomes. *Int. Rev. Cytol.*, **32**, 1–51

Flaxman, B. A. (1972). Growth *in vitro* and induction of differentiation in cells of basal cell cancer. *Cancer Res.*, **32**, 462–69

Fleischmajer, R. and Billingham, R. E. (Editors). (1968.) *Epithelial–Mesenchymal Interactions*. Baltimore: Williams and Wilkins

Forbes, J. F. and Morris, P. J. (1970). Leucocyte antigens in Hodgkin's disease. *Lancet*, **ii**, 849–51

Foulds, L. (1969). *Neoplastic Development*. Vol. 1. London and New York: Academic Press

Fox, M. and Wahman, G. E. (1968). Etiology of the compensatory renal response. Observations on the role of the lymphoid system. *Invest. Urol.*, **5**, 521–38

Franks, L. M. (1954). Latent carcinoma of the prostate. *J. Pathol. and Bacteriol.*, **68**, 603–616

Franssila, K. O. (1973). Is the differentiation between papillary and follicular thyroid carcinoma valid? *Cancer*, **32**, 853–64

Fraser, G. R. (1962). Our genetical 'load'. A review of some aspects of genetical variation. *Ann. Human Genet., London*, **25**, 387–415

Fraser, G. R. and Friedmann, A. I. (1967). *The Causes of Blindness in Childhood*. Baltimore: The Johns Hopkins Press

Fraumeni, J. F. Jr. (1974). Family studies in Hodgkin's disease. *Cancer Res.*, **34**, 1164–65

Fraumeni, J. F. Jr. and Thomas, L. B. (1967). Malignant bladder tumours in a man and his three sons. *J. Amer. Med. Ass.*, **201**, 507–509

Freedman, L. R., Blackard, W. G., Sagan, L. A., Ishida, M. and Hamilton, H. B. (1965). The epidemiology of diabetes mellitus in Hiroshima and Nagasaki. *Yale J. Biol. and Med.*, **37**, 283–99

Freeman, J. and Ravdin, I. S. (1959). Polyps and pigment in the Peutz–Jeghers syndrome. *New Eng. J. Med.*, **253**, 958–61

Freire-Maia, A. (1960). Smoking and PTC sensitivity. *Ann. Human Genet.*, **24**, 333–41

Frenster, J. H. (1965). A model of specific derepression within interphase chromatin. *Nature, London*, **206**, 1269–70

Friberg, L., Cederlöf, R., Lorich, U., Lundman, T. and de Faire, U. (1973). Mortality in twins in relation to smoking habits and alcohol problems. A study on the Swedish Twin Registry. *Arch. Environ. Health*, **27**, 294–304

Friberg, L., Kaij, L., Dencker, S. J. and Johnsson, E. (1959). Smoking habits of monozygotic and dizygotic twins. *Brit. Med. J.*, **i**, 1090–92

Fujii, T. and Mizuno, T. (1969). The relation between wound repair process and early changes of skin carcinogenesis. *Proc. Japan. Acad.*, **45**, 925–30

Furth, J. (1953). Condition and autonomous neoplasms: a review. *Cancer Res.*, **13**, 477–492

Furth, J. (1963). Influence of host factors on the growth of neoplastic cells. *Cancer Res.*, **23**, 21–34

Furth, J. (1969). Pituitary cybernetics and neoplasia. *Harvey Lectures, Series* **63**, 47–71. New York: Academic Press, Inc.

Furth, J. and Clifton, K. H. (1966). Experimental pituitary tumours. In: *The Pituitary Gland*, Vol. II, pp. 460–97. Editors: G. W. Harris and B. T. Donovan. London: Butterworths

Gallagher, H. S. and Martin, J. E. (1969). The study of mammary carcinoma by mammography and the whole organ sectioning. *Cancer*, **23**, 855–73

Gardner, E. J. (1951). Genetic and clinical study of intestinal polyposis, predisposing factor for carcinoma of colon and rectum. *Amer. J. Human Genet.*, **3**, 167–76

Gardner, E. J. and Plenk, H. P. (1952). Hereditary pattern for multiple osteomas in a family group. *Amer. J. Human Genet.*, **4**, 31–6

Gardner, E. J. and Richards, R. C. (1953). Multiple cutaneous and subcutaneous lesions occurring simultaneously with hereditary polyposis and osteomatosis. *Amer. J. Human Genet.*, **5**, 139–47

Garfinkel, L., Craig, L. and Seidman, H. (1959). An appraisal of left and right breast cancer. *J. Nat. Cancer Inst.*, **23**, 617–31

Gartler, S. M., Ziprowski, L., Keakowski, A., Ezra, R., Szeinberg, A. and Adam, A. (1966). Glucose-6-phospate dehydrogenase mosaicism as a tracer in the study of hereditary multiple trichoepithelioma. *Amer. J. of Human Genet.*, **18**, 282–87

Gates, R. R. (1946). *Human Genetics*, 2. New York: Macmillan

Gaze, R. M. (1967). Growth and differentiation. *Ann. Rev. Physiol.*, **29**, 59–86

General Register Office (1957). Studies on Medical and Population Subjects. No. 13. London: HMSO

Gilman-Sachs, A. and Knight, K. L. (1972). Identification and genetic control of two rabbit high-density lipoprotein allotypes. *Biochem. Genet.*, **7**, 177–91

Ginzburg, L., Schneider, K. M., Dreizin, D. N. and Levinson, C. (1956). Carcinoma of the jejunum occurring in a case of regional enteritis. *Surgery*, **39**, 347–51

Glober, G. A., Cantrell, E. G., Doll, R. and Peto, R. (1971). Interaction between ABO and Rhesus blood groups, the site of origin of gastric cancers, and the age and sex of the patient. *Gut*, **12**, 570–73

Glucksman, A. (1963). Carcinogenesis. In: *Cellular Basis and Aetiology of Late Somatic Effects of Ionizing Radiation*. Editor: R. J. C. Harris, pp. 121–33. London: Academic Press

Goldblatt, M. W. (1958). Occupational carcinogenesis. *Brit. Med. Bull.*, **14**, 136–40

Gorlin, R. J., Vickers, R. A., Kelln, E. and Williamson, J. J. (1965). The multiple basal-cell nevi syndrome. *Cancer*, **18**, 89–104

Goss, R. J. (1965). Kinetics of compensatory growth. *Quart. Rev. Biol.*, **40**, 123–46

Grabar, P. (1957). The problem of auto-antibodies. An approach to a theory. *Texas Rep. on Biol. and Med.*, **15**, 1–16

Grabar, P. (1959). Auto-antigenicity. In: *Recent Progress in Microbiology*, pp. 170–180. Editor: G. Tunevall. Oxford: Blackwell Scientific Publications

Graham, J. B., Graham, R. M. and Schueller, E. F. (1964). Preclinical detection of ovarian cancer. *Cancer*, **17**, 1414–32

Graham, S., Levin, M. L., Lilienfeld, A. M., Schuman, L. M., Gibson, R., Dowd, J. E. and Hemplemann, L. (1966). Preconception intrauterine and postnatal radiation as related to leukemia. *Nat. Cancer Inst. Monograph*, **19**, 347–71

Graham, S. and Lilienfeld, A. M. (1958). Genetic studies of gastric cancer in humans. *Cancer*, **11**, 945–58

Gray, L. H. (1965). Radiation biology and cancer. In: *Cellular Radiation Biology*, 7–25. Baltimore, Maryland: Williams and Wilkins Co.

Green, H. N. (1954). An immunological concept of cancer: a preliminary report. *Brit. Med. J.*, **ii**, 1374–80

Green, H. N., Anthony, H. M., Baldwin, R. W. and Westrop, J. W. (1967). *An Immunological Approach to Cancer*. London: Butterworths

Greenwald, P., Kirmss, V., Polan, A. K. and Dick, V. S. (1974). Cancer of the prostate among men with benign prostatic hyperplasia. *J. Nat. Cancer Inst.*, **53**, 335–39

Grey, H. M., Kohler, P. F., Terry, W. D. and Franklin, E. C. (1968). Human monoclonal γG-cryoglobulins with anti-γ-globulin activity. *J. Clin. Invest.*, **47**, 1875–84

Griem, M. L., Meier, P. and Dobben, G. D. (1967). Analysis of morbidity and mortality of children irradiated in fetal life. *Radiology*, **88**, 347–9

Grisham, J. W. (1962). Morphologic study of deoxyribonucleic acid synthesis and cell proliferation in regenerating rat liver: autoradiography with thymidine-H^3. *Cancer Res.*, **22**, 842–9

Grobstein, C. (1964). Cytodifferentiation and its controls. *Science*, **143**, 643–50.

Grobstein, C. (1967). Mechanisms of organogenetic tissue interaction. *Nat. Cancer Inst. Monograph*, **26**, 279–99

Gross, L. (1951). Pathogenic properties and 'vertical' transmission of the mouse leukaemia agent. *Proc. Soc. Exp. Biol. and Med.*, **78**, 342–8

Gross, L. (1970). *Oncogenic Viruses*. Oxford: Pergamon Press

Gross, L. (1974). Facts and theories on viruses causing cancer and leukemia. *Proc. Nat. Acad. Sci., USA*, **71**, 2013–17

Grover, N. B., Bloch, M. and Gross, J. (1970). Computer analysis of growth of rats. *Growth*, **34**, 145–52

Gsell, O. R. and Abelin, T. (1972). Cigar- and pipe-smoking in relation to lung cancer and excess mortality. *J. Nat. Cancer Inst.*, **48**, 1795–1803

Gurdon, J. B. and Laskey, R. A. (1970). The transplantation of nuclei from single cultured cells into enucleate frogs' eggs. *J. Embryol. and Exp. Morphol.*, **24**, 227–48

Gutierrez, R. M. and Williams, R. J. (1968). Excretion of ketosteroids and proneness to breast cancer. *Proc. Nat. Acad. Sci., USA*, **59**, 938–43

Haagensen, C. D. (1971). *Diseases of the Breast*. 2nd Edition. London, Toronto: Philadelphia, W. B. Saunders Co.

Haenszel, W. and Dawson, E. A. (1965). A note on mortality from cancer of the colon and rectum in the United States. *Cancer*, **18**, 265–72

Haenszel, W. and Kurihara, M. (1968). Studies of Japanese migrants. I. Mortality from cancer and other diseases among Japanese in the United States. *J. Nat. Cancer Inst.*, **40**, 43–68

Haenszel, W., Kurihara, M., Segi, M. and Lee, R. K. C. (1972). Stomach cancer among Japanese in Hawaii. *J. Nat. Cancer Inst.*, **49**, 969–88

Haenszel, W., Loveland, D. B. and Sirken, M. G. (1962). Lung cancer mortality as related to residence and smoking histories. I. White males. *J. Nat. Cancer Inst.*, **28**, 947–1001

Haenszel, W. and Taeuber, K. E. (1964). Lung cancer mortality as related to residence and smoking histories. II. White females. *J. Nat. Cancer Inst.*, **32**, 803–38

Hagstrom, R. M. and Baker, T. D. (1968). Primary hepatocellular carcinoma in three male siblings. *Cancer*, **22**, 142–50

Hagstrom, R. M. and Ho, Y. C. (1972). Family cancers among cases of primary liver cancer. *Cancer*, **29**, 1264–67

Hakama, M. (1969). The peculiar age-specific incidence curve for cancer of the breast—Clemmesen's hook. *Acta Pathol. et Microbiol. Scand.*, **75**, 370–74

Halazun, J. F., Kerr, S. E. and Lukens, J. N. (1972). Hodgkin's disease in three children from an Amish kindred. *J. Pediat.*, **80**, 289–91

Hale, J. F. (1968). Tumours of the thymus. *Proc. Roy. Soc. Med.*, **61**, 871–74

Hall-Craggs, E. C. B. (1968). The effect of experimental epiphysiodesis on growth in length of the rabbit's tibia. *J. Bone and Joint Surg.*, **50-B**, 392–400

Hall-Craggs, E. C. B. (1969). The effect of epiphysial stapling on growth in length of the rabbit's tibia and femur. *J. Bone and Joint Surg.*, **51-B**, 359–65

Hamerton, J. L. (1964). Lyonisation of the X chromosome. *Lancet*, **i**, 1222–3.

Hamerton, J. L. (1968). Significance of sex chromosome derived heterochromatin in mammals. *Nature, London*, **219**, 910–14

Hammond, E. C. (1966). Smoking in relation to death rates of one million men and women. *Nat. Cancer Inst. Monograph*, **19**, 127–204

Harel, L. and Montagnier, L. (1971). Homology of double stranded RNA from rat liver cells with the cellular genome. *Nature New Biology*, **229**, 106–8

Harnden, D. G., Maclean, N. and Langlands, A. O. (1971). Carcinoma of the breast and Klinefelter's syndrome. *J. Med. Genet.*, **8**, 460–1

Harvald, B. and Hauge, M. (1963). Heredity of cancer elucidated by a study of unselected twins. *J. Amer. Med. Ass.*, **186**, 749–53

Haurowitz, F. (1950). *The Chemistry and Biology of Proteins*. New York: Academic Press

Haurowitz, F. (1963). *The Chemistry and Function of Proteins*. 2nd Edition. New York: Academic Press

Hayata, I., Kakati, S. and Sandberg, A. A. (1973). A new translocation related to the Philadelphia chromosome. *Lancet*, **ii**, 1385

Haybittle, J. L. (1959). The estimation of the proportion of patients cured after treatment for cancer of the breast. *Brit. J. Radiol.*, **32**, 725–33

Heasman, M. A. and Lipworth, L. (1966). *Accuracy of Certification of Cause of Death*. General Register Office, Studies on Medical and Population Subjects, No. 20. London: HMSO

Heath, C. W. (1972). The epidemiology of Hodgkin's disease. *Ann. Internal Med.*, **77**, 313–14

Heath, C. W. Jr., Brodsky, A. L. and Potolsky, A. I. (1972). Infectious mononucleosis in a general population. *Amer. J. Epidemiol.*, **95**, 46–52

Hems, G. (1968(a)). Susceptibility to stomach cancer. *Brit. J. Cancer*, **22**, 461–5

Hems, G. (1968(b)). Factors associating with lung cancer. *Brit. J. Cancer*, **22**, 466–73

Henle, G., Henle, W. and Diehl, V. (1968). Relation of Burkitt's lymphoma-associated Herpes-type virus to infectious mononucleosis. *Proc. Nat. Acad. Sci., USA*, **59**, 94–101

Herman, B. and Enterline, P. E. (1970). Lung cancer among the Jews and non-Jews of Pittsburgh, Pennsylvania, 1953–1967: mortality rates and cigarette smoking behaviour. *Amer. J. Epidemiol.*, **91**, 355–67

Herman, B. and Rao, M. S. (1971). Lung cancer among the Jews and non-Jews of Pittsburgh, Pennsylvania, 1953–1967: II. Medical care initiation and diagnostic procedures. *Amer. J. Epidemiol.*, **94**, 11–15

Herrold, K. McD. (1972). Survey of histologic types of primary lung cancer in US veterans. *Pathol. Annual*, **7**, 45–79

Heston, W. E., Hall, W. T., Vlahakis, G., Charney, J. and Moore, D. H. (1970). Inability to predict mammary tumorigenesis in strain A mice from presence of mammary tumour virus or antigen in the milk. *J. Nat. Cancer Inst.*, **45**, 937–40

Higginson, J. (1972). The role of geographical pathology in environmental carcinogenesis. In: *Environment and Cancer*, 24th Symposium on Fundamental Cancer Research, pp. 69–92. Baltimore: Williams and Wilkins

Hill, C. S. Jr., Ibanez, M. L., Samaan, N. A., Ahearn, M. J. and Clark, R. L. (1973). Medullary (solid) carcinoma of the thyroid gland: an analysis of the M. D. Anderson Hospital experience with patients with the tumor, its special features and its histogenesis. *Medicine*, **52**, 141–71

Hirayama, T. (1967). *Smoking in relation to the Death Rates of 265 118 Men and Women in Japan*. National Cancer Center, Tokyo Research Institute, Epidemiology Division

Hirayama, T. (1972). Huge Japanese study adds to smoking-death link. Reported in: *J. Amer. Med. Ass.*, **222**, 654–5

Hirsch, H. R. (1974). The multistep theory of ageing: relation to the forbidden clone theory. A theoretical article. *Mechanisms of Ageing and Develop.*, **3**, 165–72

Hirshaut, Y., Cohen, M. H. and Stevens, D. A. (1973). Epstein–Barr virus antibodies in American and African Burkitt's lymphoma. *Lancet*, **ii**, 114–16

Hoffmann, D. C. and Brooke, B. N. (1970). Familial sarcoma of bone in a polyposis coli family. *Dis. Colon and Rectum*, **13**, 119–20

Hoi-Sen, Y. (1972). Is subline differentiation a continuing process in inbred strains of mice? *Genet. Res., Cambridge*, **19**, 53–9

Holcomb, H. S. and Meigs, J. W. (1972). Medical absenteeism among cigarette, and cigar and pipe smokers. *Arch. Environ. Health*, **25**, 295–300

Holtfreter, J. (1948). Concepts on the mechanism of embryonic induction and its relation to parthenogenesis and malignancy. *Symposia of the Soc. Exp. Biol.*, No. II, Growth in Relation to Differentiation and Morphogenesis, 17–49

Holtfreter, J. (1955). Studies on the diffusibility, toxicity and pathogenic properties of the 'inductive' agents derived from dead tissues. *Exp. Cell Res.*, Suppl. 3, 188–203

Hood, L., Eichmann, K., Lackland, H., Krause, R. M. and Ohms, J. J. (1970). Rabbit antibody light chains and gene evolution. *Nature, London*, **228**, 1040–44

Horne, R. C., Payne, W. A. and Fine, G. (1963). The Peutz–Jeghers syndrome. *Arch. Pathol.*, **76**, 29–37

Horowitz, I. and Enterline, P. E. (1970). Lung cancer among the Jews. *Amer. J. Public Health*, **60**, 275–82

Horrobin, D. F. (1975). Ideas in biomedical science: reasons for the foundation of medical hypotheses. *Med. Hypotheses*, **1**, 1–2

Horsfall, F. L. Jr. (1966). Unifying concept of the origin of cancer. *Med. Clinics N. America*, **50**, 869–74

Howel-Evans, W., McConnell, R. B., Clarke, C. A. and Sheppard, P. M. (1958). Carcinoma of the oesophagus with keratosis palmaris et plantaris (tylosis): a study of two families. *Quart. J. Med.*, NS27, 413–29

Howell, M. A. (1973). Colonic and stomach cancers: opposing aetiologies? *Lancet*, **ii**, 1338

Huang, R. C. and Huang, P. C. (1969). Effect of protein-bound RNA associated with chick embryo chromatin on template specificity of the chromatin. *J. Mol. Biol.*, **39**, 365–78

Huebner, R. J. (1961). Cancer as an infectious disease. In: *The Harvey Lectures*, 1960–1961, **56**, 45–62

Huebner, R. J. and Todaro, G. J. (1969). Oncogenes of RNA tumor viruses as determinants of cancer. *Proc. Nat. Acad. Sci.*, USA, **64**, 1087–94

Huggins, C., Wiseman, S. and Reddi, A. H. (1970). Transformation of fibroblasts by allogeneic and xenogeneic transplants of demineralized tooth and bone. *J. Exp. Med.*, **132**, 1250–58

Hulse, E. V., Mole, R. H. and Papworth, D. G. (1968). Radiosensitivities of cells from which radiation-induced skin tumours are derived. *Int. J. Radiat. Biol.*, **14**, 437–44

Humble, J. G., Jayne, W. H. W. and Pulvertaft, R. J. V. (1956). Biological interaction between lymphocytes and other cells. *Brit. J. Haematol.*, **2**, 283–94

Humphrey, L. J. and Swerdlow, M. A. (1962). Relationship of benign breast disease to carcinoma of the breast. *Surgery*, **52**, 841–46

Humphrey, L. J. and Swerdlow, M. A. (1968). Large duct epithelial hyperplasia and carcinoma of the breast. *Arch. Surg.*, **97**, 592–4

Humphries, A. L., Shepperd, M. H. and Peters, H. J. (1966). Peutz–Jeghers syndrome with colonic adenocarcinoma and ovarian tumor. *J. Amer. Med. Ass.*, **197**, 296–8

Hyman, R. A., Voges, V. and Finby, N. (1973). Bilateral hypernephroma. *Amer. J. Roentgenol., Radium Therapy and Nucl. Med.*, **117**, 104–07

Inglis, K. (1936). *Paget's Disease of the Nipple and its Relation to Surface Cancers and Precancerous States in General.* London: Oxford University Press

Ishmaru, T., Hoshino, T., Ichimaru, M., Okada, H., Tomiyasu, T., Tsuchimoto, T. and Yamamoto, T. (1971). Leukemia in atomic bomb survivors, Hiroshima and Nagasaki, 1 October 1950–30 September 1966. *Radiat. Res.*, **45**, 216–33

Izuo, M., Okagaki, T., Richart, R. M. and Lattes, R. (1971). Nuclear DNA content in hyperplastic lesions of cystic disease of the breast with special reference to malignant alteration. *Cancer*, **28**, 620–7

Jablon, S. (1973). Comments on 'The carcinogenic effects of low level radiation. A reappraisal of epidemiologists' methods and observations.' *Health Physics*, **24**, 257–8

Jablon, S. and Kato, H. (1970). Childhood cancer in relation to prenatal exposure to atomic-bomb radiation. *Lancet*, **ii**, 1000–3

Jackson, A. W., Muldal, S., Ockey, C. H. and O'Connor, P. J. (1965). Carcinoma of male breast in association with the Klinefelter's syndrome. *Brit. Med. Journal*, **i**, 223–225

Jackson, D. (1968). Genes and dental caries. *Proc. Roy. Soc. Med.*, **61**, 265–9

Jackson, D. and Burch, P. R. J. (1969). Dental caries as a degenerative disease. *Gerontologia*, **15**, 203–16

Jackson, D. and Burch, P. R. J. (1970). Dental caries: distribution, by age-group, between homologous (right-left) mesial and distal surfaces of human permanent maxillary incisors. *Arch. Oral Biol.*, **15**, 1059–67

Jacobs, B. B. (1974). Immunologic modification: a basic survival mechanism. *Science*, **185**, 582–87

Jacobsen, O. (1946). *Heredity in Breast Cancer: A Genetic and Clinical Study of Two Hundred Probands*. London: H. K. Lewis and Co. Ltd.

Jaeger, W. (1951). Gibt es Kombinationsformen der verschiedenen Typen angeborener Farbensinnstörungen? *Albrecht v. Graefes Arch. für Ophthalmol.*, **151**, 229–48

Jaeger, W. (1952). Werden die angeborenen Störungen des Rotgrünsinns ausnahmslos rezessive-geschlechtsgebunden vereht? *Albrecht v. Graefes Arch. für Ophthalmol.*, **152**, 379–84

Jeejeebhoy, H. F. (1970). The effect of heterologous anti-lymphocyte serum on lymphocytes of thymus and marrow origin. *J. Exp. Med.*, **132**, 963–75

Jeghers, H., McKusick, V. A. and Katz, K. N. (1949). Generalized intestinal polyposis and melanin spots of oral mucosa, lips, digits. Syndrome of diagnostic significance. *New Eng. J. Med.*, **241**, 993–1005; 1031–36

Jehle, H. L. (1963). Intermolecular forces and biological specificity. *Proc. Nat. Acad. Sci.*, *USA*, **50**, 516–24

Jehle, H. (1969(a)). Charge fluctuation forces in biological systems. *Ann. N.Y. Acad. Sci.*, **158**, 240–55

Jehle, H. (1969(b)). Remarks on the problem of morphogenetic movements in the development of embryos. *Int. J. Quantum Chem.*, **IIIS**, 75–82

Jehle, H., Yos, J. M. and Bade, W. L. (1958). Specificity of charge fluctuation forces. I. *Physical Rev.*, **110**, 793–800

Jelinek, W. and Darnell, J. E. (1972). Double-stranded regions in heterogeneous nuclear RNA from HeLa cells. *Proc. Nat. Acad. Sci.*, *USA*, **69**, 2537–41

Jensen, R. D. and Miller, R. W. (1971). Retinoblastoma: epidemiologic characteristics. *New Eng. J. Med.*, **285**, 307–11

Jensen, R. D., Norris, H. J. and Fraumeni, J. F. (1974). Familial arrhenoblastoma and thyroid adenoma. *Cancer*, **33**, 218–23

Jereb, B. (1971). Bilateral nephroblastoma. *Acta Radiolog.*, **10**, 417–26

Johnson, K. N., Buoen, L. C., Brand, I. and Brand, K. G. (1970). Polymer tumorigenesis: clonal determination of histopathological characteristics during early preneoplasia; relationships to karyotype, mouse strain and sex. *J. Nat. Cancer Inst.*, **44**, 785–93

Joly, D. J., Lilienfeld, A. M., Diamond, E. L. and Bross, I. D. J. (1974). An epidemiologic study of the relationship of reproductive experience to cancer of the ovary. *Amer. J. Epidemiol.*, **99**, 190–209

Juberg, R. C. and Jones, B. (1970). The Christchurch chromosome (Gp-). Mongolism, erythroleukemia and an inherited Gp- chromosome (Christchurch). *New Eng. J. Med.*, **282**, 292–97

Jukes, T. H. and Gatlin, L. (1971). Recent studies covering the coding mechanism. In: *Prog. in Nucleic Acid Res. and Mol. Biol.*, **11**, 303–50

Kafuko, G. W. and Burkitt, D. P. (1970). Burkitt's lymphoma and malaria. *Int. J. Cancer*, **6**, 1–9

Kahn, H. A. (1966). The Dorn Study of smoking and mortality among US veterans: report on eight and one-half years of observation. *Nat. Cancer Inst. Monograph*, **19**, 1–125

Kahn, L. B. and Donaldson, R. C. (1970). Multiple primary melanoma. Case report and a study of tumor *in vitro. Cancer*, **25**, 1162–69

Kaplan, H. S. and Smithers, D. W. (1959). Auto-immunity in man and homologous disease in mice in relation to malignant lymphomas. *Lancet*, **ii**, 1–4

Kaplan, L. and Cole, S. L. (1965). Fraternal primary hepatocellular carcinoma in three male adult siblings. *Amer. J. Med.*, **39**, 305–11

Kaplan, L., Katz, A. D., Ben-Isaac, C. and Massry, S. G. (1971). Malignant neoplasms and parathyroid adenoma. *Cancer*, **28**, 401–7

Kaplan, M. H., Armstrong, D. and Rosen, P. (1974). Tuberculosis complicating neoplastic disease. *Cancer*, **33**, 850–8

Kashgarian, M. and Dunn, J. E. Jr. (1970). The duration of intraepithelial and preclinical squamous cell carcinoma of the uterine cervix. *Amer. J. Epidemiol.*, **92**, 211–22

Katzenellenbogen, I. and Sandbank, M. (1966). Malignant melanoma in twins. *Arch. Dermatol.*, **94**, 331–2

Keith, L. and Brown, E. (1971). Epidemiologic study of leukemia in twins (1928 to 1969). *Acta Genet. Med. et Gemellolog.*, **20**, 9–22

Keller, A. K. (1973). Histology, survivorship and related factors in the epidemiology of eye cancers. *Amer. J. Epidemiol.*, **97**, 386–93

Kellermann, G., Shaw, C. R. and Luyten-Kellermann, M. (1973). Aryl hydrocarbon hydroxylase inducibility and bronchogenic carcinoma. *New Eng. J. Med.*, **289**, 934–47

Kennedy, A. (1972). Lung cancer in young adults. *Brit. J. Dis. of the Chest*, **66**, 147–54

Kennedy, B. J. (1970). Cyclic leukocyte oscillations in chronic myelogenous leukemia during hydroxyurea therapy. *Blood*, **35**, 751–60

Kern, W. H. and Brooks, R. M. (1969). Atypical epithelial hyperplasia associated with breast cancer and fibrocystic disease. *Cancer*, **24**, 668–75

Kern, W. H. and Mikkelsen, W. P. (1971). Small carcinomas of the breast. *Cancer*, **28**, 948–55

Kessler, I. I. (1972). Epidemiologic studies of Parkinson's disease. III. A community-based survey. *Amer. J. Epidemiol.*, **96**, 242–54

Kimball, R. F. and Perdue, S. W. (1967). Comparison of mutagenesis by X-rays and triethylene melamine in *Paramecium*, with emphasis on the role of mitoses. *Mutation Res.*, **4**, 37–50

Kissmeyer-Nielsen, F. (1971). Reported at Symposium: HL-A System and Tissue Typing. First Meeting European Division, International Society of Haematology, Milan

Klein, G. (1971). Immunological studies on Burkitt's lymphoma. *Post. Med. J.*, **47**, 141–155

Klein, J. C. (1974). Evidence against a direct carcinogenic effect of x-rays *in vitro. J. Nat. Cancer Inst.*, **52**, 1111–16

Klein, W. H., Murphy, W., Attardi, G., Britten, R. J. and Davidson, E. H. (1974). Distribution of repetitive and non-repetitive sequence transcripts in HeLa mRNA. *Proc. Nat. Acad. Sci., USA*, **71**, 1785–89

Knight, K. L. and Dray, S. (1968(a)). Identification and genetic control of two rabbit α_2-macroglobulin allotypes. *Biochemistry*, **7**, 1165–71

Knight, K. L. and Dray, S. (1968(b)). Contributions of allelic genes to the formation of individual α_2-macroglobulin molecules. *Biochemistry*, **7**, 3830–35

Knudson, A. G. Jr. (1971). Mutation and cancer. Statistical study of retinoblastoma. *Proc. Nat. Acad. Sci., USA*, **68**, 820–23

Koller, P. C. (1957). The genetic component of cancer. Chapter 10 in: *Cancer*, **1**, pp. 335–403. Editor: R. W. Raven. London: Butterworths

Lacey, J. C. Jr. and Pruitt, K. M. (1969). Origin of the genetic code. *Nature, London*, **223**, 799–804

Laiken, S., Printz, M. P. and Craig, L. C. (1971). Studies on the mode of self association of tyrocidin B. *Biochem. and Biophys. Res. Commun.*, **43**, 596–600

Laird, A. K. (1964). Dynamics of tumour growth. *Brit. J. Cancer*, **18**, 490–502

Laird, A. K. (1965). Dynamics of tumour growth: comparison of growth rates and extrapolation of growth curve to one cell. *Brit. J. Cancer*, **19**, 278–91

Laird, A. K., Tyler, S. A. and Barton, A. D. (1965). Dynamics of normal growth. *Growth*, **29**, 233–48

Lala, P. K. (1972). Age-specific changes in the proliferation of Ehrlich ascites tumor cells grown as solid tumors. *Cancer Res.*, **32**, 628–36

Lane, N., Kaplan, H. and Pascal, R. R. (1971). Minute adenomatous and hyperplastic polyps of the colon: divergent patterns of epithelial growth with specific associated mesenchymal changes. *Gastroenterology*, **60**, 537–51

Lane-Brown, M. M. and Melia, D. F. (1973). A genetic diathesis to skin cancer. *J. Invest. Dermatol.*, **61**, 39–41

Lane-Brown, M. M., Sharpe, C. A. B., Macmillan, D. S. and McGovern, V. J. (1971). Genetic predisposition to melanoma and other skin cancers in Australians. *Med. J. Australia*, **i**, 852–53

Lane-Claypon, J. E. (1930). Cancer of the lip, tongue and skin. *Reports on Public Health and Medical Subjects No. 59*. London: Ministry of Health

Langård, S. and Norseth, T. (1975). A cohort study of bronchial carcinoma in workers producing chromate pigments. *Brit. J. Indust. Med.*, **32**, 62–5

Lashof, J. C. and Stewart, A. (1965). Oxford survey of childhood cancers. Progress Report III: Leukaemia and Down's syndrome. *Monthly Bull. Min. of Health*, **24**, 136–143

Lautrop, H. (1971). Epidemics of parapertussis. 20 years' observations in Denmark. *Lancet*, **i**, 1195–98

Lawrence, J. S. (1961). Prevalence of rheumatoid arthritis. *Ann. Rheum. Dis.*, **20**, 11–17

Leckband, E. and Boyse, E. A. (1971). Immunocompetent cells among mouse thymocytes: a minor population. *Science*, **172**, 1258–60

Leduc, E. H. (1964). Regeneration of liver. In: *The Liver: Morphology, Biochemistry, Physiology*, pp. 63–89. Editor: C. Rouiller, Vol. 2. New York: Academic Press

Lee, F. I. (1971). Carcinoma of the gastric antrum in identical twins. *Post. Med. J.*, **47**, 622–24

Lee, P. N. and O'Neill, J. A. (1971). The effect both of time and dose applied on tumour incidence rate in benzopyrene skin painting experiments. *Brit. J. Cancer*, **25**, 759–770

Leelawongs, N. and Regan, C. D. J. (1968). Retinoblastoma: a review of ten years. *Amer. J. Ophthalmol.*, **66**, 1050–60

Lehane, D. E. (1970). A seroepidemiologic study of infectious mononucleosis. The development of EB virus antibody in a military population. *J. Amer. Med. Ass.*, **212**, 2240–42

Leng, N. and Felsenfeld, G. (1966). The preferential interactions of polylysine and polyarginine with specific base sequences in DNA. *Proc. Nat. Acad. Sci., USA*, **56**, 1325–32

Leong, G. F., Grisham, J. W., Hole, B. V. and Albright, M. L. (1964). Effect of partial hepatectomy on DNA synthesis and mitosis in heterotopic partial autografts of rat liver. *Cancer Res.*, **23**, 1496–1501

Levin, W. C., Houston, E. W. and Ritzmann, S. E. (1967). Polycythemia vera with Ph¹ chromosomes in two brothers. *Blood*, **30**, 503–12

Levine, S., Pictet, R. and Rutter, W. J. (1973). Control of cell proliferation and cyto-differentiation by a factor reacting with the cell surface. *Nature New Biology*, **246**, 49–52

Lewis, A. C. W. and Davison, B. C. C. (1969). Familial ovarian cancer. *Lancet*, **ii**, 235–37

Lewison, E. F. and Neto, A. S. (1971). Bilateral breast cancer at the Johns Hopkins Hospital. *Cancer*, **28**, 1297–1301

Li, F. P. and Fraumeni, J. F. Jr. (1969). Soft-tissue sarcomas, breast cancer, and other neoplasms. A familial syndrome? *Ann. Internal Med.*, **71**, 747–52

Li, F. P., Fraumeni, J. F. and Dalager, N. (1973). Ovarian cancers in the young. *Cancer*, **32**, 969–72

Li, F. P., Rapoport, A. H., Fraumeni, J. F. and Jensen, R. D. (1970). Familial ovarian carcinoma. *J. Amer. Med. Ass.*, **214**, 1559–61

Liber, A. F. (1950). Ovarian cancer in mother and five daughters. *Arch. Pathol.*, **49**, 280–90

Liebman, E. (1947). The trephocytes and their functions. *Experientia*, **111**, 442–51

Lilien, J. E. (1969). Towards a molecular explanation for specific cell adhesion. *Curr. Topics in Develop. Biol.*, **4**, 169–95

Lilienfeld, A. M. (1956). The relationship of cancer of the female breast to artificial menopause and marital status. *Cancer*, **9**, 927–34

Lilienfeld, A. M. (1965). Formal discussion of genetic factors in the aetiology of cancer: an epidemiologic view. *Cancer Res.*, **25**, 1330–35

Linden, G., Dunn, J. E. Jr., Hom, P. H. and Mann, M. (1972). Effect of smoking on the survival of patients with lung cancer. *Cancer*, **30**, 325–28

Linder, D. and Gartler, S. M. (1965). Glucose-6-phosphate dehydrogenase mosaicism: utilization as a cell marker in the study of leiomyomas. *Science*, **150**, 67–9

Lindstrom, D. M. and Dulbecco, R. (1972). Strand orientation of simian virus 40 transcription in productively infected cells. *Proc. Nat. Acad. Sci., USA*, **69**, 1517–20

Ling, L.-N., Horikawa, M. and Fox, A. S. (1970). Aggregation of dissociated cells of *Drosophila* embryos. *Develop. Biol.*, **22**, 264–81

Lockhart-Mummery, H. E. (1934). *Diseases of the Rectum and Colon and their Treatment.* Baltimore: William Wood

Lockhart-Mummery, H. E. (1967). Intestinal polyposis: the present position. *Proc. Roy. Soc. Med.*, **60**, 381–88

Lombard, H. L. and Snegireff, L. S. (1959). An epidemiological study of lung cancer. *Cancer*, **12**, 406–13

Loutit, J. F. (1962). Immunological and trophic functions of lymphocytes. *Lancet*, **ii**, 1106–08

Lynch, H. T. (1967). *Hereditary Factors in Carcinoma.* Berlin, Heidelberg and New York: Springer-Verlag

Lynch, H. T. (1969). Skin, heredity and cancer. *Cancer*, **24**, 277–88

Lynch, H. T. and Krush, A. J. (1968). Heredity and malignant melanoma: implications for early cancer detection. *Canad. Med. Ass. J.*, **99**, 17–21

Lynch, H. T. and Krush, A. J. (1971). Cancer family 'G' revisited: 1895 to 1970. *Cancer*, **27**, 1505–11

Lynch, H. T., Krush, A. J., Lemon, H. M., Kaplan, A. R., Condit, P. T. and Bottomley, R. H. (1972). Tumor variation in families with breast cancer. *J. Amer. Med. Ass.*, **222**, 1631–35

Lynch, H. T., Shaw, M. W., Magnuson, C. W., Larsen, A. L. and Krush, A. J. (1966). Hereditary factors in cancer. Study of two large Midwestern kindreds. *Arch. Internal Med.*, **117**, 206–12

Lyon, M. F. (1961). Genetic action in the X-chromosome of the mouse (*Mus. Musculus L*). *Nature, London*, **190**, 372–73

McConnell, R. B. (1966). *The Genetics of Gastro-intestinal Disorders*. London: Oxford University Press

McCormick, J. N., Nelson, D., Tunstall, A. M. and James, K. (1973). Association of α-macroglobulins with lymphoid cells. *Nature New Biology*, **246**, 78–91

McCredie, J. A., Inch, W. R., Kruuv, J. and Watson, T. A. (1965). The rate of tumor growth in animals. *Growth*, **29**, 331–47

McCurdy, P. R. (1968). Discussion of: The genetics of glucose-6-phosphate dehydrogenase deficiency. In: *Hereditary Disorders of Erythrocyte Metabolism*, pp. 121–4. Editor: E. Beutler. New York and London: Grune and Stratton

MacDougall, I. P. M. (1964). The cancer risk in ulcerative colitis. *Lancet*, **ii**, 655–58

McGrath, E. J., Gall, E. A. and Kessler, D. P. (1952). Bronchiogenic carcinoma, a product of multiple sites of origin. *J. Thorac. Surg.*, **24**, 271–83

McKusick, V. A. (1962). Genetic factors in intestinal polyposis. *J. Amer. Med. Ass.*, **182**, 271–77

McKusick, V. A. (1966). *Mendelian Inheritance in Man*. Baltimore: The Johns Hopkins Press

MacMahon, B. (1966). Epidemiology of Hodgkin's disease. *Cancer Res.*, **26**, 1189–1200

MacMahon, B. (1972). Susceptibility to radiation-induced leukaemia? *New Eng. J. Med.*, **287**, 144–45

McPhedran, P., Heath, C. W. and Lee, J. (1969). Patterns of familial leukemia. Ten cases of leukemia in two interrelated families. *Cancer*, **24**, 403–07

Macklin, M. T. (1959). Comparison of the number of breast cancer deaths observed in relatives of breast-cancer patients and the number expected on the basis of mortality rates. *J. Nat. Cancer Inst.*, **22**, 927–51

Macklin, M. T. (1960). Inheritance of cancer of the stomach and large intestine in man. *J. Nat. Cancer Inst.*, **24**, 551–71

Maddock, C. R. (1966). Environment and heredity factors in carcinoma of the stomach. *Brit. J. Cancer*, **20**, 660–69

Maldague, P. (1969). Comparative study of experimentally induced cancer of the kidney in mice and rats with X-rays. In: *Radiation-induced Cancer*, pp. 439–58. Vienna: International Atomic Energy Agency, ST1/PUB/228

Mallet-Guy, P., Ferddi, J., Eicholz, L. and Michoulier, J. (1966). Étude expérimentale de la neurectomie pér-artère-hépatique. I. Effets de la résection du 'pédicule nerveux antérieur' sur le foie normal. *Lyon Chirurg.*, **51**, 45–62

Martz, E. and Steinberg, M. S. (1972). The role of cell–cell contact in 'contact' inhibition of cell division: a review and new evidence. *J. Cell. Physiol.*, **79**, 189–210

Mayer, T. C. and Fishbane, J. L. (1972). Mesoderm–ectoderm interaction in the production of the agouti pigmentation pattern in mice. *Genetics*, **71**, 297–303

Mayneord, W. V. (1968). Radiation carcinogenesis. *Brit. J. Radiol.*, **41**, 241–50

Melvin, J. B. (1968). The localization of mitotic figures in regenerating mouse liver. *Anat. Rec.*, **160**, 607–18

Melvin, K. E. W., Miller, H. H. and Tashjian, A. H. Jr. (1971). Early diagnosis of medullary carcinoma of the thyroid gland by means of calcitonin assay. *New Eng. J. Med.*, **285**, 1115–20

Metcalf, D. (1964). Functional interactions between the thymus and other organs. In: *The Thymus*, pp. 53–72. Editors: V. Defendi and D. Metcalf. Philadelphia: The Wistar Institute Press

Metzger, H. (1969). Myeloma proteins and antibodies. *Amer. J. Med.*, **47**, 837–44

Mihm, M. C. Jr., Clark, W. C. Jr. and From, L. (1971). The clinical diagnosis, classification and histogenetic concepts of the early stages of cutaneous malignant melanomas. *New Eng. J. Med.*, **284**, 1078–82

Miller, R. W. (1969). Delayed radiation effects in atomic bomb survivors. *Science*, **166**, 569–74

Mintz, B. (1971). Genetic mosaicism *in vivo*: development and disease in allophenic mice. *Federation Proc.*, **30**, 935–43

Mintz, B. and Slemmer, G. (1969). Gene control of neoplasia. 1. Genotypic mosaicism in normal and preneoplastic mammary glands of allophenic mice. *J. Nat. Cancer Inst.*, **43**, 87–95

Mirra, A. P., Cole, P. and MacMahon, B. (1971). Breast cancer in an area of high parity: São Paulo, Brazil. *Cancer Res.*, **31**, 77–83

Mirzabekov, A. D., Lastity, D., Levina, E. S. and Bayev, A. A. (1971). Localization of two recognition sites in yeast valine tRNA I. *Nature New Biology*, **229**, 21–22

Miyakawa, Y., Tanigaki, N., Kreiter, V. P., Moore, G. E. and Pressman, D. (1973). Characterization of soluble substances in the plasma carrying HL-A alloantigenic activity and HL-A common antigenic activity. *Transplantation*, **15**, 312–19

Modan, B. (1965). Polycythemia. A review of epidemiological and clinical aspects. *J. Chronic Dis.*, **18**, 605–45

Modan, B., Kallner, H., Zemer, D. and Yoran, C. (1971). A note on the increased risk of polycythemia vera in Jews. *Blood*, **37**, 172–76

Moertel, C. G. Dockerty, M. B. and Baggenstoss, A. H. (1961(a)). Multiple primary malignant neoplasms. II. Tumors of different tissues or organs. *Cancer*, **14**, 231–37

Moertel, C. G., Dockerty, M. B. and Baggenstoss, A. H. (1961(b)). Multiple primary malignant neoplasms. III. Tumors of multicentric origin. *Cancer*, **14**, 238–48

Moertel, C. G. and Elveback, L. R. (1969). The association between salivary gland cancer and breast cancer. *J. Amer. Med. Ass.*, **210**, 306–8

Mole, R. H. (1974). Antenatal irradiation and childhood cancer: causation or coincidence? *Brit. J. Cancer*, **30**, 199–208

Moolten, F. L. and Bucher, N. L. R. (1967). Regeneration of rat liver: transfer of humoral agent by cross circulation. *Science*, **158**, 272–74

Moore, R., Tsukada, Y., Regelson, W., Pickren, J. W. and Bross, I. D. J. (1965). Synchronous tumors in patients with multiple primary cancers. *Cancer*, **18**, 1423–30

Morganti, G., Gianferrari, L., Cresseri, A., Arrigoni, G. and Lovati, G. (1956(a)). Recherches clinico-statistiques et génétiques sur les néoplasies de la prostate. *Acta Genet. et Statist. Med., Basel*, **6**, 304–5

Morganti, G., Gianferrari, L., Cresseri, A., Arrigoni, G. and Lovati, G. (1956(b)).

Recherches clinico-statistiques et génétiques sur les néoplasies de la vessie. *Acta Genet. et Statist. Med., Basel,* **6**, 306–7

Mori, W. (1971). A geopathological study on malignant melanoma in Japan. *Pathol. et Microbiol.,* **37**, 169–80

Morley, A. A. (1966). A neutrophil cycle in healthy individuals. *Lancet,* **ii**, 1220–22

Morley, A. A., Baikie, A. G. and Galton, D. A. G. (1967). Cyclic leucocytosis as evidence for retention of normal homoeostatic control in chronic granulocytic leukaemia. *Lancet,* **ii**, 1320–23

Mortimer, R., Brustad, T. and Cormack, D. V. (1965). Influence of linear energy transfer and oxygen tension on the effectiveness of ionizing radiations for induction of mutations and lethality in *Saccharomyces cerevisiae. Radiation Res.,* **26**, 465–82

Mosbech, J. and Videbaek, A. (1950). Mortality from and risk of gastric carcinoma among patients with pernicious anaemia. *Brit. Med. J.,* **ii**, 390–94

Moscana, A. A. (1963). Studies on cell aggregation: demonstration of materials with selective cell-binding activity. *Proc. Nat. Acad. Sci., USA,* **49**, 742–47

Moscana, A. A. and Moscana, M. H. (1952). The dissociation and aggregation of cells from organ rudiments of the early chick embryo. *J. Anat.,* **86**, 287–301

Mosier, H. D. and Jansons, R. A. (1970). Effect of X-irradiation of selected areas of the head of the newborn rat on growth. *Radiation Res.,* **43**, 92–104

Muir, E. G., Yates Bell, A. J. and Barlow, K. A. (1967). Multiple primary carcinomata of the colon, duodenum and larynx associated with kerato-acanthomata of the face. *Brit. J. Surg.,* **54**, 191–95

Muller, H. J. (1922). Variation due to change in the individual gene. *Amer. Natur.,* **56**, 32–50

Muller, H. J. (1941). Résumé and perspectives of the symposium on genes and chromosomes. *Cold Spring Harbor Symposia on Quant. Biol.,* **9**, Genes and Chromosomes. Structure and Organization. 290–308

Muller, H. J. (1951). Radiation damage to the genetic material. *Sci. in Prog.,* **7**, 93–165

Murray, P. D. F. and Huxley, J. S. (1925). Self-differentiation in the grafted limb-bud of the chick. *J. Anat., London,* **59**, 379–84

Nakashima, T. and Fox, S. W. (1972). Selective condensation of aminoacyl adenylates by nucleoprotenoid microparticles. *Proc. Nat. Acad. Sci., USA,* **69**, 106–8

Nash, D. J. (1970). Organ weight response of inbred and hybrid mice following X-irradiation at four weeks of age. *Growth,* **34**, 75–86

Nasim, A. and Auerbach, C. (1967). The origin of complete and mosaic mutants from mutagenic treatment of single cells. *Mutation Res.,* **4**, 1–14

National Board of Health and Welfare (1970(a)). Cancer Incidence in Sweden 1966. Stockholm

National Board of Health and Welfare (1970(b)). Cancer Incidence in Sweden 1967. Stockholm

National Board of Health and Welfare (1971(a)). Cancer Incidence in Sweden 1959–1965. Stockholm

National Board of Health and Welfare (1971(b)). Cancer Incidence in Sweden 1968. Stockholm

Nefzger, M. D., Quadfasel, F. A. and Karl, V. C. (1968). A retrospective study of smoking in Parkinson's disease. *Amer. J. Epidemiol.,* **88**, 149–58

Neiman, R. S., Rosen, P. J. and Lukes, R. J. (1973). Lymphocyte-depletion Hodgkin's disease. A clinicopathological entity. *New Eng. J. Med.,* **288**, 751–55

Nelson, D. H. (1962). Spontaneous regression of cancer. *Clin. Radiol.,* **13**, 138–40

Newell, G. R. and Waggoner, D. E. (1970). Cancer mortality and environmental temperature in the United States. *Lancet*, i, 766–68

Newton, R. E. (1902). Glioma of retina. A remarkable family history. *Austral. Med. Gaz.*, **21**, 236–7

Nielsen, M. and Goldschmidt, E. (1968). Retinoblastoma among offspring of adult survivors in Denmark. *Acta Ophthalmol.*, **46**, 736–41

Nijkamp, H. J. J., Bφvre, K. and Szybalski, W. (1971). Regulation of leftward transcription in the J-b2-*att* region of coliphage lambda. *Molec. and General Genet.*, **111**, 22–34

Nordling, C. O. (1952). Cancer theories and cancer statistics. *Nord. med.*, **47**, 817–20

Nordling, C. O. (1953). A new theory on the cancer-inducing mechanism. *Brit. J. Cancer*, **7**, 68–72

Nordling, S., Miettinen, H., Wartiovaara, J. and Saxén, L. (1971). Transmission and spread of embryonic induction. I. Temporal relationships in transfilter induction of kidney tubules *in vitro. J. Embryol. and Exp. Morphol.*, **26**, 231–52

Nφrgaard, O. (1971). Three cases of multiple myeloma in which the preclinical asymptomatic phases persisted throughout 15 to 24 years. *Brit. J. Cancer*, **25**, 417–22

Novak, E. R. and Woodruff, J. D. (1967). *Gynecologic and Obstetric Pathology*. 6th edition. Philadelphia and London: W. B. Saunders

Novick, A. and Szilard, L. (1950). Experiments with the chemostat on spontaneous mutations of bacteria. *Proc. Nat. Acad. Sci., USA*, **36**, 708–19

Nowell, P. C. and Hungerford, D. A. (1961). Chromosome studies in human leukemia. II. Chronic granulocytic leukemia. *J. Nat. Cancer Inst.*, **27**, 1013–35

Oettle, A. G. (1956). The incidence of primary carcinoma of the liver in the Southern Bantu. I. Critical review of the literature. *J. Nat. Cancer Inst.*, **17**, 249–80

Oettle, A. G. and Higginson, J. (1956). The incidence of primary carcinoma of the liver in the Southern Bantu. II. Preliminary report on incidence in Johannesburg. *J. Nat. Cancer Inst.*, **17**, 281–87

Ohno, S. (1967). *Sex Chromosomes and Sex-linked Genes*. Berlin: Springer-Verlag

Old, L. J., Stockert, E., Boyse, E. A. and Kim, J. H. (1968). Antigenic modulation loss of TL antigen from cells exposed to TL antibody. Study of the phenomenon *in vitro. J. Exp. Med.*, **127**, 523–39

Onuigbo, W. I. B. (1971). The diagnosis of lung cancer in the nineteenth century. *Brit. J. Dis. Chest*, **65**, 119–24

Oppenheim, B. E., Griem, M. L. and Meier, P. (1974). Effects of low-dose prenatal irradiation in humans: analysis of Chicago lying-in data and comparison with other studies. *Radiation Res.*, **57**, 508–44

Oppenheim, B. E., Griem, M. L. and Meier, P. (1975). The effects of diagnostic X-ray exposure on the human fetus: an examination of the evidence. *Radiology*, **114**, 529–534

Oppenheimer, B. S., Oppenheimer, E. T., Stout, A. P., Willhite, M. and Danishefsky, I. (1958). The latent period in carcinogenesis by plastics in rats and its relation to the presarcomatous stage. *Cancer*, **11**, 204–13

Order, S. E. and Waksman, B. H. (1969). Cellular differentiation in the thymus. *Transplantation*, **8**, 783–800

Orgel, L. E. (1963). The maintenance of the accuracy of protein synthesis and its relevance to ageing. *Proc. Nat. Acad. Sci., USA*, **49**, 517–21

Orr, J. W. (1958). The mechanism of chemical carcinogenesis. *Brit. Med. Bull.*, **14**, 99–101

Osgood, E. E. (1957). A unifying concept of the etiology of the leukemias, lymphomas, and cancer. *J. Nat. Cancer Inst.*, **18**, 155–6

Osgood, E. E. (1959). Regulation of cell proliferation. In: *The Kinetics of Cellular Proliferation*, pp. 282–8. New York: Grune and Stratton, Inc.

Osgood, E. E. (1964). The etiology of leukemias, lymphomas and cancers. *Geriatrics*, **19**, 208–21

Osgood, E. E. (1965). Polycythemia vera: age relationship and survival. *Blood*, **26**, 243–56

Owen, L. G., Fliegelman, M. T., Jetton, R. L. and Musgrave, J. W. (1974). Seasonal variation of basal cell epitheliomas in Kentucky. *Arch. Dermatol.*, **109**, 205–6

Papadrianos, E., Haagensen, C. D. and Cooley, E. (1967). Cancer of the breast as a familial disease. *Ann. Surg.*, **165**, 10–19

Passey, R. D. (1962). Some problems of lung cancer. *Lancet*, **ii**, 107–12

Patt, H. M. and Maloney, M. A. (1972). Bone formation and resorption as a requirement for marrow development. *Proc. Soc. Exp. Biol. and Med.*, **140**, 205–7

Paul, D., Leffert, H., Sato, G. and Holley, R. W. (1972). Stimulation of DNA and protein synthesis in fetal-rat liver cells by serum from partially hepatectomized rats. *Proc. Nat. Acad. Sci., USA*, **69**, 374–77

Pauling, L. and Delbruck, M. (1940). The nature of the intermolecular forces operative in biological processes. *Science*, **92**, 77–9

Pearson, K. D., Wells, S. A. and Keiser, H. R. (1973). Familial medullary carcinoma of the thyroid, adrenal pheochromocytoma and parathyroid hyperplasia. *Radiology*, **107**, 249–56

Pegrum, G. D., Balfour, I. C., Evans, C. A. and Middleton, V. L. (1970). HL-A antigens on leukaemic cells. *Brit. J. Haematol.*, **19**, 493–8

Pelc, S. R. (1965). Correlation between coding-triplets and amino acids. *Nature, London*, **207**, 597–99

Pellegrino, M. A., Pellegrino, A. and Kahan, B. D. (1970). Solubilization of fetal HL-A antigens. A preliminary report. *Transplantation*, **10**, 425–30

Pellié, C., Briard, M.-L., Feingold, J. and Frézal, J. (1973). Parental age in retinoblastoma. *Humangenetik*, **20**, 59–62

Peniston, W. H. and McBride, C. M. (1970). Carcinoma in the other breast. *Southern Med. J.*, **63**, 1400–4

Penrose, L. S. (1961). Mutation. Chapter 1 in: *Recent Advances in Human Genetics*, pp. 1–18, Editors: L. S. Penrose and H. L. Brown. London: J. and A. Churchill Ltd.

Pernis, B., Chiappino, G., Kelus, A. S. and Gell, P. G. H. (1965). Cellular localization of immunoglobulin with different allotypic specificities in rabbit lymphoid tissues. *J. Exp. Med.*, **122**, 853–75

Petit, P., Cauchie, Ch. (1973). Philadelphia chromosome by translocation. *Lancet*, **ii**, 94

Phillips, T. L. and Leong, G. F. (1967). Kidney cell proliferation after unilateral nephrectomy as related to age. *Cancer Res.*, **27**, 286–92

Pierce, G. B. and Wallace, C. (1971). Differentiation of malignant to benign cells. *Cancer Res.*, **31**, 127–34

Pike, M. C. and Doll, R. (1965). Age at onset of lung cancer: significance in relation to effect of smoking. *Lancet*, **i**, 665–8

Pike, M. C., Williams, E. H. and Wright, B. (1967). Burkitt's tumor in the West Nile district of Uganda 1961–66. *British Medical Journal*, **ii**, 395–9

Piraino, F. F., Brown, E. M. and Krumbiegel, E. R. (1970). Outbreak of Hong Kong influenza in Milwaukee, winter of 1968–69. *Public Health Reports*, **85**, 140–50

Pirrotta, V., Chadwick, P. and Ptashne, M. (1970). Active form of the two coliphage repressors. *Nature, London*, **227**, 41–4

Platt, R. (1955). Clonal ageing and cancer. *Lancet*, **i**, 867

Plattner, G. and Oxorn, H. (1973). Familial incidence of ovarian dermoid cysts. *Canad. Med. Ass. J.*, **108**, 892–93

Pollack, R. E., Green, H. and Todaro, C. J. (1968). Growth control in cultured cells: selection of sublines with increased sensitivity to contact inhibition and decreased tumor-producing ability. *Proc. Nat. Acad. Sci., USA*, **60**, 126–33

Post, R. H. (1965). Breast cancer, lactation and genetics. *Eugen. Quart.*, **13**, 1–29

Potworowski, E. F. and Nairn, R. C. (1968). Lymphoid-specific antigen: distribution and behaviour. *Immunology*, **14**, 591–7

Pour, P. and Ghadirian, P. (1974). Familial cancer of the esophagus in Iran. *Cancer*, **33**, 1649–52

Prehn, R. T. (1974). Immunomodulation of tumor growth. *Amer. J. Pathol.*, **77**, 119–26

Price, C. H. C. (1961). Osteogenic sarcoma. An analysis of survival and its relationship to histological grading and structure. *J. Bone and Joint Surg.*, **43B**, 300–13

Ptashne, M. (1967). Specific binding of the λ phage repressor to λDNA. *Nature, London* **214**, 232–4

Quan, S. H. Q. and Castro, E. B. (1971). Papillary adenomas (villous tumours): a review of 215 cases. *Dis. Colon and Rectum*, **14**, 267–80

Raff, M. C. (1970). Two distinct populations of peripheral lymphocytes in mice distinguished by immunofluorescence. *Immunology*, **19**, 637–50

Reed, T. E. and Neel, J. V. (1955). A genetic study of multiple polyposis of the colon (with an appendix deriving a method of estimating relative fitness). *Amer. J. of Human Genet.*, **7**, 236–63

Registrar General (1958). *Statistical Review of England and Wales, 1956, Part III. Commentary.* London: HMSO

Registrar General (1968). *Statistical Review of England and Wales, 1967, Part I, Tables, Medical.* HMSO, London

Reid, J. D. (1965). Duodenal carcinoma in the Peutz–Jeghers syndrome. Report of a case. *Cancer*, **18**, 970–7

Reidy, J. A., Lingley, J. R., Gall, E. A. and Barr, J. S. (1947). The effect of roentgen irradiation on epiphyseal growth. II. Experimental studies upon the dog. *J. Bone and Joint Surg.*, **29**, 853–73

Rigdon, R. H. and Kirchoff, H. (1953). Smoking and cancer of the lung—let's review the facts. *Texas Reports on Biol. and Med.*, **11**, 715–27

Riley, J. F. (1959). *The Mast Cells.* Edinburgh and London: E. and S. Livingstone Ltd.

Riley, J. F. (1966). Mast cells and cancer in the skin of mice. *Lancet*, **ii**, 1457–9

Riley, J. F. (1968). Mast cells, co-carcinogenesis and anti-carcinogenesis in the skin of mice. *Experientia*, **24**, 1237–8

Riley, W. T. (1973). Amino acid sequences and double-stranded messages—a means of directing the site of mutation? *J. Theoret. Biol.*, **40**, 285–300

Robbins, R. (1967). Familial multiple myeloma: the tenth reported occurrence. *Amer. J. Med. Sci.*, **254**, 848–50

Rockwell, S. and Kallman, R. F. (1972). Growth and cell population kinetics of single and multiple KHT sarcomas. *Cell and Tissue Kinet.*, **5**, 449–57

Roed-Petersen, B. (1971). Cancer development in oral leukoplakia. Follow-up of 331 patients. *J. Dent. Res.*, **50**, 711

Roed-Petersen, B., Bánóczy, J. and Pindborg, J. J. (1973). Smoking habits and histological characteristics of oral leukoplakias in Denmark and Hungary. *Brit. J. Cancer*, **28**, 575–79

Roels, F. (1969). Influence of homogenates on compensatory renal hyperplasia: inconsistency of results. In: *Compensatory Renal Hypertrophy*. Editors: W. W. Nowinski and R. J. Gross. London: Academic Press

Röller, M.-R., Owen, S. P. and Heidelberger, C. (1966). Studies on the organ culture of human tumors. *Cancer Res.*, **26**, 626–37

Rook, G. A. W. and Webb, H. E. (1970). Antilymphocyte serum and tissue culture used to investigate role of cell-mediated response in viral encephalitis in mice. *Brit. Med. J.*, **iii**, 210–12

Rosdahl, N., Larsen, S. O. and Clemmesen, J. (1974). Hodgkin's disease in patients with previous infectious mononucleosis: 30 years' experience. *Brit. Med. J.*, **ii**, 253–6

Rose, N. R. and Bonstein, H. S. (1970). Trachea-specific antigens in normal and malignant human tissues. *Clin. Exp. Immunol.*, **7**, 355–64

Rose, S. M. (1958). Failure of self-inhibition in tumors. *J. Nat. Cancer Inst.*, **20**, 653–64

Rosen, B. J., Smith, T. W. and Bloch, K. J. (1967). Multiple myeloma associated with two serum M components, γG type K and γA type L. *New Eng. J. Med.*, **277**, 902–7

Rosenberg, S. A. and Kaplan, H. S. (1966). Evidence for an orderly progression in the spread of Hodgkin's disease. *Cancer Res.*, **26**, 1225–31

Rosenblatt, M. B. (1969). The increase in lung cancer: epidemic or artifact? *Med. Counterpoint*, **1**, 29–39

Rosenblatt, M. B., Teng, P. K., Kerpe, S. and Beck, I. (1971(a)). Causes of death in 1000 consecutive autopsies. *N.Y. State J. Med.*, **71**, 2189–93

Rosenblatt, M. B., Teng, P. K., Kerpe, S. and Beck, I. (1971(b)). Prevalence of lung cancer: disparity between clinical and autopsy certification. *Med. Counterpoint*, **3**, 53–9

Roswit, B., Patno, M. E. and Rapp, R. (1968). The survival of patients with inoperable lung cancer: a large scale randomized study of radiation therapy versus placebo. *Radiology*, **90**, 688–97

Rothman, K. J. and Monson, R. R. (1973). Epidemiology of trigeminal neuralgia. *J. Chronic Dis.*, **26**, 3–12

Rowe, W. P. (1965). A survey of the tumor virus problem from an epidemiologic standpoint. *Cancer Res.*, **25**, 1277–82

Rowland, R. E., Failla, P. M., Keane, A. T. and Stehney, A. F. (1970). Some dose-response relationships for tumor incidence in radium patients. *Radiological Physics Division Annual Report* ANL-7760 Part II *Biology and Medicine*, pp. 1–18. Argonne, Illinois: Argonne National Laboratory

Rowland, R. E., Failla, P. M., Keane, A. T. and Stehney, A. F. (1971). Tumor incidence for the radium patients, pp. 1–8. In: *Radiological Physics Division Annual Report* ANL-7860 Part II *Biology in Medicine*. Argonne, Illinois: Argonne National Laboratory

Rowley, J. D. (1973). A new consistent chromosomal abnormality in chronic myelogenous leukaemia identified by quinacrine fluorescence and Giemsa staining. *Nature, London*, **243**, 290–3

Royal College of Physicians (1971). *Smoking and Health Now*. London: Pitman Medical and Scientific Publishing Co. Ltd.

Russell, J. G. B. (1970). Obstetric radiology. *Brit. J. Hosp. Med.*, **3**, 601–5

Russell, J. G. B. and Richards, B. (1971). A review of pelvimetry data. *Brit. J. Radiol.*, **44**, 780–4

Russell, W. L. (1964). In: *Genetics Today*. Proceedings XIth International Congress on Genetics, The Hague, The Netherlands. Oxford: Pergamon Press

Russell, W. L. (1965). Studies in mammalian radiation genetics. *Nucleonics*, **23**, 53–6 and 62

Ruttenberg, M. A., King, T. P. and Craig, L. C. (1966). The chemistry of tyrocidine. VII. Studies on association behavior and implications regarding conformation. *Biochemistry*, **5**, 2857–64

Ryan, G. M. (1962). Carcinoma *in situ* of the Fallopian tube. *Amer. J. Obstet. and Gynecol.*, **84**, 198

Ryskov, A. P., Saunders, G. F., Farashyan, V. R. and Georgiev, G. P. (1973). Double-helical regions in nuclear precursor of mRNA (pre-mRNA). *Biochim. et Biophys. Acta,* **312**, 152–64

Saetren, H. (1956). A principle of auto-regulation of growth. Production of organ specific mitose-inhibitors in kidney and liver. *Exp. Cell Res.*, **11**, 229–32

Saetren, H. (1963). The organ-specific growth inhibition of the tubule cells of the rat's kidney. *Acta Chem. Scand.*, **17**, 889

St. Arneault, G., Nagel, G., Kirkpatrick, D., Kirkpatrick, R. and Holland, J. F. (1970). Melanoma in twins. *Cancer*, **25**, 672–7

Sakai, A. (1970). Humoral factor triggering DNA synthesis after partial hepatectomy in the rat. *Nature, London*, **228**, 1186–7

Samaan, N. A., Hickey, R. C., Stratton Hill, C., Medellin, H. and Gates, R. B. (1974). Parathyroid tumors: preoperative localization and association with other tumors. *Cancer*, **33**, 933–9

Saneyoshi, M. and Nishimura, S. (1971). Selective inactivation of amino acid acceptor and ribosome-binding activities of *Escherichia coli* tRNA by modification with cyanogen bromide. *Biochim. et Biophys. Acta*, **246**, 123–31

Sanger, R., Race, R. R., Tippet, P., Gavin, J., Hardisty, R. M. and Dubowitz, V. (1964). Unexplained inheritance of the Xg groups in two families. *Lancet*, **i**, 955–6

Savage, D. (1956). A family history of uterine and gastro-intestinal cancer. *Brit. Med. J.*, **ii**, 341–3

Schappert-Kimmijser, J., Hemmes, G. D. and Nijland, R. (1966). The heredity of retinoblastoma. *Ophthalmol.*, **151**, 197–213

Scheike, O. and Visfeldt, J. (1973). Male breast cancer. 4. Gynecomastia in patients with breast cancer. *Acta Pathol. Microbiol.*, *Scand.*, **A81**, 359–65

Scheike, O., Visfeldt, J. and Petersen, B. (1973). Male breast cancer. 3. Breast carcinoma in association with the Klinefelter syndrome. *Acta Pathol. Microbiol. Scand.*, **A81**, 352–358

Scherer, H. J. (1940). Cerebral astrocytomas and their derivatives. *Amer. J. Cancer*, **40** 159–98

Schiller, H. M. and Silverberg, S. G. (1971). Staging and prognosis in primary carcinoma of the Fallopian tube. *Cancer*, **28**, 389–95

Schimmel, P. R., Uhlenbeck, O. C., Lewis, J. B., Dickson, L. A., Eldred, E. W. and Schreier, A. A. (1972). Binding of complementary oligonucleotides to free and aminoacyl transfer ribonucleic acid synthetase bound transfer ribonucleic acid. *Biochemistry*, **11**, 642–6

Schlesinger, M. and Hurvitz, D. (1968). Serological analysis of thymus and spleen grafts. *J. Exp. Med.*, **127**, 1127–37

Schoch, E. P. Jr. (1963). Familial malignant melanoma. *Arch. Dermatol.*, **88**, 445–56

Schoenberg, B. S., Greenberg, R. A. and Eisenberg, H. (1969). Occurrence of certain multiple primary cancers in females. *J. Nat. Cancer Inst.*, **45**, 15–32

Schottenfeld, D. and Berg, J. (1971). Incidence of multiple primary cancers. IV. Cancers of the female breast and genital organs. *J. Nat. Cancer Inst.*, **46**, 161–70

Schottenfeld, D., Berg, J. W. and Vitsky, B. (1969). Incidence of multiple primary cancers. II. Index cancers arising in the stomach and lower digestive systems. *J. Nat. Cancer Inst.*, **43**, 77–86

Schottenfeld, D., Lilienfeld, A. M. and Diamond, H. (1963). Some observations on the epidemiology of breast cancer among males. *Amer. J. Public Health*, **53**, 890–897

Schubert, D. and Cohn, M. (1970). Immunoglobulin biosynthesis. V. Light chain assembly. *J. Molec. Biol.*, **53**, 305–20

Schubert, D., Roman, A. and Cohn, M. (1970). Antinucleic acid specificities of mouse myeloma immunoglobulins. *Nature, London*, **225**, 154–8

Schutz, L. and Mora, P. T. (1968). The need for direct cell contact in 'contact' inhibition of cell division in culture. *J. Cell. Physiol.*, **71**, 1–6

Schwartz, A. D., Padash-Zadeh, M., Lee, H. and Swaney, J. J. (1974). Spontaneous regression of disseminated neuroblastoma. *J. Pediat.*, **85**, 760–3

Schwartz, D., Flamanti, R., Lellouch, J. and Denoix, P. F. (1961). Results of a French survey on the role of tobacco, particularly inhalation, in different cancer sites. *J. Nat. Cancer Inst.*, **26**, 1085–1108

Scott, L. (1955). Bilateral Wilms's tumour. *Brit. J. Surg.*, **42**, 513–16

Sedlis, A. (1961). Primary carcinoma of the Fallopian tube. *Obstet. Gynecol. Survey*, **16**, 209–26

Segi, M., Fukushima, I., Fujisaku, S., Kurihara, M., Saito, S., Asano, K., Magaike, H. and Kamoi, M. (1957). An epidemiological study of cancer in Japan. *Gann*, **48** (Suppl.), 1–63

Segi, M. and Kurihara, M. (1964). *Cancer Mortality for Selected Sites in 24 Countries*, No. 3 (1960–61). Sendai, Japan: Tohoku University School of Medicine

Segi, M. and Kurihara, M. (1966). *Cancer Mortality for Selected Sites in 24 Countries*, No. 4 (1962–63). Sendai, Japan: Tohoku University School of Medicine

Sehrt, E. (1904). *Beiträge zur Kenntnis des primären Lungencarcinoma*. Leipzig: George

Seltser, R. and Sartwell, P. E. (1966). The influence of occupational exposure to radiation on the mortality of American radiologists and other medical specialists. *Amer. J. Epidemiol.*, **81**, 2–22

Seltzer, C. C. (1963). Morphologic constitution and smoking. *J. Amer. Med. Ass.*, **183**, 639–45

Seltzer, C. C. (1967). Constitution and heredity in relation to tobacco smoking. *Ann. N.Y. Acad. Sci.*, **142**, 322–30

Seltzer, C. C. (1972). Differences between cigar and pipe smokers in healthy White veterans. *Arch. Environ. Health*, **25**, 187–91

Sen, L. and Borella, L. (1975). Clinical importance of lymphoblasts with T markers in childhood acute leukemia. *New Eng. J. Med.*, **292**, 828–32

Shands, W. C., Dockerty, M. B. and Bargen, J. A. (1952). Adenocarcinoma of the large intestine associated with chronic ulcerative colitis: clinical and pathological features of 73 cases. *Surgery, Gynec. Obstet.*, **94**, 302–10

Shearer, W. T., Atkinson, J. P., Frank, M. M. and Parker, C. W. (1975). Humoral immunostimulation. IV. Role of complement. *J. Exp. Med.*, **141**, 736–52

Shedd, D. P., von Essen, C. F. and Connelly, R. R. (1968). Cancer of the pharynx in Connecticut, 1935 to 1959. *Cancer*, **21**, 706–13

Shields, J. W. (1972). *The Trophic Function of Lymphoid Elements*. Springfield, Illinois: C. C. Thomas

Shine, I. and Allison, P. R. (1966). Carcinoma of the esophagus with tylosis. *Lancet*, **i**, 951–3

Shore, F. J., Robertson, J. S. and Bateman, J. L. (1973). Childhood cancer following obstetric radiography. *Health Physics*, **24**, 258–60

Sievers, M. L. (1973). Unusual comparative frequency of gastric carcinoma, pernicious anemia, and peptic ulcer in southwestern American Indians. *Gastroenterol.*, **65**, 867–76

Sigel, B., Baldia, L. B., Brightman, S. A., Dunn, M. R. and Price, R. I. M. (1967). The effect of blood flow reversal on the site of liver cell formation. *Gastroenterol.*, **52**, 1142 (Abstract)

Silver, W. K. and Gasser, D. L. (1973). The genetic divergence of sublines as assessed by histocompatibility testing. *Genetics*, **75**, 671–7

Silverstone, H. and Searle, J. H. A. (1970). The epidemiology of skin cancer in Queensland: the influence of phenotype and environment. *Brit. J. Cancer*, **24**, 235–52

Simon, J., Peters, G., Blinzinger, K., Magrath, D. and Boulger, L. (1970). The pathogenic role of the inflammatory reaction in poliomyelitis. Immuno-fluorescence, electron microscopic and virological studies with type 3 poliovirus. *Experientia*, **25**, 1241–1242

Simpson, D. P. (1963). Hepatic regeneration and hyperplasia. *Med. Clinics N. Amer.* **47**, 765–77

Singer, A. M., Bennett, R. C., Frydenberg, H., Russell, I. S. and Chan, D. P. S. (1972). Carcinoma of the breast in women aged between 35 and 45 years. *Med. J. Austral.*, **i**, 1200–2

Singer, M. (1952). The influence of the nerve in regeneration of the amphibian extremity *Quart. Rev. Biol.*, **27**, 169–200

Slaney, G. and Brooke, B. N. (1959). Cancer in ulcerative colitis. *Lancet*, **ii**, 694–8

Slaughter, D. P., Southwich, H. M. and Smejkal, W. (1953). 'Field cancerization' in oral stratified squamous epithelium. Clinical implication of multicentric origin. *Cancer*, **6**, 963–8

Slavkin, H. C., Bringas, P., Cameron, J., Le Baron, R. and Bavetta, L. A. (1969). Epithelial and mesenchymal cell interactions with extracellular matrix material *in vitro*. *J. Embryol. Exp. Morphol.*, **22**, 395–405

Smith, F. E., Henly, W. S., Knox, J. M. and Lane, M. (1966). Familial melanoma, *Arch. Internal Med.*, **117**, 820–3

Smith, W. G. (1958). Multiple polyposis, Gardner's syndrome and desmoid tumors. *Dis. Colon Rectum*, **1**, 323–32

Smith, W. G. and Kern, B. B. (1973). The nature of the mutation in familial multiple polyposis: papillary carcinoma of the thyroid, brain tumors, and familial multiple polyposis. *Dis. Colon Rectum*, **16**, 264–71

Smithers, D. W. (1953). Facts and fancies about cancer of the lung. *Brit. Med. J.*, **i**, 1235–9

Smithers, D. W. (1960). *A Clinical Prospect of the Cancer Problem*. Edinburgh: E. and S. Livingstone

Smithers, D. W. (1962). Cancer: an attack on cytologism. *Lancet*, **i**, 493–9

Smithers, D. W. (1962). Spontaneous regression of tumours. *Clin. Radiol.*, **13**, 132–7

Smithers, D. W. (1964). *On the Nature of Cancer in Man*. Edinburgh: E. and S. Livingstone

Smithers, D. W. (1967). Hodgkin's disease. *Brit. Med. J.*, **ii**, 263–8

Smithers, D. W. (1969). Maturation in human tumours. *Lancet*, **ii**, 949–52

Soll, L. (1974). Mutational alterations of tryptophan-specific transfer RNA that generate translation suppressors of the UAA, UAG and UGA nonsense codons. *J. Molec. Biol.*, **86**, 233–43

Spencer, I. W. F. and Coster, M. E. E. (1969). The epidemiology of gastro-enteritis in infancy. Part I. *S. African Med. J.*, **43**, 1391–7

Spencer, R. P. and Coulombe, M. J. (1966). Quantitation of hepatic growth and regeneration. *Growth*, **30**, 277–84

Sperry, R. W. (1963). Chemoaffinity in the orderly growth of nerve fiber patterns and connections. *Proc. Nat. Acad. Sci., USA*, **50**, 703–10

Spielhoff, R. (1971). The specificity of the regulation of organ growth: the effect of tissue extracts on the incorporation of tritiated thymidine in liver and kidney. *Proc. Soc. Exp. Biol. Med.*, **138**, 43–6

Squires, C. and Carbon, J. (1971). Normal and mutant glycine transfer RNAs. *Nature New Biology*, **233**, 274–7

Stampfer, M., Rosbash, M., Huang, A. S. and Baltimore, D. (1972). Complementarity between messenger RNA and nuclear RNA from HeLa cells. *Biochem. Biophys. Res. Communic.*, **49**, 217–24

Staszewski, J. (1974). Cancer of the upper alimentary tract and larynx in Poland and in Polish-born Americans. *Brit. J. Cancer*, **29**, 389–99

Steinberg, M. S. (1962). On the mechanism of tissue reconstruction by dissociated cells. III. Free energy relations and the reorganization of fused, heteronomic tissue fragments. *Proc. Nat. Acad. Sci., USA*, **48**, 1769–76

Steinmuller, D. (1971). A reinvestigation of epidermal transplantation during chemical carcinogenesis. *Cancer Res.*, **31**, 2080–4

Stell, P. M. (1972). Smoking and laryngeal cancer. *Lancet*, **ii**, 617–19

Stevens, R. and Williamson, A. (1973(a)). Translational control of immunoglobulin synthesis. I. Repression of heavy chain synthesis. *J. Molec. Biol.*, **78**, 505–16

Stevens, R. and Williamson, A. (1973(b)). Translational control of immunoglobulin synthesis. II. Cell-free interaction of myeloma immunoglobulin with mRNA. *J. Molec. Biol.*, **78**, 517–25

Stevenson, G. T. and Straus, D. (1968). Specific dimerization of the light chains of human immunoglobulin. *Biochem. J.*, **108**, 375–82

Stewart, A. (1969). Private communication to author

Stewart, A. and Kneale, G. W. (1968). Changes in the cancer risk associated with obstetric radiography. *Lancet*, **i**, 104–7

Stewart, A. and Kneale, G. W. (1970(a)). Radiation dose effects in relation to obstetric X-rays and childhood cancers. *Lancet*, **i**, 1185–8

Stewart, A. and Kneale, G. W. (1970(b)). Age-distribution of cancers caused by obstetric X-rays and their relevance to cancer latent periods. *Lancet*, **ii**, 4–8

Stewart, G. T. (1968). Limitations of the germ theory. *Lancet*, **i**, 1077–81

Stocks, P. (1953). A study of the age-curve for cancer of the stomach in connection with a theory of the cancer-producing mechanism. *Brit. J. Cancer*, **7**, 407–17

Stocks, P. (1966). Recent epidemiological studies of lung cancer mortality, cigarette smoking and air pollution, with discussion of a new hypothesis of causation. *Brit. J. Cancer*, **20**, 595–623

Stocks, P. (1970). Cancer mortality in relation to national consumption of cigarettes, solid fuel, tea and coffee. *Brit. J. Cancer*, **24**, 215–25

Sullivan, P. W. and Salmon, S. E. (1972). Kinetics of tumor growth and regression in IgG multiple myeloma. *J. Clin. Invest.*, **51**, 1697–1708

Surgeon General's Report (1971). *Health Consequences of Smoking*. US Department of Health, Education, and Welfare. Washington, DC: US Government Printing Office

Swanbeck, G. (1971). Aetiological factors in squamous cell skin cancer. *Brit. J. Dermatol.* **85**, 394–6; and private communication

Swanbeck, G. and Hillstrom, L. (1969). Analysis of aetiological factors in squamous cell skin cancer of different locations. 1. The lower limbs. *Acta Derm.-Venereol., Stockholm*, **49**, 427–35

Swanbeck, G. and Hillstrom, L. (1970). Analysis of etiological factors of squamous cell skin cancer of different locations. 2. The arm and the hand. *Acta Derm.-Venereol., Stockholm*, **50**, 350–4

Swanbeck, G. and Hillstrom, L. (1971). Analysis of etiological factors of squamous cell skin cancer of different locations. 4. Concluding remarks. *Acta Derm.-Venereol., Stockholm*, **51**, 151–6

Swedish Cancer Registry (1971). *Cancer Incidence in Sweden 1959–1965*. Stockholm.

Sybesma, J. Ph. H. B., Borst-Eilers, E., Holtzer, J. D., Moes, M., Pielage, E. and De Planque, B. A. (1972). HL-A antigens in Hodgkin's disease and other lymphomas. *Vox Sanguinis*, **22**, 319–24

Sylvén, B. (1969). Factors produced by tumour cells which contribute to the death of cancer patients. *Gazzetta Sanit.*, **18**, 1–8

Szybalski, W. (1970). Various controls of transcription in coliphage lambda. In: *RNA Polymerase and Transcription*, pp. 209–17, Editor: L. Silvestri. Amsterdam: Holland Publishing Co.

Szybalski, W., Bøvre, K., Fianot, M., Guha, A., Hradecna, Z., Kumar, S., Lozeron, H. A., Maher, S. R. V. M., Nijkamp, H. J. J., Summers, W. C. and Taylor, K. Transcriptional controls in developing bacteriophages. *J. Cell. Physiol.*, **74**, Suppl. 1, 33–70

Tarin, D. (1968). Further electron microscopic studies on the mechanism of carcinogenesis: the specificity of the changes in carcinogen-treated mouse skin. *Int. J. Cancer* **3**, 734–42

Tarin, D. (1969). Fine structure of murine mammary tumours: the relationship between epithelium and connective tissue in neoplasms induced by various agents. *Brit. J. Cancer*, **23**, 417–25

Tarin, D. (1972(a)). Tissue interactions in morphogenesis, morphostasis and carcinogenesis. *J. Theoret. Biol.*, **34**, 61–72

Tarin, D. (Editor) (1972(b)). *Tissue Interactions in Carcinogenesis*. London and New York: Academic Press

Temin, H. M. (1971). Guest Editorial. The protovirus hypothesis: Speculations on the significance of RNA-directed DNA synthesis for normal development and for carcinogenesis. *J. Nat. Cancer Inst.*, **46**, 3–7

Temin, H. M. (1972). The RNA tumor viruses–background and foreground. *Proc. Nat. Acad. Sci. USA*, **69**, 1016–20

Temin, H. M. (1974). On the origin of the genes for neoplasia: G. H. A. Clowes memorial lecture. *Cancer Res.*, **34**, 2835–41

Theodor, J. L. (1970). Distinction between 'self' and 'not-self' in lower invertebrates. *Nature, London*, **227**, 690–92

Thiessen, E. U. (1974). Concerning a familial association between breast cancer and both prostate and uterine malignancies. *Cancer*, **34**, 1102–7

Thomas, C. B. and Cohen, B. H. (1960). Comparison of smokers and nonsmokers. I. A preliminary report on the ability to taste phenylthiourea (PTC). *Bull. Johns Hopkins Hospital*, **106**, 205–14

Thomas, C. B., Fargo, R. and Enslein, K. (1970). Personality characteristics of medical students as reflected by the strong vocational interest test with special reference to smoking habits. *Johns Hopkins Med. J.*, **127**, 323–35

Thomas, D. B. (1973). An epidemiologic study of carcinoma *in situ* and squamous dysplasia of the uterine cervix. *Amer. J. Epidemiol.*, **98**, 10–28

Thomson, R. Y. and Clarke, A. M. (1965). Role of portal blood supply in liver regeneration. *Nature, London*, **208**, 392–93

Thorling, K. (1973). Familial Hodgkin's disease. Occurrence in two brothers. *Danish Med. Bull.*, **20**, 61–3

Threlfall, G., Cairnie, A. B., Taylor, D. M. and Buck, A. T. (1966). Effect of whole-body X-irradiation on renal compensatory hypertrophy. *Radiation Res.*, **27**, 559–65

Tiilikainen, A., Kaakinen, A. and Amos, D. B. (1970). The separation of genetically different lymphocyte populations *in vitro*. *Transplantation*, **10**, 361–65

Till, J. E. and McCulloch, E. A. (1964). Repair processes in irradiated mouse hemato-poieitic tissue. *Ann. N.Y. Acad. Sci.*, **114**, Art. 1, 115–25

Todaro, G. J., Lazar, G. K. and Green, H. (1965). The initiation of cell division in a contact-inhibited mammalian cell line. *J. Cell. Comparative Physiol.*, **66**, 325–33

Todd, G. F. (1972). *Statistics of Smoking in the United Kingdom*. 6th Edition. London: Tobacco Research Council

Todd, G. F. and Mason, J. I. (1959). Concordance of smoking habits in monozygotic and dizygotic twins. *Heredity*, **13**, 417–44

Tokuhata, G. K. (1964). Familial factors in human lung cancer and smoking. *Amer. J. Public Health*, **54**, 24–32

Tokuhata, G. K. (1973). Cancer of the lung: host and environmental interaction. In: *Cancer Genetics*. Editor: H. T. Lynch. In press

Tokuhata, G. K. and Lilienfeld, A. M. (1963(a)). Familial aggregation of lung cancer among hospital patients. *Public Health Reports, Washington*, **78**, 277–83

Tokuhata, G. K. and Lilienfeld, A. M. (1963(b)). Familial aggregation of lung cancer in humans. *J. Nat. Cancer Inst.*, **30**, 289–312

Torre, D. (1968). Multiple sebaceous tumors. *Arch. Dermatol.*, **98**, 549–51.

Toth, S. E. (1967). Tissue compatibility in regenerating explants from the colonial marine hydroid *Hydractinia echinata* (Flem.). *J. Cell Physiol.*, **69**, 125–32

Traviesco, C. R. Jr., Knoepp, L. F. Jr. and Hanley, P. H. (1972). Multiple adenocar-cinomas of the colon and rectum. *Dis. Colon Rectum*, **15**, 1–6

Tunstall, A. M. and James, K. (1974). Preliminary studies on the synthesis of alpha$_2$-macroglobulin by human lymphocytes *in vitro*. *Clin. Exp. Immunol.*, **17**, 697–701

Turkington, R. W. (1965). Familial factor in malignant melanoma. *J. Amer. Med. Ass.* **192**, 77–82

Tyers, G. F. O., Steiger, E. and Dudrick, S. J. (1969). Adenocarcinoma of the small intestine and other malignant tumors complicating regional enteritis: case report and review of the literature. *Ann. Surg.*, **169**, 510–18

Tyler, A. (1947). An auto-antibody concept of cell structure, growth and differentiation. *Growth*, **10**, Smith Symposium Supplement, 7–19

Tyler, A. (1960). Clues to the aetiology, pathology, and therapy of cancer provided by analogies with transplantation disease. *J. Nat. Cancer Inst.*, **25**, 1197–229

Tyler, A. (1962). A developmental immunogenetic analysis of cancer. In: *Biological Interactions in Normal and Neoplastic Growth*. Boston: Little, Brown and Co. (Inc.)

Ungar, H. (1949). Familial carcinoma of the duodenum in adolescence. *Brit. J. Cancer*, **3**, 321–30

United Nations Scientific Committee (1972). *Ionizing Radiation: Levels and Effects. Volume II: Effects*, p. 428. New York: United Nations

Upton, A. C., Conte, F. B., Hurst, G. S. and Mills, W. A. (1956). The relative biological effectiveness of fast neutrons, x-rays and gamma rays for acute lethality in mice. *Radiation Res.*, **4**, 117–31

Upton, A. C., Jenkins, V. K. and Conklin, J. W. (1964). Myeloid leukaemia in the mouse. In: *Physical Factors and Modification of Radiation Injury. Ann. N.Y. Acad. Sci.*, **114**, Art. 1, pp. 189–201

Urist, M. R. (1965). Bone: formation by autoinduction. *Science*, **150**, 893–9

Vaillier, D. (1974). Growth stimulating factors found in diffusion chambers implanted in tumor-bearing mice. *J. Int. Res. Communic. Med. Sci.*, **2**, 1208

Vakil, D. V. and Morgan, R. W. (1973). Etiology of breast cancer. I. Genetic aspects. *Canad. Med. Ass. J.*, **109**, 29–32

Van Den Brenk, H. A. S., Orton, C., Stone, M. and Kelly, H. (1974). Effects of x-radiation on growth and function of the repair blastema (granulation tissue). I. Wound contraction. *Int. J. Radiation Biol.*, **25**, 1–19

Van Duuren, B. L., Sivak, A., Katz, C. and Melchionne, S. (1969). Inhibition of tumor induction in two-stage carcinogenesis on mouse skin. *Cancer Res.*, **29**, 947–52

Van Peperzeel, H. A. (1972). Effects of single doses of radiation on lung metastases in man and experimental animals. *Eur. J. Cancer*, **8**, 665–75

Van Scott, E. J. and Reinertson, R. P. (1961). The modulating influence of stromal environment on epithelial cells studied in human autotransplants. *J. Invest. Dermatol.*, **36**, 109–17

Van Wayjen, R. G. A. and Linschoten, H. (1973). Distribution of ABO and rhesus blood groups in patients with gastric carcinoma, with reference to its site of origin. *Gastroenterology*, **65**, 877–83

Vasiliev, J. M., Olshevskaja, L. V., Raikhlin, N. T. and Ivanova, O. J. (1962). Comparative study of alterations induced by 7,12-dimethylbenz[α]anthracene and polymer films in the subcutaneous connective tissue of rats. *J. Nat. Cancer Inst.*, **28**, 515–59

Veale, A. M. O. (1965). *Intestinal Polyposis. Eugenics Laboratory Memoirs, No. 40*. London: Cambridge University Press

Verhest, A. and Van Schoubroeck, F. (1973). Philadelphia–chromosome–positive pre-leukaemic state. *Lancet*, **ii**, 1386

Veronesi, U., Cascinelli, N. and Preda, F. (1971). Prognosis of malignant melanoma according to regional metastases. *Amer. J. Roentgenol.*, **111**, 301–9

Viadana, E., Cotter, R., Pickren, J. W. and Bross, I. D. J. (1973). An autopsy study of metastatic sites of breast cancer. *Cancer Res.*, **33**, 179–81

Vianna, N. J., Greenwald, P., Davies, J. N. P. (1971). Extended epidemic of Hodgkin's disease in high-school students. *Lancet*, **i**, 1209–11

Videbaek, A. and Mosbech, J. (1954). Genetic causal factors in cancer of the stomach. *Dan. Med. Bull.*, **1**, 189–93

Virolainen, M. (1964). Mitotic response in liver autograft after partial hepatectomy in the rat. *Exp. Cell Res.*, **33**, 588–91

Vodopick, H., Rupp, E. M., Edwards, C. L., Goswitz, F. A. and Beauchamp, J. J. (1972). Spontaneous cyclic leukocytosis and thrombocytosis in chronic granulocytic leukemia. *New Eng. J. Med.*, **286**, 284–90

Wachtel, L. W. and Cole, L. J. (1965). Abscopal effects of whole-body X-irradiation on compensatory hypertrophy of the rat kidney. *Radiation Res.*, **25**, 78–91

Wachtel, L. W., Cole, L. J. and Rosen, V. J. Jr. (1966). Abscopal and direct effects of whole-body X-irradiation in weanling rats: kidney mitotic activity and DNA-content after uninephrectomy. *International J. Radiation Biol.*, **10**, 75–82

Wachtel, L. W., Phillips, T. L. and Cole, L. J. (1966). Systemic factor in recovery of rat kidney from X-irradiation: thymidine-H^3 incorporation studies. *Radiation Res.*, **28**, 647–56

Waggoner, D. E. and Newell, G. R. (1971). Regional convergence of cancer mortality rates over time in the United States, 1940 to 1960. *Amer. J. Epidemiol.*, **93**, 79–83

Walach, N. and Horn, Y. (1973). The incidence of cancer in married couples. *J. Amer. Med. Ass.*, **226**, 201

Walford, R. L. (1970). Antibody diversity, histocompatibility systems, disease states and ageing. *Lancet*, **ii**, 1226–9

Walford, R. L., Finkelstein, S., Neerhout, R., Konrad, P. and Shanbrom, E. (1970). Acute childhood leukaemia in relation to the HL-A human transplantation genes. *Nature, London*, **225**, 461–2

Walker, P. M. B. (1968). How different are the DNAs from related animals? *Nature, London*, **219**, 228–32

Wallace, D. C., Exton, L. A. and McLeod, G. R. C. (1971). Genetic factor in malignant melanoma. *Cancer*, **27**, 1262–6

Wang, A.-C., Wang, I. Y. F., McCormick, J. N. and Fudenberg, H. H. (1969). The identity of light chains of monoclonal IgG and monoclonal IgM in one patient. *Immunochemistry*, **6**, 451–9

Warner, N. E. (1969). Lobular carcinoma of the breast. *Cancer*, **23**, 840–6

Warner, N. L., Mackenzie, M. R. and Fudenberg, H. H. (1971). Antibody activity of a monoclonal macroglobulin. *Proc. Nat. Acad. Sci., USA*, **68**, 2846–51

Warthin, A. S. (1913). Heredity with reference to carcinoma as shown by the study of the cases examined in the Pathological Laboratory of the University of Michigan, 1895 to 1913. *Arch. Internal Med.*, **12**, 546–55

Waterhouse, J. A. H. (1974). *Cancer Handbook of Epidemiology and Prognosis*. Edinburgh and London: Churchill Livingstone

Weinstein, I. B. (1963). Comparative studies on the genetic code. *Cold Spring Harbor Symp. Quant. Biol.*, **28**, 579–80

Weir, J. A. (1973). Cancer of the colon in South Saskatchewan. A population study. *Cancer*, **31**, 616–20

Weiss, P. (1958). Cell contact. *Int. Rev. Cytol.*, **7**, 391–423

Weiss, P. A. (1947). The problem of specificity in growth and development. *Yale J. Biol. and Med.*, **19**, 235–78

Weiss, P. A. (1950). Perspectives in the field of morphogenesis. *Quart. Rev. Biol.*, **25**, 177–98

Weiss, P. A. and James, R. (1955). Skin metaplasia *in vitro* induced by brief exposure to vitamin A. *Exp. Cell Res.*, Suppl. **3**, 381–94

Weiss, P. A. and Kavanau, J. L. (1957). A model of growth and growth control in mathematical terms. *J. Gen. Physiol.*, **41**, 1–47

Weiss, W., Boucot, K. R., Seidman, H. and Carnahan, W. J. (1972). Risk of lung cancer according to histologic type and cigarette dosage. *J. Amer. Med. Ass.*, **222**, 799–801

Weisz, P. B. (1951). A general mechanism of differentiation based on morphogenetic studies in ciliates. *Amer. Naturalist*, **85**, 293–311

Welch, C. E. and Hedberg, S. E. (1965). Colonic cancer in ulcerative colitis and idiopathic colonic cancer. *J. Amer. Med. Ass.*, **191**, 815–18

Weller, C. V. (1941). The inheritance of retinoblastoma and its relationship to practical eugenics. *Cancer Res.*, **1**, 517–35

Wellings, S. R. and Jensen, H. M. (1973). On the origin and progression of ductal carcinoma in the human breast. *J. Nat. Cancer Inst.*, **50**, 1111–18

Westermark, B. (1971). Proliferation control of cultivated human glia-like cells under 'steady-state' conditions. *Exp. Cell Res.*, **69**, 259–64

Westlund, K. (1970). Distribution and mortality time trend of multiple sclerosis and some other diseases in Norway. *Acta Neurolog. Scand.*, **46**, 455–83

Widdowson, E. M. (1970). Harmony of growth. *Lancet*, **i**, 901–5

Williams, E. D., Brown, C. L. and Doniach, I. (1966). Pathological and clinical findings in a series of 67 cases of medullary carcinoma of the thyroid. *J. Clin. Pathol.*, **19**, 103–13

Williams, E. H., Day, N. E. and Geser, A. G. (1974). Seasonal variation in onset of Burkitt's lymphoma in the West Nile District of Uganda. *Lancet*, **ii**, 19–22

Williams, J. P. and Knudsen, A. (1965). Peutz–Jeghers syndrome with metastasizing duodenal carcinoma. *Gut*, **6**, 179–84

Willis, R. A. (1960). *Pathology of Tumours*. 3rd Edition. London: Butterworths

Willis, R. A. (1967). *Pathology of Tumours*. 4th Edition. London: Butterworths

Wilson, D. A. and Thomas, C. A. Jr. (1974). Palindromes in chromosomes. *J. Molec. Biol.*, **84**, 115–44

Wilson, H. V. (1908). On some phenomena of coalescence and regeneration in sponges. *J. Exp. Zool.*, **5**, 245–58

Winick, M. and Coscia, A. (1968). Cortisone-induced growth failure in neonatal rats. *Pediatric Res.*, **2**, 451–55

Woese, C. R. (1962). Nature of the biological code. *Nature, London*, **194**, 1114–15

Woese, C. R. (1965). Order in the genetic code. *Proc. Nat. Acad. Sci., USA*, **54**, 71–5

Woese, C. R. (1967). *The Genetic Code, The Molecular Basis for Genetic Expression*. New York, Evanston and London: Harper and Row

Woese, C. R. (1969). Models for the evolution of codon assignments. *J. Molec. Biol.*, **43**, 235–40

Woese, C. R., Dugre, D. H., Saxinger, W. C. and Dugre, S. A. (1966). The molecular basis for the genetic code. *Proc. Nat. Acad. Sci., USA*, **55**, 966–74

Wolf, N. S. and Trentin, J. J. (1968). Hemopoietic colony studies. V. Effect of hemopoietic organ stroma on differentiation of pluripotent stem cells. *J. Exp. Med.*, **127**, 205–14

Wood, P. H. N. (1971). Rheumatic complaints. *Brit. Med. Bull.*, **27**, 82–8

Woodruff, J. D. and Pauerstein, C. J. (1969). *The Fallopian Tube: Structure, Function, Pathology and Management*. Baltimore: Williams and Wilkins

Wooldridge, W. R. and Frerichs, J. B. (1971). Multiple adenoid squamous cell carcinoma. *Arch. Dermatol.*, **104**, 202–6

Woolf, C. M. (1958). A genetic study of carcinoma of the large intestine. *Amer. J. Human Genet.*, **10**, 42–7

Woolf, C. M. (1960). An investigation of the familial aspects of carcinoma of the prostate. *Cancer*, **13**, 739–44

Woolner, L. B., Beahrs, O. H., Black, B. M., McConahey, W. M. and Keating, F. R. Jr. (1961). Classification and prognosis of thyroid carcinomas. A study of 885 cases observed in a thirty-year period. *Amer. J. Surg.*, **102**, 354–87

Wynder, E. L. (1955). Neoplastic diseases. In: *The Biologic Effects of Tobacco: With Emphasis on the Clinical and Experimental Aspects*. Editor: E. L. Wynder. Boston: Little, Brown and Co. (Inc.)

Wynder, E. L., Bross, I. J. and Hirayma, T. (1960). A study of the epidemiology of cancer of the breast. *Cancer*, **13**, 559–601

Wynder, E. L., Lemon, F. R. and Bross, I. J. (1959). Cancer and coronary artery disease among Seventh Day Adventists. *Cancer*, **12**, 1016–28

Wyse, E. P., Hill, C. S., Ibanez, M. L. and Clark, R. L. (1969). Other malignant neoplasms associated with carcinoma of the thyroid: thyroid carcinoma multiplex. *Cancer*, **24**, 701–8

Yaniv, M., Folk, W. R., Berg, P. and Soll, L. (1974). A single mutational modification of a tryptophan-specific transfer RNA permits aminoacylation by glutamine and translation of the codon UAG. *J. Molec. Biol.*, **86**, 245–60

Yerushalmy, J. (1971). The relationship of parents' cigarette smoking to outcome of pregnancy—implications as to the problem of inferring causation from observed associations. *Amer. J. Epidemiol.*, **93**, 443–56

Yerushalmy, J. (1972). Infants with low birth-weight born before their mothers started to smoke cigarettes. *Amer. J. Obstet. Gynecol.*, **112**, 277–84

Yos, J. M., Bade, W. L. and Jehle, H. (1957). Specificity of the London–Eisenschitz Wang force. *Proc. Nat. Acad. Sci.*, *USA*, **43**, 341–6

Zelen, M. (1968). A hypothesis of the natural history of breast cancer. *Cancer Res.*, **28**, 207–10

Zervas, J. D., Delamore, I. W. and Israels, M. C. G. (1970). Leucocyte phenotypes in Hodgkin's disease. *Lancet*, **ii**, 634–5

Zippin, C., Cutler, S. J., Reeves, W. J. and Lun, D. (1971). Variation in survival among patients with acute lymphocytic leukemia. *Blood*, **37**, 59–72

Index